MEDICAL TRANSCRIPTION

Second Edition Revised

BLANCHE ETTINGER, Ed.D.
Bronx Community College
of the City University of New York

ALICE G. ETTINGER, RN, MSN, CPNP
Division of Pediatric Hematology-Oncology
Saint Peter's University Hospital, New Brunswick, New Jersey

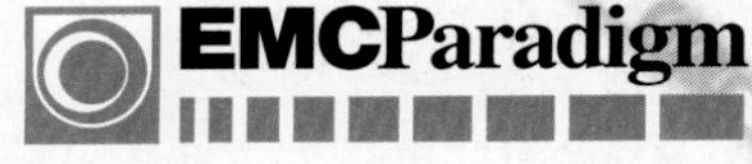

Developmental Editors Christine Hurney and Jim Patterson, RN, BSN
Editorial Assistant Susan Capecchi
Indexer Terry Casey
Copy Editor Kay Savoie
Cover and Text Designer Leslie Anderson
Desktop Production Parkwood Composition
Illustrator Precision Graphics

Publishing Management Team
George Provol, Publisher; Janice Johnson, Director of Product Development; Tony Galvin, Acquisitions Editor; Lori Landwer, Marketing Manager; Shelley Clubb, Electronic Design and Production Manager.

Photo Credits
Cover image Lightscapes/The StockMarket; **151** (top) CORBIS; (bottom) courtesy of Welch Allyn, Inc.; **152** Laureen Wilson/Custom Medical Stock Photo; **153** Custom Medical Stock Photo; **176** (bottom) courtesy of Welch Allyn, Inc.; **201** (bottom) SuperStock; **338** Michael English/Custom Medical Stock Photo.

Library of Congress Cataloging-in-Publication Data
Ettinger, Blanche.
Medical transcription / Blanche Ettinger, Alice G. Ettinger.--2nd ed., rev
p. cm.
Includes index.
ISBN 0-7638-2010-5 (text)
1. Medical transcription. I. Ettinger, Alice G., 1943- II. Title.

R728.8.E88 2004
653'.18--dc21 2001059767

Text ISBN 0-7638-2010-5
Order # 01611

Care has been taken to verify the accuracy of information presented in this book. The authors, editors, and publisher, however, cannot accept responsibility for errors or omissions or for consequences from application of the information in this book and make no warranty, expressed or implied, with respect to its content.

Trademarks Some of the product names used in this book have been used for identification purposes only and may be trademarks or registered trademarks of their respective manufacturers.

Published by EMCParadigm
875 Montreal Way
St. Paul, MN 55102
(800) 535-6865
E-mail: educate@emcp.com
Web site: www.emcp.com

Printed in the United States of America.

10 9 8 7 6 5 4 3 2

Brief Contents

Contents

Contents

Contents

Preface

Medical Transcription, Second Edition Revised by Blanche Ettinger and Alice G. Ettinger has been updated to align with the AAMT Book of Style Second Edition and is designed to develop workplace-ready transcriptionists and medical language specialists. Complete instruction in the technique and skills of transcription is provided as well as direct instruction in essential medical terminology, editing and proofreading guidelines, and report formats.

There are three core learning principles in this program.

- Mastery of editing and proofreading skills in the context of authentic medical documents is emphasized.
- Vocabulary terms, definitions, and pronunciations are presented in the context of each medical specialty, and the difficult terms included in the transcription activities are highlighted.
- Students learn by working with authentic medical documents. Each of the over 110 dictated documents in this program originated as an authentic dictated report, with only the names changed to protect confidentiality. Style and format align with American Association for Medical Transcription (AAMT) and Joint Commission on Accreditation of Healthcare Organizations (JCAHO) guidelines.

How This Text Is Organized

Medical Transcription, Second Edition Revised is divided into two parts:

- Part I Preparing to Transcribe
- Part II Transcribing for the Specialties

The chapters within Part I provide important foundation material necessary for success as a medical transcriptionist. Chapter 1 discusses the career opportunities and role of the medical transcriptionist along with the essential knowledge and skills required to perform successfully and gives an overview of the most common medical reports. Ethical and legal issues and cultural diversity sections are expanded for this new edition. Chapter 2 provides a medical terminology review which includes a new section explaining pain assessment. Chapter 3 provides an extensive grammar, word usage, and style review that reinforces basic language rules and teaches the special guidelines favored by the American Association for Medical Transcription (AAMT).

The chapters within Part II allow students to develop transcription skills in the context of specific specialties. Chapters within this section are organized by specialty and are presented in the order that is customary for the performance of a physical examination, i.e., cephalocaudal—head to toe. Since the physician generally begins with an assessment of the skin, dermatology is the first specialty addressed.

An extensive group of appendixes provide reference information on common drugs, laboratory values, and abbreviations and symbols. In addition, Appendix A provides an optional endocrinology job simulation exercise. Appendix B provides tips on finding a job as a medical transcriptionist.

How Chapters Are Organized

Each specialty chapter begins with a section that explores the structure and function, physical assessment, diseases and conditions, and common tests and surgical procedures appropriate to the specialty chapter.

Preface

In the Building Language Skills section of each specialty chapter, the text-workbook uses a systematic approach to enhance the student's medical vocabulary. The exercises in this section of the chapter place special emphasis on learning root words, combining forms, prefixes, and suffixes. Five exercises, including a particularly challenging one on combining word forms, help develop a thorough knowledge of medical terms. The sixth exercise provides an opportunity to develop proofreading skills which will apply directly to speech/voice recognition documents as well as traditional transcription editing.

In the Building Transcription Skills section, students are presented with a model document. They are to key the document, and then proofread it against the model shown in the book. After this practice, the students move on to transcribing actual dictations based on real-life patients. A series of reports follows, each one of increasing difficulty.

In the Assessing Transcription Skills section of each chapter, students are asked to demonstrate their mastery of the terminology, editing/proofreading, and document transcription skills. This testing opportunity includes dictation/transcription practice.

Resources for the Instructor

In addition to suggested course syllabus information, the Instructor's Guide on CD that accompanies *Medical Transcription, Second Edition Revised* includes answers for all end-of-chapter exercises as well as model answers for all dictations. All dictation recordings are available in digital format on a CD-ROM as well as on analog cassettes. Supplementary instructional materials are available on the Internet Resource Center, including model answers, quizzes, study aids, report templates, and general course planning information.

In addition to the many professional colleagues and staff members who made contributions to this program, the authors would like to thank the editorial team at Paradigm Publishing as well as the following reviewers and contributors for their expert advice and opinions.

Barbara Fortuna, EdD, RHIA
Miami Dade Community College
Miami, FL

Phyllis McElhinney, M.Ed.
East Central College
Union, MO

Susan Osborne, RHIA
Dyersburg State Community College
Dyersburg, TN

Ann Haber Stanton, CMT
Stanton Associates
Rapid City Regional Hospital
Rapid City, SD
Career Learning Center of the Black Hills
Rapid City, SD

Julie Wood
Tulsa Community College, Metro Campus
Tulsa, OK

The authors and editorial staff welcome your feedback on this text and its supplements. Please reach us by clicking the "Contact Us" button at www.emcp.com.

Part I

PREPARING TO TRANSCRIBE

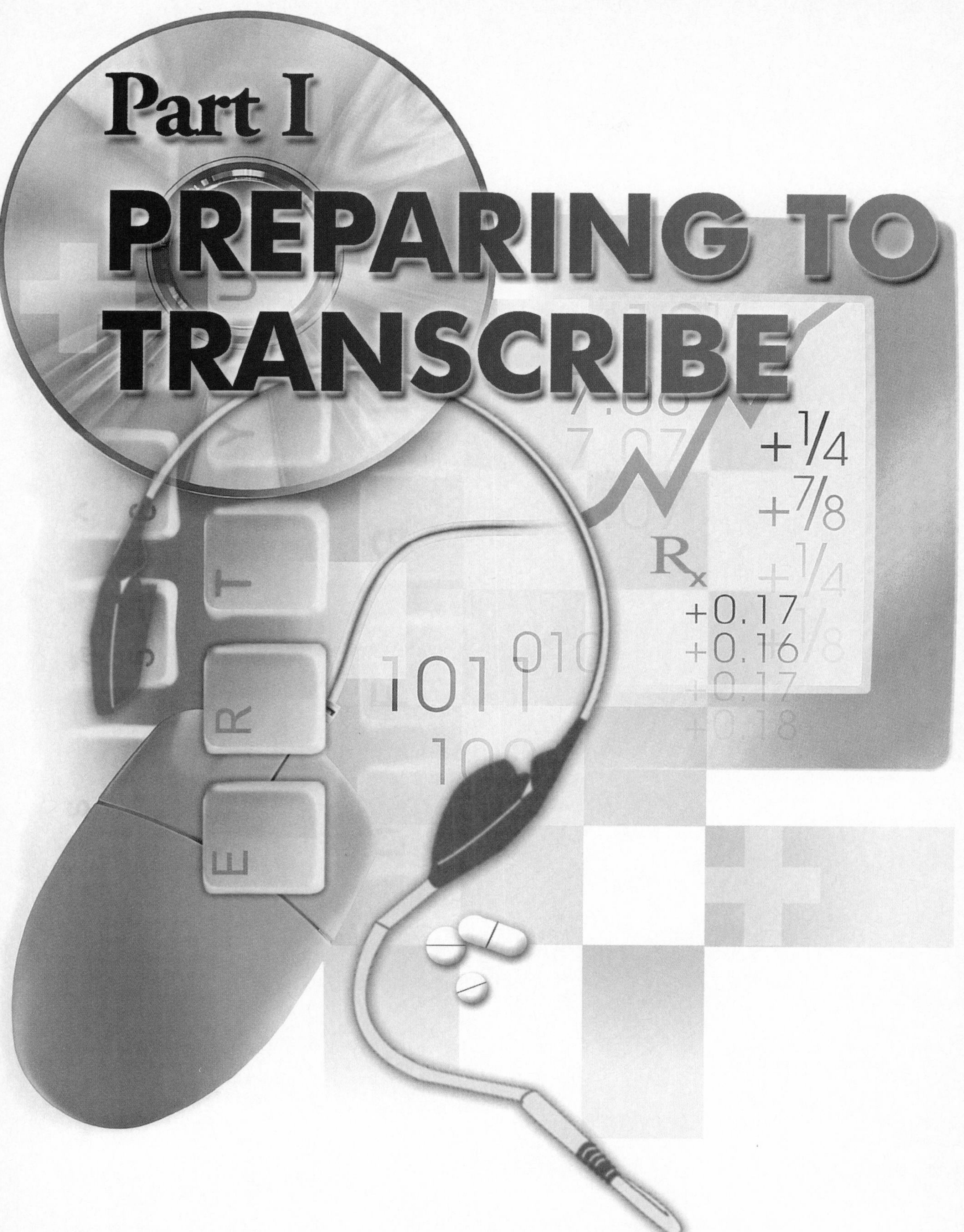

1

The World of Medical Transcription

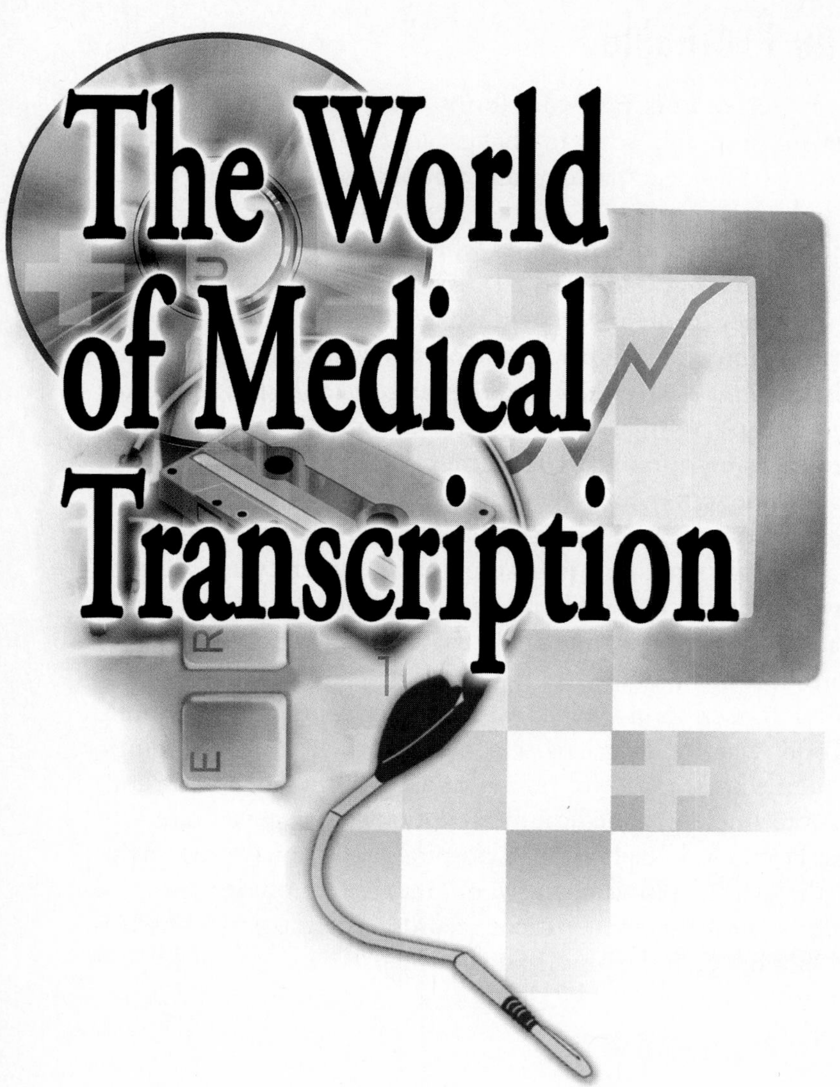

Medical transcription is one of many growing professions in the health-care industry. It offers challenge and interest as well as flexible career paths. This specialty is particularly suited to individuals who like to work independently, learn continuously, pay close attention to detail, and produce a perfect product.

OBJECTIVES

- Examine the overall job environment, types of careers, and future opportunities in the field of medical transcription.
- Explain why the medical transcriptionist is a multi-skilled professional by studying the job expectations and performance standards required by industry.
- Evaluate your own aptitude and personal attributes and assess your readiness for careers in medical transcription.
- Describe the purpose and information contained on the most common types of reports transcribed.
- Explore the issues and importance of record confidentiality and release of information.

Overview of the Profession

The word *transcription* is created from two word forms: *trans* and *scriba.* The prefix *trans* means across, beyond, through, so as to change; *scriba* means official writer. From this definition comes the meaning for transcription: to change the spoken word to the written word.

Transcription had its beginnings in early times when few people could read or write and scribes were hired to copy and interpret the spoken word. Their job was considered important since they frequently transcribed legal and sacred orations into written documents that became the rules and principles by which the society governed its members. Their work provides us with a rich heritage of historical records that portrayed life in their era.

The specialty of medical transcription had its beginnings in the early 1900s when medical stenographers became scribes for physicians who originally had maintained all of their own records. These medical stenographers helped lighten the load for busy physicians by manually documenting all of their patient interactions. Because the technology we have today was not available, medical stenographers frequently had to follow physicians during rounds, frantically trying to hear and record every word for medical record documentation.

The career of medical transcription evolved with the development of dictating equipment during World War I. Physicians were able to dictate their findings, modes of treatment, and medical reports for transcription without face-to-face contact. Today, with current technology, a medical transcriptionist may never have contact with any dictators. From local neighborhood hospitals and clinics to transcription services around the world, physicians rely on medical transcriptionists to provide accurate documentation for their patient records. The medical transcriptionist serves as a vital link between the physician and the patient.

Growth in Medical Transcription

With the rapid growth in healthcare industries, employment in the medical transcription profession is expected to grow at a much faster rate than the average for other industries. The rapid growth of medical transcriptionists counterbalances the decline of stenographers. Also, with the constant expansion of technology and the organizational restructuring throughout the nation, the secretary's role has widened and secretaries, who also transcribe dictated medical documents, now perform new responsibilities that were formerly reserved for the managerial and professional staff. Similarly, medical assistants are assuming tasks that were formerly completed by secretaries in physicians' offices. The medical transcriptionist who works in an office practice generally is the professional who translates and edits recorded dictation by physicians and other healthcare providers regarding patient assessment and treatment. The transcriptionist working in a hospital setting or at home may transcribe radiologic, pathologic, surgical, and other more technical dictation.

The rate of growth in healthcare industries is also due to increased specialization in medical treatment and technological advances in the diagnosis and treatment of disease. Many specialty areas in healthcare are providing job opportunities for qualified individuals. The demand for medical transcriptionists is expected to increase even further because of the increasing medical needs of the aging population.

It is anticipated that with the advancement of voice/speech recognition technology, discussed later in this chapter, there will be a need for medical transcriptionists who are skilled in reviewing and editing electronically transcribed drafts for accuracy. Growing numbers of transcriptionists will also be required to amend patients' files, discover discrepancies in medical records, and edit documents for proper grammar.

Employment Opportunities

Medical transcription is a field with many possibilities and areas for advancement. As a professional, multi-skilled medical worker, the medical transcriptionist can choose from a variety of employment options. You can work in a hospital transcription or medical records department; or you can work in a radiology, pathology, or emergency department. You might also find employment in a physician's office, medical clinic, professional medical group practice, outpatient clinic, rehabilitation center, medical transcription service, home office, laboratory, psychiatric center, insurance company, medical research center, or other facility. Medical transcriptionists can work in specialty areas, too. You may choose a specialty which is of interest to you or work initially in a hospital setting and learn many different phases of medicine.

In addition to having a wide choice in work environments, medical transcriptionists also have several career options. You can continue your education to pursue a management/leadership role. You can become an instructor, service owner, proofreader, or editor. Once you have medical transcription experience, you may opt to become independent. You may want to establish your own company or work at home using your own equipment, including word processor, dictation system, modem, and fax machine.

Whatever route you take, here's some important advice: The more knowledge and skills you acquire relevant to the medical field, the greater your opportunities. There is a common misconception about the degree of difficulty in doing medical transcription. Medical transcription is more than listening to someone's voice and typing what you hear. You have to acquire a great deal of knowledge and experience to do the job well. Recognizing the important role medical transcriptionists play in patient care and understanding all of the duties that the job entails will help you get a good start in the field.

The Medical Transcriptionist's Role in Patient Care

As a medical transcriptionist (MT), you have an important role as a member of the healthcare team. According to the American Association for Medical Transcription (AAMT), the professional organization for medical transcriptionists, an MT is "...a medical language specialist who interprets and transcribes dictation by physicians and other healthcare professionals regarding patient assessment, workup, therapeutic procedures, clinical course, diagnosis, prognosis, etc., in order to document patient care and facilitate delivery of healthcare services." In essence, MTs transfer the physician's spoken words via tape recorder or digital dictation system into typewritten legal documents. These documents describe the historical and factual data about events leading up to and surrounding patient care and treatment, the outcome of the illness or condition, and the details surrounding release from the hospital.

Some of the most commonly transcribed medical documents include office notes, history and physical examinations, consultations, operative reports, correspondence, discharge summaries, pathology and radiology reports, and laboratory reports. Because these documents become the foundation for a patient's healthcare, the medical transcriptionist's main responsibility is to produce impeccably accurate reports. A medical transcriptionist also may be responsible for record maintenance, i.e., keeping logs of daily work, printing, charting or delivering medical reports, training, providing administrative support, and evaluating equipment.

Personal Attributes of the Medical Transcriptionist

Successful medical transcriptionists share certain traits that allow them to fulfill their duties. A Bell South speaker at a national conference indicated the importance of accountability on the job, dealing with diverse individuals, being flexible and adaptable, and willing to assume responsibility when necessary. Table 1.1 lists the common traits of medical transcriptionists. Many of these attributes relate to skills that you can develop even if you do not have them now.

TABLE 1.1 Traits of Medical Transcriptionists

Medical transcriptionists . . .
are fascinated by the medical profession, with a special interest in medical language and its usage
listen carefully to people
use keyboarding skills
understand computer technology
have good memory retention skills
have excellent spelling skills
have investigative minds and know how to use references to research and find correct terms
are committed to quality performance and accuracy in all tasks
are self-disciplined, detail-oriented, and independent
are dedicated to professional development and enthusiastically committed to learning
are not afraid to ask questions when uncertain of the situation
understand the medical, legal, and ethical issues related to confidentiality

In addition to the attributes listed in Table 1.1, job advertisements for medical transcriptionists might request the following attributes for their applicants.

- acute-care medical transcription experience
- familiarity with laboratory terminology
- excellent organizational abilities
- "can-do" attitude
- self-starter
- proficiency and ease with computers

Required Knowledge and Skills

Medical transcription requires practical, detailed knowledge of many aspects of healthcare and healthcare records. The transcriptionist uses a headset and transcribing machine to listen to dictated documents. The keyboarding skill required for many positions is at least 50 words per minute. Many jobs require 60 words per minute or more. Some experienced machine transcriptionists transcribe up to 78–90 words per minute. Familiarity with a variety of reports about emergency room visits, chart summaries, surgical procedures, and diagnostic imaging studies is necessary for the transcriptionist. To produce accurately transcribed documents, the transcriptionist must know the language of medicine—anatomy and physiology, diagnostic procedures and treatment, and medical jargon and abbreviations. The dictator reviews and signs the document, which will then become part of the patient's permanent record.

Job opportunities for medical transcriptionists are shown in Appendix B (Medical Transcriptionist Job Search) and are listed on the Internet. These opportunities require skills shown in Table 1.2. While on the job, the transcriptionist continues to learn and improve skills, acquires new knowledge and ways of helping society, and takes pride in a job well done.

TABLE 1.2 Medical Transcriptionist Job Skills

strong knowledge of MS Word and word processing, MS Excel
certification (optional but recommended)
medical terminology
pharmacology
clinical notes
emergency room notes
note-taking
medical billing
customer service
scheduling of appointments and procedures
answering multi-line phones for a medical facility

Professional Certification

The main purpose behind certification is to protect the health, safety, and welfare of the worker and the public. However, setting uniform standards helps organizations understand the criteria for entry level work performance and helps employers hire the right person for the right job. Being able to demonstrate that you have met or exceed the standards helps you get jobs.

In the area of medical transcription, according to the *Occupational Outlook Handbook,* opportunities would be best for those who earn an associate degree or who achieve certification from the American Association for Medical Transcription (AAMT). To become certified, you must fulfill a set of requirements or satisfy a set of standards. The certification standards, available at www.aamt.org, spell out how much and what type of education or training a person must possess and on what basis his or her ability will be judged.

Professional Principles of Transcription

Throughout this text you will be learning and developing the skills involved in high-quality transcription, including recognizing and understanding medical terminology; proofreading and editing for correct word useage and the mechanics of punctuation and capitalization; and keying medical reports in the correct format and style. As you develop your abilities, keep in mind the cardinal goals shared by the best professional medical transcriptionists: accuracy, speed, confidentiality, and ethical behavior.

Increase Speed While Striving for Accuracy

To get a job, you will need to have high-level keyboarding skills. During your course of study, try to steadily increase your speed. This depends on the integration of two levels of skill: (a) keyboarding ability and (b) your growing knowledge base. A medical transcriptionist can only key as fast as the dictated word can be heard, spelled correctly, researched, and fit into context. Your instructor may establish speed criteria to meet as you complete this beginning course. Having realistic goals that approximate industry standards can help you focus, evaluate your progress, and improve.

Unless your document is accurate, a fast typing speed is useless. A medical transcriptionist should always strive for accuracy first and then work toward speed. Learn from your mistakes, ask for help, and apply your own creativity and curiosity as you research answers to questions. Remember that each dictated report becomes a legal document as well as a medical record on which the care and treatment of the patient is based. Because records play such an important role in patient care communication, it is important to correct any errors identified after the report has been transcribed. Each employer has specific procedures and guidelines to correct, change, or add information.

Maintain Confidentiality

Confidentiality is a legal requirement when working in the healthcare profession. MTs also have a moral responsibility to keep all patient record information confidential. They must protect the privacy of patients by not discussing patient information with anyone and by making sure that only those people authorized to see a patient's record have access to it. The medical transcriptionist should be careful when faxing or delivering reports and should not leave a modem on when stepping away from a machine. Also, the medical transcriptionist should make sure that the computer screen cannot be viewed by outsiders. Table 1.3 provides guidelines for ensuring that information in the computer is kept confidential. In addition, no identifying information on a patient should leave a medical transcriptionist's place of employment. The patient's authorization must be received for disclosure of any information to a third party, including the patient's insurance company. A release form must specify the information to be released, to whom, and the purpose. Maintaining patient privacy also means that medical transcriptionists should access chart information only as necessary to provide for the accuracy of the document.

Check your hospital or workplace policy for complete confidentiality guidelines. Frequently, an employer will ask a new MT employee to sign a confidentiality agreement. Violation may result in termination or prosecution. Even if you work from home, you are bound by the principle of confidentiality.

Follow Ethical Guidelines

When working in a medical environment, employees must maintain ethical standards in accordance with the law. Ethics relate to moral action and a personal code of conduct, and individuals are expected to conform to professional standards of personal integrity. Behaving ethically means conducting oneself in a manner that will bring dignity and honor to one's profession and person. It means that no matter what is happening in your personal life, you remain objective and expend your best effort with each report. It also means that you respect the dignity of patients and provide considerate care and communication through your work habits so as not to cause a patient harm.

Behaving ethically also means refusing to participate in unethical practices and

TABLE 1.3 Computer Guidelines to Ensure Confidentiality

Restrict the access of outside sources to your computerized database.
Never divulge your password unless the office manager requests it.
Do not walk away from the terminal while online.
Ensure that adequate security precautions are in place to safeguard data and the system.
Make backup files and store them securely elsewhere in case of fire, burglary, or other events that could threaten the records.

Source: *Medical Assisting: A Commitment to Service.* Published by Paradigm Publishing Inc. © 2002.

refusing to conceal them. Medical transcriptionists need to recognize the levels of authority and know when to seek information about protocol or procedure.

Appreciate Cultural Diversity

America's health in the 21st Century must wrestle successfully with equity among the young and the aged and among social and ethnic groups.

—Lincoln Chen, 2020 Vision: Health in the 21st Century
Institute of Medicine
25th Anniversary Symposium

One of the biggest challenges facing America is the rapidly changing society—an older and more diverse population. As Americans age, their lifespan will continue to increase as well. With the increasing ethnic and racial diversity, the challenges of dealing with this diversity will become more pronounced, especially in those areas with a higher concentration of these populations.

Medical professionals and staff will need to become knowledgeable of various backgrounds, cultural and language differences, and ethnic values. Healthcare workers must learn to communicate effectively with individuals from diverse backgrounds so that each individual is treated with trust and respect.

Healthcare providers need to become familiar with some of the communication barriers that may be present with persons who are of different ethnic groups and/or have English as a second language.

- Words in some countries have different meaning from those in the United States.
- Some American terms are familiar only to native speakers (e.g. *egg on* for *provoke*).
- Gestures may have different meanings. Americans give a firm handshake. Asians find this kind of handshake offensive and prefer a gentle grip.
- A smile is considered positive and friendly; however, in some African cultures, it represents a weakness.
- Americans use eye contact to indicate interest, attentiveness, and trustworthiness. Because they feel that direct eye contact is impolite and disrespectful, Koreans and Japanese use indirect eye contact.
- Some foreign expressions have found their way into the English language, such as "Hasta la vista, Baby."

The diversity of the population challenges the medical transcriptionist to understand a variety of cultures and differences in language and speech patterns. It is important not only to recognize and become familiar with various cultures but also to be able to communicate with the dictator regarding unknown or confusing terminology.

Getting Started

If you are not familiar with the process of medical transcription, deciding where to begin can be a bit overwhelming. As with learning any new skill, it is helpful to begin by familiarizing yourself with the steps in the process, the resources and equipment you will need, and how you will use those materials. As you learn, be patient and give yourself time to become comfortable with this unique way of interpreting and communicating medical information.

Transcription Equipment

MTs use a variety of transcription programs and word processing equipment. Your instructor will explain and demonstrate the particular type of equipment you will use. All transcriber systems, however, have earphones, a foot pedal, and some operational features in common.

Earphones Your earphones plug into a transcriber, allowing you to hear dictation. Earphones consist of three parts: a chinband, a cord, and a driver. The driver connects the chinband to the cord. With the earpieces in the ears and the chinband near the chin, the cord hangs downward and plugs into the transcriber. This plug may be on the side or on the front of the machine. If you are having trouble hearing with your earphones, one of the first things to check is the earphone cord. It can be worn or cracked and may need replacement.

Earphones are available in a variety of styles. Some have rigid chinbands and others are more pliable. Earpieces also vary from those that fit into the ear snugly, to earpieces padded with sponges, to earpieces that look like small microphones and rest on the inside of the external ear canal. Earphone choice is a matter of personal preference, but whichever earphones you select, you may find that fitting something into the ear for a couple of hours at a time requires some getting used to.

Before you start to play a tape, check the volume and position it at a comfortable range. In situations where you have used the speaker feature to listen to dictation out loud—for example, if you have asked another person to help you decipher a difficult word—remember to turn down the volume after you have finished.

Another point to remember: Earphones collect debris and wax. If they are used by more than one student, they should be sterilized between uses. You may also clean them with rubbing alcohol. Some earpieces unscrew to allow for cleaning from the inside. Use cotton swabs to reach into small areas.

Foot Pedal The foot pedal allows you to keep your hands free for keyboarding. A foot pedal consists of two parts: the pedal and the cord. Pressing the foot pedal causes the transcriber to play. As soon as you release the pedal with your foot, the machine stops. If you press on the foot pedal and nothing happens, check the cord connection to make sure it is plugged firmly into the transcriber.

Foot pedals are available in a variety of styles. With most models, the center of the foot pedal is the position to press for play; fast forward is on the left; and rewind is on the right. Some foot pedals have only two options: right for play and left for rewind. There is no fast forward on this type of foot pedal.

Look closely at your foot pedal to see which side is which, or test it with your foot. Usually the pedal will have printed instructions on where the positions are. Some models have a knob underneath that allows you to adjust the amount of tension on the foot pedal. Turn your foot pedal over and check to see if it has this extra feature.

Transcriber Features The transcriber is the device that makes it possible to transform voice recordings into transcript or printed documents. Table 1.4 lists the features that appear on most machines.

Tapes Standard cassette transcribers play standard audio tapes. There are also microcassette transcribers and minicassette transcribers. When you insert a cassette, make sure the side you wish to play is top side up.

TABLE 1.4 Transcriber Features

ON/OFF button or POWER: This is used to turn the transcriber on and off. Usually there is some type of light to indicate that the power is on. If this light does not come on, check your power source to make sure your machine is plugged in.
INDEX COUNTERS: Some transcribers have an index counter that measures the length of dictation on a cassette. This is a useful tool in finding the correct dictation or in scanning cassettes. The index counter may be an indicator strip and a flashing light or numbers that roll forward or backward as you play the tape. As you fast forward, rewind, stop, or play a tape, the light will move, indicating the minutes of dictation by the numbers on the index counter. You can press the clear button next to the index counter to stop the light from flashing or press the reset button to set the counter to zero. Some transcribers are set up to scan, or mark, each separate dictation, or *seizure*. The term *seizure* is coined from the way the report is dictated onto the cassettes. Physicians dictate by telephoning from their office or home to the hospital. They dial a special number that *seizes* the transcribing equipment. As the tape is scanned, it is being rewound. At the end of every dictation series, you can hear a beep or a blip. At this point, the index counter lights up and marks where the dictation ends for each series on the control strip. When you play the tape, you will be able to see how much dictation remains. You can tell if you are near the beginning, halfway through, or almost finished.
AUTO PLAYBACK/AUTO REWIND: This feature allows you to replay a word or a string of words. Using an auto backspace button on the bottom of the transcriber, set the adjustment to whatever is comfortable for you. With a digital dictation system, this adjustment may have to be made via a computer system. Allowing a little repeat at the beginning is usually helpful to ensure that you are not missing any words. When you begin transcription, your adjustment may be on or near the maximum amount of replay. Make an effort to lessen the amount of replay as you become more experienced.

(continues)

TABLE 1.4 Transcriber Features (Continued)

SPEAKER: Use the speaker button to listen to dictation out loud or to play the tape for someone to listen to. If your transcriber does not have a speaker button, just remove your headphone cord from the transcriber to activate the speaker feature.
EJECT: The eject button opens the cassette door. Press it to place or remove a cassette.
SPEED CONTROL: You can increase or decrease the speed control while you are learning. Try to match the dictation speed to your transcription speed. The voice should not sound distorted, but natural.
VOLUME CONTROL: Some physicians speak loudly while others are difficult to hear. Increase or decrease the volume to compensate for a louder or softer voice.
TONE: This feature mutes or accentuates consonants (treble/bass) for nasal tones or a stuttering style of dictation.
ERASE: This feature allows you to clear or erase tapes. Be careful with this button to make sure you do not erase dictation before it is transcribed.

Voice/Speech Recognition Systems

Voice/speech recognition software is a rapidly evolving technology that has the potential to change a medical transcriptionist's role. When using this software, the doctor or other medical specialist dictates into a computer system and the dictation software transcribes the dictation directly onto the computer screen. While it is possible for the doctor or medical specialist to edit the dictation through voice commands or keyboard input, it will be the role of the transcriptionist to edit and prepare the final reports for these electronically transcribed documents. It is the transcriptionist who is a language expert and specialist and who knows and applies proper formatting, correct grammar usage, punctuation, and capitalization.

Voice/speech recognition systems do not replace the transcriptionist; however, they do magnify the transcriptionist's editing role, while eliminating the original transcription function. Voice/speech recognition technology increases the productivity of the transcriptionist by eliminating the need to transcribe the dictation. The transcriptionist's primary activity is in editing the dictation that is transcribed by the voice/speech recognition software. The transcriptionist begins the editing process by accessing the transcribed document at the transcriptionist's work station. Then, the transcriptionist uses voice commands or the computer keyboard to make necessary changes.

Proofreading in this type of environment, even with grammatical and spell checking software, is a critical skill. Words that have been incorrectly transcribed by the voice/speech recognition software may be words that appear in the dictionary. These words must be identified and corrected by the transcriptionist. For example, the doctor might have dictated "Ann Mitchell" and the voice/recognition software might transcribe that as "an Mitchell."

Voice recognition capability has been around for over 50 years; however, in the last five to six years, tremendous strides have been made to improve the software so that it is user friendly, relatively easy to master, and remarkably accurate. Some of the voice recognition systems, such as Dragon Systems from L & H, Inc. and IBM Voice Via Gold software, contain dictionaries for medical terminology. This feature greatly improves the accuracy of the transcription of voice dictation by doctors and medical specialists.

Until the year 2001, the term *voice recognition* denoted that the user (in this case the doctor and the transcriptionist, if she/he used voice input for editing) had to train the system to understand that user's dictation. The software, as a matter of fact, learns the user's voice, accent, and personal way of speaking. The initial training activity took thirty minutes to one hour of time. Once an individual trained the system, every time that user dictated into the system, it continually upgraded that person's voice and speech mannerisms profile so that the accuracy of the transcription improved.

Prior to the year 2001, speech recognition represented software that did not have to be trained. This type of software required more powerful computer equipment and a more sophisticated level of software. In 2001, Microsoft released Office XP that included a component for "Speech Recognition" in Word and Excel. The user still has to train the system to understand that person's voice and speech mannerisms. The proofreading exercises throughout the text force students to concentrate on meaning and language usage, which is indispensable when producing quality document generated from voice/speech recognition technology.

Transcription Ergonomics

Medical transcription is a sedentary occupation. Working at a computer for long periods of time can produce sore muscles, headaches, eyestrain, tension, and fatigue. The good news is that you can arrange your workstation and develop specific habits that will relieve physical and mental stress.

Eyes Take short, frequent breaks to rest your eyes. The American Optometric Association recommends a 10-minute break for every hour or two spent staring at a computer screen. Or take 30-second microbreaks to focus on distant objects, squeeze your shoulders, stretch your back, and shake your arms. If you wear glasses, tinted lenses may reduce glare from the screen. Move your monitor away from the window or use drapes, blinds, or an antiglare screen. Adjust your contrast and brightness levels to suit your comfort level. Select screen colors that are restful for your eyes. Computer workers blink at one-fifth the normal rate while they are watching the screen, causing dry, scratchy eyes. The solution? Make a conscious effort to blink more often, or moisten your eyes with cool water or a tear substitute (sold at drugstores).

Ears Prevent ear infections by keeping your earphones clean and not allowing others to use them. Work in a quiet environment and cover printers to reduce noise.

Hands and Wrist Computers originally were built for speed, not comfort, but as carpal tunnel syndrome and other repetitive motion injuries are becoming a major problem in the workplace, keyboards are being redesigned. A new popular design is the split keyboard, which is slanted to accommodate the natural position of the hands as opposed to a straight, flat keyboard that does not support the wrists. Alternatively, you can purchase a wrist rest. The support provided by this inexpensive device may also alleviate back pain caused by tensing the muscles around the shoulders. Taking frequent breaks and exercising will also help.

Posture Adjust your workstation to your body. Be creative. Heighten or lower your chair and provide support for your lower back with a lumbar cushion, a rolled up towel, or a small, thin, firm pillow. Use a foot rest such as a footstool. Adjust screen height, the angle of your screen, and the distance between you and your screen. Adjust your table or desk height if possible. Check computer supply catalogs for trays that swing out and offer height options for your keyboard.

Lifestyle Changes Fatigue and discomfort are major contributors to decreased production and errors. Find an outside activity to relieve tension caused by stress. Eat a varied, nutritious diet, exercise regularly, and get enough sleep to improve your alertness, thinking, and comfort both on and off the job.

Using Reference Materials

One resource that is indispensable for the transcriptionist is a reference library. Books should be up to date. Later printings or editions of the source book may have significant differences.

Although the list of available books is enormous, experienced transcriptionists generally agree that only a few are essential for the beginning transcriptionist.

The following references are types of must-have books that provide general information on medical terminology, language style, drug names, and technical terms. As you encounter new specialties in your work, you will want to add specialty-specific books to your collection—for example, OB/GYN (obstetrics/gynecology) words, neurology words, or radiology/oncology words.

If you do not find an answer in one book, go to another. Books on medical equipment words and books of medical phrases have many of the same category entries, but a specific suture, for example, may only be listed in one of them.

Medical Dictionary A medical dictionary is the medical transcriptionist's primary reference, providing a complete alphabetical listing of terms and their definitions, pronunciation keys, and word origin information. Take time to explore your dictionary, especially the appendices in the back and user's guide in the front. Medical dictionaries also include anatomy charts, which can be helpful sources for terms that sound mumbled. For example, if you know that the dictator is talking about a muscle in the face but you do not recognize even the first sound in the term, looking at the chart may suggest a word that sounds like what the dictator has said. Some medical dictionaries are available in electronic form. This format allows quick access and the capability of creating a database of words for instant access and spell checking.

Drug Book Your drug book will be your resource that gets the most wear and tear. You can look up drugs by their generic name, trade name, and sometimes indication or usage. This is an excellent source when verifying drug spelling, dosages, and indications. Your drug book will often have lab values, abbreviations commonly used in medical orders, chemotherapy regimens, and a list of sound-alike words in the appendices.

Medical Style Guide A medical style guide provides information on report formats and the use of abbreviations, numbers, capital letters, and punctuation. The standard guide is the *AAMT Book of Style* published by the Association for Medical Transcription; however, there are several other style books available. Check with the institution and/or dictator for a specific reference.

Medical Word Book/Medical Phrase Index You should be able to find just about anything you are looking for in a medical word book/medical phrase index—if you have a pretty good idea of how to spell it. If you can make out part of a phrase but not all of it, you can look it up by the word(s) you are able to hear because of the cross-referencing feature. This type of book does not contain definitions or pronunciations, only correct spelling of words.

Abbreviations and Acronyms Reference You will run into many abbreviations in transcription. Always look up the abbreviation to make sure it is correct and fits into the context of what you are transcribing. If you cannot decipher a word or phrase but can understand some of the syllables, check to see if it is an acronym or abbreviation.

Medical Equipment/Surgical Words Book A medical equipment/surgical words book lists specific equipment names—especially trade names, e.g., *McLean clamp*—and surgical terminology that you will not likely find elsewhere, e.g., *Lempert incision.*

Laboratory Word Book In a laboratory word book, you will find laboratory reference range values, eponymic diseases and syndromes, and—especially helpful—laboratory test names.

Eponym Book Eponyms are adjectives. They are instrument, disease, or procedure names usually derived from the last name of the person who developed the procedure or designed the instrument. An example is *Parkinson's disease.* An eponym reference book lists these names alphabetically. The AAMT recommends dropping the possessive ('s) with eponyms.

Online Resources On the Internet you can find reference information and chat forums that will help you become more knowledgeable on the job. With a Web browser, you can search for information on any topic that interests you, including medical specialties, new drugs, transcription productions, and directories of physician names. The following Web sites may be especially useful.

- American Association for Medical Transcription (AAMT): www.aamt.org
- American Cancer Society: www.cancer.org

- American Medical Association: www.ama-assn.org
- Keeping Abreast of Medical Transcription (KAMT): www.wwma.com/kamt
- Medlineplus, a service of the national Library of Medicine: www.nlm.nih.gov/medlineplus
- Medical Transcription Daily: www.mtdaily.com
- Medical Transcription Monthly: www.mtmonthly.com
- Medicine Net.com: www.medicinenet.com
- National Institutes of Health: www.nih.gov

Medical transcriptions have created a lively and mutually supportive online community where you can find others who have similar interests and questions. For example, within a chat forum, a medical transcriptionist may pose a question about the use of hyphens. Or, someone else might ask for help finding the spelling of certain terms or physicians' names. Over the Internet, you can get advice and information from hundreds of working medical transcriptions quickly and easily. Be careful, however, about accepting information as correct unless you can verify it in a reference source.

Nonmedical References Additional nonmedical resources that provide essential information include a standard English dictionary and an English language reference manual.

Transcribing, Proofreading, and Editing Tips

As you learn to transcribe medical documents, you will be integrating the skills of using language correctly; choosing the proper medical terms based on what you hear dictated; applying your knowledge of the mechanics of punctuation, capitalization, abbreviations, and spelling; and formatting medical reports according to healthcare industry standards. Initially, you may experience some frustration dealing with the challenges of this demanding area of study. But these challenges should be balanced with the satisfaction of knowing you will one day play a critical role in an important area of people's lives. As a medical transcriptionist, you will provide essential services and support to physicians and personnel who count on you to communicate medical information. You become a partner in the vital business of caring for people's health. For this reason, it is very important that you check your work with careful proofreading and editing.

The Transcription Process

The steps in the transcription process are listed below. As you review the steps, create a mental picture of each one to help you learn the entire sequence.

1. Place all the information and materials you need at your workstation.
2. Position the headset, transcriber, and foot control in the desired location and make sure the components are connected to the unit.

3. Check that the transcription unit is turned on and ready to go.
4. Insert the cassette or CD-ROM.
5. Reset the indicator strip to estimate the length of the document.
6. Adjust the volume and speed controls as necessary.
7. Listen to all of the instructions.
8. Transcribe the dictation, using the process of "listen, stop, key." Listen to a single sentence or phrase (whatever number of words you can mentally retain and repeat to yourself), pause the tape, then key the words. Leave spaces for words you cannot hear or do not understand.
9. Carefully proofread the document and correct as many errors as you can. Use your reference materials to help you identify missing words.
10. Print the final document.
11. Review document a final time. Does document include proper format, spelling, and punctuation? Does the document make sense (a prostatectomy would not be done on a female patient)?

Editing Documents from Dictation

There are many times that the medical transcriptionist will need to edit while transcribing. However, an important caveat is that the intent must not be changed.

Some simple rules-of-thumb for editing include:

- Add punctuation.
- Make a word singular or plural if it is dictated incorrectly.
- Correct subject-verb agreement.
- Choose one tense when the dictator uses different tenses throughout the document unless the dictator is distinguishing between past and present events.
- Correct improper articles such as *a* and *an* before words beginning with a vowel or vowel sound.
- Check your references and if you cannot find a particular word, or if the word appears to be a combination of two or more words or word forms, query the dictator.

Many medical terms and drug names sound alike. When attempting to identify a term in a dictation, you may be tripped up because the word is spelled differently than it sounds. Table 1.5 provides some tips and examples for discerning similar sounds in words that sound alike.

Whole syllables, not just single letters, are sometimes confused. Table 1.6 provides some alternative spellings for some hard-to-discern word beginnings and endings. Syllables that begin a word are shown with a hyphen at the end. Syllables that end a word are shown with a hyphen before them.

Dealing with Jargon and Clipped Sentences

Individual dictation styles vary from very formal to informal. Some dictators use recurring phrases and terms that reflect their own speech patterns, culture, and geographic area. Some phrases are commonly used in medical writing even though they may contain sentence fragments. As you gain experience, you will become familiar with medical jargon. It is important to adhere to departmental guidelines and style, as well as physician preference, when deciding about acceptable sentence structure.

It is acceptable to use clipped sentences or fragments in portions of the medical report if they have been dictated that way. This typically applies to the physical examination, review of systems, and laboratory data sections.

Again, if you make corrections and make a complete sentence from a fragment, be consistent and make sure the sentences make sense and the original meaning or intent has not been changed.

TABLE 1.5 Tips for Discerning Similar Sounds in Dictation

If you hear...	also consider...	Examples
c	k and g	Kufs disease, guanine
f	ph	phacocyst, farnesol
i (short *i* as the first or second sound)	e, a, and y	enalapril, indoluria, Restoril
y	j	Jungian analysis
k	c, ch	kaliuresis, chiasm
m	n	modal, nodal, naproxen
n	m, pn, gn, mn, kn, cn	nacreous, macrocyte, pneumonia, gnathic, mnemic, knismogenic, cnemis
s	z, c, ps	zymoscope, ciliary, pseudopsia
t	b, p, pt, ct, v	popliteal, ptosis, vinculum
z	x	Xylocaine, Xanax, xanthiuria, Zaglas ligament
	s	seromuscular, Szent-Gyorgyi reaction

TABLE 1.6 Tips for Discerning Word Parts in Dictation

If you hear...	also consider...	If you hear...	also consider...
-able	-ible	ny-	gn-, n-
-air	-are, -aer	para-	peri-, pero-
-ance	-ence	per-	par-, pir-, por-, pur-, pre-, pro-, pru-, pyr-
-ant	-ent	peri-	para-, pero-
ante-	anti-	pre-	per-, pra-, pri-, pro-, pru-
-cer	-cre	si-	psi-, ci-
-cks, -gz	-x	super-	supra-
dis-	dys-	-tion	-sion, -cion, -cean, -cian
-ei	-ie	-tious	-seous, -scious
-ere	-ear, -eir, -ier	-ture	-teur
fizz-	phys-	we-	whe-
hyper-	hypo-	wi-	whi-
inter-	intra-	zi-	xy-
-is	-us, -ace, -ice		
-le	-tle, -el, -al		

Styles of Writing

There are many styles of medical writing. Many caregivers will use a formal style for correspondence, consults, and chart notes. Other caregivers will use an informal style with incomplete sentences, especially for chart notes, progress notes, and consult notes. Styles vary also.

Professional journals have a style that they require for all submitted articles. If you transcribe an article to be submitted to a professional journal, the dictator will probably give you the punctuation style required. However, you might ask the dictator to lend you a copy of the journal, or you can borrow an issue from the library. Also, style specifications for each professional journal are available online at the Web site of the particular journal.

While there are several stylebooks, it is important that you follow the direction of the person for whom you work. You must have flexibility, especially if you have several different dictators, each one using a different style. Most of all, be consistent within each document that you transcribe. For instance, if the dictator prefers that you not use a comma before the *and* or *or* when using compounds, be sure to use that style throughout the entire document.

Dealing with Dictator Accents

Transcribing reports dictated by persons with accents may be difficult, especially for a new MT. The difficulty may be compounded by the addition of extra sounds at the ends of words or by the thickness of the accent.

As a general rule, do not second-guess the dictator who speaks English as a second language. Try to retain the basic style that is dictated, but edit for obvious errors as noted above. Some general suggestions include:

- Listen to the dictation once from beginning to end, transcribing all of the words you can without stopping or replaying the tape.
- Key a symbol, such as an asterisk or ampersand, for every word, phrase, or sentence that you cannot decipher.
- Go through the tape a second time using the word processing Find and Replace feature for the symbol. Fill in whatever you can, as you become familiar with the sounds and patterns of the accent.
- Keep a record of the words and phrases you did not understand and refer to this when you are unsure of what you are hearing. Save copies of past reports that may help you decipher subsequent reports.

Proofreading Methods

Each transcriptionist develops successful methods to proofread his/her work. As you gain experience in the field, you too will determine your particular style. There are several tips that you should consider, but you should always proofread as you type and then again when you have completed the document. Replay the tape and read the typed document on the screen, keeping in mind the following bulleted points. Then, print the document and review again.

- As you listen to the document, does the grammar sound correct? Are all sentences complete where warranted? Do the nouns and pronouns match the verb in number? Are the tenses consistent throughout?
- Consider if the punctuation is correct. Are the commas, semicolons, and colons used correctly?
- Check your document with the Spell Check feature and review for sound-alike words.
- Pay particular attention to numbers to avoid possible keying errors.
- Use the View Page feature to look at the entire page of your document. Does the format look correct and consistent throughout? Have you filled in any blank spaces?

Evaluating Your Work

The Performance Comparison chart (Figure 1.1) is a practical and simple way of examining and evaluating your language skills, knowledge of terminology, listening ability, proofreading competency, editing power, and concentration. A template of

Name ______________________________ Date ____________

Error Categories	Model Document		Report __		Report __		Report __	
	No.	Description	No.	Description	No.	Description	No.	Description
Transcription Errors								
Word Omission								
Wrong Word								
Spelling Errors								
Format or Style Errors								
Capitalization Errors								
Usage/Grammar Errors								
Punctuation Errors								
Abbreviation Errors								
Errors with Numbers								
Transcription Blanks								
Speed Performance (WAM)								

Document Analysis

1. Where did you make most of your errors when you keyed from hard copy? ____________
2. Where did you make most of your errors when you transcribed the document? ____________
3. Analyze your transcription errors and list the kinds of listening errors you made: ____________

   ____

   ____

4. What words or phrases caused you difficulty? ______________________________

   ____

FIGURE 1.1

Performance Comparison Chart

This chart will help you track your progress by comparing your sight-keyed version of the model document with transcriptions of the taped dictation in each chapter in Part II.

this chart is included on the Internet Resource Center (IRC) that accompanies this text. This chart will help you identify, categorize, and track patterns of transcription errors. By using this tool, you will eventually internalize the quality standards by which your transcription work will be judged in the workplace.

In Chapters 4 through 15, you will study the terminology used in the discipline covered and follow up by doing exercises to indicate your strengths and weaknesses in editing and proofreading. The quality of your transcribed reports relies on your ability to proofread and edit medical documents. To prepare for actual transcription work, you will study and key the model medical document in each chapter. Next, determine the number of errors you made in keying this document, and enter the information in the space allocated in the Performance Comparison chart. Then, transcribe the reports in the Patient Studies section of the chapter. For at least three of the reports, categorize and document the types of errors you made. Then, answer the document analysis questions at the bottom of the chart. With continuous practice and assessment, the quality of your work will improve.

When turning in transcribed documents to your instructor for grading, use the Performance Report chart (Figure 1.2) as a cover sheet. Transcribed documents will be evaluated based on their mailability as well as other criteria identified by your instructor.

Working with Medical Records

A medical record is a permanent compilation of written documents that provide information and insight into a patient's life and health history. Many healthcare professionals contribute reports and information to this record. Since patient care is multidisciplinary, and order and organization are important in communication, the healthcare industry has developed specific policies, procedures, and guidelines that determine how evaluations and treatments are documented in the medical record.

Medical Record Formats

Medical records appear in standard formats to help medical professionals organize and access information about a patient. These standard formats give the medical transcriptionist a tool for easy keying of a concise record that allows rapid scanning and quick retrieval of information by any member of the healthcare team.

Problem Oriented Medical Record In the 1960s, the healthcare industry developed a record-keeping method that has helped to standardize information and make it quickly accessible to all practitioners and in medical databases. The problem oriented medical record (POMR) is a method of record-keeping centered around the patient's specific health problems. This system provides a logical, systematic analysis of the relevant data. For team members, it allows effective communication that focuses on a problem list, or statements of the patient's health-related problems as addressed by various healthcare disciplines. Additions to the list are made by any healthcare professional.

Name ______________________________ Date ____________

Report Number	Date Completed	Document Processing Speed (If Available)	Instructor Comments	Document Appraisal M=Mailable MC=Mailable w/corrections NM=Not Mailable
				M MC NM
				M MC NM
				M MC NM
				M MC NM
				M MC NM
				M MC NM
				M MC NM
				M MC NM
				M MC NM

Comments ______________________________

____

____

____

FIGURE 1.2
Performance Report Chart
Use this chart as a cover sheet when handing in transcribed reports for grading.

The POMR system divides the medical record into four main sections: the database, the problem list, the plan, and the progress notes.

1. Database: This is the section of the chart where all information about the patient's history and current health status is recorded and continuously updated. The database contains input from many sources and includes past and current physical examination results, x-ray and test data, social and occupational histories, and any other information about the patient.

   In the database is the history and physical (H&P), a two-part report documenting the patient's medical history and the findings of a complete physical examination. Hospitals require that an H&P be performed for each patient within a few hours of admission, and physicians may not be allowed to perform surgical or major procedures unless a record of the current H&P is included in the patient's chart or has been dictated.
2. Problem List: This is a numbered list of the patient's problems, which may include a specific diagnosis, a symptom, an abnormal test result, or other health problem. The problem list serves as a basis for the plan of care and includes areas for observation, diagnosis, treatment and/or management, and patient and family education. All problems are identified from physiologic, psychosocial, economic, occupational, and other standpoints. Usually each problem is assigned a number to simplify charting and understanding by all practitioners.
3. Plan: The plan is a description of what actions will be taken to address the various active items on the problem list. A separate plan is noted for each identified problem. Plans include a notation of who might carry out each plan and traditionally includes the areas of diagnosis, treatment, and patient education.
4. Progress Notes: This section contains documentation of observations, assessments, care plans, orders, and other relevant information for all members of the healthcare team. Placing all progress notes in one section of the chart provides easy access for anyone providing care to the patient and encourages coordination of care through effective communication.

The SOAP format is used to simplify documentation and make charting more effective. Caregivers use the abbreviations S, O, A, and P to identify the following parts of the document.

- **S**ubjective: the patient's description of the problem
- **O**bjective: the laboratory data and/or other information observed in the physical examination
- **A**ssessment: an evaluation of the information gathered to produce a diagnosis
- **P**lan: the details of what will be done to address the diagnosis and related problems

The SOAP format of charting is so efficient and so well understood among healthcare professionals that many hospitals and offices use it for progress notes even if they have not adopted the entire POMR system.

Narrative-Style Charting An alternative to the POMR is the traditional narrative style chart. In this method, information is organized according to its source (e.g., physicians, nurses, and therapists). Because data are not grouped by type-specific information in these charts, quick retrieval of information may be difficult and documents may contain repetition.

How Records Are Used

Medical records are used to provide:

- a means of communication for patient treatment and care;
- justification for insurance and compensation purposes;
- a means to support research and education, monitoring medical treatments that are successful and those that need improvement;
- statistics for planning how to best use future resources;
- objective documentation of care or evidence to protect the legal interests of the hospital, physician, and the patient in a court of law.

Legal Issues Surrounding Medical Records Although each hospital or physician establishes specific rules and procedures regarding medical records, there are general guidelines for handling patient information. These rules have been developed in the courts through years of litigation.

Retention The period of retention of medical records is governed by state and local laws. It is typically seven to ten years for original records. Some institutions keep their records indefinitely.

Ownership of Document and Content Medical records that are created in a healthcare facility are considered to belong to that particular facility, as the facility owns the paper on which the record is written. However, the patient owns the information contained in the record. Access to the record is regulated by federal and individual state law.

Release of Information Medical transcriptionists should not release information related to patient care; however, there are some instances where release of information can be accomplished legally. All requests should be processed according to the institution's release-of-information guidelines with the emphasis on confidentiality. There can be no disclosure to any unauthorized person. If there is any doubt whatsoever about releasing information, the medical transcriptionist should not release the information but rather should refer the request to the proper authority. Security of patient records, both computer records and paper records, is very important.

Medicolegal issues that relate to medical records vary from state to state. On the job, you will need to familiarize yourself with the policy manual or office procedure manual detailing your employer's rules for the release of information. If you have questions, consult your supervisor, your employer, or your employer's legal consultant.

Legal Terms Regarding Release of Information Table 1.7 lists some important legal terms with which a medical transcriptionist should become familiar.

Important Components of Medical Records

The hospital record is composed of several types of reports, notes, and documents. Each hospital medical record provides information for one admission for one individual patient. Table 1.8 provides a list of the basic reports that may be contained in the medical record of an inpatient. The discussion that follows details further information about the contents of these reports.

TABLE 1.7 Important Legal Terms

writ
a written order issued by a court or judicial officer commanding a specified person to perform or refrain from performing a specified act.

subpoena
a writ commanding a specified person to appear in court or else serve a penalty for failure to appear. A subpoena of medical records must be honored because it is a legal document.

subpoena duces tecum
(Latin term "in his possession"): a writ commanding a person to produce in court certain specified documents or evidence.

right of privacy
the right to be let alone and free from unwarranted publicity and to withhold personal information from public scrutiny if so desired.

privileged communication
information that may be disclosed only with the patient's permission.

nonprivileged information
this type of information can be disclosed without the patient's permission and usually relates to admission/discharge, treatment dates, name and address of the patient, and name of the individual who accompanied the patient to the hospital or physician's office.

privileged information
any and all information that can only be disclosed with the patient's permission.

breach of confidential communication
the unauthorized release of patient information.

invasion of the right of privacy
needless investigation into another's personal affairs where there is no valid reason to do so, in a way to cause public embarrassment or humiliation to that person.

libel
a written statement or graphic portrayal made or given to a third party that damages a reputation or subjects a person to ridicule.

slander
a witnessed statement that damages a reputation or subjects a person to ridicule.

defamation
slander or libel.

TABLE 1.8 Basic Medical Reports

Report	Contents
Summary Sheet (Face Sheet)	Contains patient demographics and authorization for treatment. If the patient was admitted from the Emergency Room (ER), the Emergency Department Report may be found here or within the History and Physical section.
History and Physical	May include the Emergency Department Report.
Physician Orders	Includes instructions to the healthcare team for the patient's treatment and care.
Diagnostic Report	May include the following, or they may be listed separately. Laboratory and Delivery Report Radiology Report Electrocardiogram/Echocardiogram Pathology Report
Operative Report	Includes a separate report for the Recovery Room record.
Progress Notes (Chart Notes)	May include the following or they may be listed separately. Nurse Notes Social Service Notes
Consultation Request or Letter	No additional contents
Discharge Summary	No additional contents
Autopsy Report	May include lab reports

History and Physical When a patient enters a healthcare system, the physician or examiner generates a comprehensive document called a history and physical (H&P), which becomes the foundation for the medical record. This two-part report documents the patient's medical history, the immediate problem that prompted the patient to seek help, a social and family history, and the findings of a complete physical exam. The primary purpose of the history and physical is to help the physician determine the diagnosis(es), the basis for the patient's care and treatment.

For the history portion (called *subjective* information since it is supplied by the patient), the examiner interviews the patient, asking first for the reason of the visit (called the *Chief Complaint*). This is followed by questions about childhood illnesses and all previous diseases, surgical procedures, medications, immunizations, and allergies. Also included are questions about parents' and siblings' state of health. Finally, the physician asks the patient questions about all the body systems in a cephalocaudal (head-to-toe) order.

The second part of the report is the complete physical examination (called *objective* information because the physician observes it), which also is conducted in cephalocaudal order. Other objective information includes vital statistics and general appearance.

Concluding the entire report is the physician's impression or diagnosis and a plan of care. Figure 1.3 displays a sample history and physical.

Operative Report The operative report describes a surgical or other invasive procedure. Whenever a surgical procedure is done in a hospital, outpatient center, or clinic, an operative report should be recorded in the medical record. The operative report is illustrated and discussed in Chapter 6.

Discharge Summary The discharge summary summarizes the reason a patient was admitted to the hospital, a short history and a sequential listing of events and treatment that occurred during the patient's hospitalization, and a final diagnosis(es) upon release from the hospital. See Chapter 7 for an illustration and discussion of the discharge summary.

Chart Note The chart notes, also called progress notes or office visits, are brief reports that document the findings from each examination of the patient. The chart note/office visit is featured in Chapter 4.

Consultation Request or Letter The consultation request or letter documents the findings of a specialist requested to see the patient of an attending physician to offer a second opinion. See Chapter 5 for an illustration and explanation of the consultation letter.

Radiology Report Radiology reports describe findings and interpretations from x-rays or special diagnostic studies performed in a radiology department. They list a radiologic diagnosis by the radiologist who reviews the films or test results. The radiology report is featured in Chapter 8.

Pathology Report The pathological report describes disease-related findings from a sample of tissue. This report is illustrated and explained in Chapter 9.

Autopsy Report The autopsy report is also a pathological report requested by the attending physician or a coroner to determine a patient's cause of death. Also called a post-mortem, this report is featured in Chapter 15.

Guidelines for Preparing and Managing Medical Records Four major medical organizations have developed guidelines for preparing and managing medical records:

- American Association for Medical Transcription (AAMT), a nonprofit professional corporation for medical transcriptionists and MT students that administers a certification exam and publishes a medical report style guide as well as a journal for members.

PATIENT: Raymond Cheever
DATE: 7/10/XX
HOSPITAL NO: 93-22-17
PHYSICIAN: Harry Washington, MD

CHIEF COMPLAINT: Severe pain in the left hip.

HISTORY OF PRESENT ILLNESS: The patient is a 57-year-old white male who is admitted from the emergency department with hypertension, hyperglycemia, and greater trochanteric bursitis.

The patient has been under treatment for greater trochanteric bursitis with Lortab and Naprosyn. He returns today because of increasing left hip pain.

In the emergency room, he was noted to be significantly hypertensive and hyperglycemic. He is unaware of having a history of either.

ALLERGIES: No medicine allergies.

PRESENT MEDICATIONS
1. Lortab 7.5 mg q.d.
2. Naprosyn 375 mg q.d.

PAST MEDICAL HISTORY: Negative.

SURGICAL HISTORY: Tonsils and adenoids removed in early childhood.

SOCIAL HISTORY: The patient does not smoke at present. He stopped smoking 6 to 7 years ago; he smoked an average of a pack per day for many years. He denies ethanol use. He is married. He has 2 children, who are alive and in good health. He works as a plant manager for a chemical company.

FAMILY HISTORY: Mother is alive and in good health. His father is deceased secondary to complications of black lung and asthma. He has 2 brothers and 1 sister. He thinks his sister has a history of hypertension.

(continued)

FIGURE 1.3
Sample History and Physical Report

HISTORY AND PHYSICAL
PATIENT: Raymond Cheever
HOSPITAL NO: 93-22-17
DATE: 7/10/XX
Page 2

REVIEW OF SYSTEMS: A full review of systems was negative. He states that his weight has been stable in the past year. He denies polyuria, polydipsia, or polyphagia.

PHYSICAL EXAMINATION
GENERAL: Well-developed, well-nourished male in no acute distress.
VITAL SIGNS: Blood pressure 200/104. Repeat, after rest and pain medication, was 170/96. The pulse was 72. Respiratory rate was 18 and labored. Patient refused to be weighed at this time because of pain.
HEENT: Pupils were somewhat constricted, but fundi were visualized minimally. No hypertensive retinopathy, exudates, hemorrhages, or papilledema were noted. Oral examination revealed no ulcerations, erosions, or masses.
NECK: Supple, without lymphadenopathy. The carotid upstrokes were brisk and equal bilaterally, without bruits. Thyroid nonpalpable.
CHEST: Chest was clear to auscultation in all fields.
CARDIOVASCULAR: Regular rate and rhythm, without murmurs, thrill, gallop, or click.
ABDOMEN: Abdomen nontender and nondistended, without masses, organomegaly, guarding, tenderness, or rebound.
EXTREMITIES: Without clubbing, cyanosis, or edema. Peripheral pulses were intact, with good upstrokes. Palpation of the left hip did reveal tenderness, although the patient did report it was much improved after analgesia.

LABORATORY DATA: Review of a Chem-7 revealed a blood sugar of 201. His urinalysis revealed greater than 1000 glucose. CBC revealed a hemoglobin of 16.3 and hematocrit of 50. White count was 14.7. Platelets were 291,000. Differential was essentially within normal limits.

IMPRESSION
1. Marked hypertension.
2. Asymptomatic hyperglycemia with glycosuria.
3. Left greater trochanteric bursitis.

(continued)

FIGURE 1.3
Sample History and Physical Report (Continued)

HISTORY AND PHYSICAL
PATIENT: Raymond Cheever
HOSPITAL NO: 93-22-17
DATE: 7/10/XX

Page 3

PLAN
1. Admit.
2. Orthopedic consultation.
3. Endocrinology consultation.
4. Cardiology consultation.

____

Harry Washington, MD

HW/XX
D: 07/10/XX
T: 07/11/XX

FIGURE 1.3
Sample History and Physical Report (Continued)

- Joint Commission on Accreditation of Healthcare Organizations (JCAHO), a nongovernmental agency that offers a voluntary healthcare accreditation process for hospitals. Part of the accreditation process requires compliance with JCAHO's standards for the kinds of information entered into the medical record, the completeness of medical reports, abbreviation systems, and turnaround times for report dictation and transcription.
- American Medical Association (AMA), the professional organization for physicians. This group has developed several medicolegal forms that hospitals use regularly, including a variety of patient consent forms.
- American Health Information Management Association (AHIMA), formerly known as the American Medical Record Association. This organization has developed broad guidelines for the development and distribution of patients' medical record information, including positions on the patient's right of access.

Each chapter of this text features a medical document type and presents the AAMT and JCAHO style, format, and content guidelines for transcribing that document. Follow these guidelines to learn the generally accepted report formats. When you are on the job, however, consider the guidelines a starting point. In all cases, it is the dictator of the report who has the final word on style. Medical transcriptionists must follow their employers' special style preferences.

Using Templates

A document or form that will be used in the future as a framework for other documents can be created and saved as a template or as a master form. Templates are created to ensure consistency in information processing and standardization in reporting. Templated forms are created so that anyone who fills in the form is working on a copy of the document, not the original. The original is the template document and is saved as a protected document. In this way, a form or template is used over and over again without changing the original form. Template documents can include headings, text boxes, check boxes, and lists. Figure 1.4 is an example of a template.

As you work through the text, you will find that a specialized type of medical report is featured in each chapter. Also, there are other types of reports within each chapter. When transcribing the chapter reports, use the templates provided. These templates correspond to the model documents and standard formats of the various reports. During the transcription process, you will be prompted to key the dictated information after the headings. In some cases, forms may need to be modified and you may find that headings may need to be added or changed. Be aware that each institution will have its own templates and letterhead stationery. Those provided here are merely suggestions for different report types.

LIFETIME ANNUITY INSURANCE APPLICATION

FIRST APPLICANT

Name:
Address:
Date of Birth:
Occupation:

SECOND APPLICANT

Name:
Address:
Date of Birth:
Occupation:

1. During the past 3 years, have you for any reason consulted a doctor or been hospitalized?

   First Applicant: Yes No
   Second Applicant: Yes No

2. Have you ever been treated for or advised that you had any of the following: heart, lung, nervous, kidney, or liver disorder; high blood pressure; drug abuse, including alcohol; cancer or tumor, AIDS, or any disorder of your immune system; diabetes?

   First Applicant: Yes No
   Second Applicant: Yes No

These answers are true and complete to the best of my knowledge and belief. To determine my insurability, I authorize any health care provider or insurance company to give any information about me or my physical or mental health.

FIRST APPLICANT'S SIGNATURE ____________________

SECOND APPLICANT'S SIGNATURE ____________________

FIGURE 1.4
Sample Template
The shaded areas of this template can be filled in, but the other copy is not changed.

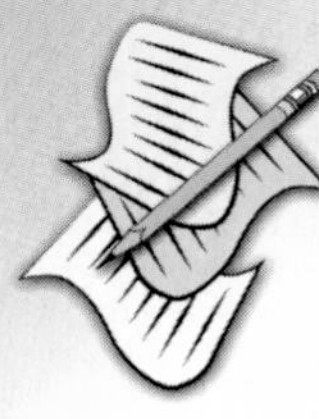

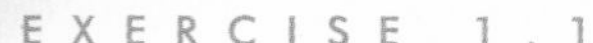

EXERCISE 1.1

Issues for Discussion

1. In the future, transcriptionists may not hear the dictator's voice but instead receive electronic files of reports that the computer "transcribed" from voice input.
   - How would this scenario change your job as a medical language specialist?
   - How would your job remain the same?
2. What types of errors in transcribed documents are the most critical from the patient's perspective? From the hospital's perspective? How do you think transcriptionists learn they have made an important error?
3. Think about the job requirements for speed and accuracy. Name two medical situations where a fast turnaround between dictation and transcription may be critical to a patient's care.
4. Review the list of personal attributes needed on the job and then think about what type of employment setting you prefer (home business, clinical, hospital). Which of the personal traits listed are most needed for the job setting you prefer? Evaluate your strengths and weaknesses in each of these areas.

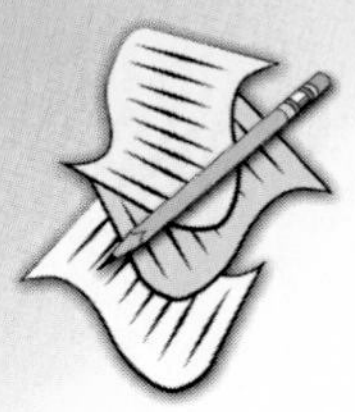

EXERCISE 1.2

Editing a Document Created on Voice/Speech Recognition Software

The paragraph that follows was dictated and transcribed using voice/speech recognition software. Edit it to include making corrections in punctuation and the context and re-key it.

HISTORY OF PRESENT ILLNESS. Mr. Carr is a 40 year old mail admitted to Riverside medical center for treatment of deep vein thrombophlebitis in his left lower extremity. Mr. Carr has always been healthy, has never been hospitalized, and has had no medical problems until recently. About six weeks ago, he developed a superficial thrombophlebitis of the left low extrimity. He was treated for this without incident and scenes to improve. About one week ago, he was trying to get back into shape and started working out on a treadmill. He noted some discomfort in his left calf, which she had attributed to muscle pain and continued his exercise. All over the past 24 hours, the left of lower extremity has become more painful and swollen. He was seen by doctor Winston at the Riverside medical center and a Doppler ultrasound was performed demonstrating clear evidence of deep venous thrombosis. He is now admitted for treatment of that condition. He has not had any undue shortness of breath, nor has he had any polyp petitions, cough, or chest pain. The notes that he usually runs a rapid Paul's in the range of 80 or 90.

Transcription Practice 1.A — Employee Healthcare Program

This letter explains the employee healthcare program provided to the Marathon Health Services company.

REPORT 1.1

- Preferred format will vary by agency, but AAMT prefers block format.

Transcription Practice 1.B — Administrative Medical Assistant Position

A position as administrative medical assistant is open at River Oak Medical Center. Ms. Anita Brooks, a student at Winthrop College, is being recommended by Mr. Peter Harris, Director of Placement.

REPORT 1.2

- Inside addresses will be spelled out by dictator.
- CPT codes are used in medical billing.
- Check the spelling of the various disciplines used in the dictation.
- Listen for these names:
  Winthrop College
  Harley Association

Transcription Practice 1.C — Health Care Seminars Announcement

The Ohio Health Care Treatment Center, The Women's Club of Danbury, and Springfield Hospital have joined forces to offer health-related seminars. Residents of the community are invited to attend. No entrance fee is required; however, individuals interested in attending must register in advance.

REPORT 1.3

- Leave four blank lines after the dateline to personalize the letter, if desired.
- Madeline Delroy, a medical assistant, is the dictator.
- Use the spell check and proofread carefully for sentence structure, meaning, capitalization, and punctuation.

Transcription Practice 1.D — Emerging Trends in Alternative Medicine

Changes are occurring in conventional medicine, and alternative therapies are being used by a percentage of the population. Facilities that use conventional medicine are now starting to evaluate alternative therapies. This report cites a number of approaches being used for healthcare.

REPORT 1.4

- Use solid caps when keying sideheadings.
- Leave a space before and after a sideheading.
- Check the meaning of terms with which you may not be familiar.
  concerted
  comprehensive
  impacting
  alternative therapies
  self-hypnotic
  vital signs
  vertebrae
  holistic

2

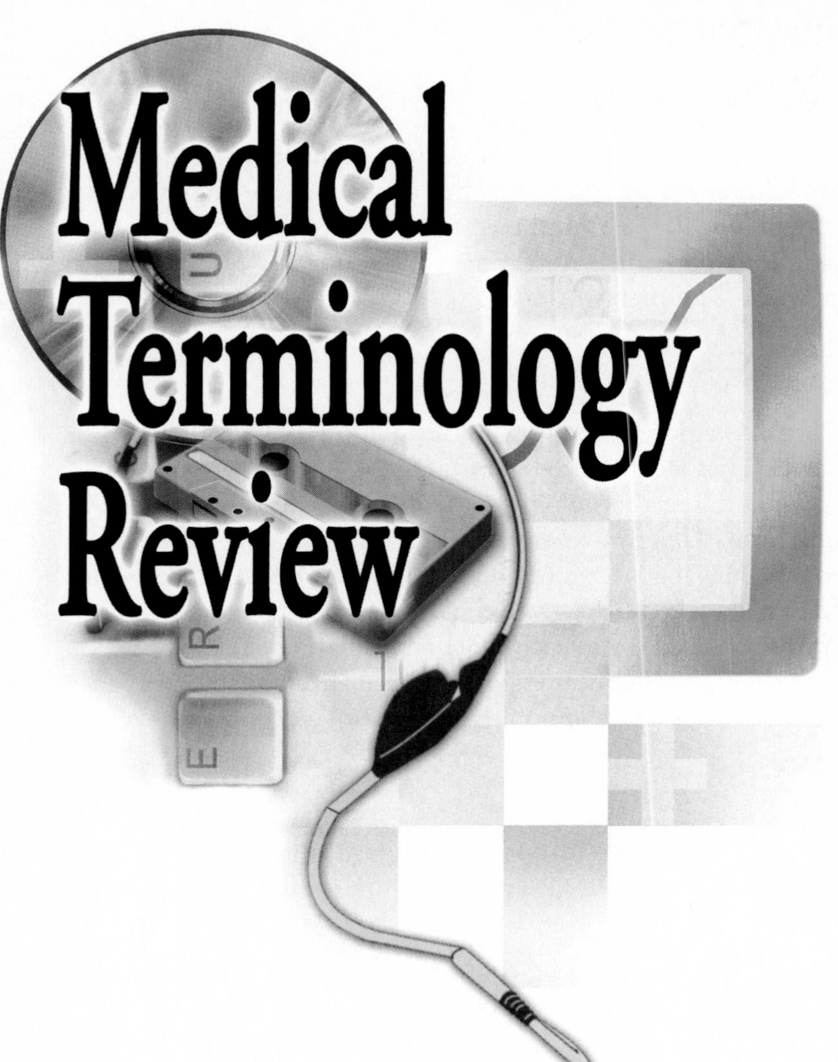

The field of medicine has a specialized language with an enormous vocabulary of words identifying diseases, medical processes and procedures, body structures, and body systems. A solid knowledge of medical terms is essential for working in a healthcare environment.

OBJECTIVES

- Acquire basic knowledge of medical terms and their elements.
- Learn how the elements of terminology can be interchanged to meet specific needs.
- Become familiar with physicians' terms that map the human body.
- Learn the directional and positional terms used in diagnosis.
- Recognize the diagnostic importance of color and pain sensations and modern medical imaging procedures.

Word Parts and How They Are Combined

A prerequisite for learning medical transcription is a course in medical terminology. In that course you learned many words and how they are used. Most importantly, you learned word parts and how they are combined to form a complete term. In the following tables you will find a brief review of some common root words, suffixes, combining vowels and forms, and prefixes.

Root Words and Combining Forms

Root words provide the foundation of the medical term and are the source of its meaning. Each body system has a core of root words that will be provided in each of the sections of this book. Adding a combining vowel to a root word creates a word part called a combining form. These vowels make it easier to spell and pronounce medical terms and serve as links for root words when more than one root is needed to form the term. Additionally, a combining vowel may be used to join a root word and a suffix. Root words may be added to each other and function equally to serve as the foundation or contribute to the meaning of the original root. Table 2.1 provides a list of common root words and combining forms that you should know.

Prefixes

A prefix is a word part that comes before the root and begins the term. Prefixes further modify the root or roots; they often give an indication of direction, time, or orientation.

Suffixes

A suffix provides an ending that modifies and gives specific meaning to the root word. The suffixes presented in Tables 2.3, 2.4, and 2.5 are grouped by type: general; conditions, symptoms, or diagnoses; and procedures. Many of the anatomic and physiologic terms for each body system include one of the general suffixes, while names of conditions and diagnoses tend to use one of the condition-related suffixes that indicate disease actions. A special group of suffixes for procedures relate to some type of surgical cutting.

Suffixes are also used to create plural forms of words. In medical terminology, plural word forms can be confusing unless you understand one simple aspect: some plural terms are formed on the basis of Greek and Latin rules, while others are formed using English language rules. In English, plurals usually are constructed by simply adding *s* or *es* to the singular form (the plural of vein is veins). With Latin- and Greek-based words, plurals are formed by adding an ending based on the ending of the singular form (*stria,* meaning a discolored stripe on the skin, becomes *striae* as a plural). Singular words ending in *um* take an *a* in the plural form (*diverticulum,* a pouch or sac that has developed within the gut or bladder, becomes *diverticula* as a plural). Words ending in *nx* take an *nges* ending as plurals (*larynx,* part of the throat, becomes *larynges*).

TABLE 2.1 Common Root Words and Combining Forms

Root Word	Combining Form	Meaning
abdomin-	*abdomin/o*	abdomen
angi-	*angi/o*	vessel
bacteri-	*bacteri/o*	bacteria
bi-	*bi/o*	life (Greek derivation)
carcin-	*carcin/o*	cancer; cancerous
cardi-	*cardi/o*	heart
cephal-	*cephal/o*	head
cyst-	*cyst/o*	sac or cyst containing fluid; urinary bladder
cyt-	*cyt/o*	cell
electr-	*electr/o*	electricity
enter-	*enter/o*	intestines
fibrin-	*fibrin/o*	fiber
gnath-	*gnath/o*	jaw
gynec-	*gynec/o*	woman, female
hem-	*hem/o*	blood
hemat-	*hemat/o*	blood
hepat-	*hepat/o*	liver
irid-	*irid/o*	iris
kerat-	*kerat/o*	keratin (a protein)
lip-	*lip/o*	fat
mast-	*mast/o*	breast
necr-	*necr/o*	death
nephr-	*nephr/o*	kidney
onc-	*onc/o*	tumor
path-	*path/o*	disease
pelv-	*pelv/o*	pelvic
radi-	*radi/o*	x-rays
ren-	*ren/o*	renal, the kidney
sarc-	*sarc/o*	flesh
sial-	*sial/o*	saliva, salivary glands
thromb-	*thromb/o*	clot
trache-	*trache/o*	trachea
uter-	*uter/o*	uterus

TABLE 2.2 Common Prefixes

Prefix	Meaning	Example
a-	without, not	apnea—without breathing
an-		anhydrous—without water
ab-	away from	abnormality—away from normal
ad-	toward, to, near	adduction—toward the center
ambi-	both	ambidextrous—use of both hands
ante-	before	antepartum—before labor or childbirth
pre-		prenatal—before birth
pro-		procephalic—anterior part (before) of the head
anti-	against; opposed to	antibiotic—against bacteria
contra-		contraindication—opposed to a certain treatment
auto-	self	autoimmune—immunity to self
bi-	two (Latin derivation); both	bilateral—both sides
di-		didactylism—condition of two digits on a hand or foot
bio-	life	biology—study of life
brady-	slow	bradycardia—slow heart rate
circum-	around; circular movement	circumorbital—around the orbit (eye)
peri-		pericardium—around the heart
con-	with or together	consanguineous—with blood (common ancestry)
sym-		symbiotic—with life
syn-		synergy—with energy
de-	not; from; down	decalcify—removal of calcium
dia-	across or through	diathermy—through heat
trans-		transurethral—across the urethra
dis-	apart; separate	disease—separate from ease
dys-	faulty; painful; difficult	dysuria—painful urination
e-	out; away	efferent—conduction away from
ec-		ectomorphic—away from form
ex-		excrete— separate, cast out
ecto-	outside	ectoderm—outer layer of skin
exo-		exothermic—release of heat
extra-		extracellular—outside the cell
en-	inside; within	enclosed—contained within
endo-		endocardium—innermost layer (lining) of the heart
intra-		intra-abdominal—within the abdomen

(continues)

TABLE 2.2 Common Prefixes (Continued)

Prefix	Meaning	Example
epi-	upon	epigastric—upon (above) the stomach
eu-	normal or good	eupnea—normal breathing
hemi-	half	hemicardia—half of the heart (right or left)
semi-		semilunar—half moon
hyper-	above or excessive; extreme	hyperkalemia—excess potassium (in the blood)
hypo-	deficient; below	hypoglycemia—low blood sugar
infra-	under; below	inframammary—below the breast
sub-		subdural—below the dura mater
inter-	between	intercellular—between cells
mal-	bad	malaise—bad comfort; discomfort
meso-	middle	mesophlebitis—inflammation of the middle layer of the wall of a vein
meta-	beyond; after; change	metastasis—extension of disease from one part of the body to another
micro-	small	microcardia—small heart
mono-	one	mononuclear—one nucleus
uni-		unilateral—one side
neo-	new	neonatal—new birth
pachy-	thick	pachyderma—thick skin
pan-	all	panimmunity—immune to all diseases
para-	abnormal; alongside; beside	paracystic—alongside the bladder
per-	through	percutaneous—through the skin
poly-	many	polycythemia—many red blood cells
multi-		multidisciplinary—many areas of study
post-	after	postmortem—after death
quadri-	four	quadriplegic—paralysis of all four limbs
tetra-		tetradactylism—condition of only four digits on a hand or foot
re-	again or back	resorb—absorb again
retro-	backward or behind	retroflexion—backward bending
sub-	under, below	subvaginal—below the vagina
super-	above or excessive	superficial—near the surface
supra-	outside or beyond	suprascleral—outside the sclera
tachy-	fast	tachycardia—rapid heart rate
tri-	three	trigeminy—three abnormal heartbeats
ultra-	beyond, excessive	ultrasonic—excessive sound

TABLE 2.3 Most Commonly Used General Suffixes

Suffix	Meaning	Example
-ac	pertaining to	hemophiliac—pertaining to an individual with hemophilia
-al		temporal—pertaining to the temporal lobe of the brain
-ar		clavicular—pertaining to the clavicle
-ry		sensory—pertaining to the senses
-eal		esophageal—pertaining to the esophagus
-ic		gastric—pertaining to the stomach (gastrum)
-ose		adipose—relating to fat
-ous		cutaneous—pertaining to the skin
-tic		spermatic—pertaining to sperm
-blast	immature	osteoblast—immature bone cell
-cyte	cell	osteocyte—bone cell
-e	noun marker (indicates this form of the word is a noun)	melanocyte—pigment-producing skin cell
-gram	record	electroencephalogram—record of brain activity
-graph	instrument for recording	electroencephalograph—instrument for recording brain activity
-graphy	process of recording	electrocardiography—process of recording the electrical activity of the heart
-meter	instrument for measuring	arthrometer—instrument for measuring motion in a joint
-metry	process of measuring	arthrometry—process of measuring joint motion
-iatric	treatment	psychiatric—treatment of the psyche
-iatry	study of	psychiatry—study of the psyche
-logy		urology—study of urine
-logist	one who specializes in the the treatment or study of	cardiologist—one who specializes in the treatment or study of the heart
-icle	small	ventricle—small pouch or cavity, particularly within the heart or brain
-ole		arteriole—small artery
-ula		macula—small spot
-ule		pustule—small lesion (pimple) with pus
-ium/-eum	tissue or structure	periosteum—structure surrounding bone
-ize	make; use; subject to	anesthetize—subject to anesthesia
-ate		impregnate—make pregnant
-or	one who	medicator—one who gives medicine
-poiesis	formation	erythropoiesis—formation of red blood cells
-scope	instrument for examining	cystoscope—instrument for examining the bladder
-scopy	examination	cystoscopy—examination of the bladder
-stasis	stop or stand	hemostasis—stop bleeding

TABLE 2.4 Suffixes Related to Conditions, Symptoms, or Diagnoses

Suffix	Meaning	Example
-algia *-dynia*	pain	myalgia—muscle pain arthrodynia—pain in a joint
-cele	pouch, sac, or hernia	cystocele—hernia of the bladder
-emesis	vomit	hyperemesis—excessive vomiting
-emia	condition of blood	anemia—condition of insufficient iron in the blood
-form *-oid*	like or resembling	vermiform—resembling vermin osteoid—resembling bone
-genic *-genesis*	beginning, origin, or production	pyogenic—production of pus pathogenesis—origin of disease
-ia *-ism*	condition of	dysuria—condition of painful urination hirsutism—condition of excessive hair
-iasis	formation of; presence of	lithiasis—formation of stone
-itis	inflammation	tendinitis—inflammation of a tendon
-lysis	breaking down	hemolysis—breaking down of blood
-malacia	softening	osteomalacia—softening of bone
-megaly	enlargement	cardiomegaly—enlargement of the heart
-oma	tumor	osteoma—tumor of bone
-osis	condition;	psychosis—condition of the psyche
-penia	abnormal reduction; lack of	leukocytopenia—abnormal reduction of white blood cells
-phage *-phagia* *-phagy*	eat; devour	macrophage—large cell that devours geophagia—eating dirt aerophagy—swallowing air
-phile *-philia*	attraction for; love for	pedophile—abnormal adult attraction to children hemophilia—attraction for blood
-phobia	fear of	photophobia—fear of light
-plasia	formation	dysplasia—faulty formation
-pnea	breathing	apnea—without breathing
-ptosis	drooping; falling or downward displacement	mastoptosis—drooping breast
-rrhage *-rrhagia* *-rrhagic*	to burst forth	hemorrhage—bursting forth of blood hemorrhagia—condition of bleeding hemorrhagic—relating to condition of bleeding
-rrhea	discharge or flow	amenorrhea—absence of menstrual flow
-rrhexis	rupture or breaking	trichorrhexis—breaking of hair
-spasm	involuntary contraction	laryngospasm—involuntary contraction of the larynx
-trophy	development	hypertrophy—excess development (enlargement)
-y	condition or process of	ambulatory—process of ambulation (walking)

TABLE 2.5 Suffixes Related to Procedures

Suffix	Meaning	Example
-centesis	puncture to remove fluid	amniocentesis—puncture of the amniotic membrane to remove fluid
-desis	binding	arthrodesis—binding of a joint
-ectomy	excision; surgical removal	splenectomy—removal of the spleen
-pexy	surgical suspension or fixation	uteropexy—surgical fixation of the uterus
-plasty	surgical repair or reconstruction	hernioplasty—surgical repair of a hernia
-rrhaphy	suture	myorrhaphy—suture of muscle
-stomy	surgical creation of an artificial opening	colostomy—creation of an artificial opening in the colon
-tomy	incision	tracheotomy—incision into the trachea
-tripsy	crushing	lithotripsy—crushing of stones

The rules do not apply consistently, however, and for that reason the best strategy is to memorize the plural spelling for each new word you learn. Whenever you are uncertain of the correct plural form of a term, consult your medical dictionary. Table 2.6 lists some of the common plural forms.

TABLE 2.6 Frequently Used Plural Forms

Singular	Ending	Plural
apex	*-ex/-ices*	apices
appendix	*-ix/-ices*	appendices
bacterium	*-ium/-ia*	bacteria
cardiopathy	*-y/-ies*	cardiopathies
condyloma	*-a/-ata*	condylomata
diagnosis	*-is/-es*	diagnoses
fungus	*-us/-i*	fungi
phenomenon	*-on/a*	phenomena
thorax	*-ax/-aces*	thoraces
vertebra	*-a/-ae*	vertebrae

Suggestions for Learning Medical Terms

In each specialty chapter in Part II of this text, a list of vocabulary terms that relate to the specialty is provided, along with their definitions and a pronunciation key. Words that are included in the transcription activities are highlighted in order to help you focus your study of these terms.

Every vocabulary word that may be difficult to pronounce is displayed with a phonetic pronunciation. As is common in dictionaries, the words are broken into syllables (indicated by hyphens), and **boldface** letters indicate which syllable(s) should receive the emphasis when you say the word out loud. Note also that the word's part of speech is included in parentheses—for example, (n) for noun and (adj) for adjective; pl stands for plural. The letters and letter combinations in Table 2.7 represent specific sounds in the phonetic pronunciations provided throughout this text.

TABLE 2.7 Phonetic Pronunciation Chart

Symbol	Pronunciation
a	the short a as in can
ay	the long a as in cane
ah	a as in father
ai	ai as in fair
ar	ar as in far
aw	a as in fall
e	the short e as in pen
ee	the long e as in me
i	the short i as in pin
I	the long i as in pine
o	the short o as in not
O	the long o as in note
oo	oo as in food
or	or as in for
ow	ow as in cow
oy	as in boy
u	the short u as in run
yoo	the long u as in cube
zh	s as in casual

As you study each chapter's vocabulary list, follow these suggestions for learning and expanding your vocabulary.

1. Read and study each word for pronunciation and meaning.
2. Write each unfamiliar word from the list on a notecard, write the definition or a paraphrase of the definition on the back, and draw a simple picture to help you learn the word.
3. Study the pronunciation, spelling, and definition of each word on your notecard, then key each word twice for reinforcement. Check the spelling.
4. Add the terms to your word processor's spell checker.

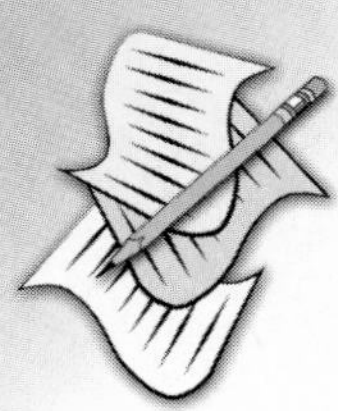

EXERCISE 2.1

What Can it Mean?

Give the definition for each of the following word parts.

Suffixes

1. -iasis __________
2. -emesis __________
3. -phile__________
4. -malacia __________
5. -itis __________
6. -oid__________
7. -trophy __________
8. -rrhea__________
9. -ptosis__________
10. -phobia__________

Prefixes

11. tri- __________
12. pre-__________
13. brady-__________
14. auto-__________
15. dys-__________
16. syn-__________
17. bio-__________
18. ambi-__________
19. anti- __________
20. an- __________

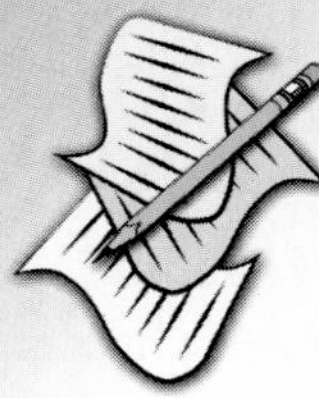

EXERCISE 2.2

Name that Part

Divide each of the following terms into prefixes, combining forms, and suffixes. Then define each term. You may need to look up some of the terms in a medical dictionary.

	Word Parts	Definition of Term
1. abdominocentesis	____________________	____________________
2. angiogram	____________________	____________________
3. melanocyte	____________________	____________________
4. carditis	____________________	____________________
5. cephalgia	____________________	____________________
6. cytorrhexis	____________________	____________________
7. dysuria	____________________	____________________
8. osteocyte	____________________	____________________
9. epigastric	____________________	____________________
10. esophageal	____________________	____________________
11. fibroid	____________________	____________________
12. gastric	____________________	____________________
13. hemigastrectomy	____________________	____________________
14. intracranial	____________________	____________________
15. urology	____________________	____________________

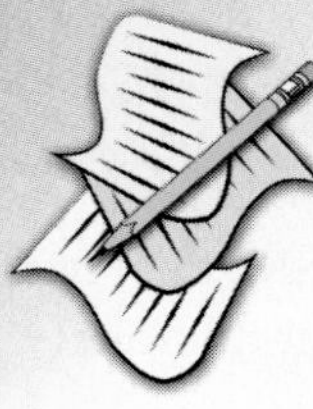

E X E R C I S E 2 . 3

Here's the Answer. What's the Question?

In the following exercises, write a question using a medical term for each definition (What is ....?). Some of the word parts are provided. Use the tables in this chapter and a medical dictionary as needed.

Diagnostic and Procedural Terms

hyper-	-otomy	mast-
-itis	-ectomy	-ptosis
-oma	-megaly	-phagy
oste-	-genic	neo-

1. excess development or enlargement ______
2. origin of or producing pus ______
3. inflammation of a tendon ______
4. bone tumor ______
5. enlargement of the heart ______
6. swallowing (eating) air ______
7. drooping breast ______
8. incision into the trachea ______
9. removal of the spleen ______
10. immediately after birth ______

Medical Specialties

cardi- dermat- nephr- gastroenter- neur-

11. study of the heart ______
12. study of skin ______
13. study of the kidneys ______
14. study of the digestive system ______
15. study of nerves ______

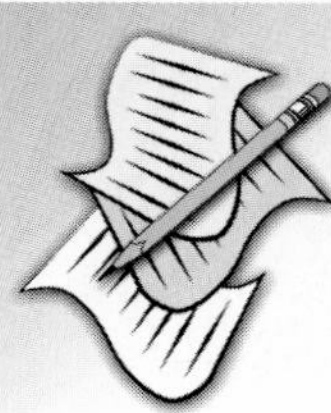

E X E R C I S E 2 . 4

Matching Singulars and Plurals

Circle the proper noun in each sentence. Indicate whether the proper term is singular or plural.

1. When the physician examined the patient, he heard (rhonchi/rhonchus) in the lower lung fields.
2. The x-ray revealed obstruction in each of the (broncus/bronchi).
3. After using the inhaler, the patient's (alveolus/alveoli) were cleared.
4. It was clear to see the single (hypha/hyphae) under the microscope.
5. The patient was infected with two types of (fungus/fungi).
6. The infant's left (naris/nares) was occluded.
7. The 3rd thoracic (vertebra/vertebrae) was injured in the accident.
8. The students reviewed the x-rays and became familiar with observing different sizes of (thorax/thoraces/thoraxes) of hundreds of patients.
9. There were lesions noted at both of the (apex/apices/apexes) of the lungs.
10. When looking at the eyes, the examiner notes whether the (conjunctiva/conjuctivae) in each eye is clear.

Anatomical Terms That Map the Human Body

The human body is a living organism from the tiniest microscopic cell to the large systems that work together to make the body function. There are medical terms used to describe every part of the body—each cell, cavity, region, division—providing a map of the exact place and structure of that part. This section will describe the terms that are used to depict these elements and where they are located.

Levels of Organization

After the cell was defined as the unit of life in the human body, researchers could picture the way groups of cells make up a tissue, a group of tissues make up a body organ, and the organs make up functional systems such as the nervous system, the gastrointestinal system, the urinary system, and others. This concept is known as the *levels of organization* (see Figure 2.1). Note that each level becomes larger, or more complex, than the one below it.

As a foundation for your study of body systems, you will learn the general, whole-body terminology that you need to build your vocabulary of individual body system words. The terms related to cells and tissues and their structure are found in this book's pathology reports. Surgical reports contain terms related to tissues and organs.

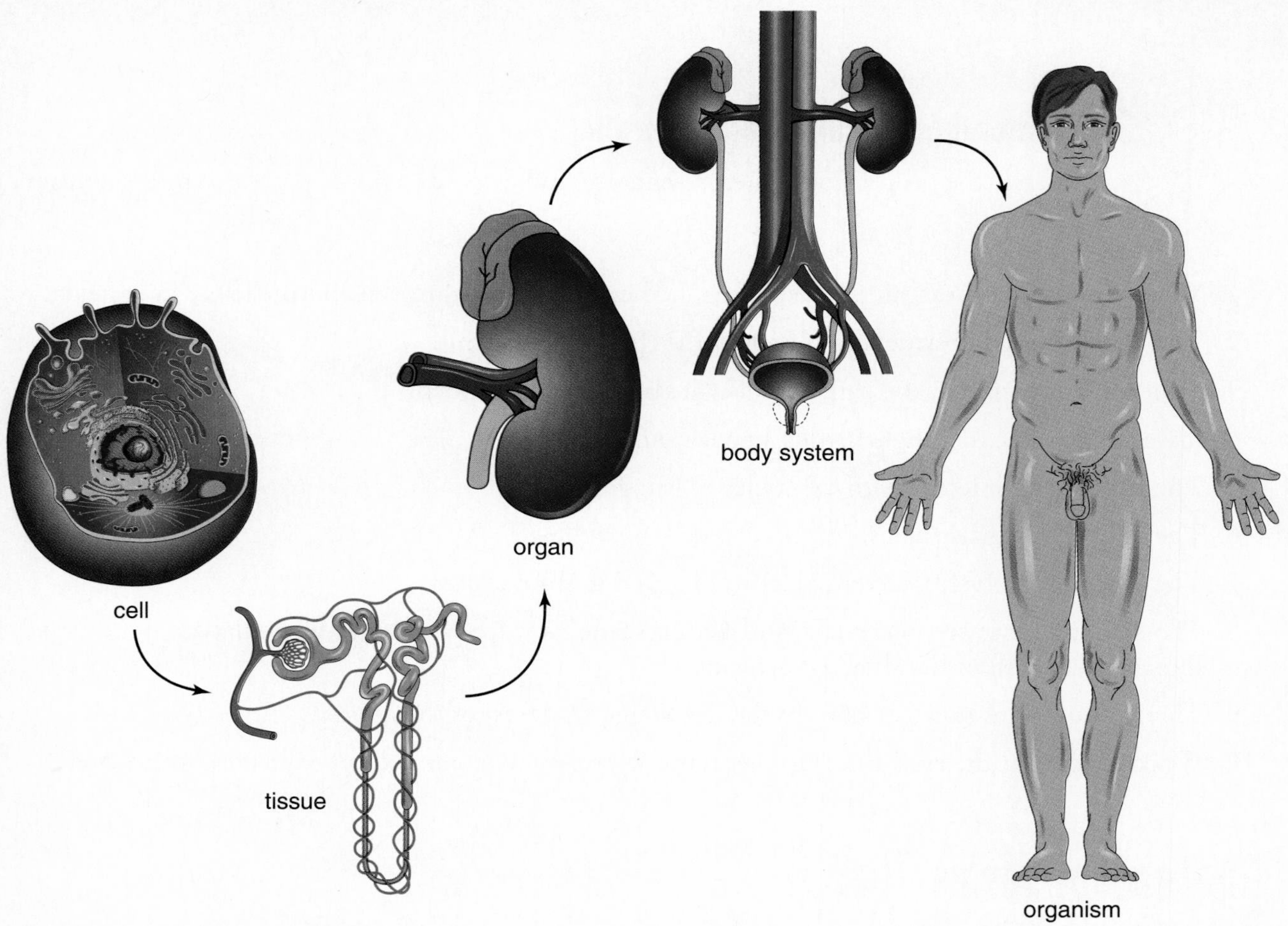

FIGURE 2.1
Levels of Organization

Cells Cytology is the study of cells, including their origin, structure, functions, and pathology. (You may recall that the combining form *cyt/o* means "cell" and the suffix *-logy* means "study of.") The cell is the basic unit of all living things and is the smallest unit capable of independent life and reproduction (see Figure 2.2). All cells have certain similarities, but cells in the human body are highly specialized. Each has its own distinct outer membrane that maintains the cell and controls passage of materials into and out of the cell.

Inside the membrane is a substance that early scientists called protoplasm (*protos* = first or original; *plasma* = substance). Thanks to the discipline of microbiology (*micro-* = small; *bio-* = life; *-logy* = study of), we now know that this substance (cytoplasm) is actually a collection of structures—called organelles—in a thick, fluidlike matrix. The organelles perform various activities that help maintain the cell and assist with cell reproduction.

The interior of the cell also contains the nucleus, a structure that controls activities of the cell and contains genetic material necessary for reproduction. DNA, or deoxyribonucleic acid, is a chemically complex substance that determines the heritable characters and the makeup and functioning of the cell. The interior of a cell may also contain food particles (such as fat and starch), pigment granules, and spe-

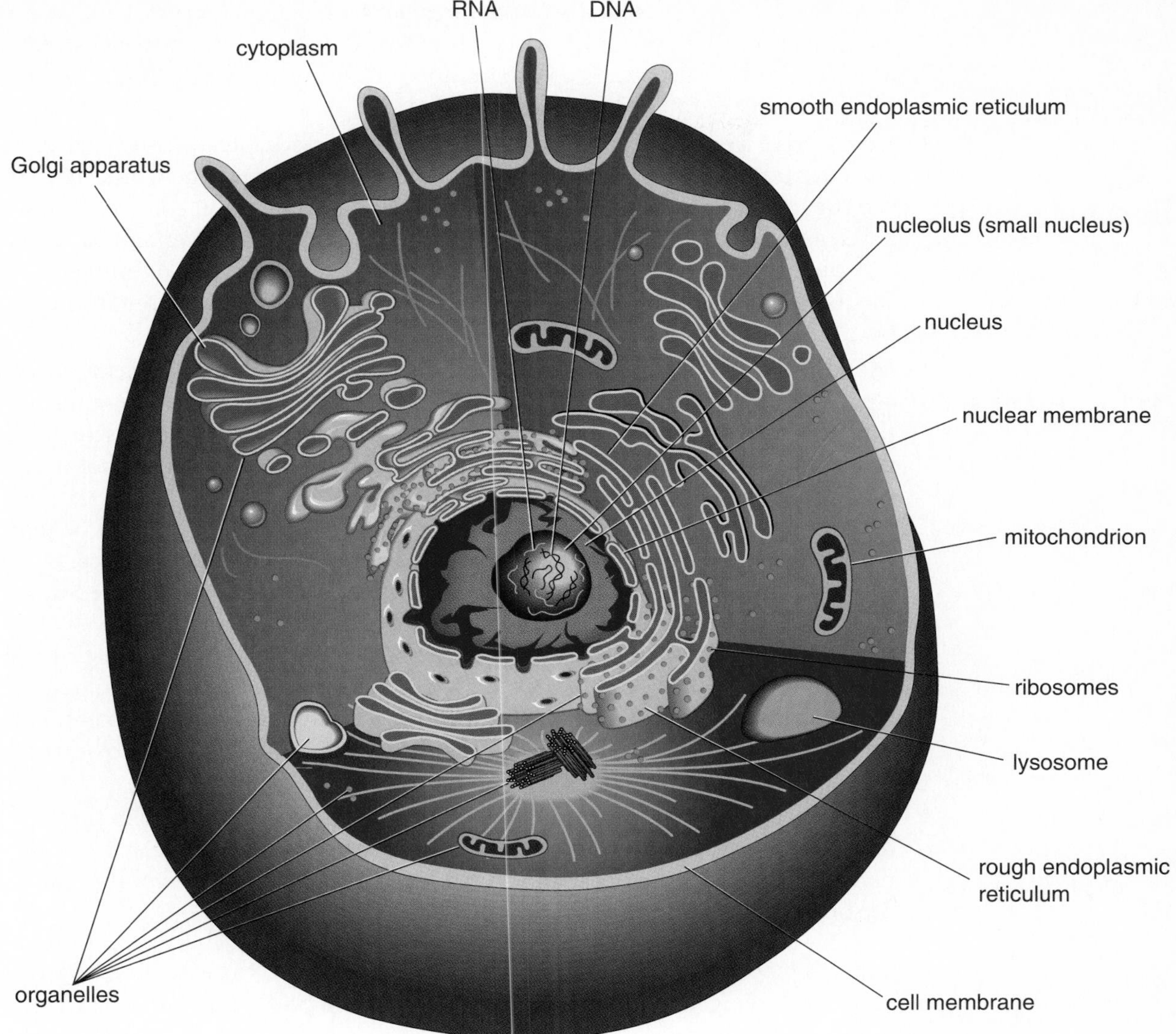

FIGURE 2.2
Cell Structure

cial complexes of protein and vitamins. Humans consist of billions of cells that are grouped together and arranged to form tissues.

Tissues A collection of specialized cells with similar structures and functions forms a tissue. A nonliving material called intercellular matrix joins the cells and fills the spaces between them. The matrix contains special substances, such as electrolytes, salts, and fibers, that give the tissue unique characteristics. Histology is a branch of science specializing in the microscopic study of tissues. There are four basic types of tissue—epithelial, connective, muscle, and nerve—and the entire body is made up of combinations of these tissues.

- **Epithelial Tissue** Epithelial tissue (*epi-* = upon or over) is found throughout the body and makes up the covering of external and internal surfaces. The skin and the linings of the digestive system, urinary system, and respiratory system are all epithelial tissue. Histologists recognize several types of epithelial tissue and classify them according to the number of cell layers and the shape and other characteristics of the surface layer.

- **Connective Tissue** Connective tissue is the most widespread tissue type in the human body. It forms bones, cartilage, tendons, and ligaments. Connective tissue provides a framework for the body, holds organs in place, connects body parts, and allows for movement of joints. It also supports nerves and capillaries and plays an important role in the body's immune system. Fat, or adipose tissue, is a type of connective tissue that provides for storage of energy in the body and insulates against heat loss.
- **Muscle Tissue** There are three types of muscle tissue: smooth, skeletal or striated, and cardiac. The main function of muscle tissue is contraction, and the three muscle tissue types are categorized as voluntary (under the conscious control of the individual) or involuntary (individual has little or no control over the movement).

  Smooth muscle, which is involuntary, is found in the walls of hollow internal structures—such as the intestines, bladder, blood vessels, and uterus. Skeletal muscle is voluntary and makes up the muscles that are attached to—and move—bones and joints. It is also called striated muscle because, viewed through a microscope, it appears to have stripes, or striae. When seen close up, cardiac muscle tissue also appears to have some striae, but the heart muscle is involuntary (not under conscious control). Found only in the heart, cardiac muscle is specialized to conduct the electrical impulses that cause the heart to contract rhythmically.
- **Nervous Tissue** Nervous tissue makes up the nerves and is specialized to conduct nerve impulses. Its cells are similar to those in cardiac or skeletal muscle tissue; it comprises the brain and spinal cord, in addition to nerves throughout the body.

Organs These four tissue types—epithelial, connective, muscle, and nervous—combine in varying ways to produce organs, essential body structures that work in harmony within body systems and carry on the specialized functions of a living human. Examples of organs are the heart, liver, pancreas, lungs, stomach, and spleen. Internal organs of the body are called viscera and are located in the various body cavities. Not all organs are internal, and not all are as localized as the heart or liver. For example, sweat glands, hair, and skin are all considered body organs.

Body Systems A body system is composed of several related organs that work together to perform a complex function. The concept of levels of organization provides scientists with a useful tool for thinking about how all parts of the body function and how the functions are interrelated. The chapters in Part II are organized by the medical specialty which refers to each body system.

Body Cavities and Regions

The medical language includes sets of terms commonly used to identify both general and specific areas of the body: body cavities, abdominopelvic regions and quadrants, and spinal column divisions. These terms are used in both verbal and written communication and may accompany diagrams. Table 2.8 lists the major body cavities and the organs or structures they contain. Figures 2.3–2.5 illustrate the terms for cavities and regions. Table 2.9 lists important terms and abbreviations.

Divisions of the Spinal Column

The back is divided into five regions, corresponding with the divisions of the spinal column, or vertebral column (see Figure 2.6): cervical, thoracic, lumbar, sacral or sacrum, and coccygeal or coccyx. The vertebral column consists of a series of bony structures called vertebrae that encase and protect the spinal cord. There are a total of 24 separate vertebrae (vertebra is the singular form), with two sets of fused parts—five fused parts are in the sacrum and four are in the coccyx. Physicians use these divisional terms to identify problems with the spine and resulting impairments

TABLE 2.8 Body Cavity Structures

Body Cavity	Structures
abdominal/abdominopelvic	stomach, liver, gallbladder, spleen, pancreas, small and large intestines
cranial cavity	brain
pelvic cavity	ureters, urinary bladder, urethra female: uterus, ovaries, fallopian tubes, vagina male: prostate gland, seminal vesicles, ejaculatory duct, vas deferens
spinal cavity	spinal cord
thoracic cavity	lungs, esophagus, trachea, bronchial tubes, thymus gland, aorta, heart

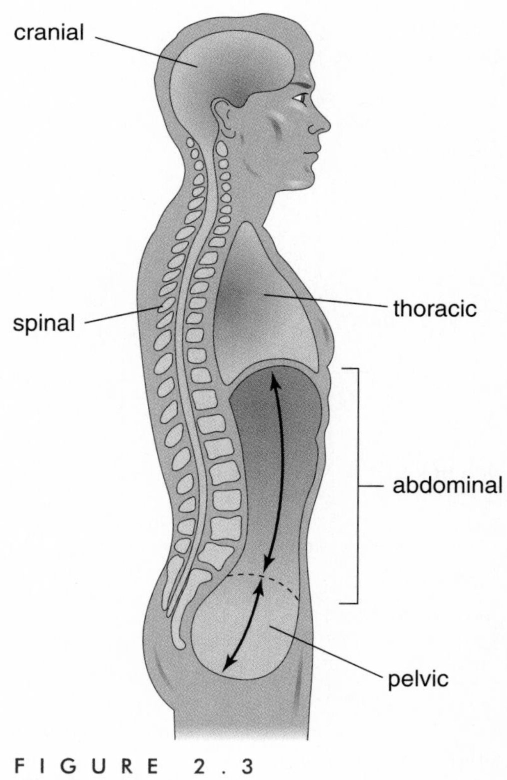

FIGURE 2.3
Body Cavities

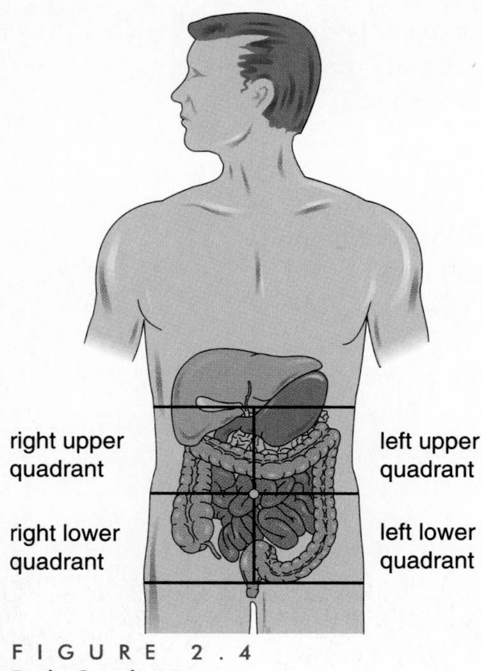

FIGURE 2.4
Body Quadrants

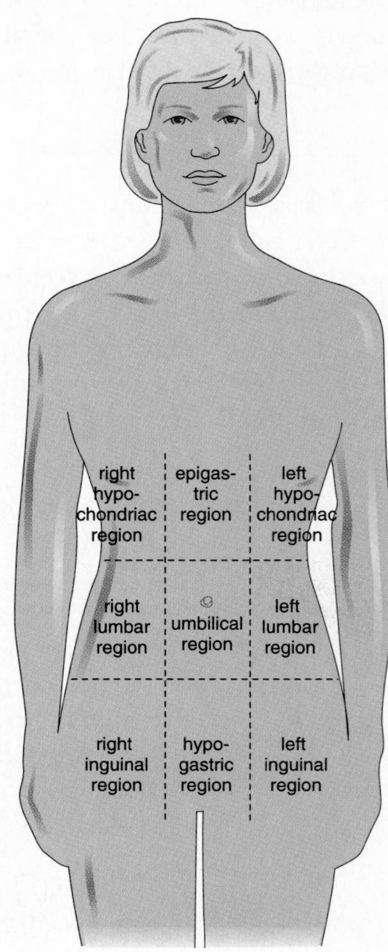

FIGURE 2.5
Abdominopelvic Regions

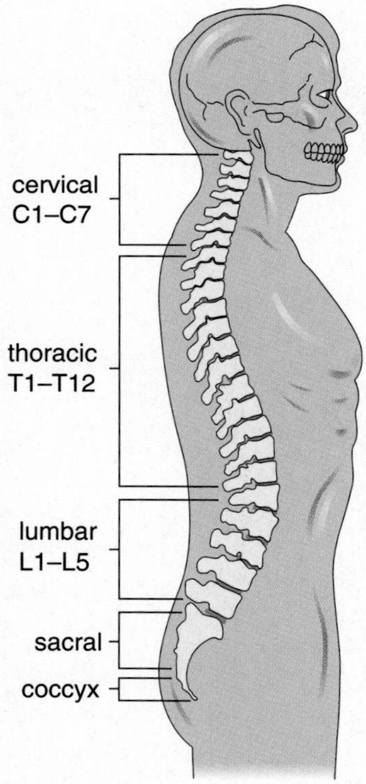

cervical C1–C7
thoracic T1–T12
lumbar L1–L5
sacral
coccyx

FIGURE 2.6
Spinal Column Regions

in function. For example, a major spinal cord lesion in the thoracic region (T1–T12) might tell a doctor that the patient is paraplegic (paralyzed in the lower half of the body). Table 2.10 lists the spinal divisions, their location, number of vertebrae, and the abbreviation.

TABLE 2.9 Abdominopelvic Regions or Quadrants and Abbreviations

right hypochondriac	upper right beneath the ribs
left hypochondriac	upper left beneath the ribs
epigastric	upper middle over the stomach
right lumbar	right middle near the waist (in back only)
left lumbar	left middle near the waist (in back only)
umbilical	around the navel
hypogastric	lower middle under the navel
right inguinal	right side near the groin
RUQ	right upper quadrant (includes liver, gallbladder, duodenum, head of pancreas, right kidney and adrenal, hepatic flexure of colon, part of ascending and transverse colon)
RLQ	right lower quadrant (includes cecum, appendix, female: right ovary and tube, male: right ureter and right spermatic cord)
LUQ	left upper quadrant (includes stomach, spleen, left lobe of liver, body of pancreas, left kidney and adrenal, splenic flexure of colon, part of transverse and descending colon)
LLQ	left lower quadrant (includes part of descending colon, sigmoid colon, female: left ovary and tube, male: left ureter and left spermatic cord)

TABLE 2.10 The Vertebrae

Spinal Division	Region of the Back	Number of Vertebrae	Abbreviation
cervical	neck	7	C (C1–C7)
thoracic	chest	12	T (T1–T12)
lumbar	loin	5	L (L1–L5)
sacral, sacrum	lower back	5 fused parts	S (S1–S5)
coccygeal, coccyx	tailbone	4 fused parts	

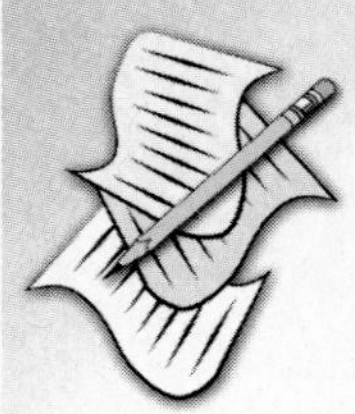

EXERCISE 2.5

State Your Position

Provide definitions for the following positional and directional terms.

1. cephalic ____________________
2. ventral ____________________
3. dorsal ____________________
4. medial ____________________
5. distal ____________________
6. bilateral ____________________
7. plantar ____________________
8. superficial ____________________
9. parietal ____________________
10. visceral ____________________

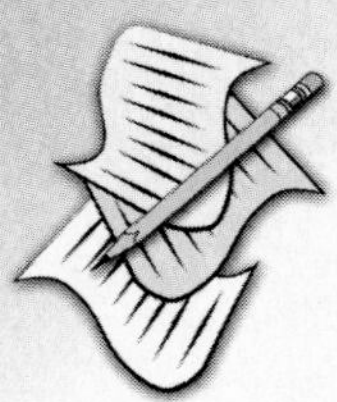

EXERCISE 2.6

Here's the Answer. What's the Question?

Provide the correct terms for the following definitions. Write your answer as a question (What is. . .?).

1. bending of a joint ____________________
2. straightening of a joint ____________________
3. movement toward the midline of the body ____________________
4. movement away from the midline of the body ____________________
5. turned outward ____________________

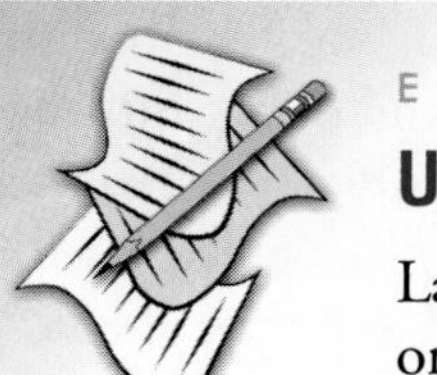

EXERCISE 2.7

Use Your X-Ray Vision

Label the diagram with the appropriate cavity name. Then list the major organ or organs contained within each body cavity.

1. cranial cavity
2. spinal cavity
3. thoracic cavity
4. abdominal cavity

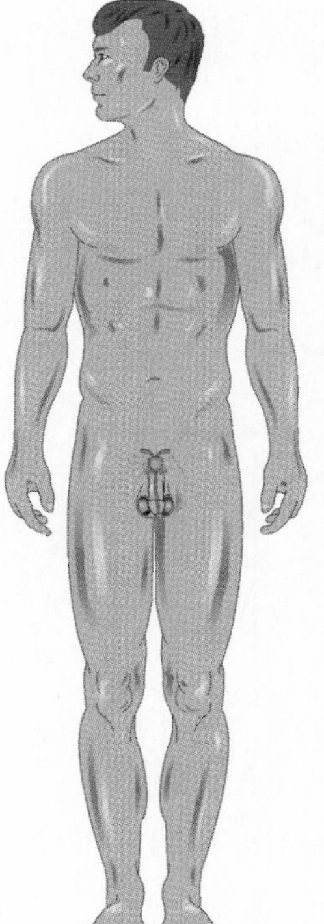

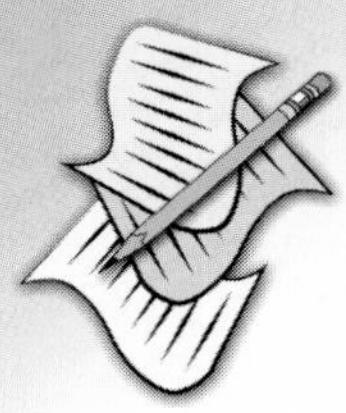

EXERCISE 2.8

Back Up What You Say

Identify the spinal division and region of the back that contain the following vertebrae

1. C4
2. C7
3. T3
4. T5
5. T9

Diagnostic Terms To Assess the Human Body

The language of medical communication includes words that describe the function of the human body as well as the physical parts. There are terms that describe the color of things seen in the body. It is also necessary to understand what the patient is feeling when there are problems that cause pain or discomfort. Further assessment is often needed through the science of medical imaging which provides an inside look at the cavities, tissues, bones, and internal organs.

Directional and Positional Terms

Medical personnel use assumed positions and reference points to communicate about the human body. Anatomic position is used as a reference position in medical communication and assumes that the patient is standing, facing forward, with arms at the sides, palms out, legs straight, and feet flat on the floor with toes pointed forward. Figure 2.7 illustrates this orientation. Imagining a person in anatomic position gives uniform reference points for anyone describing areas of the body. The directional terms provided in Table 2.11 are part of the core medical vocabulary that is used to communicate about every body system.

Directional Planes Another set of terms that serve to describe the body and its parts are directional planes. The directional planes are imaginary cuts slicing through the body at various points and in various directions. Figure 2.8 illustrates the three planes.

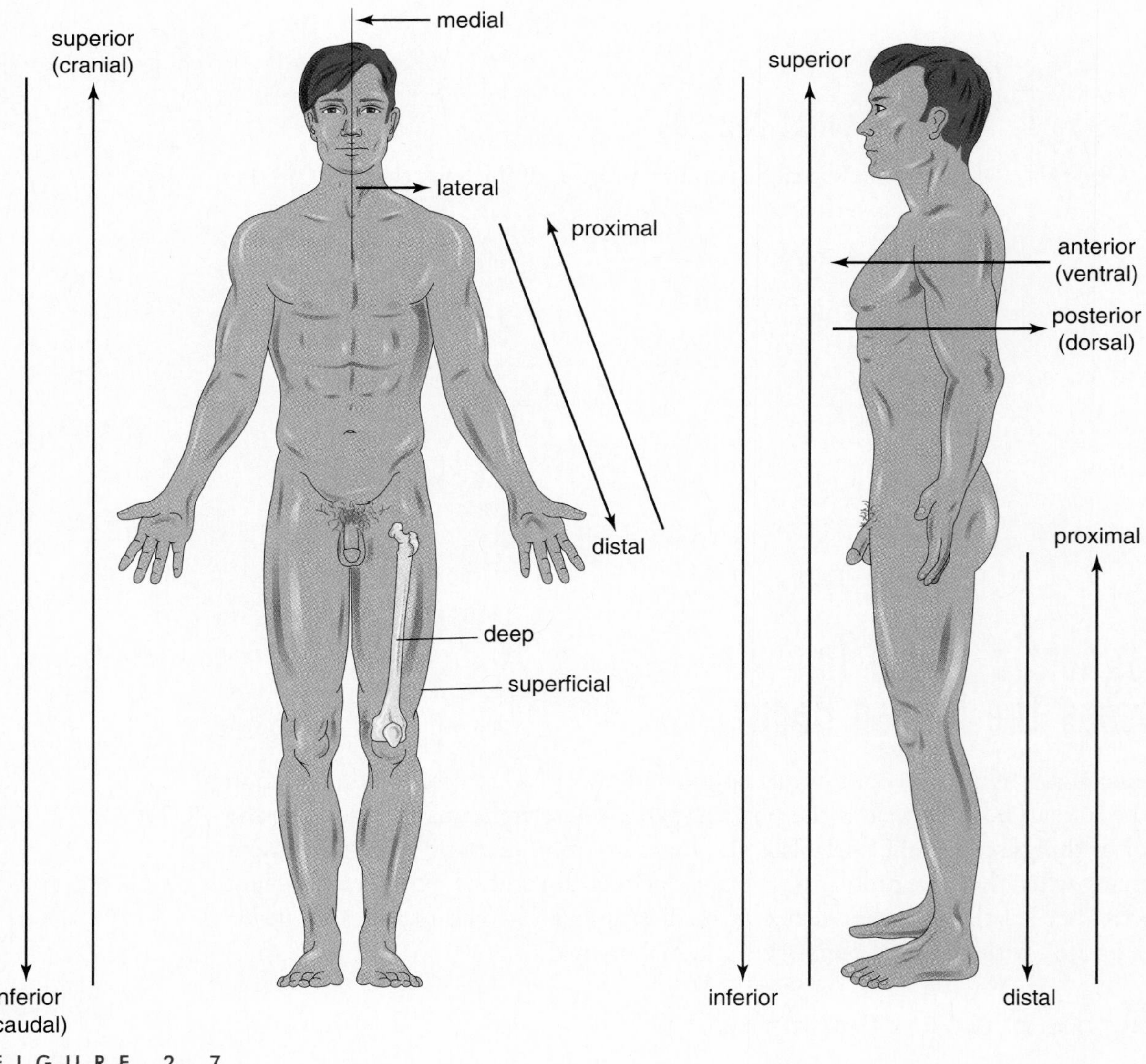

FIGURE 2.7
Anatomic Position

TABLE 2.11 Directional Terms

Term	Definition
superior or cephalic	toward the head, the surface, or the upper portion of the body The heart is superior to the diaphragm.
inferior or caudal	toward the feet or lower portion of the body, The kidneys are inferior to the adrenal glands.
anterior or ventral	toward the front of the body The sternum is anterior to the vertebral column.
posterior or dorsal	toward the back The scapulae (shoulder blades) are posterior to the mammary glands.
medial	toward the midline or center of the body or structure; inner The nose is medial to the cheekbone.
lateral	to the side of the body or structure The axilla (armpit) is on the lateral aspect of the chest, where the arm and chest join.
proximal	near the center of the body or structure The shoulder is proximal to the elbow.
distal	away from the body The distal portion of the femur (thigh bone) is closer to the knee than to the hip.
bilateral	pertaining to both sides of the body or structure The kidneys are positioned bilaterally in the lower back.
unilateral	pertaining to only one side of the body or structure The heart is positioned unilaterally, on the left side of the chest.
palmar	pertaining to the palm of the hand The palmar surface of the hand may be heavily creased.
plantar	pertaining to the sole of the foot The plantar surface of the foot is subject to thickening of the skin.
deep	toward the interior The heart is deep within the chest.
superficial	near the surface A scratch on the skin is superficial.
parietal	the wall of a hollow organ or a body cavity The parietal peritoneum lines the abdominal cavity.
visceral	the inner covering of the surface of an organ or body cavity The visceral peritoneum covers the stomach and other organs of the abdominal cavity.

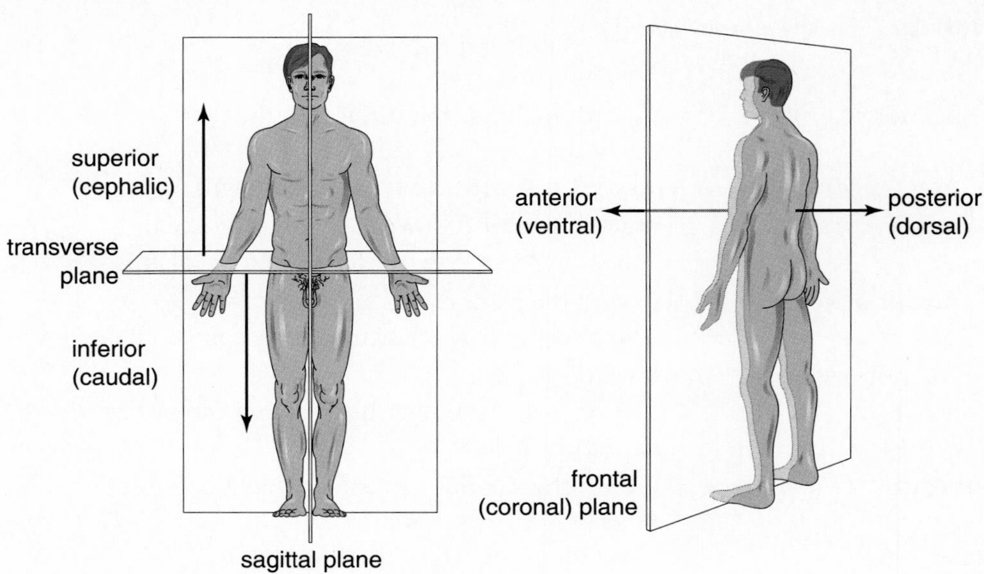

FIGURE 2.8
Body Planes

1. The sagittal plane divides the body into two parts lengthwise (right vs. left), though not necessarily into halves. The term *midsagittal plane* refers to the sagittal plane dividing the body into equal parts, or halves.
2. The frontal (or coronal) plane divides the body into front and back sections from top to bottom. The front side is referred to as anterior or ventral, and the back side is called posterior or dorsal.
3. The transverse plane is also called the horizontal plane. It runs parallel to the floor, dividing the body into upper and lower portions. The upper portion is called superior or cephalic; the lower portion is referred to as inferior or caudal.

Movement Terms The terms in Table 2.12 describe opposite actions or movements of body parts. Study Figure 2.9 as you read the definitions.

Combining Forms Referring to Color

Combining forms referring to color are used in many areas of science and medicine. Dermatologists apply them to skin lesions, cytologists use them to discuss various cell types, and all physicians employ them to describe both normal and abnormal conditions with color terms. Table 2.13 shows the combining forms for color-related terms and gives examples of medical words based on those terms. Figure 2.10 provides examples of the colors.

TABLE 2.12 Movement Terms

Term	Definition
flexion	bending of a joint When the hand is placed on the chest, the elbow is flexed.
extension	straightening of a joint When the hand is resting beside the thigh, the elbow is extended.
abduction	away from the midline of the body When the legs are spread apart, they are abducted.
adduction	toward the midline of the body When the legs are positioned together, they are adducted.
eversion	turned outward When the feet are everted, they point outward. (This term is frequently used to describe the movement of turning the eyelid outward to expose the inner side.)
inversion	turned inward When a foot is turned inward, it is inverted.

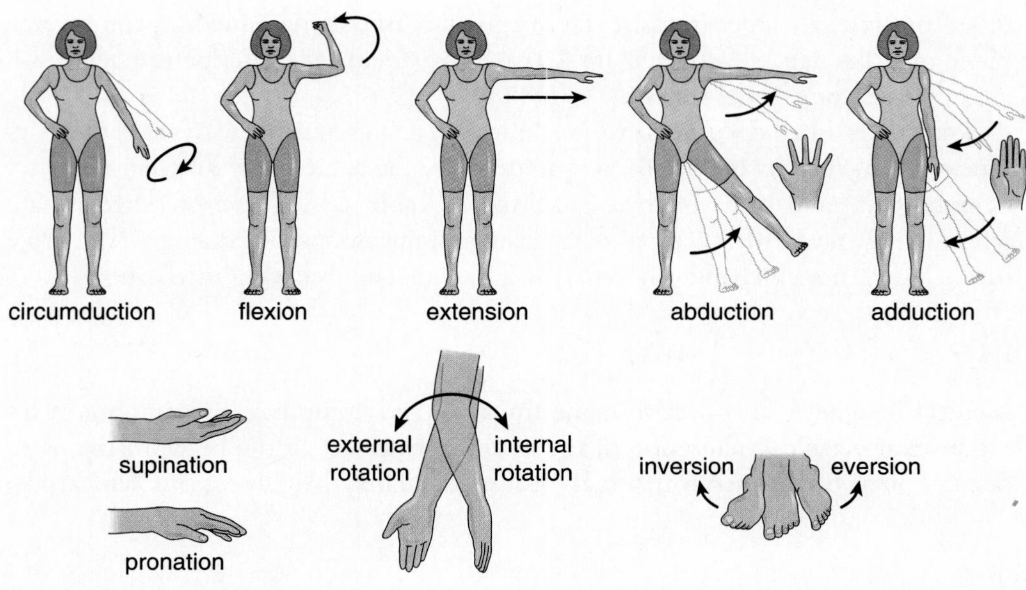

FIGURE 2.9
Skeletal Muscle and Joint Movements

TABLE 2.13 Color Combining Forms

Combining Form	Translation	Example
cyan/o	blue	cyanosis: bluish discoloration of skin due to lack of oxygen
erythr/o	red	erythrocyte: red blood cell
leuk/o	white	leukocyte: type of white blood cell
melan/o	black	melanin: pigment portion of the skin
purpur/o	purple	purpura: a condition characterized by hemorrhaging into the skin, causing purple lesions
xanth/o	yellow	xanthopsia: an abnormal visual condition in which all objects appear yellow

Pain Assessment

Surveys show that over two-thirds of all American workers, or more than 80 million people, suffer from some sort of pain every year. Additionally, about 15 million Americans working full time suffer from chronic pain—the ongoing or recurring pain that lasts 6 months or longer. These statistics have forced healthcare professionals to look closely at pain in their patients—asking questions about pain that they may be experiencing, relief measures taken, and providing adequate pain relief.

Today pain is considered the fifth vital sign, along with temperature, respirations, pulse or heart rate, and blood pressure. It is considered a subjective vital sign, and thus it is not as easily measured as the other vital signs. However, when the patient is experiencing pain, there may be an increase in respirations, heart rate, and/or blood pressure. In order to assist the caregiver in assessing a patient's pain, several different scales can be used (Figure 2.11). The patient will describe the degree of pain by using one of the scales.

Some transcribed documents will include pain as an assessment as well as the pain intervention taken by the healthcare professional. There are many different terms to describe pain, and some of these are listed in Table 2.14. Descriptive terms can reflect the character (description) of the pain and the amount (frequency). The drug list included in each chapter in Part II will include pain-relieving medications.

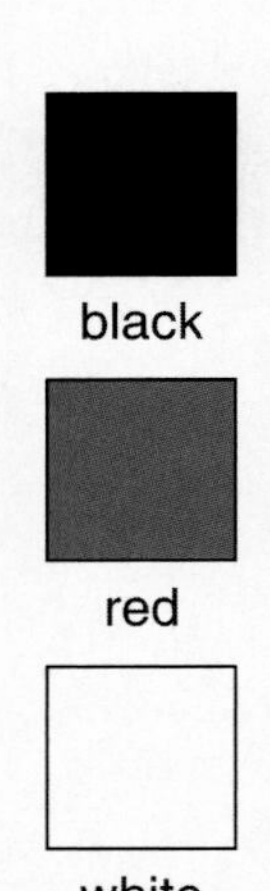

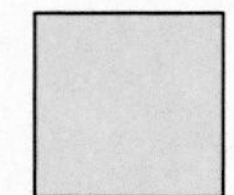

FIGURE 2.10
Color Names

Medical Imaging Terms

Medical imaging is a collective name for x-ray and computerized scanning techniques that permit visualization of the internal structures of the body. In the past, doctors often had to perform surgery just to accurately diagnose a problem inside the body. Advances in medical imaging have made it possible for physicians to view refined, detailed pictures of the body's interior without touching a scalpel. The new equipment and techniques have revolutionized medicine and have made diagnosis more accurate and safer for the patient.

Medical imaging results often appear in medical records as part of the diagnostic work. In hospital patient charts, there may be a separate section for medical imaging reports; in the problem-oriented medical record format, these reports appear in the database section. Although the report, or radiologist's interpretation of the pictures, is physically part of the medical record, the films themselves are usually stored separately from the chart. These films can be damaged or destroyed by exposure to certain substances and environmental conditions, so proper storage is essential. Generally, films are stored in the radiology or medical imaging department. Sometimes a physician requests that old films be retrieved for reinterpretation or comparison with more recent films.

Radiologic imaging includes conventional x-rays and fluoroscopy, sonography (or ultrasound), computed tomography (CT), and magnetic resonance imaging (MRI). In some instances, the term *nuclear medicine* denotes the branch of medicine that uses radioactive emissions to produce images of the body for diagnosing and treating various illnesses.

Radiology Radiology is the study of x-rays or other imaging modalities to screen for or diagnose abnormalities. X-ray films are produced by exposing sensitized film to the energy waves from an x-ray generator (a cathode ray tube). When part of the

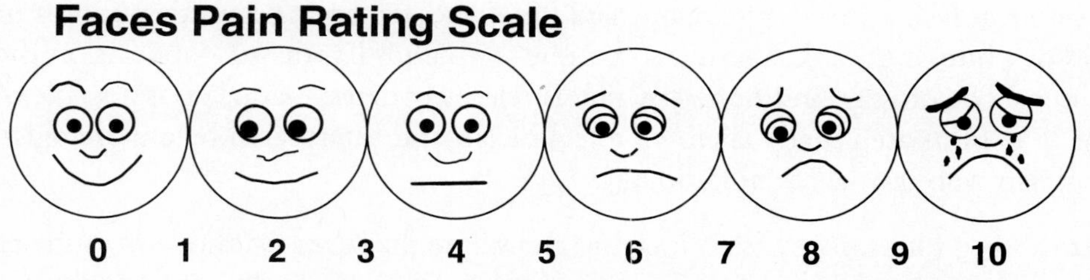

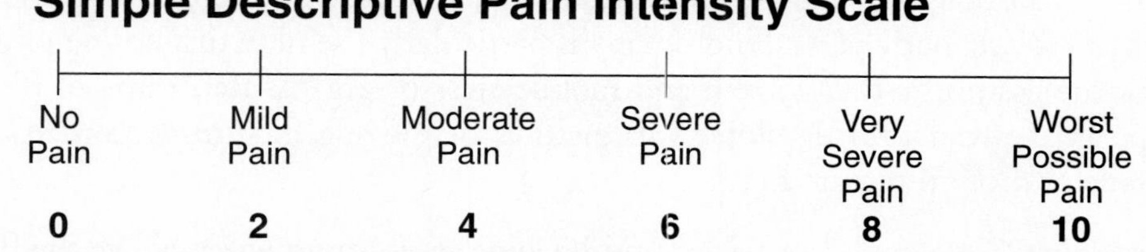

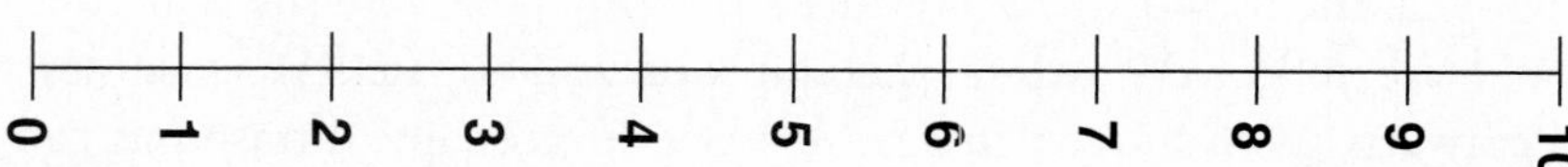

FIGURE 2.11
Pain Scale

TABLE 2.14 Terms to Describe Pain

Term	Definition
ache (achy, aching)	a dull, steady pain
continuous	a pain that does not stop
discomfort (uncomfortable)	a feeling of being uncomfortable
dull	blunted; not sharp; not acute
intense	strong, sharp
intermittent	not continuous; stopping and starting
severe	strong, extreme
sharp	a pain that has a stabbing quality; usually described in one particular spot
stabbing	a pain that may be sharp in quality and stopping and starting
throbbing	a dull, steady pain with an intermittent exacerbation occurring periodically

body is positioned between an x-ray source and sensitized film, the result is an image—actually a shadow—of that body part. Radiographs appear in various shades of black, white, and gray. The areas where x-rays strike the film directly appear black, whereas areas where the x-rays are blocked (by tissues of varying densities) appear in shades of white or gray. As a result, soft tissue—which is less dense—appears on the film as a shade of gray, and bone—which is relatively dense—appears as a shade of white. The films are usually taken by a technician and interpreted by a radiologist, a physician who specializes in radiology.

Fluoroscopy Fluoroscopy is an imaging technique that uses a cathode ray tube to allow an observer to view a moving image. It is very similar to the traditional x-ray process, except that x-ray images are typically still, whereas fluoroscopy can provide images of moving body parts. Fluoroscopy is particularly useful in diagnosing problems of the gastrointestinal system and mobile areas or organs. Recording of fluoroscopy images can provide either still pictures or moving pictures (recorded on videotape or motion picture film).

Sonography Sonography, or ultrasound imaging, uses sound waves above the frequency that can be heard by the human ear to produce images of body structures. A transducer (a device that produces the ultrasound waves) is placed over the body part to be imaged; the sound waves produced partially penetrate the structure to be examined and are reflected back to the transducer. The transducer senses these echoes and converts them into an image. As with fluoroscopy, ultrasound can produce a moving image, and that image can be recorded as a still or moving picture.

Computed Tomography Computed tomography (CT) is a medical imaging technique that uses computer interpretations of x-rays to produce images of structures

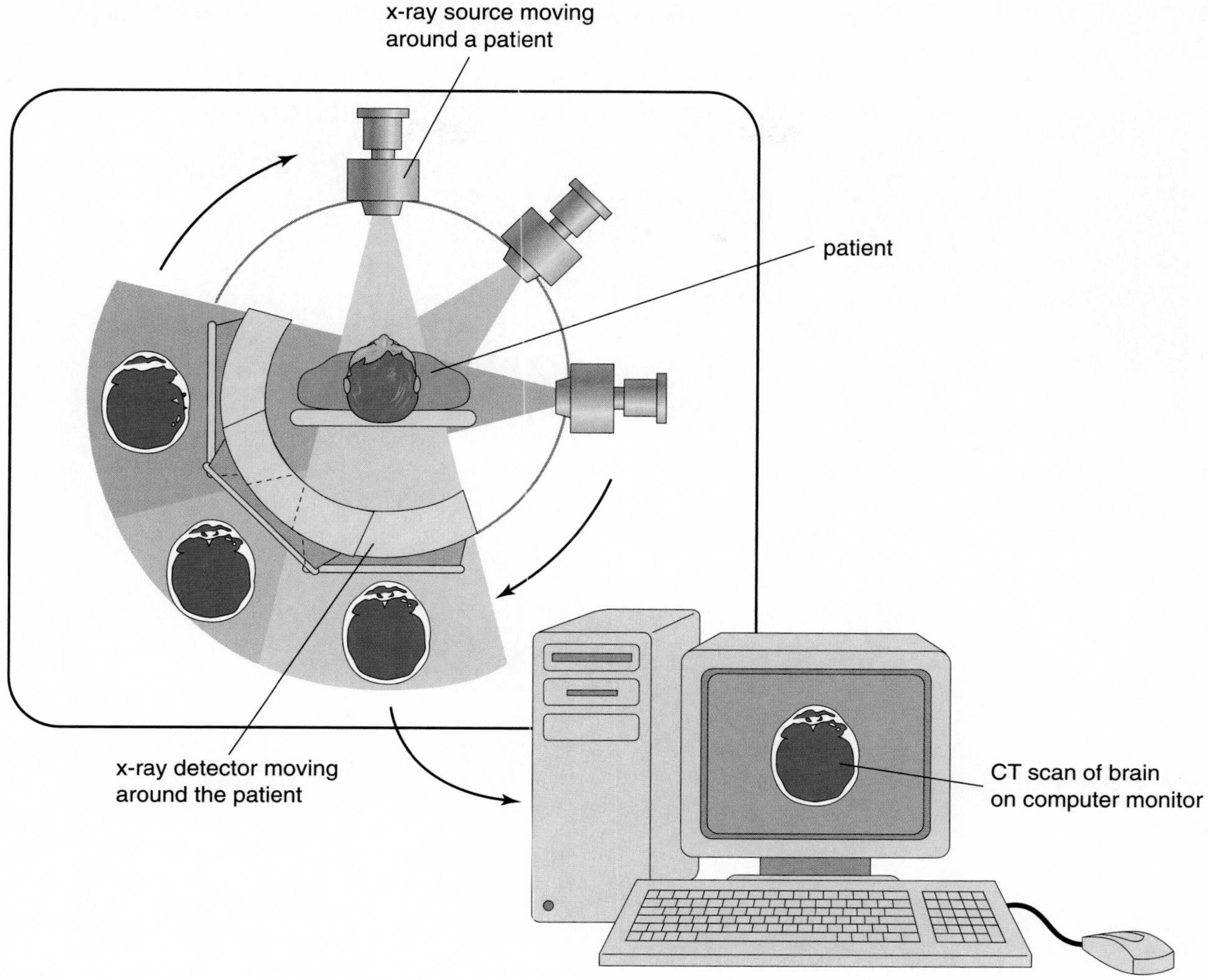

FIGURE 2.12
CT Scan

inside the body (see Figure 2.12). The body area is scanned in layers, using x-rays to penetrate the various structures. The computer calculates the densities of the structures from the x-rays and displays the results as an image. Comparing the scans of many layers of a body area produces a highly accurate representation of that area. Sometimes it is necessary to use a contrast medium, or dye, in conjunction with CT scanning to more accurately visualize the area. Positron emission tomography (PET) is a variation of computed tomography.

Magnetic Resonance Imaging Magnetic resonance imaging (MRI), also called nuclear magnetic resonance (NMR), creates images from computer interpretations of the body's response to a strong magnetic field (see Figure 2.13). The patient is placed within the magnetic field, and the responses of the body's hydrogen atoms in the area being scanned are assessed by a computer to produce a highly accurate three-dimensional image. Since MRI is a noninvasive procedure, as are many of the imaging techniques, it is possible to gather a great deal of information with minimal risk to the patient.

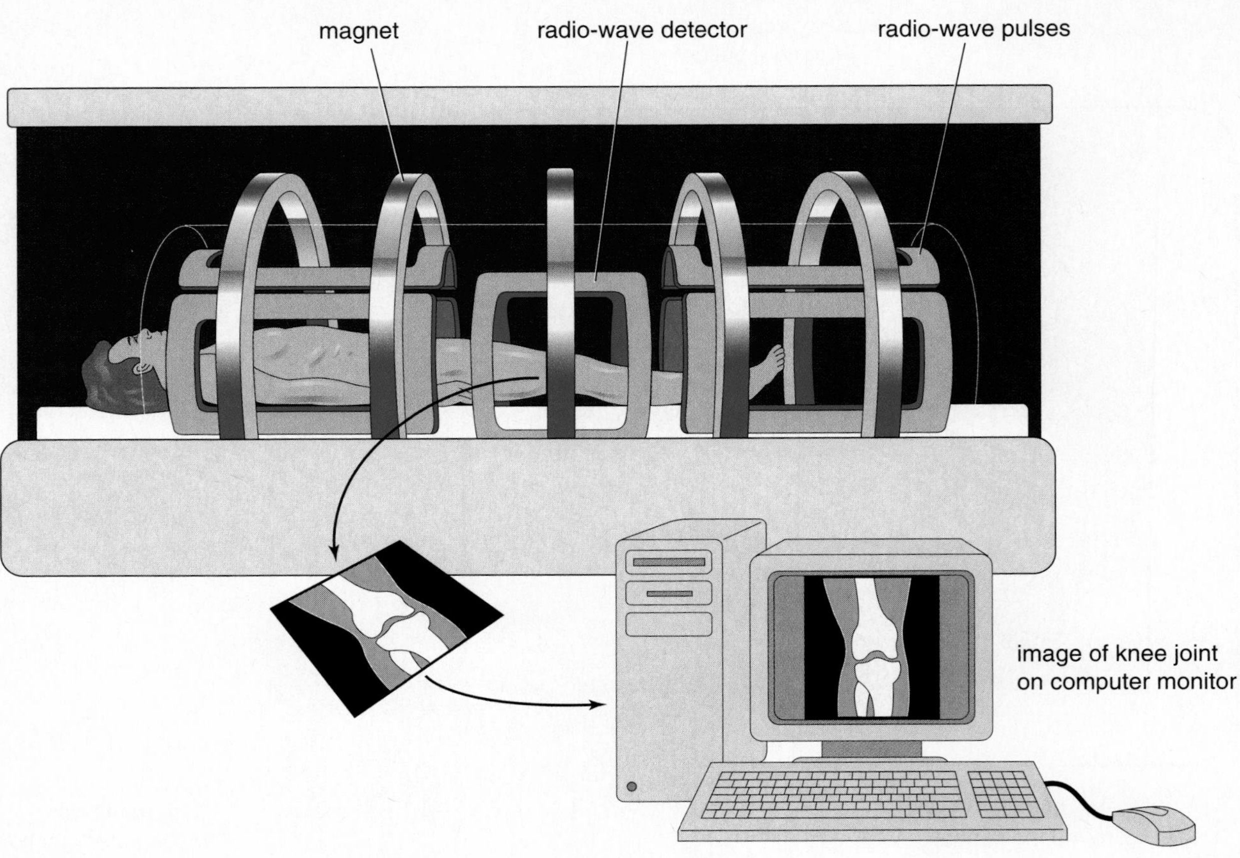

FIGURE 2.13
MRI

Table 2.15 lists common terms associated with radiology, nuclear medicine, and diagnostic imaging. Notice that most of the procedural and diagnostic test terms contain the suffixes *-graphy* (process of recording) or *-gram* (record).

TABLE 2.15 Terms Associated with Radiology and Nuclear Medicine

Materials and Equipment Terms	
barium	contrast medium or dye, frequently used to provide enhanced images of body structures
film	thin sheet of cellulose coated with light-sensitive chemicals used to take photos or x-rays
gray	international unit of measurement of ionizing radiation
radioactive	emitting radiation energy
radiogram	image on x-ray film
radioisotope	radioactive form of an element
roentgen	unit of exposure to radiation (obsolete: replaced by the gray)
shield	device used to protect against radiation
transducer	device for converting energy from one form to another

(continues)

TABLE 2.15 Terms Associated with Radiology and Nuclear Medicine (Continued)

Diagnostic Procedure Terms	
angiocardiography	process of viewing the heart and blood vessels by injecting radiopaque dye into circulating blood and exposing the chest to x-rays
angiography	process of recording a vessel (through the use of radiopaque dye and x-rays)
bronchography	process of viewing the bronchus (radiograph examination of the bronchus or bronchi)
cholangiogram	radiograph examination of the bile ducts
cholecystogram	radiograph examination of the gallbladder
echogram	examination of body structures using ultrasound imaging techniques
echocardiogram	examination of the heart using ultrasound imaging
fluoroscopy	examination of body tissues and deep structures by use of fluoroscope
lymphangiograph	radiograph of lymphatic vessels
myelograph	radiograph of the spinal cord
pyelograph	radiograph of the kidney and ureter
radiograph	image produced by ionizing radiation (x-rays) and radiation sensitive film
radioimmunoassay	measurement of antigen-antibody interaction using radioactive substances
radiotherapy	treatment of disease using radium; treatment for some cancers
salpingograph	radiograph of fallopian tubes
sonogram	image produced by sound waves reflected off of body structures (examination of a part of the body using sound waves)
tomograph	radiograph exam whereby the x-ray source is moved to view layers or slices of the body
ultrasonography	imaging technique that uses sound waves to study a portion of the body
Directional Terms in Medical Imaging	
anteroposterior	front to back (direction of x-rays passing through the chest when the patient is in a standard radiograph examination position)
axial	pertaining to around an axis

(continues)

TABLE 2.15 Terms Associated with Radiology and Nuclear Medicine (Continued)

Directional Terms in Medical Imaging (Continued)	
lateral decubitus	lying on the side
posteroanterior	from back to front (direction of x-rays)
General Terms in Medical Imaging	
radiologist	physician who specializes in use of x-rays; interprets radiographs
radiopaque	describing materials (such as lead) that are able to block x-rays
roentgenology	alternate term for x-ray technology
scan	repeated recording of emissions from radioactive substances onto a photographic plate in one specific area of the body
scintiscan	image created by gamma radiation, indicating concentration within the body
sonolucent	permitting the passage of ultrasound waves
tagging	attachment of radioactive material to a substance that can be traced as it moves through the body
therapeutic	treatment of disease
uptake	absorption of radioactive substance into tissue

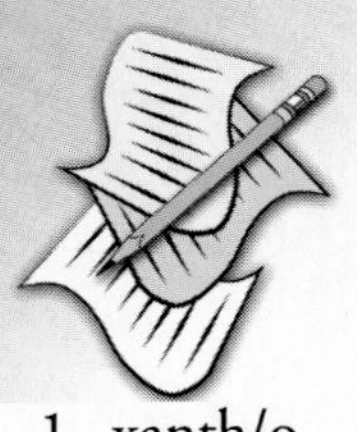

EXERCISE 2.9

Color Me . . .

Give the correct color indicated by each of the following word parts.

1. xanth/o ______________________
2. leuk/o ______________________
3. cyan/o ______________________
4. erythr/o ______________________
5. melan/o ______________________

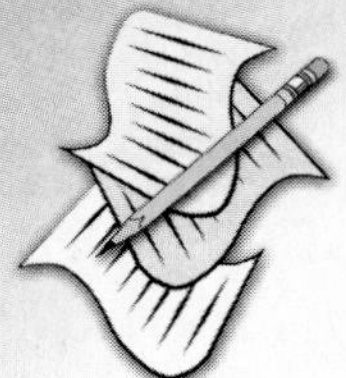

EXERCISE 2.10

This Is a Pain

Choose the descriptive term that best completes the following sentences.

severe	continuous	sharp
discomfort	intense	intermittent
dull	stabbing	
ache	throbbing	

1. Mr. Alverex went to the dentist because he had a tooth ________.
2. The migraine headache was described as intense pain with an intermittent, sharp ________ pain occurring several times during each hour.
3. Surgical pain is usually ________ and without relief until pain medication is given.
4. There was a blunted, ________ quality to the pain of the sprained muscle.
5. A strong, sharp pain is also described as ________.
6. A pain that is not continuous is ________.
7. The difference between a ________ pain and a stabbing pain is that the former is pulsating and the later is very sharp, intermittent, and usually felt in one spot.
8. If a person describes a feeling of being uncomfortable, it is described as ________.
9. A pain that has a stabbing quality, usually in one particular area is ________.
10. Very strong, extreme pain is described as ________.

EXERCISE 2.11

Scan Artist

Define each of the following medical imaging terms.

1. radioactive ________________________________
2. transducer ________________________________
3. echocardiogram ________________________________
4. fluoroscopy ________________________________
5. radiopaque ________________________________
6. sonolucent ________________________________
7. anteroposterior ________________________________
8. sonogram ________________________________
9. cholangiogram ________________________________
10. pyelography ________________________________

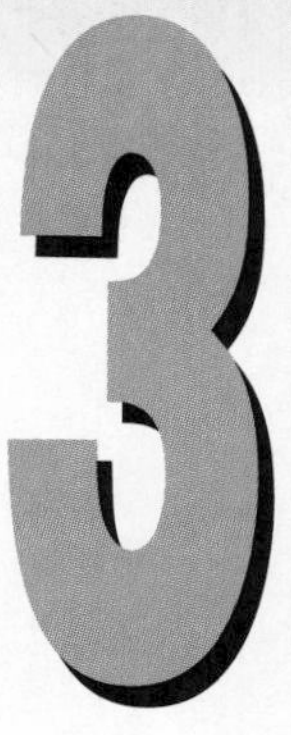

Perfecting Your Editing Skills

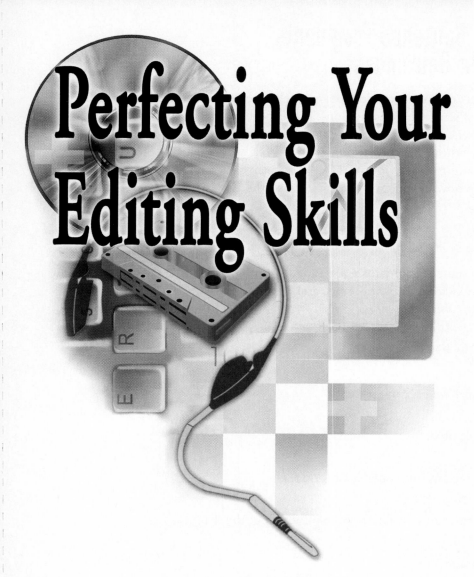

Communication among medical personnel takes a number of forms—oral, dictated, written, and transcribed. For the good of the patient, the transmission of information must be accurate, concise yet detailed, and prompt. Mutual understanding of procedures and terms is paramount.

In this chapter, you will perfect your use of words and your understanding of grammar and construction. These skills will help you edit and proofread medical reports for correct language, punctuation, format, and clarity of meaning. As you become familiar with these basics, you will have a deeper understanding of the way a medical transcriptionist contributes to the well-being of the patient.

OBJECTIVES

- Use medical terms correctly according to the context and purpose of the communication.
- Become familiar with writing resources and the vocabulary of general and specialty reference materials.
- Start to learn the format of various types of medical documents, beginning with the simplest reports.
- Transcribe dictation requiring concentration and listening skills.
- Edit medical reports to conform with AAMT style guidelines.
- Proofread and correct transcripts to produce error-free documents.

Repairing Sentence Fragments and Run-On Sentences

One of the most common trouble spots in workplace documents such as letters and reports is faulty sentence construction. These problems take the form of either incomplete sentences (sentence fragments) or run-on sentences (two sentences that "run together" without the correct punctuation separating them). To be able to correct fragments and run-ons, you must know what makes a sentence complete. You also must know how to punctuate a sentence so the reader knows where it begins and ends.

What Is a Sentence?

Every complete sentence contains a subject and a verb and expresses a thought. The subject is generally a noun or pronoun, and the verb always expresses some action or state of being (*am, was, will be,* etc.).

> Bill worked.
> s v
>
> Dr. Brown will see the patient.
> s v
>
> You look tired.
> s v
>
> My physician is unavailable on Fridays.
> s v
>
> The patient and his family were informed of the diagnosis.
> s s v
>
> [compound subject]
>
> A corporate healthcare facility seeks a full-time medical transcriptionist.
> s v

Sometimes the subject is implied but not stated. In the following sentence, for example, the subject *you* is understood.

> Have a nice day.
> v
>
> Follow up with me next week.
> v
>
> Create a letterhead for all medical documents.
> v

Fragments

A fragment is a group of words that expresses a partial thought and leaves the reader puzzled. It is not a complete sentence.

WRONG:	The patient was instructed that if he develops a fever over 101° or if he has increasing abdominal pain. [This is a long dependent clause. What is missing is important information detailing what the patient should do in these situations.]
CORRECT:	The patient was instructed to call the doctor's answering service if he develops a fever over 101° or if he has increasing abdominal pain.
WRONG:	After the lecture, the applause of the audience. [This sentence is not complete. Information referring to the quality of the lecture and impact on the audience is needed.]
CORRECT:	The audience applauded the speaker for a wonderful, informative lecture.

Run-On Sentences

A run-on sentence consists of two sentences that are not separated by punctuation. If the second sentence is closely related, use a semicolon to connect them. Otherwise, key them as two individual sentences, each ending with a period (or a question mark or exclamation mark).

WRONG:	The patient's condition gradually improved on intravenous antibiotic therapy the speech therapist saw the patient in consultation.
CORRECT:	The patient's condition gradually improved on intravenous antibiotic therapy. The speech therapist saw the patient in consultation.
WRONG:	Some companies may have alternative work schedules the employee is given a choice.
CORRECT:	Some companies may have alternative work schedules; the employee is given a choice.

Exceptions to the Rules in Medical Reports

Certain sections of medical reports may contain incomplete sentences. For example, a doctor may dictate laboratory values that do not have to be written in sentence form. The physical examination may or may not be in sentence form.

LABORATORY DATA: WBC 5500 with 45 segmented neutrophils, 15 basophils, 5 eosinophils, 17 monocytes.

Heart: Regular rate and rhythm. No murmurs, rubs, or gallops.

Narrative dictation (for example, the history of present illness) must be in complete sentences. When historical items are placed in a formal list, however, they do not have to be in complete sentences.

PAST MEDICAL HISTORY
1. Status post coronary artery bypass grafting 5 years ago.
2. Bilateral hip pain.
3. History of hypertension, under good control on medical therapy.

Outpatient chart notes are less formal than other types of dictation and may be dictated in clipped sentences. A doctor may dictate without using subjects and articles. These notes should be transcribed as dictated. Such a note might look like this.

> Seen for postoperative visit. Doing well. Wound healing, without signs of infection. Sutures removed. Will be seen again in 2 weeks. May return to work after that time.

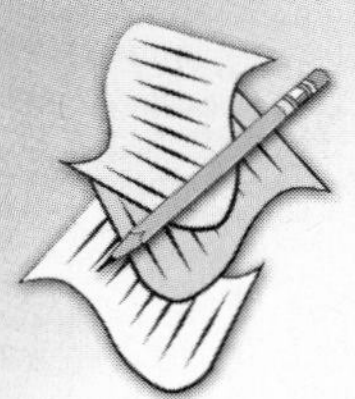

EXERCISE 3.1

Editing for Correct Punctuation

Read the following sentences and decide if any are run-on sentences or sentence fragments. Create complete sentences by combining groups of words or by changing the punctuation, then key the corrected sentences. Remember that as a transcriptionist, you must remain as true as possible to the original dictation while correcting obvious errors.

1. The patient's wife called 911 and the paramedics arrived some 10 minutes later to find the patient in a semiconscious state with an irregular heart rhythm the exact nature of which is unknown.
2. Strict sterile precautions must be taken. Using only autoclaved instruments and adequate skin preparation.

3. Medications Lasix 20 mg per morning Micro-K 10 mEq twice per day Cardizem 30 mg per day Isordil 20 mg twice per day.
4. The patient was extubated and noted to have purulent sputum and purulent urine and blood and urine cultures were positive for Klebsiella pneumoniae therefore the patient was started on gentamicin.
5. The patient was seen in routine follow-up. Six months since the last examination.
6. After informed consent was obtained the patient was brought to the operating room where general anesthesia was established and the lower abdomen was prepared and draped in the usual sterile fashion and an incision made just below the umbilicus.
7. The patient should apply the zinc oxide ointment directly to the lesions as often as needed to cool the burning sensation making sure she washes her hands before and after the application.
8. The patient is a 17-year-old female. A known IV drug abuser. She presents today to the emergency department she has an infected area on her left arm. The area is red and tender.
9. On examination the head shows no deformities the nose and throat are clear the neck has no adenopathy the chest is clear with normal breath sounds the abdomen is soft and nontender extremities are normal skin shows no rash or redness.
10. This 35-year-old Hispanic male presented today with a 1-cm laceration of the right hand at the web space between the middle and ring fingers.

Creating Subject-Verb Agreement

The subject and verb of a sentence must match in number and person. Singular verbs require singular subjects, and plural verbs require plural subjects. Use first-person verbs with first-person subjects *(I, we),* second-person verbs with second-person subjects *(you),* and third-person verbs with third-person subjects

> I am confused.
> s v
>
> [singular subject and verb]
>
> You are an excellent student.
> s v
>
> [The pronoun *you* can be either singular or plural in meaning, but it always takes a plural verb.]
>
> The patient and her husband are discussing the procedure.
> s s v
>
> [plural subject and plural verb]
>
> Individuals who share a job must have similar work values and be able to
> s v v
>
> cooperate with each other.
>
> [plural subject and compound verb]

The two firms who were competitors have decided to merge.
S V

[plural subject and plural verb]

Note: Sometimes a subject "looks" plural but functions as one unit and is singular in meaning. This is a collective noun. Be sure you use a singular verb(s) in such cases.

I&D was performed.
S V

[The procedure involves two steps, but together they make up ONE procedure; therefore this subject is singular.]

Pediatrics is her specialty.
S V

[Even though pediatrics has an *s*, it is the name of a single specialty and therefore requires a singular verb.]

Note: A collective noun may also be singular in form but represents a group of individuals or things; therefore, it acts individually and takes a plural verb.

The committee were in disagreement on the plans for the new building.
S V

Complicating Factor: Inverted Order Sentences

Sentences are usually written with the subject before the verb. However, sometimes the sentence is inverted, meaning that the verb comes first. This can cause some confusion in achieving subject-verb agreement. Many of these sentences begin with *Here* or *There*.

There is no reason to delay treatment.
V S

Outside the restaurant, there was a crowd waiting to be seated.
V S

There was no tenderness to palpation.
V S

Here are the patients' files that doctors need to keep.
V S

Here are my reasons for declining the position.
V S

Complicating Factor: Intervening Words and Phrases

In complicated sentences, first identify the verb and then the subject(s) of that verb. Then be sure you choose a singular verb for a singular subject or a plural verb for a plural subject. Disregard the parts of the sentence that come between the subject and the verb.

> A verbal report (s) of the biopsies was requested (v).
>
> Resection (s) of the malignant tumors was carried out (v).
>
> The patient (s), along with his family, is (v) pleased with the outcome of his surgery.
>
> The tornado (s) that occurred in Texas caused (v) a lot of damage.
>
> The celebration (s) that was planned for the couple was held (v) at the Botanical Gardens.

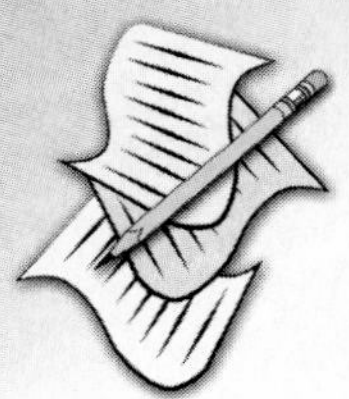

EXERCISE 3.2

Editing for Subject-Verb Agreement

Read the following discharge summary section and circle the correct verbs from the choices in parentheses. Then key the report using correct subject-verb combinations.

SUBJECTIVE: The patient, a 56-year-old female with multiple medical problems, (presents/present) to the ophthalmology outpatient clinic with 24 hours of tearing and irritation of both eyes. Vision in both eyes (seems/seem) unimpaired. She has no history of allergies or URIs and (does/do) not wear contact lenses.

She has a thick mucous discharge in both eyes, which (causes/cause) the lashes to stick together. She denies any history of trauma to the eyes and no previous history of similar symptoms (is/are) noted.

OBJECTIVE: In each eye the conjunctiva (is/are) grossly inflamed and injected. There (is/are) moderate chemosis and some lid edema. Traces of mucopurulent discharge (is/are) noted on the eyelashes. Examination with Tetracaine and fluorescein (reveals/reveal) no corneal abrasion. Funduscopic and slit-lamp exam (is/are) entirely normal.

ASSESSMENT: Acute bacterial conjunctivitis OU.

PLAN: The patient, with her sister in attendance, (was/were) instructed to use sulfonamide ophthalmic solution 2 drops OU q.i.d. Techniques of careful handwashing and hygiene (was/were) explained to the patient. The patient will return if her symptoms (does/do) not improve.

Creating Agreement between Pronouns and Antecedents

Remember that a pronoun takes the place of a noun in a sentence. Words such as *she, he, it, they, us, them, I,* and *you* are pronouns.

Pronouns must agree in person, number, and gender with the nouns they represent, which are called antecedents. In the sentences below, the pronoun is highlighted and the antecedents are underscored.

> The patient reports that his headaches have been increasing.
>
> The physician dictated the report and sent it to the transcriptionist.
>
> Transcriptionists know they must keep their skills sharp.
>
> Holly keeps her problems to herself.
>
> Either Josephine or Maria will submit her findings of the survey.
>
> Josephine and Maria agreed to discuss their findings with the group.

The pronouns *this, that, these,* and *those* must also agree with the nouns they modify.

this procedure	these procedures
that medication	those medications

The pronouns *them* and *their* are plural forms. Do not use these pronouns for singular meanings. When gender is not known, try to create a sentence that does not require the awkward construction of *his/her.*

WRONG:	The patient should be asked to empty their bladder prior to the test.
CORRECT:	The patient should be asked to void prior to the test.
WRONG:	If the child completes the assignment, praise them for their efforts.
CORRECT:	Praise children for their efforts in completing their assignments.

Pronouns as Subject or Object

A pronoun can represent a subject or an object. That is, the pronoun can be either the performer of an action or the recipient of the action. Subject pronouns are *I, you, he, she, it, we,* and *they.* Object pronouns are *me, you, him, her, it, us,* and *them.*

A predicate is either a verb or group of words that tells something about the action or state of being of the subject of the sentence. A predicate always has a verb and may also include helping verbs such as *has* or *have.*

Pronoun/Subject Agreement

Most people do not have difficulty achieving pronoun agreement in simple sentences that contain one pronoun in the predicate, e.g., Bill dislikes *me.* However, problems do come about when a sentence contains multiple nouns and pronouns, e.g., Bill dislikes *he/him* and *I/me.* To select the correct pronoun, simplify the sentence by looking only at the verb and the pronoun in question. Your ear should help you make the right choice.

> dislikes *he* or *him*? correct choice: dislikes him
>
> dislikes *I* or *me*? correct choice: dislikes me
>
> Bill dislikes him and me.

The three supervisors usually meet monthly to review their productivity. [This is a complete sentence. The words *usually* and *monthly* describe the verb *meet.* The complete predicate consists of the verb and all of the other words.]

Who versus Whom

Use the pronoun *who* for the subject of a verb; use *whom* for the object of a verb.

> Who has the first appointment?
> s v
>
> Whom did you assign to the emergency room?
> o v s v

In sentences or questions that contain a who/whom dilemma, substitute *he* for *who* and *him* for *whom* and then trust your ear.

> Who will deliver these reports? [He will deliver these reports].
>
> James will deliver these reports to whom? [James will deliver these reports to him.]

Myself, Himself, and Other Reflexive Pronouns

Reflexive pronouns are formed by adding *-self* or *-selves* to a personal pronoun(s). *Myself, yourselves, herself,* etc. are reflexive pronouns, meaning that they must reflect back to a noun or pronoun within that same sentence (*Mikey* wrapped the gift all by *himself.*) Many dictators mistakenly refer to themselves as myself instead of me (He was seen by *myself* in the clinic). Do not use a reflexive in a sentence when a simple personal pronoun is appropriate. (He was seen by *me* in the clinic.)

WRONG:	The surgery was conducted by Dr. Jones, Dr. Roberts, and *myself.*
CORRECT:	The surgery was conducted by Dr. Jones, Dr. Roberts, and me.
WRONG:	The physician who had a middle ear infection treated *her.*
CORRECT:	The physician who had a middle ear infection treated *herself.*
WRONG:	The executive board discussed the issues among them.
CORRECT:	The executive board discussed the issues among *themselves.* [The executive board acted as individuals, not as a single unit.]

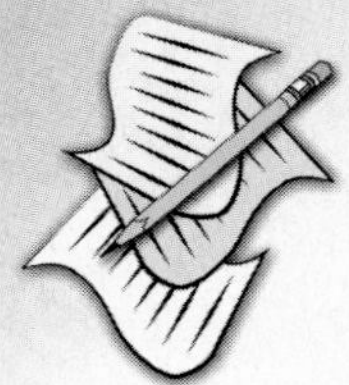

EXERCISE 3.3

Editing for Agreement of Pronouns and Antecedents

Read each sentence and circle the pronoun in parentheses that correctly completes the meaning.

1. The patient and (I/me) have discussed the options for treatment.
2. (Who/whom) is my first patient today?
3. I will ask the nurse to arrange for my partner or (I/me) to see the child tomorrow.
4. A patient (who/whom) has a cholesteatoma may present with unilateral hearing loss.
5. The receptionist should always ask a new patient if (he or she/they) brought (his or her/their) records.
6. Do not assume that patients know how (his or her/their) medications are to be taken.
7. Both tympanic membranes were noted to be bulging, and (its/their) color was bright red.
8. This patient, (who/whom) I consider to be reliable, says that he was treated poorly by your department.
9. Please call if Dr. Adams or (I/me) can be of help.
10. A patient with chronic tonsillitis often has to have (his or her/their) throat cultured.

Punctuating with Commas, Semicolons, and Colons

In a spoken conversation, meaning is conveyed through tone of voice, gestures, and pauses. We pause and change the inflection in our voices to clarify meaning. In written language, punctuation marks serve as "road signs" for readers. Punctuation clarifies meaning and prevents confusion.

Commas: To Introduce

Use a comma to set off an introductory word or phrase.

> Fortunately, the records were located.
>
> Because his temperature spiked, the patient was not cleared for discharge.
>
> Due to her rapid deterioration, the patient was transferred to the intensive care unit.
>
> When Mr. Johnson arrived, we met with the attorneys to discuss the terms of the will.

TIP: A sentence that is in the natural order (subject followed by verb and modifiers) does not contain an introductory clause and does not need an introductory comma.

> I confirmed the patients' appointments for next week before leaving the office.
>
> Your first-aid kit should be readily accessible in the event of a medical emergency.
>
> We will replace the desk light although the warranty is no longer in effect.

When a sentence is out of the natural order (inverted), a comma is needed to help the reader identify the important information of the sentence.

> Before leaving the office, I confirmed the patients' appointments for next week.
>
> In the event of a medical emergency, your first-aid kit should be readily accessible.

Be careful to place introductory phrases close to the word they modify; otherwise, your sentence may be grammatically incorrect and/or cause confusion to readers.

UNCLEAR:	After pausing the tape, the operative report was completed.
CLEAR:	After pausing the tape, he completed the operative report.
CLEAR:	To arrive on time, we will have to leave at 8 a.m.

Commas: To Separate

Coordinate conjunctions *(and, but, or, nor, for, so)* join two main clauses into one sentence. Use a comma immediately before the coordinate conjunction. Remember that a main clause contains a subject, verb, and complement and can stand alone. (A complement completes the sense of the verb and explains or describes the subject.) The main clause is also called an independent clause.

The patient was prepared and draped in the usual sterile orthopedic fashion, and the tourniquet was inflated to 250 mmHg.

The patient has had intermittent confusion, so the home health nurse was assigned to dispense the patient's medications.

I do not know how long it will last, but the patient has stopped smoking.

We investigated several locations for the conference, but we selected the facility that would attract the largest number of members.

If the main clauses are very short, you may omit the comma.

The wound was cleaned and a dressing was applied.

In a series of three or more items, use a comma before the conjunction.

The patient's past medical history is significant for coronary artery disease, insulin-dependent diabetes mellitus, and peptic ulcer disease.

Dr. Johnson sees outpatients on Mondays, Wednesdays, and Fridays.

You will find paper, disks, and CDs in the storage room.

The supervisor read the reports, selected several for presentation, and assigned grades.

Use a comma between consecutive adjectives that equally modify the same noun if the *and* is omitted.

She is a kind, dedicated nurse. [She is a kind and dedicated nurse].

Tomorrow will be a sunny, warm spring day. [Tomorrow will be a sunny and warm spring day.]

Do not use a comma between two adjectives if you would not use *and.* Test this by saying the adjectives in a different order and insert *and* between them.

> The patient is an elderly white female. [We would not say she is an elderly *and* white female].

When placing commas, be sure you do not separate the subject from the verb. Even if the subject is several words long, it must not be separated from the verb by a comma.

WRONG:	Patients who are afraid of hospitals and doctors because of past painful experiences, need to be given an extra dose of compassion.
CORRECT:	Patients who are afraid of hospitals and doctors because of past painful experiences need to be given an extra dose of compassion.

Commas: To Enclose

Use commas to set off nonessential or interrupting words or phrases from the rest of the sentence.

> I will graduate, unless I fail my chemistry class, next year.
>
> The dose, at least according to my calculations, is 12.5 mg per hour.
>
> The number of Internet users, according to the latest statistics, will continue to increase in the next decade.

TIP: Think of commas that enclose as parentheses. By enclosing information in commas, you are telling the reader that the information is not vital to the meaning of the sentence.

Do not use commas to set off essential or restrictive words or phrases that give a clear meaning to the sentence.

> The lady whose car I backed into was understanding and willing to settle for damages. [The essential clause indicated which lady's car was damaged.]

Semicolons

Semicolons are used in two situations: (1) to join two independent clauses and (2) to separate items in a series that has internal commas. Use one space after a semicolon in medical documents.

Use a semicolon to join two closely related independent clauses that are not joined by a coordinating conjunction *(and, or, but, nor).* Note that the clauses could also stand alone as sentences.

We have given you clear instructions; be sure to follow them explicitly.

When independent clauses are joined by *however, therefore,* etc., use a semicolon before the conjunctive adverb and a comma after it.

The patient has continued to take the medication; however, his condition has not improved.

Use a semicolon to separate items in a series when one or more of those items contains an internal comma.

He has written books about antique automobiles, specifically the Model T; sports trivia, his favorite topic; and outdoor cooking.

I have lived in Phoenix, Arizona; Portland, Oregon; and Seattle, Washington.

Colons

Colons are the neon signs of punctuation, alerting the reader to important information. Most commonly, they are used with report headings and in ratios.

Use a colon (and one space) after a report heading but only if the information follows on the same line. Capitalize the first letter after the heading.

HISTORY: The patient is a . . . .

Use a colon to express a ratio. Do not key a space before or after the colon.

The ECG revealed a 2:1 block.

Xylocaine with 1:100,000 epinephrine was instilled for local anesthesia.

Use a colon after introductions to listed items such as *the following* and *as follows.*

The required skills for the job are the following: ability to communicate, knowledge of Word, and ability to work in a team.

Use a colon to separate hour and minutes when expressing time.

The meeting is scheduled for 5:30 p.m.

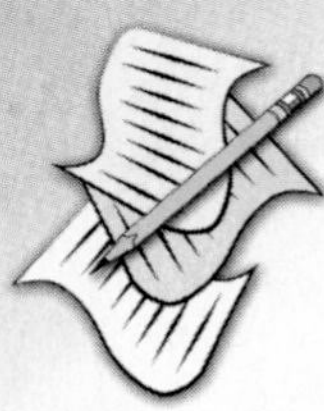

EXERCISE 3.4

Editing for Correct Punctuation

Read the following sentences and add commas, semicolons, or colons where necessary for correct meaning.

1. Since the patient has improved with conservative management we will not consider operative intervention at this time.
2. Our latest project remodeling the waiting room is going to be more expensive than we had planned.
3. Past surgeries include hysterectomy cholecystectomy and appendectomy.
4. Surprisingly the patient's condition improved.
5. Laboratory tests to be ordered include a complete blood count chemistry panel and electrolytes.
6. The risks and benefits of the procedure were explained to the patient and his wife and the patient signed the consent forms.
7. The planned surgery has a very high success rate however I explained to the patient that any surgery has an element of risk.
8. Abdomen is soft no organomegaly is noted.
9. The patient is to return to the emergency department immediately if he develops nausea fever over 100° or dramatically increased pain.
10. The patient has a history of coronary artery disease having undergone an angioplasty.
11. When testing the students should refrain from speaking.
12. After the induction of general anesthesia an endotracheal tube was placed.
13. The wound was then irrigated using normal saline and the deep muscles were closed using chromic sutures.
14. The experimental drug studies were carried out in San Diego California Denver Colorado Minneapolis Minnesota and Atlanta Georgia.
15. The patient is a young female college student.
16. Patients with AIDS who generally are underweight should receive nutritional counseling.
17. Thank you Dr. Smith for seeing this patient in pulmonary consultation.
18. Given the patient's overall debilitated condition and end-stage lung disease he wishes to be made a DNR.

Using Dashes, Quotation Marks, and Parentheses

Dashes

Use dashes to set off interrupting phrases from the rest of the sentence. They indicate a change in thought or a side comment not essential to the meaning of the sentence. Use them sparingly, especially in any type of formal document.

> Thank you for seeing Mrs. Johnson—especially on such short notice—for evaluation of her chest pain. [em dash]
>
> Many universities are focusing on online collaborative learning—it's exciting, informative, and a new approach to learning. [em dash]
>
> The project should be completed in 9–11 months. [en dash]

Note: Key dashes with no spaces before or after them. Proportional fonts such as New Times Roman include a special dash character. If you are using a monospaced font such as Courier, create a dash by keying two hyphens.

Quotation Marks

Use quotation marks to surround the exact words someone has spoken. The marks should appear in pairs, with one set at the beginning of the quote and the other at the end. The placement of other punctuation marks with quotes frequently causes confusion.

Always key a period and comma inside the quotation marks.

> The surgeon said, "We will first repair the heart valves and then deal with her coronary artery disease."
>
> "I want to go to the concert next Friday," Stephanie said.
>
> "I cannot tolerate pain," the patient complained, "but I know I need this surgery."
>
> "The new catalogs," John said, "will be available for distribution next month."

Place a colon or semicolon outside quotation marks.

> These are her "requirements": Arrive on time and attend all sessions.
>
> He said "thrombophlebitis"; I'm sure of it.
>
> The manager said, "A meeting will be held every Thursday on a monthly basis"; therefore, the supervisor needs to plan accordingly.

Place a question mark or exclamation mark outside the quotation marks if the entire sentence is a question or exclamation but inside if only the quoted words are a question or exclamation.

> Was she the physician who said, "No two surgeries are alike"?
>
> "If the pain subsides in two days," she asked, "should I continue taking the medicine?"
>
> The director asked, "How long have you been employed?" [Omit final period.]
>
> Mr. Courtney was so surprised he said, "I can't believe you finished the project!" [Omit final period.]

History and physical reports may begin with a chief complaint. If the chief complaint is dictated in first person, key it in quotation marks.

> CHIEF COMPLAINT: "I have been throwing up for two days."

If the quoted material is not a complete sentence, do not start the quote with a capital letter (unless the first word is a proper noun or an acronym).

> The patient says his left knee "doesn't feel right." [Contractions are acceptable in direct quotes but not in other dictation.]
>
> The patient said he had "some kind of x-ray test" on his back but did not know the name of the study.

Use quotation marks to draw attention to words and phrases or to designate slang, cliches, or nicknames.

> The patient's condition was "touch-and-go" for the first 24 hours but then gradually stabilized.
>
> I saw your patient Richard "Bud" Goodman for evaluation of his hypertension.

Use quotation marks to set off titles of magazine or newspaper articles and chapters of a book. The titles of magazines, newspapers, brochures, and books are placed in italics (in proportional spaced fonts such as Times New Roman) or underlined (in Courier).

All of our pregnant patients receive the *Eating For Two* brochure.

According to "Guide to a Healthy Heart," an article in the *Health Nuts* magazine, individuals who maintain a low-fat diet and who exercise regularly lower their risk of heart attack.

Parentheses

Use parentheses to enclose side thoughts or words not vital to the main idea of the sentence.

The sodium level was 131 (normal).

According to the surgery schedule (usually a reliable source), Michelle Brown will be admitted for excisional biopsy tomorrow.

Exercising on a daily basis *(swimming, walking, aerobics)* improves one's health.

Use parentheses to enclose acronyms or abbreviations.

Mr. Johnson underwent transurethral resection of the prostate (TURP) on the day of admission.

He will be referred for percutaneous transluminal coronary angioplasty (PTCA) of his right coronary artery lesion.

To become a certified public accountant (CPA), you have to pass the required examination.

Use parentheses to enclose numbers when a list is given in paragraph form.

The past history is remarkable for (1) coronary artery disease treated with PTCA; (2) diabetes mellitus, controlled on insulin therapy; and (3) hypertension, not well controlled.

If parentheses enclose a complete sentence that does not interrupt another sentence, place the period inside the parentheses.

The risks and benefits of the procedure were explained to the patient, and he opted to proceed. (The signed consent form is on the chart.)

If parentheses enclose an interrupting statement within a sentence, do not place a period inside the parentheses.

The procedure and its risks (bleeding, infection, possible need for transfusion) were explained to the patient.

His risk factors for coronary artery disease include history of smoking (he quit one year ago), positive family history, and elevated cholesterol level.

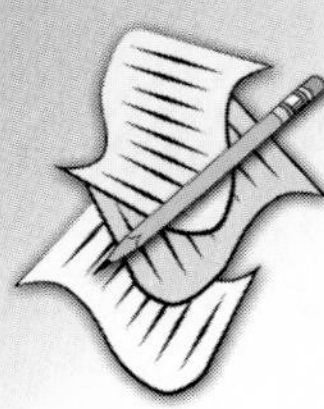

EXERCISE 3.5

Editing for Correct Punctuation

Read the following sentences from a medical report and add the appropriate special punctuation marks.

1. CHIEF COMPLAINT: I think I'm having a heart attack. [the patient's statement]
2. Gertrude Trudy Schmidt presented to my office today. [Indicate that Trudy is a nickname.]
3. Because her chest pain did not resolve with sublingual nitroglycerin, she was transported to the emergency department by a family member her son.
4. The patient states that his knee doesn't feel right when he walks. [a partial quote]
5. The patient's history has been well documented on previous admissions please see old records.
6. In accordance with his wishes, the patient was made a DNR do not resuscitate.
7. DISCHARGE DIAGNOSIS: Acute bacterial endocarditis, resolving.
8. Please set up an appointment with Dr. Edwards you can get his phone number from my secretary at your earliest convenience.
9. The patient has a history of one chronic obstructive pulmonary disease, two congestive heart failure, and three hypertension.
10. If the infection does not respond to amoxicillin, we may need to call in one of the big guns like cephalexin. [Mark the slang phrase]

Using Modifiers to Achieve Correct Meaning

Modifiers are words, phrases, and clauses that describe or tell more about another word, phrase, or clause. Good transcriptionists pay careful attention to the placement of modifiers to ensure clear meaning of sentences.

Related Words Should Be Placed Together

Place modifiers as close as possible to the words being modified.

UNCLEAR:	Examination at that time of the esophagus was negative. [What is "that time of the esophagus"?]
CLEAR:	Examination of the esophagus at that time was negative.
UNCLEAR:	The lady was a teller in the bank who wore a red suit. [The clause *who wore a red suit* modifies the noun lady.]
CLEAR:	The lady in the red suit was a teller in the bank.

Misplaced or Dangling Modifiers

Many transcription "bloopers" are caused by misplaced or dangling modifiers, particularly prepositional phrases or phrases beginning with *ing* words. These phrases are adjective phrases that modify a noun. Miscommunication occurs when the phrase is not placed next to the noun it modifies.

WRONG:	The bleeder was clamped with a hemostat, hoping to achieve hemostasis. [The phrase *hoping to achieve hemostasis* is an adjective phrase that refers to the surgeon—not to the bleeder, as is suggested in this sentence construction.]
CORRECT:	The bleeder was clamped with a hemostat in the hope of achieving hemostasis.
OR:	Hoping to achieve hemostasis, the surgeon clamped the bleeder with a hemostat.
WRONG:	The driver was referred to a doctor with a severe head injury. [The phrase *with a severe head injury* refers to the driver, not the doctor.]
CORRECT:	The driver with a severe head injury was referred to a doctor.
WRONG:	Withdrawing the instrument, polyps were encountered in the transverse colon. [Are the polyps withdrawing the instrument?]
CORRECT:	Withdrawing the instrument, I encountered polyps in the transverse colon.

Note: Be very careful when altering dictation. Reserve rewording for instances when the dictation is not clear because of the misplacement or misuse of a modifier. If you must edit, always use the dictator's original words for terms, procedures, instruments, and diseases. Too much editing can be considered tampering.

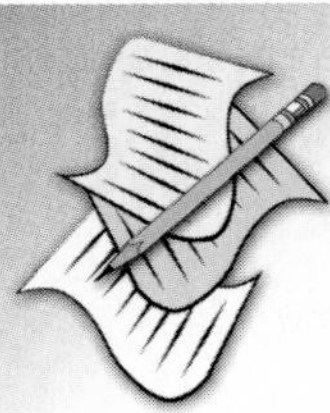

EXERCISE 3.6

Editing for Placement of Modifiers

Revise and key the following dictated sentences to show the correct use and placement of modifiers.

1. The patient was referred to a gastroenterologist who, because of increasing complaints of esophageal reflux, ordered an upper GI.
2. In the left lateral Sims position, the doctor performed the rectal examination.
3. When 3 weeks post appendectomy, she called about her husband's inflamed incision.
4. X-ray this morning of the chest revealed moderate clearing of the infiltrate.
5. After improving on antibiotic therapy, surgery was deferred.
6. At 225 pounds, her doctor instructed her to eat smaller meals and to exercise more often.
7. A curved incision was made just above the umbilicus of 3 cm.
8. Feeling very nauseous, the nurse handed the patient an emesis basin.
9. With a family history of colon polyps, screening colonoscopy will be carried out every 2 years.
10. The doctor arranged for Mr. Smith's admission. Had he notified the insurance company, reimbursement would have been greater.

Forming Plurals

The first section of this chapter reviewed the guidelines for creating agreement between subjects and verbs. The guidelines are based on the principle that plural subjects require plural verbs and singular subjects require singular verbs. Since nouns and pronouns function as subjects of sentences, it is important to know the general rules for creating the plural forms of medical terms.

Generally, most nouns are made plural by adding *s* or *es* to the singular form. The same rules usually apply to nouns in medical reports. However, many medical words and terms are of Latin and Greek origin; therefore, they do not follow the English rules. For example, the plural form of *diagnosis* is not *diagnosises;* it is *diagnoses.* Consult a medical dictionary when necessary.

Rules for Plural Forms

As you become more familiar with the medical language, forming and/or recognizing plural forms will become easier. The following rules for making plural forms will be helpful.

1. If the singular form ends in a, make the plural by adding e (vertebra–vertebrae).
2. If the singular form ends in um, change the um to a (diverticulum–diverticula).
3. If the singular form ends in us, change the us to i (fungus–fungi).
4. If the singular form ends in is, change the is to es (diagnosis–diagnoses).

5. If the singular form ends in ax or ix, change the x to ces (thorax–thoraces; cervix–cervices).
6. If the singular form ends in ex, change the ex to ices (index–indices).
7. If the singular form ends in nx, change the x to ges (pharynx–pharynges).
8. If the singular form ends in en, change the en to ina (lumen–lumina).
9. If the singular form ends in on, change the on to a (phenomenon–phenomena).
10. If the singular form ends in ma, add ta (condyloma–condylomata). Note that it is also acceptable to form plurals of these words just by adding s. (carcinoma–carcinomas).

Other Plural Forms

Very few plural forms contain an apostrophe, so do not be tempted to add one when keying a plural unless you are certain it is correct.

Some words have only a singular or plural form. The word *adnexa* means appendages or auxiliary parts (plural), usually referring to the fallopian tubes and ovaries. So if you heard "right and left adnexa nontender" in a report of a pelvic examination, you would transcribe *adnexa,* not *adnexae* or *adnexi* because there are no such words. Also, the words *feces, genitalia, menses, scabies, tongs,* and *tweezers* are always plural in use. On the other hand, the words *circulation, vision, ascites,* and *herpes* are singular in meaning. *Biceps, forceps, scissors,* and *series* are the same whether the meaning is singular or plural.

TIP: Always consider the context of the dictation when choosing the singular or plural form of a noun. For instance, if you hear "conjunctiva clear," you would transcribe this in plural form (unless the patient only has one eye or the eye exams are being dictated individually).

Forming Plural Abbreviations

Add *s* (no apostrophe) after all uppercase abbreviations.

> Serial ECGs revealed no changes.
>
> CBCs over the last six months have been abnormal.
>
> Many people select CDs to get a higher interest rate than they can in a savings account.

Add *s* to abbreviated forms such as *poly* or *seg* (polys, segs).

> White count was 5500 with 67 segs, 7 mono*s*, 2 eos.

Plural Numbers and Units of Measure

When pluralizing numbers, add *s* without an apostrophe unless the number is only one digit.

> She had her appendix removed in her 20s.
>
> Doctors have made many advances in the 1990s.
>
> 8's and 9's on Apgar scores are common.

Do not put an *s* on the end of an abbreviated unit of measure, no matter how large the value is, e.g., 1 mg or 1,000,000 mg.

> We removed 200 cc of fluid from the patient's peritoneal cavity.
>
> The incision measured 6 cm.

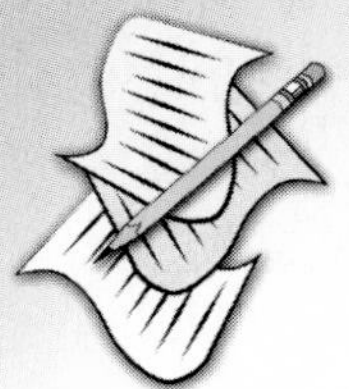

EXERCISE 3.7

Editing for Correct Plural Forms

Write the appropriate plural form on the blank line after each word.

1. fossa __________
2. prognosis __________
3. appendix __________
4. labium __________
5. datum __________
6. salpinx __________
7. uterus __________
8. ovum __________
9. criterion __________
10. foramen __________

From the choices given, write the correct plural form for each word.

11. Colonoscopy revealed multiple (diverticulum/diverticula) in the ascending colon. __________
12. Hysterosalpingogram showed right (hydrosalpinx/hydrosalpinges). __________
13. Her history of intolerance to cold led to the diagnosis of Raynaud (phenomenon/phenomena). __________

14. She was treated with ampicillin 500 (mg/mgs) q.i.d. times 10 days. ____________________
15. Delivery of the infant was achieved using (forcep/forceps). ____________________
16. James was told by his doctor that he had a (herpe/herpes) infection. ____________________
17. Examination of her cervix revealed the presence of different (fungus/fungi).
____
18. Babinskis/Babinski's were negative. ____________________
19. Serial (CBC/CBCs/CBC's) were obtained. ____________________
20. (Ascitis/Ascites) is a common condition in people with liver disease. ____________________

Using Capitals Correctly

Capitalization is a signal writers can use to tell the reader that what is capitalized is important or specialized. However, the overuse of capitals diminishes their effect and may confuse rather than help the reader. Transcriptionists need to know the basic rules of capitalization and how and when to apply them.

Proper Nouns

Capitalize formal names of persons, places, and organizations.

John A. Smith, MD	Mayo Clinic
Coronado Hospital, San Diego	the American Cancer Society

Capitalize languages and races. Do not capitalize skin color.

French	black
Caucasian	white
Mexican-American	

Capitalize days of the week, months, and holidays but not seasons.

Thursday, May 28	spring 1997
Independence Day	

Capitalize trade or brand names, but do not capitalize generic drugs.

Amoxil	amoxicillin
Cardizem	diltiazem
Xeroform dressing	

Capitalize a job title only when it precedes a name and is used as that person's title. Do not capitalize the title when it replaces or renames the person.

> Director of Education Maria Jaeb will read the announcement. [The job title precedes the name.]
>
> Maria Jaeb, education director, will read the announcement. [*Maria Jaeb* identifies the person being discussed, and *education director* gives further information about (or renames) Maria.]

Capitalize the genus but not the species of bacteria.

> Clostridium difficile
>
> Streptococcus aureus

Do not capitalize hospital department names.

intensive care unit	operating room
emergency department	neurology service

Abbreviations

Do not capitalize Latin abbreviations that deal with drug dosage *(b.i.d., a.c., p.o.)*. According to the AAMT, the correct form for Latin abbreviations is lowercase with periods between each letter.

h.s.	at bedtime	q.4h.	every four hours
a.m.	morning	q.d.	once a day
a.c.	before meals or food	q.12h.	every twelve hours
t.i.d.	three times a day	p.o.	by mouth
q.	every	p.m.	afternoon or evening
q.i.d.	four times a day	b.i.d.	twice a day

Some hospitals direct their MTs to capitalize the abbreviation NPO, which stands for *nil per os* (nothing by mouth). They want the term capitalized because it is very important information. If the term goes unnoticed in a patient's record, there could be life-threatening consequences. However, in this instance, as with other style issues, follow your employer's preference.

Abbreviate courtesy titles when they appear with complete names or with last names only *(Mr., Mrs., Ms., Dr.)*.

> Mr. Jonathan Brendel is the incoming treasurer of the organization.
>
> Mrs. Mumford will prepare the address list.

Ms. Nancy Coletti is the new supervisor.

Dr. Sanders will be glad to accept your invitation to be keynote speaker at the convention.

Spell out all other titles used with personal names *(Senator, President, Governor, Captain).*

Senator McCain

Governor George Byron

Always abbreviate *Jr.* and *Sr.* when they follow personal names.

Dr. Frank Smith, Sr.

Abbreviate *Esq.* and *MD* after a full personal name; however, never use a courtesy title before a full name.

Courtney Lorenzo, MD NOT Dr. Courtney Lorenzo, MD

Paul Mirando, Esq.

Abbreviated words used in routine correspondence and business forms are followed by a period and a space.

etc.	et cetera
vs.	versus
vol.	volume
fwd.	forward

However, when these terms are used within a sentence, use small letters with periods.

c.o.d.	This package arrived c.o.d.
e.o.m.	The invoice will be processed with other e.o.m. accounting procedures.

When expressing time, use the abbreviation *a.m.* and *p.m.*

10 a.m.

4 p.m.

Acronyms

Acronyms are abbreviations formed using the initial letters of words or phrases. Capitalize all the letters of an acronym. No periods are required.

ASHD	atherosclerotic/ arteriosclerotic heart disease	LVD	left ventricular dysfunction
LAO	left anterior oblique	CHF	congestive heart failure
		MI	myocardial infarction

Some business terms are often abbreviated when used on business forms. Note that there are no periods used with these abbreviations.

ASAP	as soon as possible
CEO	chief executive officer
COD	cash on delivery
EOM	end of month
FDIC	Federal Deposit Insurance Company
FOB	free on board
FYI	for your information

Eponyms

Eponyms are adjectives created from proper nouns. The terms usually derive from the name of the person who identified the disease, developed the protocol, or designed the instrument. The eponym itself, but not the noun, is capitalized. The possessive form (Down's syndrome) has been replaced with the nonpossessive (Down syndrome) form. This transition is occurring with all eponyms. Do not use the possessive form.

Alzheimer disease	Foley catheter
Bruce protocol	Gram stain

Note that *Parkinson disease* is capitalized, but the adjectival form parkinsonian is not.

The patient exhibited symptoms of Parkinson disease.

The patient's symptoms were parkinsonian.

Drug Allergies

The capitalization of the word *allergy* (or variations) and all letters of a drug name listed under an allergies heading attracts the reader's attention.

The patient is ALLERGIC TO MORPHINE, which causes a rash.

Document Elements

Capitalize the first letter of a formal list.

> DISCHARGE INSTRUCTIONS
> - Activities ad lib.
> - Diet as tolerated.
> - Followup will be in one week in my office.
>
> MEDICATIONS
> 1. Aspirin 325 mg 1 daily.
> 2. Hydrochlorothiazide 50 mg p.o. q.d.

Capitalize headings and the first word after a heading.

> HEENT: Pupils, equal, round, reactive to light.
> HISTORY OF PRESENT ILLNESS: The patient presents. . . .
> FAMILY HISTORY: Noncontributory.

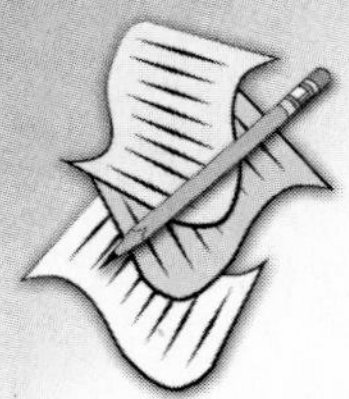

EXERCISE 3.8

Editing for Correct Capitalization

Read the following partial discharge summary and circle all capitalization errors. Then key the summary with the errors corrected.

History of present illness: willie dayton is a 55-year-old african-american who speaks french and chinese, presenting with a chief complaint of chest pain. he has been having mild chest pain since early autumn, but it has been increasing recently, especially over the holidays. he has been taking dyazide for blood pressure and also uses ibuprofen occasionally. On

(continued)

Sunday, new year's day, he called his insurance company and was referred to south side hospital. the patient presented to the emergency department for evaluation and was noted to have t wave inversions on his ecg. chest x-ray showed no pneumonia or pulmonary edema. he was given nitroglycerin sublingually times two, with resolution of his chest pain. cpk was shown to be elevated, and cardiology was called to evaluate this patient and assume his care. The patient was admitted to the intensive care unit at 0300.

past medical history: the patient has a diagnosis of early parkinson disease and is treated by a neurologist for this.

allergies: sulfa (hives).

physical examination
vital signs: blood pressure 110/95, pulse 75, respirations 18.
heent: normocephalic, atraumatic; pupils equal, round, reactive to light and accommodation. fundi clear, no av nicking. ears, nose, and throat clear.
neck: supple, no jvd, no lymphadenopathy.
chest: clear to percussion and auscultation.
heart: s1 and s2 normal. there was a grade 2/6 systolic ejection murmur heard best at the left lower sternal border.
abdomen: supple. no organomegaly or rebound tenderness.
genitalia: deferred.
extremities: no clubbing, cyanosis, or edema.

hospital course: the patient was taken to the cardiac catheterization laboratory on the morning of admission. This study revealed no areas of stenosis of the coronary arterial system. The patient was given nitroglycerin sublingually p.r.n. chest pain and was given procardia for his hypertension. His ecg normalized, and on Tuesday he was subjected to a treadmill exercise test using the modified bruce protocol. this test was interpreted by the cardiologist as showing no signs of ischemia.

the patient was discharged in excellent condition to follow up in one week with dr. smith at the south bay regional cardiac center.

discharge medications
1. procardia 10 mg q.d.
2. aspirin 325 mg 1 daily.
3. nitroglycerin sublingual p.r.n. chest pain.

Using Numbers in Word or Figure Form

Numbers are written in figures or words depending on the situation. As a basic rule, use figures to express quantities with clinical significance. Lab values, age, and values with a unit of measurement should all be expressed with arabic numerals. Otherwise spell out numbers under 10. Use figures for numbers 10 and above.

> The patient will be seen again in 3 weeks.
>
> The purchasing department ordered four computers for the new staff members.
>
> About 50 doctors attended the meeting.
>
> To become a member of our association, you need to pay an annual fee of $75.

Exceptions to the basic rule are discussed below.

First Word of a Sentence

Spell out numbers that are the first word of a sentence.

> Twelve years ago the patient had a stroke.
>
> Five new men joined the choir.
>
> Two of the lymph nodes were positive.
>
> Fifty people signed up for the show.

Large numbers spelled out at the beginning of a sentence may slow down the reader. Instead, rewrite the sentence so the number appears in a different location.

> WORDY: Forty-three thousand five hundred was his highest white count.
>
> BETTER: His highest white count was 43,500.

Units of Measurement and Lab Values

Use figures when indicating quantity with a unit of measurement or with lab values.

> Three 1-liter solutions were used.
>
> The surgeon made two 5-cm incisions.
>
> Results of the PSA revealed a mild elevation of 4.1 ng/L.

Similar Types of Data

When numbers in a sentence describe the same kind of data, express them in the same style regardless of their size.

> There were 65 lymphocytes, 2 monocytes, and 5 eosinophils.
>
> There were 12 laptop computers, 3 printers, and 2 scanners.
>
> Today the doctor saw 15 patients in the office and 5 in the hospital.
>
> Jerry had a cataract removed in the left eye 15 years ago, and 3 years later had the same procedure on the right eye.
>
> Pathology revealed 2 positive lymph nodes from the left groin and 1 positive node from the right.

Dates

The date line of a business letter should be written in full (April 20, 20XX). Use figures for short-form dates with slashes and for the day of a month.

> He has an appointment for 10/29/XX.

Use a cardinal figure when the day follows the month.

> Please arrange for surgery to be performed on October 3.
>
> Please keep July 1 open for graduation ceremonies.

A day that precedes a month should be expressed in ordinal numbers (numbers expressing place or position as in *first, second, third*) or in ordinal words.

> We have continued to follow this patient on the 5th of each month.
>
> The international business conference will be held in London from the fifth of October until the ninth.

The military and international style for expressing dates reverses the day and month, with no commas in between. Follow this format if your client or employer prefers.

> The patient was admitted on 10 April 20XX.

Age

Express ages and other vital statistics in figures.

> She is a 21-year-old, well-developed, well-nourished white female. Height 5 feet 6 inches, weight 130 pounds, blood pressure 110/70, pulse 74, respirations 18. [Note that common nonmetric units of measurement *(feet, inches, pounds)* are spelled out.]

Time

Use figures to express times of day. No zeros are required when the time falls on the hour.

> The patient will be seen at 2 p.m.
>
> Surgery is scheduled for 7 a.m.
>
> The patient expired at 11:45 p.m.
>
> The meeting will be held from 9 a.m. to 12:30 p.m.

Many medical facilities follow the military style of expressing time. Military time uses no colons, and instead of starting over at 12 noon, the clock continues to count to 2400 (stated as *twenty-four hundred hours*). If this confuses you, simply subtract 1200 to get "civilian" time, for example, 2350 - 1200 = 1150 p.m. Note the following dictated sentences and the times intended.

> The infant was delivered at fourteen forty-five. [2:45 p.m.]
>
> The last dose was given at zero three twenty hours. [3:20 a.m.]

Anatomic position may be dictated using a clock-face orientation *(o'clock).* Use figures in these expressions.

> A suspicious mass was noted at the 3 o'clock position on the left breast.
>
> The lesion appears at 12 o'clock on the right cheek.

Money

Use figures to express amounts of money. Do not include zeros in even dollar amounts.

> The patient has a $5 copay. [Not $5.00]
>
> He purchased $250 worth of equipment.

When amounts of money include millions and billions of dollars, write out *million* or *billion.* Do not add *dollars.*

> A $2.5 billion donation was given to the school.

Measurements, Mathematical Expressions, and Symbols

Use figures for measurements and ratios and in expressions involving symbols and abbreviations.

The mass on the head of the pancreas measured 2 x 3 cm. [Note that the unit of measurement is expressed only once.]

It is an 8- by 14-meter room.

or

It is an 8 x 14-m room.

The patient's height is 5 feet 6 inches and her weight is 135 pounds.

The paper measures 8 inches by 11 inches.

The incision was closed with 3-0 Prolene.

The baby's rectal temperature was 103°.

The thermostat is set at 68 degrees.

The patient has 20/50 vision in the right eye and 20/70 in the left eye.

The solution was diluted 1:50. [no space before or after the colon]

Pulses were 2+.

Express vertebral levels using a capital C, T (or D), L, or S followed by an arabic numeral, as in T2. Do not use a hyphen. Do not superscript or subscript the numeral.

Use a hyphen to express the intervertebral space (space between two vertebrae), as in L5-S1 or L2-L3.

Decimals and Fractions

Use figures to express decimals. If a decimal less than 1 is dictated, transcribe a zero before the decimal point, even if it is not dictated. When whole numbers are dictated, do not add a decimal point and zero.

DICTATED:	The patient takes digoxin point 125 mg q.d.
TRANSCRIBED:	The patient takes digoxin 0.125 mg q.d.
INCORRECT:	She was given 5.0 mg of Valium.
CORRECT:	She was given 5 mg of Valium.

If similar functions are performed by numbers in a sentence, write them uniformly.

The liquidators sell clothing for $75.50, $29.95, $55.00, and $60.00. [Note the consistent use of decimal points and places.]

When a metric measurement is dictated as a fraction, convert the fraction to a decimal. Common fractions and decimal equivalents include the following: ¼ = 0.25, ½ = 0.5, and ¾ = 0.75.

INCORRECT:	Local anesthesia was achieved using ½ percent Xylocaine.
CORRECT:	Local anesthesia was achieved using 0.5% Xylocaine.

Write fractions standing alone as words.

> At least two-thirds of the tourists were from overseas.

When a physician dictates a fraction in a general, nontechnical form, use words to express the fraction.

INCORRECT:	The upper ½ of the esophagus appeared normal.
CORRECT:	The upper one-half of the esophagus appeared normal.
INCORRECT:	The distal ⅔ of the esophagus revealed no abnormalities.
CORRECT:	The distal two-thirds of the esophagus revealed no abnormalities.

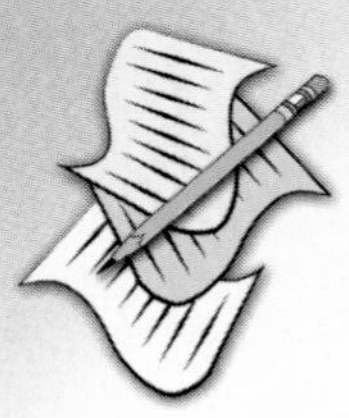

EXERCISE 3.9

Editing for Correct Use of Numbers

Edit the following discharge summary for the correct use of numbers. Circle the correct number expressions from the choices in parentheses, then key the report with the errors corrected.

DISCHARGE SUMMARY

PATIENT: Juarez, Juan
MR#: 12-34-56
DATE OF ADMISSION: (April 4 20XX; 4/4/XX)
DATE OF DISCHARGE: (April 6 20XX; 4/6/XX)

DISCHARGE DIAGNOSIS: Herniated nucleus pulposus, (L-5-S-1; L5-S1).

OPERATION PERFORMED: Right partial (L-4; L4) hemilaminectomy with excision of herniated disk.

HISTORY: This is a (fifty; 50)-year-old Hispanic male who presented with a (four; 4)-month history of progressive low back pain. Over the past (one; 1) month, he has had worsening symptoms and now has numbness, tingling, and pain radiating down his right leg.

PAST MEDICAL HISTORY: His history is significant for (two; 2) episodes of pneumonia (five; 5) years ago, and he has chronic asthma.

SOCIAL HISTORY: The patient smokes (one; 1) pack of cigarettes per day and has done so for the past (twenty; 20) years. He drinks (2 6-packs; two six-packs; two 6-packs; 2 six-packs) of beer per week.

ADMISSION MEDICATIONS
1. Theo-Dur (three hundred milligrams; 300 milligrams; 300 mg) (tid; t.i.d.; TID).
2. Proventil inhaler (two; 2) puffs (q12h; q. 12 h.; q.12h.)

DRUG ALLERGIES: CODEINE, which causes a rash.

PHYSICAL EXAMINATION
GENERAL APPEARANCE: This is a slightly obese Hispanic male appearing slightly older than his stated age of (fifty-years; 50-years; 50 years).
VITAL SIGNS: Blood pressure (one hundred twenty over sixty; 120 over 60; 120/60), pulse (eighty; 80) and regular, respirations (twelve; 12), temperature (ninety-eight degrees; 98°).
HEENT: Pupils equal and reactive to light. The left tympanic membrane was (one plus/1+) injected. Nares were patent bilaterally.
NECK: Right shotty supraclavicular lymph node approximately (two, 2) cm wide. Trachea midline.
LUNGS: Clear to percussion and auscultation.
HEART: Auscultation revealed a grade (two over six; 2 over 6; 2/6) systolic ejection murmur. PMI is at the (fifth; 5th) intercostal space.
ABDOMEN: Slightly obese, (one plus; 1 plus; 1+) tenderness in the epigastrium. Bowel sounds were present, no hepatosplenomegaly.

(continued)

DISCHARGE SUMMARY
PATIENT: Juarez, Juan
MR#: 12-34-56
DATE: 1/8/XX
Page 2

SPINE: Negative CVA tenderness. There was (two plus; 2+) tenderness in the (L-4-L-5; L4-L5) area. Straight leg raising was negative on the left, positive on the right at (forty-five; 45) degrees.
EXTREMITIES: No clubbing, cyanosis, or edema. Distal pulses were good.
NEUROLOGIC: Cranial nerves (two through twelve; II-XII; 2-12) were intact. The patient was alert and oriented (times three; x3).

LABORATORY DATA: Admission CBC revealed WBC of (5,800; 5800) with (seventy-one; 71) polys, (two; 2) bands, (one; 1) eosinophil and (twenty-six; 26) lymphs. Hemoglobin was (thirteen; 13), hematocrit (thirty-nine percent; 39 percent; 39%). BUN was (eight; 8), creatinine (point nine; .9; 0.9).

HOSPITAL COURSE: Lumbar myelogram on day of admission revealed significant disk herniation at the (L-4-L-5; L4-L5) level. The patient was taken to the operating room, where right hemilaminectomy was performed.

Postoperatively the patient had a temperature spike to (101°; one-hundred one degrees) and was started on Ancef. He had no further temperature elevations and his chest x-ray remained clear. He had good resolution of his symptoms.

The patient was discharged to home to be followed in clinic in (five; 5) days. Instructions were given for no heavy lifting. It was suggested that a (thirty, 30)-minute walk be taken daily.

DISCHARGE MEDICATIONS
1. Vicodin (one; 1) p.o. (q. three to four hours, q.3-4h.) p.r.n. pain.
2. Theo-Dur and Proventil as previously.

NS/XX
D: 1/8/XX
T: 1/10/XX

Using Abbreviations Correctly

Abbreviations are selected letters of a longer word or phrase. Abbreviations save space and may speed up communication, but they can also cause confusion and misinterpretation.

Your medical transcription library should include an abbreviations reference. Keep context in mind as you search for abbreviations to ensure that the extended form you choose is the appropriate term.

Generally, transcribe abbreviations in full capital letters without punctuation and without spaces between the letters. Short forms, such as *segs* for *segmented neutrophils* or *lymphs* for *lymphocytes,* are transcribed as dictated.

To Abbreviate or Not to Abbreviate

In medical reports, there are some areas in which abbreviations are not used even if they are dictated. Do not use abbreviations in any impression, assessment, admitting or discharge diagnosis, or preoperative or postoperative diagnosis. Do not use abbreviations in the title of the procedure for an operative report.

> DICTATED:
> ADMITTING DIAGNOSIS: S/P CVA.
>
> TRANSCRIBED:
> ADMITTING DIAGNOSIS: Status post cerebrovascular accident.
>
> DICTATED:
> PROCEDURE PERFORMED: ORIF, right hip fracture.
>
> TRANSCRIBED:
> PROCEDURE PERFORMED: Open reduction and internal fixation, right hip fracture.

Do not abbreviate any medical term that is dictated in full except for metric units of measure *(milligrams, milliliters)* preceded by a number (for example, transcribe 5 mg, *not* 5 milligrams). Metric units of measure most often appear in laboratory results and drug dosages.

Units of Measure

Use abbreviations when a numeric quantity precedes metric units of measure. Do not add *s* or *'s*.

DICTATED:	Ampicillin five hundred milligrams
TRANSCRIBED:	Ampicillin 500 mg
DO NOT USE:	Ampicillin 500 mg.; or 500 mgs; or 500 mgs.

Metric units of measure are abbreviated in technical and scientific work, in tables, and on business forms *(lb, km, mph).* Spell out units of measure in nontechnical writing.

> The broker indicated it was a 350-acre estate.
>
> The new reference manual will be a 9½- by 6-inch (or 9-1/2-by-6-inch) book.

Spell out common nonmetric units of measure, like foot, inch, ounce, and so on, except in tables. Do not use an apostrophe or quotation marks to indicate feet or inches except in tables.

> The child's height was 4 feet 2 inches.
>
> The infant weighed 8 pounds 8½ (or 8-1/2) ounces.
>
> A 5-inch incision was made.

Punctuation with Abbreviations

Usually, no punctuation is used with abbreviations. The exception is the group of Latin abbreviations that deal with medication administration. These are always keyed in lowercase with periods in between.

> b.i.d. p.r.n. q.12h.

If more than one Latin abbreviation is dictated together, put a space between the two abbreviations.

> Zantac 150 mg p.o. b.i.d.

DICTATED:	She takes Valium five milligrams p-o-b-i-d-p-r-n anxiety.
TRANSCRIBED:	She takes Valium 5 mg p.o. b.i.d. p.r.n. anxiety.

Plural Abbreviations

Abbreviations in capital letters do not require an apostrophe before the *s (WBCs, ECGs, VCRs, CDs, CPAs).* Add an apostrophe to words that could be misread (for example, CPS's). Add an *s* to short forms for laboratory terms *(lymphs, monos, segs).*

Abbreviations That Have Multiple Meanings

Do not guess. If an abbreviation with multiple meanings is dictated—for example, PT—you may or may not be able to determine the intended meaning based on the context of the report. To figure out the meaning, read the rest of the report to see if the full term has been dictated elsewhere, or look at the patient's record if you have easy access to it. If you are unsuccessful, leave the term in abbreviated form, even in a diagnosis. It is better to leave an abbreviated form that knowledgeable people will be able to interpret than to transcribe a full term that is incorrect.

If the abbreviation itself is not clear (CVP? CPT? CCP?), try the same methods as above. Again, do not guess. It is better to leave a blank than to guess incorrectly.

Shorthand Dictation

Physicians sometimes use a verbal "shorthand" for certain words or expressions that appear regularly in medical reports. For example, the terms *discharged, discontinued,* and *identified* may be dictated as "dee seed" [DC'd] and "i deed" [ID'd]. The terms should be transcribed in full:

DICTATED:	Streptococcus was ID'd on blood culture.
TRANSCRIBED:	Streptococcus was identified on blood culture.
DICTATED:	The patient was DC'd from the hospital today.
TRANSCRIBED:	The patient was discharged from the hospital today.
DICTATED:	Physical therapy was DC'd because the patient complained of severe pain.
TRANSCRIBED:	Physical therapy was discontinued because the patient complained of severe pain.

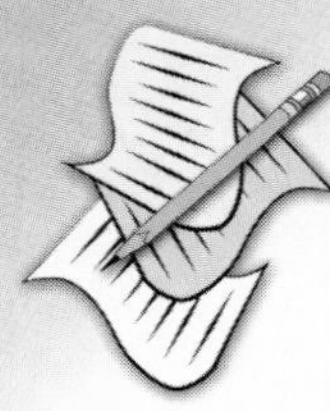

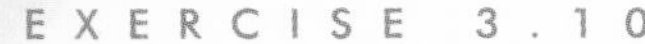

EXERCISE 3.10

Identifying Abbreviations

Use your abbreviations references, if available, to find the appropriate extended forms. Otherwise, use the abbreviations appendix at the end of the book. Then key the report with the abbreviations spelled out.

1. The patient was diagnosed with ALS, a degenerative neurologic disease commonly known as Lou Gehrig disease.
2. Because of her symptoms of left hemiparesis and confusion, Mrs. Smith was believed to have suffered a CVA.
3. An EEG, a test showing the electrical activity of the brain, was performed to rule out seizure disorder.
4. HEENT: PERRLA. Extraocular movements intact.
5. The patient suffers from weakness, paresthesias, and speech disturbances secondary to MS, a degenerative neurologic disorder.
6. The patient is alert and oriented, in NAD, resting comfortably.
7. The patient is NPO in preparation for surgery; do not serve him breakfast.
8. The infant's PKU test was positive, so he will require a diet very low in phenylalanine to prevent mental retardation.
9. The patient has had several episodes of TIAs with neurologic deficits.
10. The myelogram revealed HNP at the L3-L4 level, with a significant disk protrusion.

Using Apostrophes Correctly

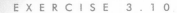

Apostrophes are used to denote omitted letters in contractions, to express a year or decade, to show possession, and to form some plurals.

Contractions

Use contracted forms in medical reports only in a direct quote; otherwise, write out the words.

DICTATED:	I don't feel the patient is improving.
TRANSCRIBED:	I do not feel the patient is improving.
DICTATED:	The patient said, "I don't feel I'm improving."
TRANSCRIBED:	The patient said, "I don't feel I'm improving."

Remember that *it's* means *it is,* while the word *its* is a singular possessive pronoun. Because *it's* is a contraction, do not use it in a medical report.

> The central venous line was placed and its ports were flushed with saline.
>
> It is important that the bandages be changed every two hours.

Whose is a relative pronoun that can function in various ways, including as a connector between a subordinate clause and a main clause. *Who's* is a contraction for the two words *who is.* Note the differences in use:

> She is a physician whose research is widely regarded as the best in the field. [*Whose* connects the subordinate clause with the main clause.]
>
> He is a new employee whose architectural interpretation for the new building was highly rated. [possessive pronoun]
>
> It is not important who's speaking at the conference, as long as the field of candidates is carefully selected. [*Who's* stands for *who is.*]
>
> Who's responsible for taking the minutes for the meeting? [*Who is* responsible?]
>
> Who said they're booking a cruise? [*They are* booking.]

Years

When a single year is expressed without the century, precede it with an apostrophe ('97). Use an apostrophe preceding expressions of decades of the century (in the '90s), but not when referring to decades of a patient's life (in his 50s).

Possessive Forms

Apostrophes indicate ownership, either literally or figuratively. When the noun is singular, add an *'s* to create the possessive.

> The patient's laboratory tests were normal. [possessive singular noun, one patient, his tests]
>
> He will be seen in one day's time. [the time belonging to one day]

Add only an apostrophe to form the possessive of singular nouns that end in *s.*

> Meredith Dobbs' car crashed down the embankment.

Some singular nouns *(Mr. Harris)* become difficult to pronounce when you add *'s* because the addition makes an extra syllable. In this case, add only an apostrophe to show possession.

> Mrs. Billings' condition is stable.

When a possessive is an abbreviation, use *'s* just as you would with a singular word.

> The HMO's policies are clear.

Add only an apostrophe to express the possessive of plural nouns that end in *s.*

> PLURAL: The *physicians'* opinions were varied. [more than one physician]
>
> PLURAL: All of the AIDS *patients'* study results were compiled. [more than one patient, their results]

Add *'s* to plural nouns that do not end in *s* to make them possessive.

> The conference dealt with children's issues.
>
> More and more, women's rights are being protected and continuing to increase.

Use *'s* after the last word in a hyphenated compound term.

> Her mother-in-law's health was failing.
>
> Her daughters-in-laws' schedules were conflicting. [the schedules of both daughters-in-law]

The AAMT style guidelines state not to use *'s* with eponymic terms (Alzheimer disease, not Alzheimer's disease). This has been widely accepted by all medical writing authorities. However, defer to the wishes of your client or employer. It should be noted, though, that eponymic surgical terms generally do not require *'s.* Without the apostrophe, *As* could be read as the word *as.*

Plurals

In some instances, *'s* forms plurals that are not possessives. For example, use *'s* to form plurals of single letters or numbers.

> Three A's, two B's, and two C's.
>
> Mind your p's and q's.
>
> He rates his pain as mostly 1's and 2's on a scale of 1–10.

However, do not use an apostrophe to form the plural of capital letter abbreviations or numbers of two characters or more.

> Serial ECGs showed no change.
>
> Her hematocrits have been in the high 30s.

Plural nouns that act as descriptive terms in the name of a company or organization may or may not require an apostrophe. Determine the organization's preference and follow their usage.

> Childrens Hospital, or Children's Hospital.

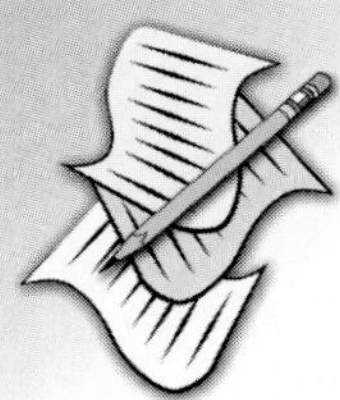

EXERCISE 3.11

Editing for Correct Apostrophe Use

Circle the letter beside each correctly written sentence below. Some items may have more than one correct answer.

1. (a) Its important to rule out malignancy in this case.
   (b) It's important to rule out malignancy in this case.
   (c) It is important to rule out malignancy in this case.

2. (a) CBC's have continued to show decreased hemoglobin and hematocrit.
   (b) CBCs have continued to show decreased hemoglobin and hematocrit.
   (c) CBCS have continued to show decreased hemoglobin and hematocrit.

3. (a) The CMT's knowledge was evident in her reports.
   (b) The CMTs knowledge was evident in her reports.
   (c) The CMTs' knowledge was evident in her reports.

4. (a) The physician who's patients' records were transferred is Dr. Che.
   (b) The physician whose patients records were transferred is Dr. Che.
   (c) The physician whose patients' records were transferred is Dr. Che.

5. (a) The patients CD4s have been decreasing.
   (b) The patient's CD4's have been decreasing.
   (c) The patient's CD4s have been decreasing.

6. (a) I don't think she will respond to more aggressive therapy.
   (b) I do not think she will respond to more aggressive therapy.
   (c) I dont think she will respond to more aggressive therapy.

7. (a) The patient whose family just arrived was discharged from the hospital today.
   (b) The patient who's family just arrived was discharged from the hospital today.

8. (a) He had an appendectomy in his '40s.
   (b) He had an appendectomy in his 40s.
   (c) He had an appendectomy in his 40's.

9. (a) She was first diagnosed with lupus in the late 80s.
   (b) She was first diagnosed with lupus in the late '80s.
   (c) She was first diagnosed with lupus in the late '80's.

10. (a) She will be followed up in 2 days time.
    (b) She will be followed up in 2 day's time.
    (c) She will be followed up in 2 days' time.

11. (a) Her son-in-laws all came to visit her.
    (b) Her sons-in-law's all came to visit her.
    (c) Her sons-in-law all came to visit her.

12. (a) Mr. Simmons's condition is stable.
    (b) Mr. Simmon's condition is stable.
    (c) Mr. Simmons' condition is stable.

Using Hyphens Correctly

Hyphens are commonly used to form compound adjectives, nouns, and verbs. In these cases, hyphens help readers understand that a combination of words has a single meaning and function in the sentence, as in the phrase *24-year-old patient.* Hyphens are also occasionally used to connect prefixes to root words, especially when an unhyphenated spelling may confuse the reader. Finally, hyphens are used in fractions and in certain medical technical terms such as L1-L2.

Using hyphens to create compounds can be complicated because so many variables are involved and because the construction of a compound may change as it becomes widely used. For these reasons, you should always consult a current dictionary when you question the spelling of a compound word. The rules below provide general guidelines.

Compound Adjectives

Compound adjectives are two or more words that work together to modify the same noun *(once-in-a-lifetime opportunity, gram-negative bacteria).* Use a hyphen to connect the words that form a compound adjective.

> The patient is a 24-year-old female. [The adjective *24-year-old* modifies female.]
>
> Lymphocytes are bacteria-fighting white blood cells. [The adjective *bacteria-fighting* modifies blood cells.]

She is a well-developed, well-nourished infant. [The adjectives *well-developed* and *well-nourished* modify infant.]

Mary had her book autographed by the well-known author. [The adjective *well-known* modifies author.]

When the compound adjective appears *after* the word it modifies, do not hyphenate the words.

The infant is well developed and well nourished.

The author who autographed Mary's book is well known.

Do not hyphenate adverb-adjective combinations. You can identify these combinations by checking if the first word ends in *ly*, which means it is an adverb. In the phrase, *a slowly enlarging lesion,* for example, *slowly* is not an adjective but an adverb, so the modifying phrase is not hyphenated.

She bought a poorly constructed house on Main Street.

Compound adjectives using the prefixes *self-* or *all-,* or the suffix *-free* should always be hyphenated, whether or not they precede a noun.

self-esteem	all-encompassing	symptom-free
self-limiting	all-inclusive	pain-free

Note: You may decide to rewrite a sentence to omit some of the hyphenated words. Do this cautiously and only when absolutely necessary.

DICTATED:	The patient has a 2-pack-per-day-times-30-year cigarette-smoking history.
TRANSCRIBED:	The patient smoked 2 packs of cigarettes per day for 30 years.

Prefixes and Suffixes

Prefixes are syllables that are added to the beginning of a word. Suffixes are syllables that are attached to the end of a word.

Do not hyphenate words with the prefix *non* unless the following element is capitalized or starts with a number. An exception is non-insulin-dependent diabetes.

nontender	non-Hodgkin lymphoma
nonnarcotic	non-A hepatitis
nonsteroidal	non-MD members
nonprofessional	non-2002 graduates

Do not hyphenate words with the prefix extra unless the word can be easily misread.

extradural	extra-large
extrapapillary	extra-apical
extraordinary	extra-base hit

Do not use a hyphen with the prefixes *anti-, bi-, dis-, tri-, uni-, co-, infra-, inter-, intra-, mid-, mini-, multi-, pseudo-, sub-, super-, supra-, ultra-, out-, over-, ante-, semi-, un-, non-, pre-, post-, pro-, trans-,* and *re-* unless the word that follows begins with the same vowel that ends the prefix: it may cause confusion and be misread. Generally, no hyphens are added when a prefix is the first element of a compound or a suffix is the last element.

PREFIX: interoffice, nonessential

SUFFIX: leadership, excitement

antiemetic	anti-inflammatory drug
antibiotic	

Do not hyphenate words with the suffix *-like* unless the word is capitalized, ends in *l* or a vowel, or has three or more syllables.

AIDS-like	slitlike
flu-like	Parkinson-like
plate-like	

Hyphenate words with the prefix *ex* when *ex* means former. Otherwise do not hyphenate.

ex-husband	excision
ex-president	expression
ex-patient	exogenous

Hyphenate words that would be misread without a hyphen. If the lack of a hyphen makes a word difficult to interpret, hyphenate the word.

re-cover (to cover again, not to return to normal)

re-create (to make again, not to play)

It was time to re-cover the chair.

Try to re-create the Titantic and enter it into the contest.

non-neoplastic

pre-clotting

Some words are so commonly used together that they are read as a unit without hyphenation. A few examples are listed below. Check your dictionary when in doubt, since there are no firm guidelines.

arterial blood gas

deep tendon reflex

jugular venous distention

low back pain

status post cellulitis

blood pressure readings

exercise tolerance test

left upper lobe

normal sinus rhythm

red cell count

Suspended Hyphens

Suspended hyphens connect two or more prefixes or adjectives to the same term. Use a suspended hyphen after each prefix or word in the series.

full- and split-thickness skin grafts

2- and 3-cm lengths

Boxes of 5-, 10-, and 15-pound books will be sent to you by FedEx.

Specific Words

The verb, adjective, and noun variations of the words *follow up* can cause confusion if not transcribed correctly.

verb:	The patient will follow up with me next week.
adjective:	He will have a followup chest film to document resolution of his pneumonia.
noun:	Followup will be with her primary physician.

Other Uses of the Hyphen

Hyphenate fractions expressed in words.

> The lower one-third of the right lung was removed.
>
> Three-fourths of my patients are nonsmokers.

Use a hyphen to express the space between two vertebrae.

> C4-C5
>
> L5-S1

Use hyphens with most suture sizes. Include the number symbol (#) if the physician dictates the word *number.*

DICTATED:	The fascia was reapproximated with three oh Vicryl.
TRANSCRIBED:	The fascia was reapproximated with 3-0 Vicryl.
DICTATED:	The skin was closed with number seven Ethibond.
TRANSCRIBED:	The skin was closed with #7 Ethibond.

In numeric and alphabetic ranges, use a hyphen in place of the word *to* if it separates two consecutive units. Use an en dash for *through* if the range indicates more than two.

> The child brought to the emergency room appeared to be 2-3 years old.
>
> The construction will take from 10–12 hours.

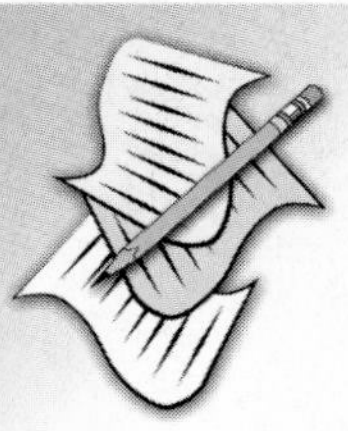

EXERCISE 3.12

Editing for Correct Use of Hyphens

Edit the following text placing hyphens where needed. Also correct those words written as two words that should be written as one word. Then key the report with the correct hyphenation and word format.

HISTORY: This 30 year old white male reported to clinic today for a routine follow up appointment, with diagnosis of HIV disease.

He was initially diagnosed in mid August 20XX. Additional diagnoses include major depression, chronic serous otitis media, chronic active hepatitis, low back pain, and headaches.

Since his previous examination, the patient has continued to have active medical problems. With regard to his HIV infection, the patient continues to have a decreasing CD4 count. He is followed by a physician in Los Angeles, and his most recent CD4 count was an absolute value of 250. The patient notes a 10 to 12 week history of increasing night sweats. The patient, at present, is on no anti retro viral therapy, having discontinued AZT therapy two months ago.

The patient also had a long recovery complicated by infection following a scar revision of his lower lip earlier this year. He also continues to be followed for his diagnosis of chronic active hepatitis. He also is followed for chronic depression, for which he is treated with Zoloft therapy. The patient continues to be affected by right sided migraine like headaches; a recent CT scan was negative for any intra cranial pathology.

FAMILY HISTORY: Non contributory.

SOCIAL HISTORY: The patient continues to work but on a part time basis. He works at home using his computer. He is a non drinker. He was a one pack per day smoker until two years ago, when he stopped.

PHYSICAL EXAMINATION: He is a slightly ill appearing white male who just turned 30 years old.
VITAL SIGNS: Temp. 97.6° F, P 80, R 20, BP 140/80.
HEENT: Pupils equal and reactive. Extra ocular movements are intact.
NECK: Mild supraclavicular adenopathy. No jugular venous distention.
LUNGS: Mild end expiratory wheezes, worse on the left.
HEART: Regular rate and rhythm. PMI is in the 5th left inter costal space at mid clavicular line.
ABDOMEN: Soft, non tender on the left with some mild right sided pain. Liver span is two finger breadths below the costal margin. Back reveals mild tenderness at the L4 L5 level. No costo vertebral angle tenderness.
GENITALIA: Normal male phallus with descended testes bilaterally. Rectal exam reveals normal anal sphincter tone with a few mild external and internal hemorrhoids. Pulses, including brachio radialis, femoral, popliteal, and dorsalis pedis, normal.

(continued)

LABORATORY DATA: White blood cell count is 4.1, hematocrit 45.5, hemoglobin 15.6, platelet count 181,000. Differential shows 52% segs, 34% lymphocytes, 12% monocytes, 2% eosinophils. The urinalysis revealed 1 to 2 white cells per high power field, otherwise normal. The liver function tests are normal. The CD4 count is 210 with a CD4 percentage of 15%. Intradermal skin testing reveals the patient to be anergic. VDRL is nonreactive.

DIAGNOSES
1. Human immuno deficiency virus infection.
2. Chronic hepatitis B.
3. History of major depression.
4. Migraine like headaches.
5. History of chronic middle ear infections.

PLAN: The patient will follow up in six months for clinic visit and repeat labs. We have discussed appropriate short and long term goals for this patient. He will continue to work part time, as he enjoys this and is having no difficulty performing his job related activities.

Part II

TRANSCRIBING FOR THE SPECIALTIES

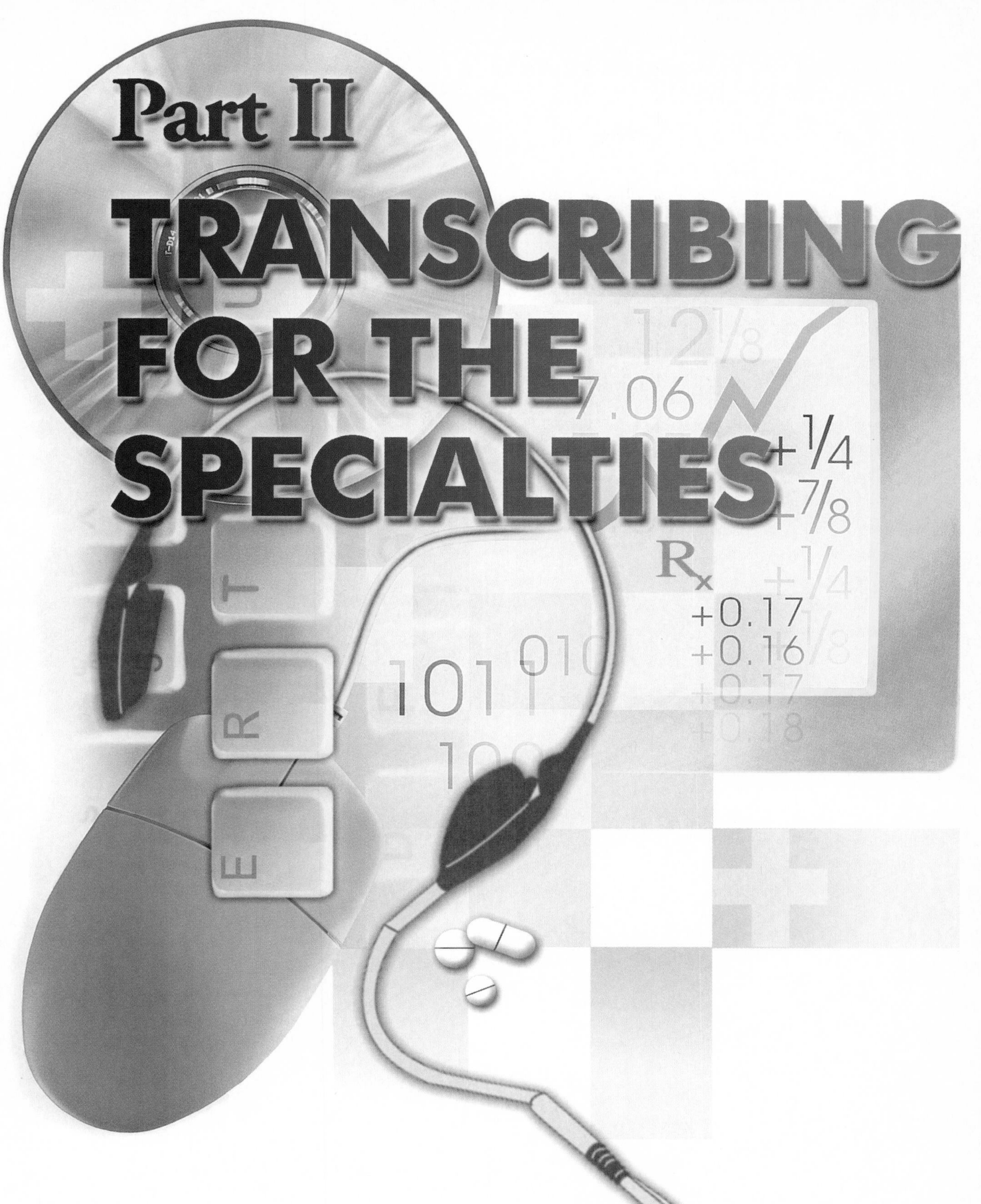

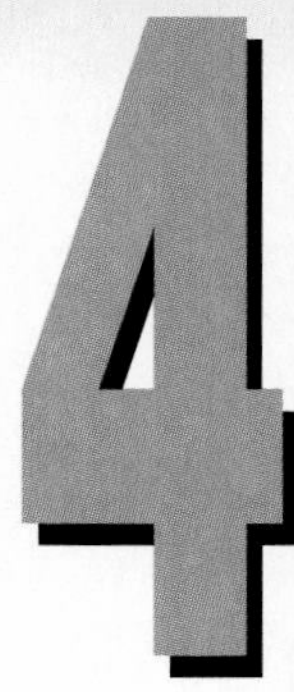

Dermatology

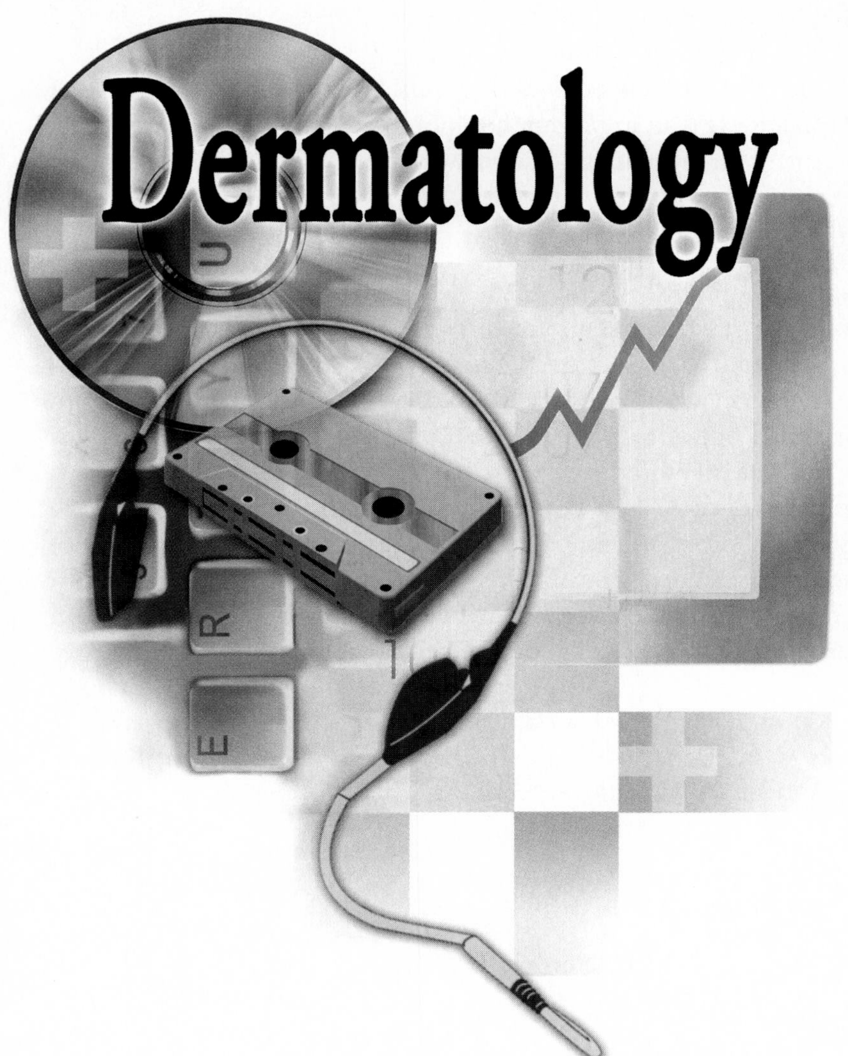

Dermatology encompasses the entire integumentary system, which includes the skin, hair, and nails. Because the skin can reflect the general health of the patient, it is the first part of the assessment by the healthcare professional.

OBJECTIVES

- Use dermatology terms correctly according to the context and purpose of the dictation.
- Select and use appropriate general and specialty reference materials.
- Key dermatology office notes of varying complexity and format.
- Transcribe authentic medical dictation requiring concentration and listening skill.
- Edit medical reports to conform with AAMT style guidelines.
- Proofread and correct transcripts to produce error-free documents.

Exploring Dermatology

The skin is the largest organ of the body and is considered the body's first line of defense against organisms. It is an important area of medical attention since approximately 5–10 percent of all ambulatory patient visits in the United States are for skin-related complaints.

Structure and Function

The skin forms a barrier between the internal organs and the outside environment. It is rich with various types of sensory nerve endings that constitute the four cutaneous senses: touch pressure (sustained touch), cold, warmth, and pain. It communicates with the external openings of the digestive, respiratory, and urogenital systems through the mucous membranes.

The skin is composed of three layers, or strata: the epidermis, the dermis, and the subcutaneous tissue, as shown in Figure 4.1. The epidermis is the external layer of the skin composed of squamous epithelial cells. These cells divide continuously, pushing the older, dead cells closer to the surface and completely replacing them every three to four weeks. The dead cells contain keratin, an insoluble, fibrous protein that comprises the horny layer of the epidermis and helps protect the body. There are different amounts of keratin in different areas of the body. The palms of the hands and soles of the feet contain more keratin than other parts of the skin. This extra thickness increases with use and results in callus formation.

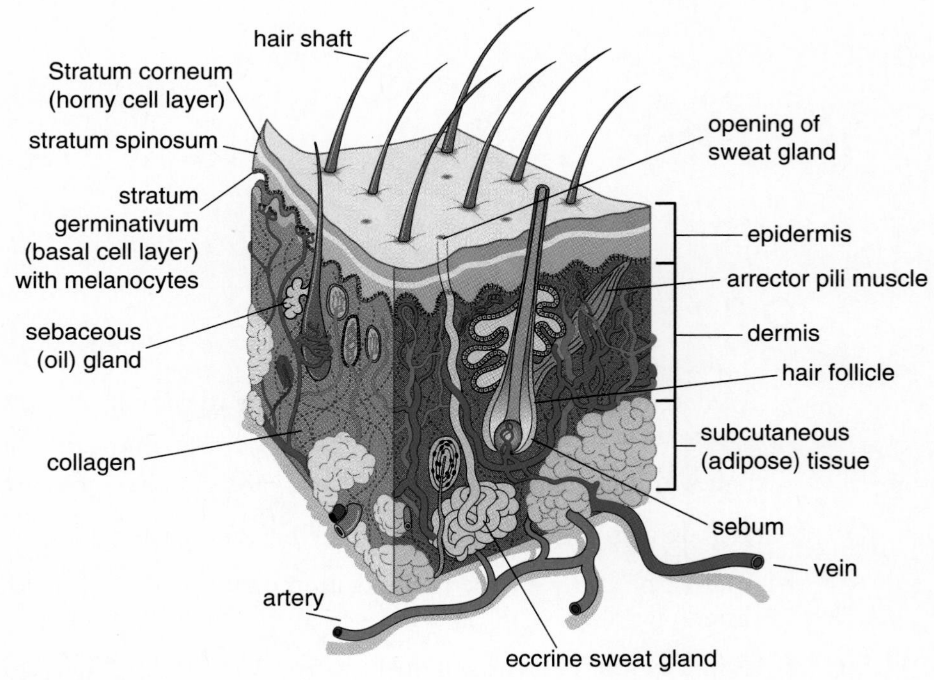

FIGURE 4.1
Anatomic Structures of the Skin

Cells within the epidermis called melanocytes produce melanin, the pigment or color of the skin. The more melanin present, the darker the skin color. Melanin can absorb ultraviolet light, protecting the person from the harmful effects of sun exposure. People with lighter skin have an increased risk of sunburn after sun exposure. On the positive side, the ultraviolet rays of sunlight react with chemicals within the skin to convert them into vitamin D, a necessary nutrient, which is absorbed through the skin.

The dermis lies immediately under the epidermis and is composed of collagen and elastic fibers, blood and lymph vessels, nerves, sweat and sebaceous glands, and hair roots. The subcutaneous layer is composed of adipose, or fat, tissue. This layer is important in the regulation of body temperature and connects the skin to the muscles and bones.

The glands of the skin are within its layers. The sebaceous glands drain an oily secretion into an area between each hair follicle and its hair shaft to make the hair soft and pliable. Sweat glands are found within the skin and are classified into two categories: eccrine and apocrine. Eccrine sweat glands are found all over the body and have ducts that open directly onto the surface of the skin. They secrete a watery fluid in response to warm temperatures and are controlled by the sympathetic nervous system (see Chapter 13). Apocrine sweat glands, which become active at puberty, secrete a substance that contains parts of the cells themselves. They produce a milky sweat that is broken down by bacteria and can cause underarm odor. Specialized apocrine sweat glands produce cerumen, the wax found in the ear.

Hair is composed of keratin. It appears all over the body except on the palms and soles. Hair grows from a root within a cavity known as a hair follicle. The follicle is located in the dermis; the hair shaft extends beyond the skin. Hair grows in two phases: a growing phase (anagen) and a resting phase (telogen). About 80 percent of the body's hair follicles on the scalp are in the anagen phase at any one time.

The nails are composed of hardened keratin. The nail grows from a root within the cuticle, a thin fold of skin at the base of the nail. Nails protect the very sensitive areas of the fingers and toes. Nail growth is relatively slow. Fingernails take about 180 days to completely regenerate; toenails take up to 18 months.

Physical Assessment

Assessment of the skin involves the entire body. The physician inspects and palpates the patient's skin, mucous membranes, hair, and nails to determine appearance, color or pigmentation, temperature, and turgor. Turgor includes motility, elasticity, and moisture or dryness. The physician notes vascularity and inspects the skin thoroughly for abnormalities or lesions (Figure 4.2).

Diseases and Conditions

Since the skin is the first line of defense protecting the inner organs of the body from outside pathogens, early diagnosis and treatment of skin disorders is essential. The most common skin problem is pruritus, or itching, which can indicate either local or systemic problems. Pruritus can cause skin breakdown from the irritation of

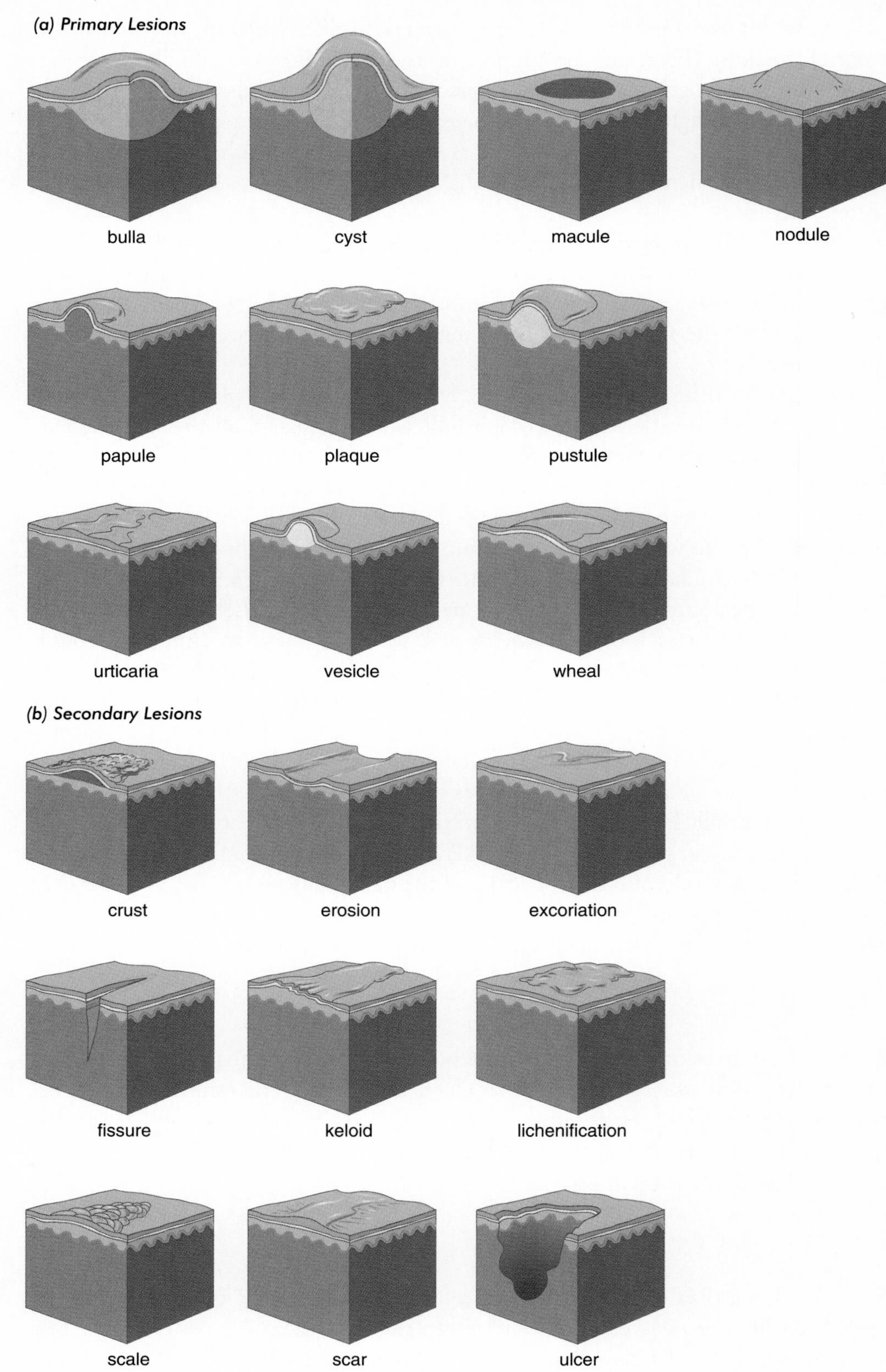

FIGURE 4.2
Common Skin Lesions

scratching. Local disorders causing pruritus include allergies to food, medications, soaps, and creams and other topical chemicals. Contact dermatitis, miliaria (prickly heat), dry skin, and poison ivy are some pruritic diseases. It is not always easy to find the cause of pruritus, but it is often necessary to determine the allergen in order to avoid further irritations.

Pruritus may be associated with urticarial and erythematous lesions. Commonly, the varicella (chickenpox) and herpes zoster (shingles) viruses may be accompanied by itching, redness, burning, and pain. Many of the "childhood" viral illnesses such as measles, rubella, and "fifth disease" display a red rash, usually without pruritus.

Several bacterial, fungal, and yeast infections cause skin eruptions. *Staphylococcus aureus* and *Streptococcus* are common bacteria found on the skin. These organisms can cause skin lesions such as folliculitis, furuncles, carbuncles, bullae, and impetigo. Ringworm is caused by the fungus known as a dermatophyte. Tinea corporis, tinea pedis, tinea manus, tinea cruris, tinea capitis, and tinea unguium are all dermatophyte infections. Candidal rashes are usually found in the groin or other areas where heat and moisture promote growth. People on antibiotic therapy or who are immunocompromised are at increased risk for *Candida* fungal infections.

Psoriasis is a chronic, noninfectious inflammatory skin disease characterized by an increase in the rate of growth of epidermal cells. Although it is one of the most common skin diseases, the exact cause is unknown. There may be a combination of genetic and environmental stimuli to precipitate the onset. The immune system, emotional stress, and seasonal and hormonal changes have been implicated in the exacerbation of psoriasis.

Common Tests and Surgical Procedures

Physicians routinely order allergy skin testing such as scratch tests, patch tests, and intradermal tests to determine which allergens are responsible for causing allergic reactions. KOH (potassium hydroxide) preparation is used to diagnose fungal infections, and Tzanck's smear is used to diagnose viral skin vesicles. In addition, the dermatologist performs three types of biopsies: excisional (complete removal of a skin lesion), incisional (partial removal of a lesion by cutting out part of the lesion), and punch (removal of a portion of skin containing a lesion by means of a special surgical instrument).

Cosmetic surgery is common today. Laser treatment to remove unwanted hair, varicose veins, and other lesions is also common. Dermabrasion and chemical peels are methods used to remove the upper skin layers in order to eradicate scars, tattoos, and fine lines.

Building Language Skills

The following tables list common dermatology terms, drugs, and abbreviations. The list of terms and definitions includes the most difficult words contained in the dictated reports in this chapter. These words are identified in GREEN type. A list of common drugs is found in Appendix D.

Medical Terms and Pharmacologic Agents

abrasion
(a-**bray**-zhun) (n) scraping away of skin or mucous membrane by friction

abscess
(**ab**-ses) (n) a pus-filled cavity, usually because of a localized infection

acne
(**ak**-nee) (n) an eruption of papules or pustules on the skin, involving the oil glands

adipose
(**ad**-i-pOz) (adj) containing fat

albinism
(**al**-bi-nizm/al-**bin**-izm) (n) a congenital lack of melanin in the skin, hair, and eyes

allergen
(**al**-er-jen) (n) a substance that produces an allergic reaction

alopecia
(al-O-**pee**-shee-a) (n) partial or total loss of hair

alopecic
(al-O-**pee**-sik) (adj) relating to alopecia

anagen
(**an**-a-jen) (n) the actively growing phase of the hair growth cycle

angioedema
(an-jee-O-e-**dee**-ma) (n) periodically recurring episodes of noninflammatory swelling

angioma
(an-jee-**O**-ma) (n) a swelling or tumor composed primarily of blood vessels; spider, strawberry, cherry angiomas

anhidrosis
(an-hI-**drO**-sis) (n) the suppression or absence of perspiration

antecubital
(an-te-**kyoo**-bi-tal) (adj) front of the elbow; often the site for drawing blood

apocrine
(**ap**-O-krin) (adj) relating to sweat glands

assessment
(as-**ses**-ment) (n) a complete evaluation of the patient; diagnosis

bedsore
(**bed**-sor) (n) an infected wound on the skin that occurs at pressure points in patients confined to bed

biopsy
(**bI**-op-see) (n) the removal of tissue and/or fluid from the body for microscopic study; the specimen obtained

bullae
(**bul**-ee) (n, pl) blisters of the skin containing clear fluid

café-au-lait spots
(kaf-ay-O-**lay** spots) (n) light brown spots of patchy pigmentation of the skin

callous
(**kal**-us) (adj) being hardened and thickened, having calluses; also feeling no emotion or sympathy.

callus
(**kal**-us) (n) thickened skin which develops at points of pressure or friction; the bony substance which develops around the broken ends of bone during healing

candidal rash
(**kan**-di-dal rash) (n) a rash which usually includes itching, a white discharge, peeling, and easy bleeding; caused by the yeastlike fungus *Candida;* common examples are diaper rash, thrush, and vaginitis

carbuncle
(**kar**-bung-kl) (n) subcutaneous, pus-filled interconnecting pockets, caused by staphylococcal infection; eventually discharges through an opening in the skin

carcinoma
(kar-si-**nO**-mah) (n) a cancerous growth or malignant tumor that occurs in epithelium (cell layers covering outside body surfaces)

caruncle
(**kar**-ung-kl) (n) small, fleshy outgrowth

cellulitis
(sel-yoo-**lI**-tis) (n) inflammation of the connective tissue caused by infection

cephalocaudal
(**sef**-a-lO-**caw**-dal) (adj) relating to the axis of the body from the head to the base of the spine

cerumen
(se-**roo**-men) (n) earwax

chancre
(**shang**-ker) (n) hard sore; the sore that develops at the site of entry of a pathogen

chloasma
(klO-**as**-ma) (n) light brown patches on the face and elsewhere; commonly associated with pregnancy

cicatrix
(**sik**-a-triks) (n) scar

circumscribed
(**ser**-kum-skrIbd) (adj) having a boundary; confined

cirrhosis
(sir-**rO**-sis) (n) a degenerative liver disease characterized by damaged cell function and impaired blood flow

collagen
(**kol**-a-jen) (n) the protein which forms the tough white fibers of connective tissue, cartilage, and bone

comedo
(**kom**-i-dO) (n) in a hair follicle or oil gland, a plug of dead cells and oily secretions; blackhead; comedones (com-i-**dO**-neez) (pl)

concussion
(kon-**kush**-un) (n) an injury resulting from violent striking or shaking, especially an injury to the brain

confluent
(**kon**-floo-ent) (adj) merging together; connecting

congenital
(kon-**jen**-I-tal) (adj) present at birth

contusion
(kon-**too**-zhun) (n) a bruise

cryosurgery
(**krI**-O-ser-jer-ee) (n) the use of extreme cold to destroy tissue

cutaneous
(koo-**tay**-nee-us) (adj) pertaining to the skin

cuticle
(**kyoo**-ti-kl) (n) the edge of thickened skin around the bed of a nail; the sheath surrounding the base of a hair follicle

cyanosis
(cI-a-**nO**-sis) (n) bluish cast to the skin and/or mucous membranes due to decreased amount of oxygen in the blood cells

dermabrasion
(**der**-ma-bray-zhun) (n) peeling of skin done by a mechanical device with sandpaper or wire brushes

dermatitis
(der-ma-**tI**-tis) (n) inflammation of skin often evidenced by itching, redness, and lesions

dermatology
(der-ma-**tol**-o-jee) (n) the study of the skin, hair, and nails

dermatophyte
(**der**-ma-tO-fIt) (n) a parasitic fungus that causes skin disease

desiccate
(**des**-i-kayt) (v) to dry out

diagnosis
(dI-ag-**nO**-sis) (n) deciding the nature of a medical condition by examination of the symptoms; diagnoses (pl)

diaphoresis
(**dI**-a-fO-ree-sis) (n) profuse perspiration or sweating

discrete
(dis-**kreet**) (adj) separate; distinct

ecchymosis
(ek-im-**O**-sis) (n) reddish or purplish flat spot on the skin; a bruise; ecchymoses (pl)

eccrine
(**ek**-rin) (adj) relating to sweat glands

eczema
(**ek**-si-ma/**eg**-ze-ma) (n) inflammatory condition of the skin characterized by blisters, redness, and itching

electrodesiccation
(el-ek-trO-de-si-**kay**-shun) (n) destruction of tissue by the use of electrical current; fulguration

electrolysis
(el-ek-**trol**-i-sis) (n) destruction of a hair follicle by passing an electrical current through it

ellipse
(el-**lipz**) (n) a conic section taken either parallel to an element or parallel to the axis of the intersected cone; an oval

ephelides
(ef-**ee**-lI-deez) (n, pl) freckles

epidermis
(ep-i-**der**-mis) (n) the top or outer layer of the skin

epinephrine
(ep-I-**nef**-rin) (n) a hormone of the adrenal medulla that acts as a strong stimulant and blood vessel constrictor

epithelial
(ep-i-**thee**-lee-al) (adj) relating to or composed of epithelium

epithelium
(ep-i-**thee**-lee-um) (n) cell layers covering the outside body surfaces as well as forming the lining of hollow organs (e.g., the bladder) and the passages of the respiratory, digestive, and urinary tracts

erythema
(er-i-**thee**-ma) (n) redness of the skin; inflammation

erythema infectiosum
(er-i-**thee**-ma in-fek-shee-**O**-sum) (n) a mild, infectious disease characterized by an erythematous rash; also called fifth disease

erythematous
(er-i-**them**-a-tus/er-i-**thee**-ma-tus) (adj) relating to or having erythema; reddened; inflamed

erythrocyte
(e-**rith**-rO-sIt) (n) mature red blood cell

erythroderma
(e-rith-rO-**der**-ma) (n) any skin condition associated with unusual redness of the skin

exanthema
(eg-zan-**thee**-ma) (n) a disease, such as measles or chickenpox, accompanied by a general rash on the skin, which may have particular characteristics specific to the disease

excisional biopsy
(ek-**sizh**-un-al **bI**-op-see) (n) surgical removal of a tissue for microscopic examination

excoriation
(eks-kO-ree-**ay**-shun) (n) a scratching or scraping injury to the skin

familial
(fa-**mi**-lee-al) (adj) pertaining to a disease or characteristic that is present in some families

fifth disease
(n) erythema infectiosum; a mild, infectious disease characterized by an erythematous rash

fistula
(**fis**-tyoo-la) (n) abnormal opening or channel connecting hollow organs or leading from an internal organ to the outside or a cavity; such as a urinary fistula

follicle
(**fol**-i-kl) (n) pouch-like cavity, such as a hair follicle in the skin enclosing a hair

folliculitis
(fol-i-kyoo-**lI**-tis) (n) inflammation of the hair follicles

fossa
(**fos**-a) (n) channel or shallow depression; fossae (pl)

fulguration
(ful-gyoo-**ra**-shun) (n) destruction of tissue by the use of electrical current; electrodessication

furuncle
(**fyoo**-rung-kl) (n) a localized, pus-forming infection in a hair follicle or gland

gangrene
(**gang**-green) (n) death of cells or tissue due to obstruction of blood supply

gland
(n) organ that secretes one or more substances not needed by the organ itself

glans
(n) the head of the penis; "glans penis"

hemangioma
(he-man-jee-**O**-ma) (n) a congenital benign tumor consisting of a mass of blood vessels

hematology
(hee-ma-**tol**-o-jee) (n) the study of blood

hemosiderin
(hee-mO-**sid**-er-in) (n) an iron-containing pigment derived from hemoglobin when red blood cells disintegrate

herpes zoster
(**her**-peez **zos**-ter) (n) a viral infection causing inflammation along the path of nerve with associated painful vesicles (blisters) on the skin above; shingles

hirsutism
(**hur**-soot-izm) (n) excessive body hair

hyperpigmentation
(hI-per-pig-men-**tay**-shun) (n) darkening of the skin due to excessive pigment in the skin

hypertrophy
(hI-**per**-trO-fee) (n) increase in size

impetigo
(im-pe-**tI**-gO) (n) a streptococcal or staphylococcal infection of the skin characterized by lesions, usually on the face, which rupture and become covered with a thick yellow crust; highly contagious

incised
(in-**sIzd**) (adj) cut with a knife

incisional biopsy
(in-**si**-zhun-al **bI**-op-see) (n) removal of part of a lesion for microscopic examination

incision and drainage
(n) commonly dictated "I and D"; procedure of cutting through an infected lesion and allowing it to drain

integumentary
(in-teg-yoo-**men**-ta-ree) (adj) relating to the skin

jaundice
(**jawn**-dis) (n) yellowish skin and whites of the eyes

keloid
(**kee**-loyd) (n) a mass of scar tissue

keratin
(**ker**-a-tin) (n) a tough, fibrous protein in skin, hair, and nails

keratosis
(ker-a-**tO**-sis) (n) a condition in which the skin thickens and builds up with excessive keratin

keratotic
(ker-a-**tot**-ik) (adj) relating to keratosis

lesion
(**lee**-zhun) (n) general term for any visible, circumscribed injury to the skin; such as a wound, sore, rash, or mass

macrophage
(**mak**-ro-fayj) (n) a large scavenger cell (phagocyte) that digests microorganisms and cell debris

macule
(**mak**-yool) (n) a small discolored spot on the skin

maculopapular
(mak-yoo-lO-**pap**-yoo-lar) (adj) describing skin lesions that are raised in the center

malformation
(mal-for-**may**-shun) (n) abnormal development or structure of the body or a part

melanin
(**mel**-a-nin) (n) naturally-occurring dark brown or black pigment found in the hair, skin, and eyes

melanocyte
(**mel**-an-O-sIt) (n) a cell that produces melanin

melanocytic
(mel-a-nO-**sit**-ik) (adj) pertaining to or composed of melanocytes

melitis
(mee-**lI**-tis) (n) inflammation of the cheek

milia
(**mil**-ee-a) (n, pl) whiteheads, due to obstruction of the outlet of hair follicles or sweat glands

miliaria
(mil-ee-**ay**-ree-a) (n) a skin eruption of small vesicles and papules; heat rash

motility
(mO-**til**-i-tee) (n) ability to move spontaneously

mycosis
(mI-**kO**-sis) (n) disease caused by a fungus

neuromuscular
(noor-O-**mus**-kyoo-lar) (adj) pertains to the muscles and nerves

nevus
(**nee**-vus) (n) congenital discoloration of the skin; birthmark or mole; nevi (pl)

obese
(o-**bees**) (adj) very fat

onycholysis
(on-ee-**kol**-i-sis) (n) loosening of the nails from their beds

papule
(**pap**-yool) (n) a small, solid, raised skin lesion, as in chickenpox

paraplegia
(par-a-**plee**-jee-a) (n) paralysis of the lower portion of the body and of both legs

paronychia
(par-O-**nik**-ee-a) (n) infected skin around the nail

pathogen
(**path**-O-jen) (n) any microorganism or substance capable of producing a disease

pemphigus
(**pem**-fi-gus) (n) a distinctive group of diseases marked by successive crops of bullae

perineum
(**per**-i-**nee**-um) (n) the external region between the urethral opening and the anus, including the skin and underlying tissues

peritoneum
(per-i-tO-**nee**-um) (n) lining of the abdominal cavity

petechia
(pe-**tee**-kee-a/pee-**tek**-ee-a) (n, sing.) tiny reddish or purplish flat spot on the skin as a result of a tiny hemorrhage within the skin (usually used in the plural form, petechiae)

petechial
(pee-**tee**-kee-al/pee-**tek**-ee-al) (adj) relating to or having petechiae

pigment
(**pig**-ment) (n) any organic coloring substance in the body

pigmented
(**pig**-men-ted) (v) colored by a pigment

presents
(pre-**sents**) (v) appears; shows; displays; the symptoms displayed are the presenting symptoms

pruritic
(pru-**ri**-tic) (adj) itching

pruritus
(proo-**rI**-tus) (n) itching skin condition

psoriasis
(sO-**rI**-a-sis) (n) chronic skin disease in which reddish scaly patches develop

punch biopsy
(punch **bI**-op-see) (n) a special instrument is used to take a small cylindrical piece of tissue for microscopic examination

pustular
(**pus**-choo-lar) (adj) relating to or having pustules

pustule
(**pus**-chool) (n) small pus-containing elevation on the skin

rhinophyma
(rI-nO-**fI**-ma) (n) enlargement of the nose from severe rosacea

rubella
(roo-**bel**-a) (n) a contagious viral disease with fever and a red rash; German measles

scabies
(**skay**-beez) (n) contagious rash with intense itching; caused by mites

scrotal
(**skrO**-tal) (adj) relating to the scrotum

scrotum
(**skrO**-tum) (n) the pouch of skin containing the testes

sebaceous
(see-**bay**-shus) (adj) relating to sebum

seborrhea
(seb-O-**ree**-a) (n) overactivity of the oil glands of the skin

sebum
(**see**-bum) (n) an oily secretion of the oil glands of the skin

sequela
(see-**kwel**-a) (n) a condition following and resulting from a disease; sequelae (pl)

serosanguineous
(**see** row sang win ess) (adj) characterized by blood and serum

Staphylococcus aureus
(staf-il-O-**kok**-us **awr**-ee-us) (n) a common species of Staphylococcus (a bacteria), present on nasal mucous membranes and skin that causes pus-producing infections

Streptococcus
(strep-tO-**kok**-us) (n) a genus of bacteria; many species cause disease in humans

subcutaneous
(sub-kyoo-**tay**-nee-us) (adj) under the skin

subjective data
(sub-**jek**-tiv **day**-tah) (n) information revealed by the patient to the health care provider

suture
(**soo**-chur) (n and v) natural seam, border in the skull formed by the close joining of bony surfaces; closing a wound with a sterile needle and thread

syndrome
(**sin**-drOm) (n) the signs and symptoms that constitute a specific disease

telogen
(**tel**-O-jen) (n) the resting phase of the hair growth cycle

texture
(**teks**-chur) (n) character, structure, and feel of parts of the body

tinea
(**tin**-ee-a) (n) fungal infection; such as tinea pedis or athlete's foot

torso
(**tor**-sO) (n) trunk of the body

turgor
(**ter**-gOr) (n) fullness; the normal resiliency of the skin

Tzanck's smear
(tsangks smeer) (n) a method to help diagnose skin lesions by the miscroscopic examination of material from them

urticaria
(er-ti-**kar**-ee-a) (n) hives; an eruption of itching red, raised lesions

urticarial
(er-ti-**kar**-ee-al) (adj) relating to or having urticaria

varicella
(var-i-**sel**-a) (n) chickenpox; a highly contagious viral disease

varicose veins
(var-I-kOs vaynz) (n) veins that become distended, swollen, knotted, tortuous, and painful because of poor valvular function

vascularity
(vas-kyoo-**lar**-i-tee) (n) the blood vessels in a part of the body

vesicle
(**ves**-i-kl) (n) blister; small, raised skin lesion containing clear fluid

vesiculopustular
(ves **ick** you low **pus** to ler) (adj) characterized by vesicles and pustules

vitiligo
(vi-ti-**lee**-gO) (n) white patches, due to loss of pigment, appearing on the skin

wheal
(hweel) (n) a raised, red circumscribed lesion usually due to an allergic reaction; usually accompanied by intense itching; welt

xanthoma
(zan-**thO**-mah) (n) yellowish nodules in or under the skin, especially in the eyelids

Xylocaine
(**zI**-lO-kayn) (n) trade name for lidocaine hydroxhloride

Abbreviations

Bx	biopsy
C&S	culture and sensitivity
derm.	dermatology
FS	frozen section
HSV-1	herpes simplex virus type 1
HSV-2	herpes simplex virus type 2
I&D	incision and drainage
KOH	potassium hydroxide
ung.	ointment
UV	ultraviolet

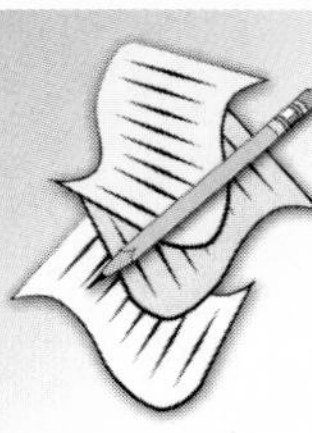

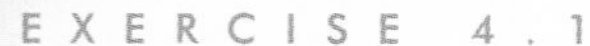

EXERCISE 4.1

Recognizing Look-Alikes and Sound-Alikes

Below is a list of frequently used words that look alike and/or sound alike. Study the meaning and pronunciation of each set of words, then read the following sentences carefully and circle the word in parentheses that correctly completes the meaning.

cirrhosis	disease of the liver
psoriasis	skin condition
discreet	cautious, careful with speech or behavior
discrete	separate, distinct; "discrete mass"
glands	organs or groups of cells that produce or secrete substances
glans	head of the penis; "glans penis"
miliaria	eruption of vesicles and papules at the sweat glands
malaria	acute blood disease caused from bite of tropical mosquito
milia	white raised "pimple" found on skin of infants
patience	ability to suppress restlessness; to be patient
patients	individuals who are receiving medical treatment
patient's	possessive form of noun patient
patient	(n) an individual who is receiving medical treatment
patient	(adj) behaving calmly
perianal	around the anus
perinatal	relating to the time shortly before and after birth
perineum	pelvic floor and associated structures
peritoneum	serous membrane lining the walls of the abdominal and pelvic cavities
vesical	(adj) relating to a bladder
vesicle	(n) blister
wheal	raised, red lesion on the skin
wheel	circular frame of hard material that can turn on an axle (as on a car)

1. We will refer the patient to the dermatologist regarding his (cirrhosis, psoriasis).
2. Due to the patient's (cirrhosis, psoriasis), we need to repeat her liver function tests.
3. It is important to be (discreet, discrete) when transcribing patient care documentation.
4. I noted a few (discreet, discrete) papular lesions on the patient's left arm.
5. The examination of the (perineum, peritoneum) shows that the patient's episiotomy is well healed.
6. A family physician sometimes sees up to 40 (patients, patient's) a day.
7. When transcribing difficult dictation, (patience, patients) is important.
8. He is having some irritations of the foreskin and (glands, glans).
9. A (vesical, vesicle) is beginning to form at the burn site.
10. Apparently she is allergic to amoxicillin because she developed pruritic (wheals, wheels) on her trunk a few hours after taking the first dose.

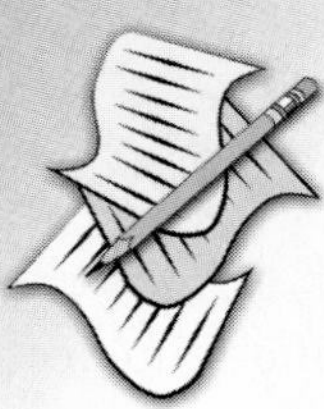

EXERCISE 4.2

Matching Sound and Spelling

The numbered list that follows shows the phonetic spelling of hard-to-spell words. Sound out the word, then write the correct spelling in the blank space provided. Each of the words can be found in the Glossary or in the drug list in Appendix D.

1. er-i-**thee**-ma ____________________
2. see-**bay**-shus ____________________
3. er-ti-**kar**-ee-a ____________________
4. **des**-i-kayt ____________________
5. al-O-**pee**-shee-a ____________________
6. **kon**-floo-ent ____________________
7. pe-**tee**-kee-a/pe-**tek**-ee-a ____________________
8. **kom**-i-dO ____________________
9. **per**-i-**nee**-um ____________________
10. eks-kO-ree-**ay**-shun ____________________
11. an-te-**kyoo**-bi-tal ____________________
12. sel-yoo-**lI**-tis ____________________
13. **ap**-O-krin ____________________
14. sO-**rI**-a-sis ____________________
15. ek-im-**O**-sis ____________________

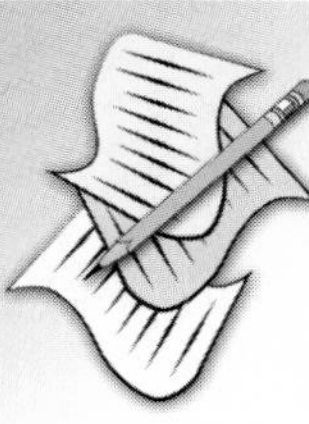

EXERCISE 4.3

Choosing Words from Context

When transcribing dictation, the medical transcriptionist frequently needs to consider the situation when determining the word that correctly completes the sentence. From the list of words below, select the term that meaningfully completes each statement.

follicle	sebaceous	erythematous
integumentary	adipose	torso
excoriations	pruritic	subcutaneous
comedo	pigment	acne
nevus	perineum	vesicle

1. He has a rash with many _______________, due to constantly scratching the area.
2. The patient is complaining of a ______________ rash and would like a medication to relieve itching.
3. He had a _______________ that opened and drained a clear fluid.
4. The ________________system is the first system noticed when the patient appears in the physician's office.
5. This ______________ on my nose has caused me much embarrassment.
6. The patient has a ______________ rash sprinkled across the nose.
7. The patient has a ______________ that she would like removed from her chin. She states it has been there since birth.
8. The _______________ shows scarring from the episiotomy performed after the birth of her first child.
9. The ______________ glands clog and cause acne.
10. The 16-year-old girl consulted the dermatologist because the over-the-counter medications she used to treat her _____________ were not effective.

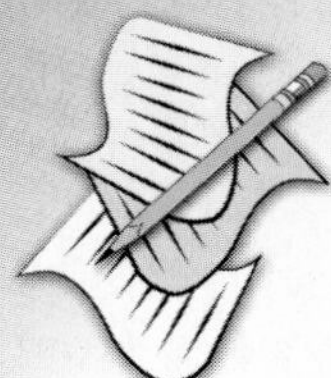

EXERCISE 4.4

Pairing Words and Meanings

From this list, locate the term that best matches each of the following definitions. Write the letter of the term in the space provided beside the definition.

A. dermatitis
B. petechiae
C. confluent
D. wheal
E. pruritus
F. hyperpigmentation
G. alopecia
H. onycholysis
I. cephalocaudal
J. ephelides
K. erythema
L. rhinophyma
M. I&D
N. urticaria
O. torso

1. patchy light brown spots in pigmentation of skin __________
2. from head to toe __________
3. loss of hair __________
4. redness __________
5. tiny reddish or purplish spots appearing on the skin resulting from tiny hemorrhages __________
6. a raised, red, circumscribed lesion __________
7. pertaining to merging of tissues, pustules, or lesions __________
8. unusual darkening of the skin __________
9. inflammation of the skin __________
10. trunk of a body __________

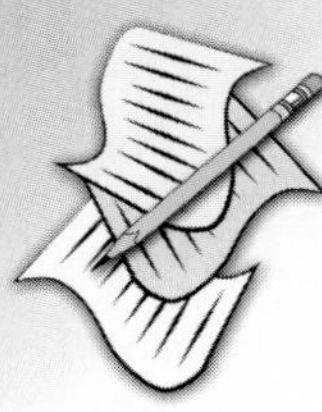

EXERCISE 4.5

Creating Terms from Word Forms

Combine prefixes, root words, and suffixes from this list to create medical words that fit the following definitions. Fill in the blanks with the words that you construct. The first word is done for you.

cephal/o	head	urtica	itchy eruption
derm/a	skin	-brasion	removal
dermat/o	skin	-cyte	cell
erythr/o	red	-ema	condition of
hemat/o	blood	-ia	condition
hyper-	above or excessive	-itis	inflammation
melen/o	black	-logy	study of
seb/o	oil	-ous	pertaining to
caudal	referring to tail	-rrhea	discharge
pigmentation	coloring	-trophy	development
tension	pressure		

1. study of skin, hair, and nails *dermatology*
2. excessive growth ______
3. redness of skin ______
4. peeling of skin with sandpaper ______
5. head to toe ______
6. skin condition associated with abnormal redness of skin ______
7. inflammation of skin ______
8. condition caused by over-activity of the sebaceous glands ______
9. red blood cell ______
10. study of the blood ______
11. a darkened skin cell ______
12. excessive pigment in the skin ______

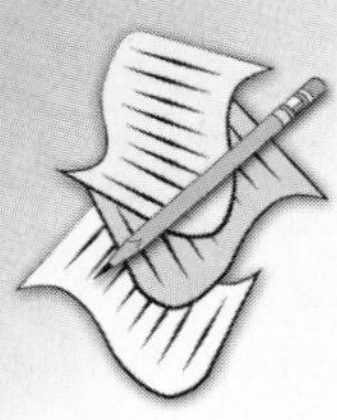

EXERCISE 4.6

Proofreading Review

As a medical transcriptionist, you are responsible for producing quality work. One of the most important skills you need to develop is proofreading, which involves checking for all types of mistakes in the document.

You must carefully read for accuracy of content, omission of words, consistency of format, English usage, spelling, punctuation, capitalization, word choice, and typographical errors. Read the following reports and look for incomplete sentences and errors in spelling and punctuation.

1. Thank you for referring Kyle Sanderson to me. This baby is truely in pain with scrotal inflammation and excoriation of the perineum. I have instituted Burow soaks to the area q.i.d., with Mycostatin ointment after each soak. If this does not clear the rash I would be concerned about an secondary infection. I would expect to see improvement within 1 week otherwise I feel the baby should be admitted to the hospital and more aggressive antifungal agents be used to clear this rash.
2. Robert is a very cooperative, gregaris youngster. Examination reveals normal vitle signs and the cuteanus lesions noted above. Aside from his nuromuculer deficit his exam was otherwise unremarcable.

Building Transcription Skills

The Office Note

An office note typically describes an office visit and becomes part of the patient's chart. Figure 4.3 is an example of an office note. Sometimes the office note may describe a minor procedure performed in the physician's office. These notes are not always written as complete sentences, although physicians frequently use the SOAP (Subjective, Objective, Assessment, Plan) format. The rules of grammar and numeral usage may not be followed precisely. Note that if the report is short, it is acceptable to add a colon after each SOAP heading and key the text on the same line.

Preparing to Transcribe

To prepare for transcribing dictation, review the tables of common dermatology terms, drugs, and abbreviations presented in the Building Language Skills section of this chapter. Then, study the format and organization of the model document shown in Figure 4.3, and key the model document. Proofread the document by comparing it with the printed version. Categorize the types of errors you made, and document them on a copy of the Performance Comparison chart provided in Chapter 1. A template of this chart is included on the IRC that accompanies this text.

1" margins → left justification; no hyphenation

single-space after colons

PATIENT NAME: Avis Smith
DATE OF VISIT: 3/31/XX format date as MM/DD/YY

double-space between headings

CHIEF COMPLAINT
Itching and rash.

double-space

SUBJECTIVE single-space from heading to following paragraph
The patient is complaining of itching and a rash that began about 3 weeks ago, starting on the hands and arms and spreading to the chest and back. Taking Benadryl at bedtime with little relief. Stated that she has tried a new perfume after her shower for the past 3 or 4 days.

double-space

OBJECTIVE
VITAL SIGNS: Temperature 98.6°, blood pressure 140/74, weight 185 pounds, height 5 feet 4 inches, heart rate 74, respirations 22.
GENERAL APPEARANCE: Obese.
HAIR: Within normal limits.
SKIN: Comedo formations on nose. Several pustular lesions on forehead. Smooth, erythematous rash over neck extending over trunk and back. There is a small hyperpigmented nevus on the right breast. There is a 2 x 3-cm cafe-au-lait spot on the lower back. There are several nevi on the buttocks. On the upper extremities, she has a confluent, erythematous rash extending to fingertips. Wheals with petechiae are noted in the antecubital fossae bilaterally.

double-space

ASSESSMENT
Contact dermatitis, secondary to allergy to perfume.

double-space

PLAN

1 space after → number and period or use a tab setting

1. Avoid use of any perfume or perfumed soap.
2. Wash or dry clean all clothing and linens that were exposed to the suspected perfume.
3. Take diphenhydramine (Benadryl) 25 mg q.6h. x 3 days.

quadruple-space

____
Julia M. Waters, MD

DR:MT ← MT stands for transcriptionist's initials; DR stands for dictator's initials
D: XX/XX/XX
T: XX/XX/XX

↑ 1 space after colons

FIGURE 4.3
Office Note

Patient Studies

Transcribe, edit, and correct each report in the following patient studies. Consult reference books for words or formatting rules that are unfamiliar.

As you work on the transcription assignment for this chapter, fill in the Performance Comparison chart that you started when you keyed the model document. For at least three of the reports, categorize and document the types of errors you made. Answer the document analysis questions on the bottom of the chart. With continuous practice and assessment, the quality of your work will improve.

After you have produced a final version of each transcribed report, complete the Performance Report cover sheet, attach it to the top of the transcripts, and submit them to your instructor for evaluation.

Patient Study 4.A — Avis Smith

Ms. Avis Smith is a 45-year-old woman who presents with a 3-week history of generalized itching and a maculopapular, erythematous rash, most prominent on the torso.

REPORT 4.1 Office Note

Patient Study 4.B — Albert Alvarez

Mr. Albert Alvarez, a 45-year-old male, was referred to dermatologist Anthony Palmer, MD, by his internist for assessment of several lesions. Although Dr. Palmer found none of the lesions suspicious, he removed them, as they were inflamed.

REPORT 4.2 Office Note

- Listen for these terms:
  excision
  keratotic papules

Patient Study 4.C

Kyle Sanderson

Ms. Sanderson's 6-month-old infant, Kyle, was referred to Dr. Palmer by the pediatrician for evaluation of a persistent rash on his scalp, behind his ears, and in the diaper area.

REPORT 4.3 Office Note

- Listen for these difficult terms:
  seborrheic (adjective) and seborrhea (noun)
  alopecic (adjective) and alopecia (noun)
  perineum
- PMD means "primary medical doctor." This fairly common medical abbreviation should be transcribed only when it is dictated. Do not change "primary medical doctor" to PMD and do not change "PMD" to primary medical doctor. The same rule applies to other abbreviations such as BP (blood pressure) and ER (emergency room).
- Drug dosages are expressed in Latin abbreviations, for example, q.i.d., which means four times a day, or b.i.d., which means twice a day. The dictator will pronounce the letters rather than say "four times a day." Transcribe the abbreviation in lowercase letters with periods and no internal spaces. See Chapter 3 for more information on capitalization rules.

Patient Study 4.D — Ramon Yates

Ramon Yates, a 45-year-old construction worker, sought medical help after he noticed a small, raised bump in his groin area.

REPORT 4.4 Office Note

- When you hear "injected with point five cee cees of one percent lidocaine with epinephrine," transcribe the amount as 0.5 cc of 1% lidocaine with epinephrine. Note that lidocaine and epinephrine are generic drug names and thus should not be capitalized. Also, see Chapter 3 for more information on numbers.
- Silver nitrate is a generic drug name and thus is not capitalized.

Patient Study 4.E — Sandra Mahoney

Recently, Ms. Mahoney visited her local clinic to have a mole removed from her forearm.

REPORT 4.5 Office Note

- Mixed numbers (a whole number plus a fraction) should be transcribed in figures, so when you hear "two and a half," key 2½. If fractions are not available, use 2-1/2.
- Steri-Strips is a brand name and thus should be capitalized. Benzoin is a generic name.

Patient Study 4.F — John Smith

John Smith is a teenager who was brought to the neighborhood health clinic after his mother noticed a small lump on his scalp while cutting his hair. He had not bumped his head or sustained any other injuries that could have caused the lump to occur.

REPORT 4.6 Office Note

- Listen for these terms:
  parietal
  angioma
- Compound modifiers made up of an adverb or an adjective and a participle, for example, well-defined and oval-shaped, require a hyphen. See Chapter 3 for a discussion of compound words.

Patient Study 4.G — Robert Charles

Robert Charles is an 8-year-old brought to the dermatology clinic for evaluation of skin lesions. His past medical history includes a familial spastic paraplegia syndrome.

REPORT 4.7 Office Note

- Listen for these terms:
  gregarious
  cutaneous
  neuromuscular
  urticaria pigmentosa
  antihistamines
  hydroxyzine
  cyproheptadine

Patient Study 4.H

Alberta Mariano

Alberta Mariano is a young woman who had been diagnosed with childhood leukemia as a young child. She presented to the dermatologist with a pigmented lesion on her left breast. Reports included are the operative and pathology reports

REPORT 4.8 Operative Report

- Listen carefully for the following terms:
  expeditiously
  sequelae
  Xylocaine
  epinephrine
  Monocryl suture
  Bacitracin

REPORT 4.9 Pathology Report

- Listen carefully for the following terms:
  nevus
  melanocytic

Using Medical References

Use the appropriate medical reference to locate the correct spelling and part of speech for the words below. (If the reference is not available, use the Glossary in this text.) Circle the correct spelling, then write a sentence using the word correctly.

1.	psoriasus	psoriasis	psoriases
2.	impetigo	impettigo	impetigoe
3.	syanosis	cyanosis	sianosus
4.	cicatricks	cickatricks	cicatrix
5.	urticaria	uticaria	urticarea
6.	pruritis	pruritus	puritus
7.	paronychia	peronychia	paronychea
8.	hirsuitism	hirsutism	hirutysm
9.	zanthoma	xanthoma	xenthoma
10.	joundice	jaundyce	jaundice
11.	asimtomatic	assimtomatic	asymptomatic
12.	neevus	nevus	nevis

Making Expert Decisions

Circle the correct word from the choices in parentheses.

1. The patient fell and sustained a (concussion/contusion) to her elbow.
2. "Mycosis" refers to a (bacterial/fungal/viral) infestation.
3. The patient underwent a skin peel, or (dermabrasion/electrolysis/fulguration), by the dermatologist.
4. The patient had a (KOH/Tzanck's smear) test because a fungal infection was suspected.
5. (A, An) (excisional/incisional/punch) biopsy was done to completely remove the lesion on the nose.
6. The patient (presence/presents) with symptoms of rubella marked by the (presence/presents) of fever, rash, mild upper respiratory symptoms, enlarged lymph nodes, and pain in the joints.
7. The (macular/papular) rash contained small raised areas that were well circumscribed.
8. The (glands/glans) of the penis showed several verrucous formations.
9. The tumor was composed of several small (discreet/discrete) masses.
10. The (vesical/vesicle) was located on the tip of the fourth digit of the right hand.
11. Robert had an (pigmented/urticarial) rash requiring antihistamine treatment.
12. Elderly patients frequently have much less (adipose/subcutaneous) tissue than obese patients.

Transcribing Professional Documents

Transcribe the document named Chapter 4 Assessment. Before you key, review the appropriate report formatting guidelines. Proofread your transcribed document and revise it until you think it is error-free.

5

Ophthalmology

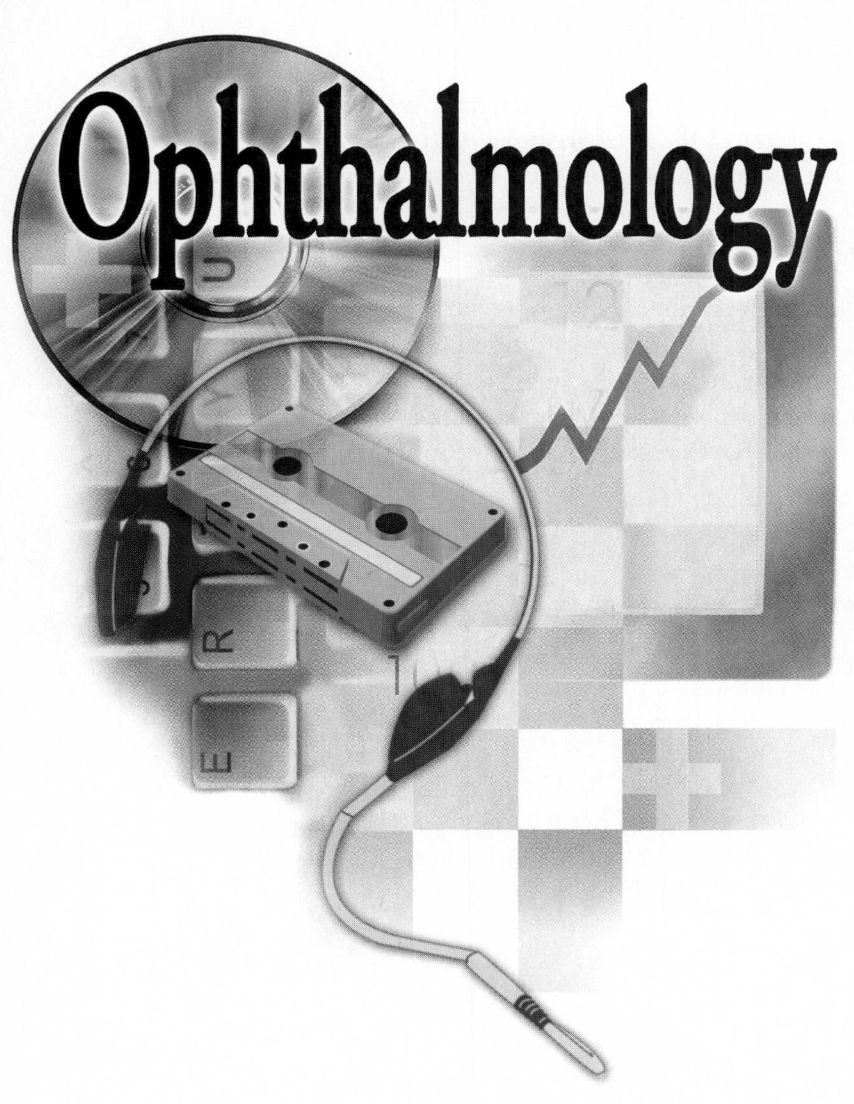

The professionals within this specialty include the ophthalmologist, the medical doctor (MD) who diagnoses and treats eye disorders; the optometrist, the doctor of optometry (OD) who specializes in refraction of the eyes to determine the extent of vision and prescribes glasses; and the optician who takes the prescription from the MD or OD, grinds the lenses, and fits the glasses.

OBJECTIVES

- Use ophthalmology terms correctly according to the context and purpose of the dictation.
- Select and use appropriate general and specialty reference materials.
- Key ophthalmology documents of varying complexity and format.
- Transcribe authentic medical dictation requiring concentration and listening skill.
- Edit medical reports to conform with AAMT style guidelines.
- Proofread and correct transcripts to produce error-free documents.

Exploring Ophthalmology

The word ophthalmology is derived from a Greek root, *oculus*, for eyeball. This specialty encompasses the study of the eyeball, along with vision, the eyelids, the eye sockets (orbits), and the related parts of the face, brain, sinuses, nose, and throat.

Structure and Function

Working in partnership with the brain, the eye is the organ of sight. Vision is possible when the retina converts light into nerve impulses.

The main parts of the eye include the sclera, cornea, lens, retina, pupil, and iris (see Figure 5.1). The sclera is the "white" of the eye, the outer protective layer of the eyeball. The cornea is the transparent center, allowing light to enter the eye and

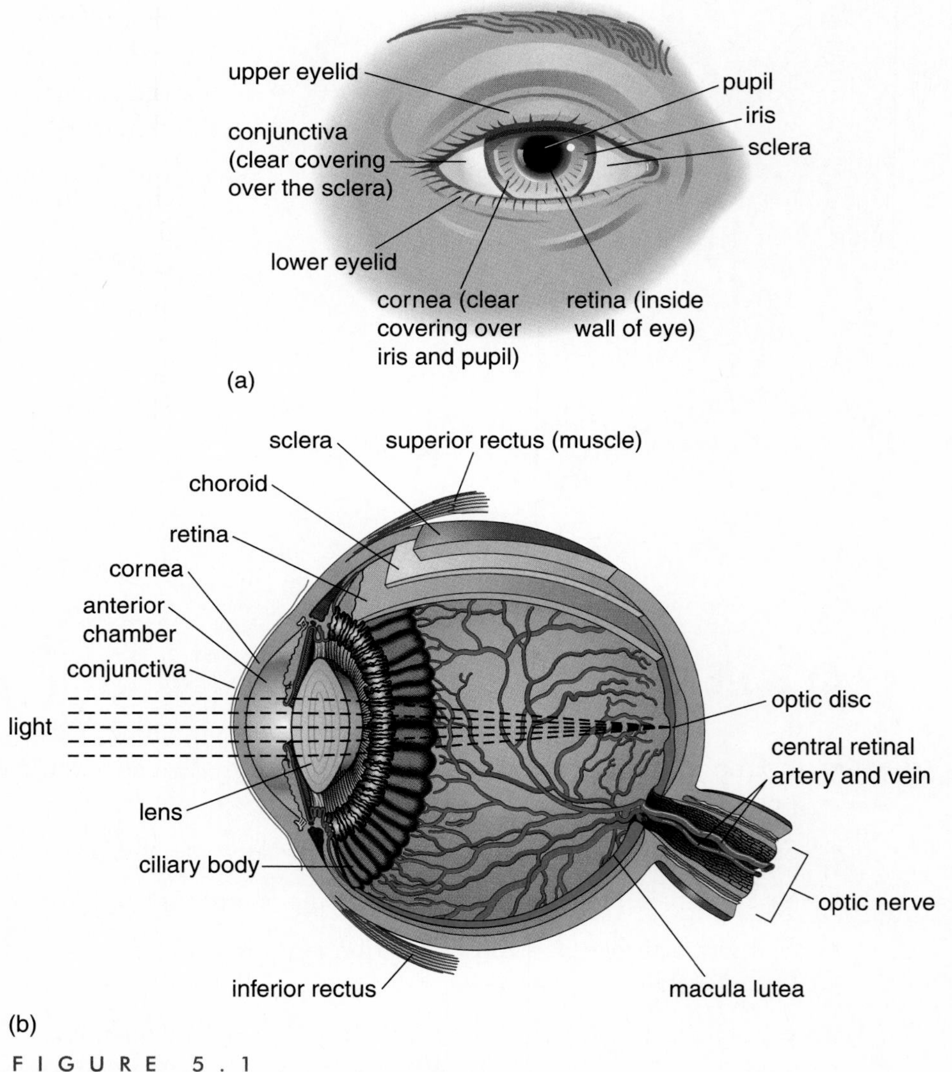

FIGURE 5.1
The Eyeball ***(a) Anterior view (b) Sagittal view***

directing it through the lens to the retina at the back of the eye. The cornea is the protective membrane at the center of the exterior eye and is important in the refractive system. The lens focuses the light; the pupil and iris control the amount of light that enters the eye.

Vision occurs when the retinas of both eyes send pictures to the brain, which merges the information into one image. Diplopia, or double vision, occurs when there is failure to merge the images.

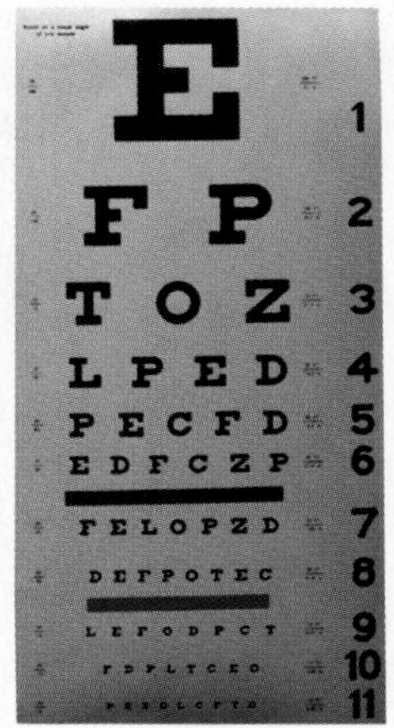

The Snellen eye chart is used to test visual acuity.

Physical Assessment

The physician assesses the eye by examining the eyeballs and surrounding structures, including the eyebrows, upper and lower eyelids, and eyelashes. The patient's eyes may reflect feelings such as pain or fear as well as the individual's general health.

After the initial observation, the physician makes a closer inspection by asking the patient to perform certain tasks to reveal facial neuromuscular coordination. The patient's squinting, blinking, raising and lowering of eyebrows, and making faces, such as a grimace, can reveal if there are any neuromuscular problems related to the eyes. These movements test the cranial nerves and are also performed by the neurologist (see Chapter 13).

There should be no pain or tenderness on palpation over the forehead, around the eye sockets, or across the lids and eyeballs. The eyeballs should feel firm, round, and bouncy to the touch.

The examination includes the observation of the sclerae, which should be white. Discolored sclerae can indicate jaundice. Very thin, blue-appearing sclerae can occur in some connective tissue disorders. The physician inspects the cornea with a light to determine if there are any irregularities, foreign bodies, or scars. The pupils are inspected for size, equal appearance, and reaction to light, an assessment that appears in the medical record as PERRLA (pupils equal, round, reactive to light and accommodation). The patient will be asked to look at the examiner's finger about 15 cm from the eyes and then look at a distant object. The pupils should narrow when looking close and widen when looking at a distance.

A Snellen, or "E," chart tests visual acuity. The chart has lines of letters with numbers on the side to represent how far a person can be from the chart to read that line. Therefore, if the patient is seated 20 feet away from the chart and can read the line marked 20 feet, the person is said to have 20/20 vision. That is the distance that a normal eye can read at 20 feet. Testing is also done to determine sight in visual fields, or peripheral vision.

The ophthalmoscope is the instrument used to look at the retina. By observing the veins and arteries directly, the examiner can check for damage associated with hypertension, diabetes and other diseases. The pupils may be dilated by means of special drops to perform a thorough examination.

The nerve fibers in the cornea make it extremely sensitive to pain. Examining the cornea requires a slit lamp that magnifies and lights up the lens, cornea, and iris. A local anesthetic is used to relieve pain during the examination. It may be necessary to use fluorescein staining to outline any epithelial defects.

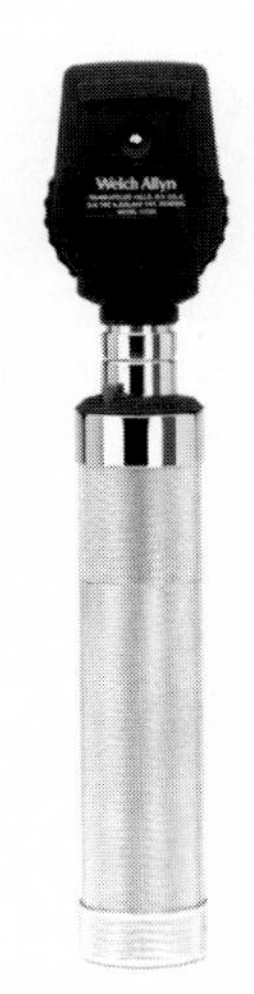

An ophthalmoscope is used to examine the retina.

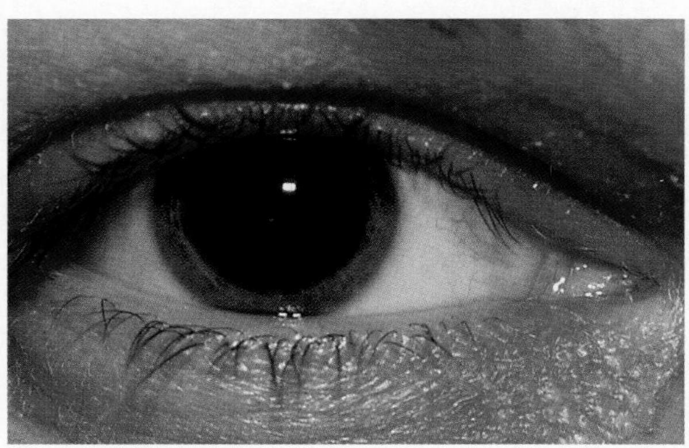

The dilated pupil remains open during the retinal examination.

Diseases and Conditions

Examination of the eye is difficult from infancy to young school age. Frequently, the physician must sedate the young patient in order to complete the examination. The diagnosis of strabismus (crossed eyes) is usually made in childhood. This condition is typically the result of a weakness in one of the muscles controlling eye movement. Diplopia (double vision) is most common and can lead to reversible amblyopia (decreased vision) if diagnosed before the age of about seven years. Other deviations of eye control include esotropia (inward turning of the eyes), exotropia (outward turning of the eyes), and hypertropia (upward squinting).

The eyelids protect the eyeball; therefore, it is important to seek medical attention when there are abnormalities of the eyelid. There can be irritation, inflammation, or infection of the eyelid, including blepharitis, an inflammation of the margins of the lid, and chalazion, a sterile granulomatous inflammation of the meibomian gland. A sty (also spelled *stye*) is an infection of the lid usually caused by *Staphylococcus aureus.*

Conjunctivitis is an inflammation of the conjunctiva and can be caused by bacterial, viral, fungal, or parasitic organisms. There is usually hyperemia (redness), discharge, tearing, itching and/or burning, and a feeling of having a foreign body present in the eye.

Trachoma, caused by the organism *Chlamydia,* is a type of conjunctivitis that affects millions of people. It is rare in the United States, but is endemic to Africa, the Middle East, and Asia. Trachoma is the world's leading cause of blindness. It is very contagious through direct contact with infected individuals or materials they have touched and possibly through insect carriers, but it can be prevented by good hygiene and education. The symptoms of this disease include inflammation, blurred vision, and increasing pain and discomfort. Treatment consists of tetracycline or sulfonamides.

Uveitis is the inflammation of the structures of the uveal tract caused by allergens, bacteria, fungi, viruses, chemicals, or eye trauma. It is characterized by pain, photophobia, blurred vision, and erythema. A physician will prescribe corticosteroid drops to reduce inflammation and proper systemic treatment to treat the underlying cause.

Corneal abrasions occur from trauma, foreign bodies, including contact lenses, or any defect to the flow of protective tears. Keratitis is an infection of the cornea and can be caused by any organism that has entered the cornea through an abrasion. Because there is easy entry of infectious agents through the eye into the body, patients with severe infectious keratitis are hospitalized and placed on antibiotic therapy.

Keratoconus is a progressive thinning of the cornea that first shows up in puberty and affects women more than men. Vision is distorted, leading to astigmatism and myopia that are difficult to correct even with eyeglasses. Surgery may be necessary to correct this problem.

Corneal transplants are performed using corneas from deceased donors. A circular blade called a trephine is used to incise the cornea. The new cornea is sutured into place. Healing may be slow because of the decreased blood supply of the cornea. A transplant eye bank has been established to make donated corneas available.

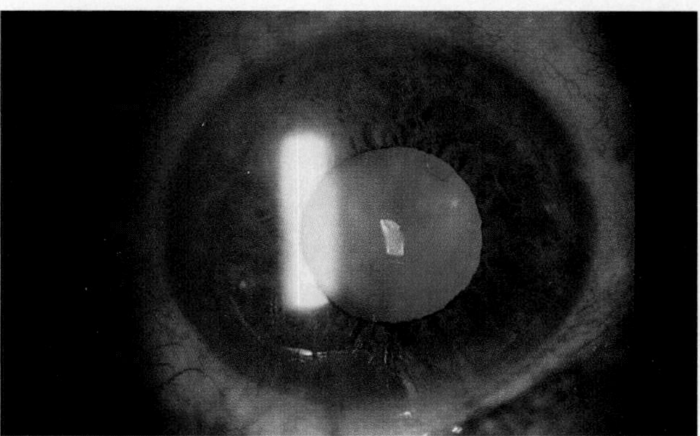

This eye's lens is clouded with a cataract. Surgical removal of the cataract is usually done as an outpatient procedure.

Over 2 million persons have been diagnosed with glaucoma in the United States. Glaucoma is one of the leading causes of blindness in the Western world, though blindness is preventable with early diagnosis and management. Glaucoma is characterized by damage to the optic nerve. Primary glaucoma is thought to be hereditary and usually affects both eyes. Secondary glaucoma, or open-angle glaucoma, often affects only one eye and is due to a build-up of pressure inside the eye. Physicians treat glaucoma with drugs that relieve the intraocular pressure (IOP) and restore the normal flow of aqueous humor.

A cataract is a clouding of the crystalline lens. The opaque lens scatters light rather than producing a fine, sharp image. Vision becomes blurred and distorted. While a cataract is usually associated with aging, it can be caused by systemic disease, such as diabetes mellitus, hypoparathyroidism, radiation exposure, or sickle C syndrome.

Retinal detachment is a separation of the neurosensory retina, or rods and cones, from the epithelial, or nourishment, layer of the retina; it results in partial or total loss of vision in the affected eye. The most common type of detachment is rhegmatogenous, or a tear-induced detachment, which occurs in 1 out of 10,000 persons between 40 and 70 years old.

Diabetic retinopathy is a common complication of diabetes mellitus. The risk for this complication increases with the duration of the diabetes.

Macular degeneration is caused by damage to the photoreceptor cells in the area of the macula. It may be hereditary and is the leading cause of severe visual impairment for people over 65 years of age.

Common Tests and Surgical Procedures

Many of the common ophthalmology tests and procedures concern the diagnosis and treatment of glaucoma. Gonioscopy, for example, is used to visualize the anterior chamber angle with a slit lamp and a goniolens, a special mirror contact lens. Gonioscopy is necessary to determine if the angle is open or closed in glaucoma. Laser surgery is the primary treatment of glaucoma and other eye disorders. Some of the laser surgical procedures include laser iridotomy, peripheral iridectomy, radial keratotomy, trabeculoplasty, and gonioplasty.

Building Language Skills

The following tables list common opthalmology terms, drugs, and abbreviations. The list of terms and definitions includes the most difficult words contained in the dictated reports in this chapter. These words are identified in GREEN type. A list of common drugs is found in Appendix D.

Medical Terms and Pharmacologic Agents

accommodation
(ah-kom-o-**day**-shun) (n) the eye's ability to focus or see

afferent
(**af**-er-ent) (adj) inward or toward a center, as a nerve; carrying a sensory impulse

amblyopia
(am-blee-**O**-pee-a) (n) decreased vision in one or both eyes; not correctable

anterior
(an-**teer**-ee-or) (adj) front of a part, organ, or structure

astigmatism
(a-**stig**-ma-tizm) (n) visual condition in which light rays entering the eye are bent unequally, preventing a sharp focus point on the retina

blepharectomy
(blef-ar-**ek**-tO-mee) (n) excision of a lesion of the eyelid

blepharitis
(blef-a-**rI**-tis) (n) inflammation of the eyelid

calcification
(kal-si-fi-**kay**-shun) (n) a hardening of tissue resulting from the formation of calcium salts within it

cataract
(**kat**-a-rakt) (n) clouding of the lens of the eye, resulting in loss of transparency

chemosis
(kee-**mO**-sis) (n) an accumulation of fluid in the eye, causing swelling around the cornea

chemotherapy
(kem-O-**thayr**-a-pee/**keem**-O-thayr-a-pee) (n) treatment of disease with drugs

choroid
(**kO**-royd) (n) a vascular membrane surrounding the eyeball, between the retina and sclera

conjunctiva
(kon-junk-**ti**-va) (n) the mucous membrane covering the front of the eyeball and inside the eyelids; conjunctivae (pl)

conjunctival
(kon-**junk**-ti-val (adj) pertaining to the conjunctiva

conjunctivitis
(kon-junk-ti-**vI**-tis) (n) inflammation of the conjunctiva

cornea
(**kor**-nee-a) (n) the outer, transparent portion of the eye through which light passes to the retina

diabetes insipidus
(dI-a-**bee**-tez in-**sip**-i-doos) (n and adj) disease caused by insufficient secretion of antidiuretic hormone (AHD) from the posterior pituitary gland

diplopia
(di-**plO**-pee-a) (n) double vision; may be monocular

enucleation
(ee-noo-klee-**ay**-shun) (n) removal of a tumor or structure as a whole, as in removal of the eyeball

epiphora
(ee-**pif**-O-ra) (n) overflow of tears

esotropia
(es-O-**trO**-pee-a) (n) a condition in which one or both eyes appear to turn inward; cross eye(s)

exophthalmos
(ek-sof-**thal**-mos) (n) protrusion of the eyeball(s)

exotropia
(ek-sO-**trO**-pee-a) (n) outward turning of one eye relative to the other

extraocular
(**ek**-stra-**ok**-yoo-lar) (adj) outside the eye

floater
(**flO**-ter) (n) spot in the visual screen when one stares at a blank wall; caused by bits of protein and other debris moving in front of the retina

fluorescein
(**floor**-ess-scene) (n) a yellow dye which glows in visible light

fundus
(**fun**-dus) (n) that part of the interior of the eyeball exposed to view through an ophthalmoscope; lowest part; fundi (pl)

funduscopic
(fun-dus-**skop**-ik) (adj) relating to funduscopy

funduscopy
(fun-dus-**kop**-ee) (n) examination of the fundus of the eye using a funduscope; ophthalmoscopy

glaucoma
(glaw-**kO**-ma) (n) disease of the eye in which intraocular pressure increases, damaging the optic nerve; can lead to blindness

Goldmann perimeter screen test
(n) assesses patient response when a light comes into view

gonioplasty
(gO-ni-O-**plas**-tee) (n) procedure that contracts the peripheral iris to eliminate contact with the trabecular meshwork

gonioscopy
(gO-ni-**O**-skOp-ee) (n) procedure that allows viewing of the anterior chamber angle using a slit lamp and a goniolens, a special mirror contact lens

histiocyte
(**hiss**-tee-O-cyte) (n) a cell that participates in the body's reaction to infection or injury; found in connective tissue

HMS drops
(ach-**em**-ess) (n) a brand name of eye drops containing Medrysone, a corticosteroid

hydrocephalic
(hI-drO-se-**fal**-ik) (adj) relating to or having hydrocephalus

hydrocephalus
(hI-drO-**sef**-a-lus) (n) increased accumulation of cerebrospinal fluid within the ventricles of the brain

hydrocephaly
(hI-drO-**sef**-a-lee) (n) the condition of having hydrocephalus

hyperopia
(hI-per-**O**-pee-a) (n) farsightedness

hypertropia
(hI-per-**trO**-pee-a) (n) a type of squint in which the eye looks upward

hypotropia
(hI-pO-**trO**-pee-a) (n) a type of squint in which the eye looks downward

infundibulum
(in-fun-**dib**-yoo-lum) (n) a funnel-shaped opening

intraocular pressure
(in-tra-**ok**-yoo-lar **presh**-er) (n) the pressure of the fluid within the eye

iris
(**I**-ris) (n) colored portion of the eye that regulates the amount of light entering through the pupil; irides (**ir**-i-deez) (pl)

keratoplasty
(**ker**-a-tO-**plas**-tee) (n) surgery on the cornea, especially transplant of a cornea

laser iridotomy
(ir-i-**dot**-O-mee) (n) cutting some of the fibers of the iris with a laser

macula
(**mak**-yoo-la) (n) small discolored spot on the retina

metastasis
(me-**tas**-ta-sis) (n) spread of a tumor from its site of origin to distant sites

metastatic
(met-a-**stat**-ik) (adj) relating to metastasis

motility
(mO-**til**-i-tee) (n) ability to move spontaneously

myopia
(mI-**O**-pee-a) (n) nearsightedness; visual defect in which parallel rays come to a focus

myelocyte
(**my**-e-lo-cyte) (n) immature granulocytic leukocyte normally found in bone marrow and present in the circulatory blood in certain diseases, e.g., myelocytic anemia

nystagmus
(nis-**tag**-mus) (n) involuntary, rhythmic oscillation of the eyeballs

oblique
(ob-**leek**) (adj) slanting

ophthalmologist
(of-thal-**mol**-o-jist) (n) a physician specializing in diseases of the eye

ocular
(**ok**-yoo-lar) (adj) concerning the eye or vision

ophthalmoscopy
(of-thal-**mos**-ko-pee) (n) procedure used to examine the optic nerve head for color, shape, and vascularization

ophthalmus
(of-**thal**-mus) (n) the eye

optic
(**op**-tik) (adj) pertaining to the eye or sight

optic chiasm
(**op**-tik **kI**-azm) (n) the point of crossing of the optic nerves

optometrist
(op-**tom**-e-trist) (n) a professional who tests visual acuity and prescribes corrective lenses

osteosarcoma
(os-tee-O-sar-**ko**-ma) (n) a tumor of the bone, usually highly malignant

palsy
(**pawl**-zee) (n) an abnormal condition characterized by partial paralysis

papilledema
(**pap**-ill-e-dee-ma) (n) edema and inflammation of the optic nerve at its point of entrance into the eyeball

papillopathy
(pap-i-**lop**-a-thee) (n) the blood supply to the optic disk and retina is obstructed; often producing low-tension glaucoma

peripheral iridectomy
(per-**if**-er-al ir-i-**dek**-tO-mee) (n) procedure that creates a hole in the iris; used to relieve high intraocular pressure

phacoemulsification
(fak-O-ee-mul-si-fi-**kay**-shun) (n) process that disintegrates a cataract using ultrasonic waves

photophobia
(fO-tO-**fO**-bee-a) (n) marked intolerance to light

platelet
(**playt**-let) (n) disc-shaped, small cellular element in the blood that is essential for blood clotting

presbyopia
(prez-bee-**O**-pee-a) (n) farsightedness associated with aging

prognosis
(prog-**nO**-sis) (n) the expected outcome of a disease

pterygium
(ter-**ij**-ee-um) (n) web eye; an outward growth of tissue of the eye

ptosis
(**tO**-sis) (n) sagging of the upper eyelid

pupil
(**pyoo**-pil) (n) the round opening in the center of the iris which opens or closes to adjust to light

pupillary
(**pyoo**-pi-layr-ee) (adj) relating to the pupil of the eye

radial keratotomy
(**ray**-dee-al ker-ah-**tot**-O-mee) (n) incision(s) in the cornea radiating out from the center

radiotherapy
(ray-dee-O-**thayr**-a-pee) (n) the treatment of disease by application of radium, ultraviolet, and other types of radiation

recession
(ree-**sesh**-un) (n) the withdrawal of a part from its normal position

rectus
(**rec**-tus) (adj) relating to the rectus muscle of the eye

referral
(ree-**fer**-al) (n) a physician's sending of a patient to another physician

reflex
(**ree**-fleks) (n) an involuntary response to a stimulus

regression
(ree-**gresh**-un) (n) returning to an earlier condition

retina
(**ret**-i-na) (n) innermost layer of the eyeball that receives images formed by the lens and transmits visual impulses through the optic nerve to the brain; composed of light-sensitive nerves

retinal hemorrhage
(**ret**-i-nal **hem**-or-age) hemorrhage of the retina

retinitis pigmentosa
(ret-in-**I**-tis pig men **toe** saw) (n) a inflammation of the retina with pigment changes, eventually leading to blindness

retinoblastoma
(**ret**-i-nO-blas-**tO**-ma) (n) malignant sarcoma or neoplasm of the retina; hereditary and generally occurring in young children

retinopathy
(ret-i-**nop**-a-thee) (n) any disorder of the retina without inflammation

retinoscopy
(ret-i-**nos**-ko-pee) (n) light beam test used to detect refractive errors

sclera
(**skle**-rah) (n) white of the eye; the tough, outer covering of the eye

sclerostomy
(skle-**ros**-tO-mee) (n) surgical formation of an opening in the sclera

scotoma
(skO-**tO**-ma) (n) a blind spot; a small area of defective vision

seed
(n) as related to oncology, it is the beginning of a tumor

seeding
(n) the local spreading of immature tumor cells

Seton procedure
(n) placing of a tube in the anterior chamber to drain fluid and decrease the intraocular pressure

slit-lamp
(n) instrument consisting of a microscope and a thin, bright beam of light; used to examine the eye

sphincterotomy
(sfink-tur-**ot**-O-mee) (n) procedure that produces cuts in the iris sphincter muscle to allow pupillary enlargement

sporadic
(spO-**rad**-ik) (adj) occurring occasionally or in isolated situations

strabismus
(stra-**biz**-mus) (n) improper alignment of eyes; crossed eye(s)

sty
(stI) (n) an infection of a marginal gland of the eyelid; stye

tangent screen test
(n) maps the field of vision using a marker

thrombocytopenia
(**throm**-bO-cy-to-**pee**-nee-a) (n) abnormal decrease in the number of blood platelets

tonometry
(tO-**nom**-et-ree) (n) a test that measures intraocular pressure

trabeculectomy
(tra-bek-yoo-**lek**-tO-mee) (n) surgical removal of a section of the cornea to decrease intraocular pressure in patients with severe glaucoma

trabeculoplasty
(tra-**bek**-yoo-lO-**plas**-tee) (n) surgical procedure that decreases intraocular pressure in open-angle glaucoma

unilateral
(yoo-ni-**lat**-e-ral) (adj) affecting or occurring on only one side

uveitis
(yoo-vee-**I**-tis) (n) inflammation of the uvea, including the choroid and the iris

viable
(**vI**-a-bl) (adj) capable of surviving; living

visual acuity
(**vizh**-yoo-al a-**kyoo**-i-tee) (n) clearness of vision, e.g., 20/20 visual acuity

vitreous humor
(**vit**-ree-us **hyoo**-mer) (adj) glassy; gelatin-like substance within the eyeball

xanthopsia
(zan-**thop**-see-a) (n) yellow vision; a condition in which everything seen appears yellowish

Abbreviations

ACC	accommodation
D	diopter
DCR	dacryocystorhinostomy
ECCE	extracapsular cataract extraction
Em	emmetropia
EOM	extraocular movements
ERG	electroretinography
ICCE	intracapsular cataract extraction
IOL	intraocular lens
IOP	intraocular pressure
L&A	light and accommodation
LASIK	laser assisted *in-situ* keratomileusis
my	myopia
OD	right eye *(oculus dexter);* doctor of optometry
OS	left eye *(oculus sinister)*
OU	both eyes *(oculus uterque)*
PAN	periodic alternating nystagmus
PERLA	pupils equal, reactive to light and accommodation
PERRLA	pupils equal, round, reactive to light and accommodation
PRK	photorefractive keratectomy
REM	rapid eye movement
ROP	retinopathy of prematurity
ST	esotropia
VA	visual acuity
VF	visual field
XT	exotropia

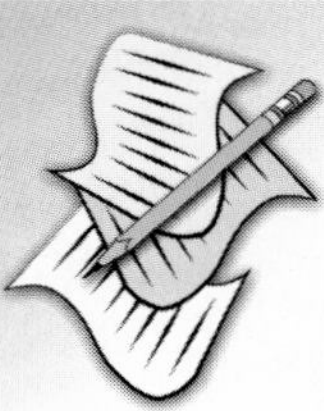

EXERCISE 5.1

Recognizing Look-Alikes and Sound-Alikes

Below is a list of frequently used words that look alike and/or sound alike. Study the meaning and pronunciation of each set of words, then read the following sentences carefully and circle the word in parentheses that correctly completes the meaning.

efferent	conducting (as a nerve) or progressing away from the center
afferent	conducting (as a nerve) or progressing toward the center

effluent	discharged fecal material
affluent	having wealth

anterior	front
inferior	below; lower
posterior	back; behind
superior	above

hyper -	(prefix) more, greater
hypo-	(prefix) less, smaller

macula	a small, yellowish spot on the retina at the back of the eye
macule	a spot discoloration or thickening of the skin

metastases	plural form of metastasis
metastasis	spread of a tumor to different parts of the body
metastasize	to invade by metastasis
metastatic	relating to metastasis

esotropia	inward turning of the eye
exotropia	outward turning of the eye

fundus	part farthest from the opening
fungus	organism

recession	withdrawal of part from its normal position
resection	cutting out part of an organ

apprise	to notify; to tell
appraise	to set a value on; to give an expert judgment of the value or merit of

1. The head is (inferior, superior) to the chest.
2. Your face is located on the (anterior, posterior) part of your body.
3. The legs are (inferior, superior) to the head.
4. The spine is (anterior, posterior) to the chest.
5. Examination of the face revealed a 1-cm (macula, macule) on the cheek.
6. Due to her (hyperthyroidism, hypothyroidism), she requires thyroid supplementation.
7. The patient's (hypertension, hypotension) is under good control on the Calan SR.
8. On ophthalmic exam, the (fundus, fungus) appeared normal.
9. This patient has metastatic colorectal carcinoma with (metastases, metastasis) diagnosed in the liver, lung, and brain.
10. The patient is status post craniotomy for removal of tumor (metastasis, metastatic).

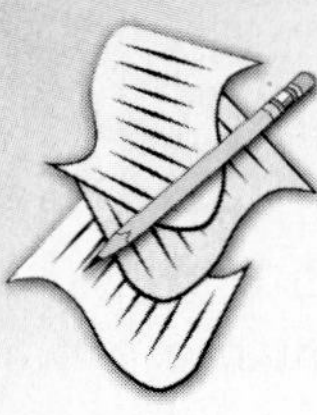

EXERCISE 5.2

Matching Sound and Spelling

The numbered list that follows shows the phonetic spelling of hard-to-spell words. Sound out the word, then write the correct spelling in the blank space provided. Each of the words can be found in the Glossary or in the drug list in Appendix D.

1. kal-si-fi-**kay**-shun__________
2. **ret**-i-nO-blas-**tO**-ma __________
3. yoo-ni-**lat**-e-ral__________
4. **pyoo**-pi-layr-ee__________
5. ob-**leek** __________
6. hI-drO-**sef**-a-lus__________
7. blef-a-**rI**-tis__________
8. **vit**-ree-us __________
9. fO-tO-**fO**-bee-a __________
10. me-**tas**-ta-sis__________
11. nis-**tag**-mus __________
12. ek-sof-**thal**-mos __________
13. **os**-tee-O-sar-**kO**-ma__________
14. pap-i-**lop**-a-thee__________
15. mO-**til**-i-tee__________

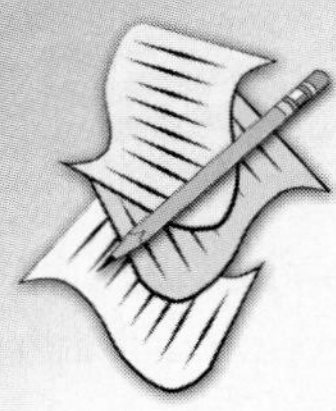

EXERCISE 5.3

Choosing Words from Context

When transcribing dictation, the medical transcriptionist frequently needs to consider the situation when determining the word that correctly completes the sentence. From the list below, select the term that meaningfully completes each of the following statements.

conjunctivitis	retinopathy	diplopia
strabismus	optic	nystagmus
radiotherapy	osteosarcoma	optic chiasm
scotoma	enucleation	epiphora
esotropia		

1. The patient is status post ______________ of the left eye, with a poorly fitted prosthesis in place.
2. The right fundus showed a flame hemorrhage superior to the ______________ nerve.
3. She had an amputation of the right leg below the knee because she was diagnosed with a malignancy called ________________.
4. She describes a blind spot in the right eye; this is most likely a ___________.
5. When you have ___________, your eyes may deviate either toward the nose or to the outside of midline.
6. The patient's allergic ________________ seems to be controlled on the antibiotic eyedrops.
7. It was recommended that Joseph have __________________ treatments to the eye, rather than have an enucleation.
8. A mild form of ____________, where the eye turns inward, can often be corrected with exercises for the eye.
9. The funduscopic exam showed no signs of ______________.
10. The MRI revealed an enhancing lesion surrounding the ______________.

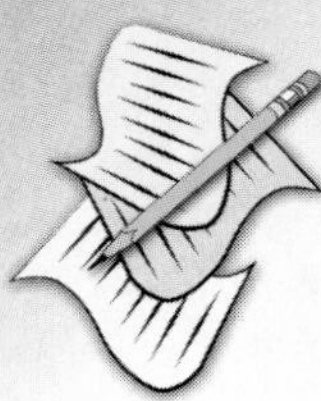

EXERCISE 5.4

Pairing Words and Meanings

From this list, locate the term that best matches each of the following definitions. Write the letter of the term in the space provided by each definition.

A.	pupillary	G.	seed	M.	nystagmus
B.	calcification	H.	funduscopy	N.	retina
C.	macula	I.	optic	0.	papilledema
D.	retinopathy	J.	hydrocephalus	P.	extraocular
E.	cornea	K.	ophthalmus	Q.	diplopia
F.	rectus	L.	amblyopia		

1. outer portion of eye through which light passes to retina __________
2. pertaining to vision __________
3. pertaining to pupil of eye __________
4. accumulation of cerebrospinal fluid within ventricles of brain __________
5. examination of the base of the eye __________
6. small, yellowish spot on retina __________
7. hardening of tissue resulting from calcium salts __________
8. beginning of a tumor __________
9. disorder of the retina __________
10. a muscle of the eye __________
11. swelling of the optic nerve in the eye __________
12. double vision __________

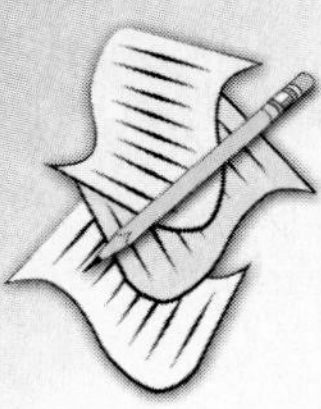

EXERCISE 5.5

Creating Terms from Word Forms

Combine prefixes, root words, and suffixes from this list to create medical words that fit the following definitions. Fill in the blanks with the words you construct.

angi/o	vessel
blephar/o	eyelid
conjunctiv/o	mucous membrane lining inner eyeball and eyelids
cyt/o	cell
extra	outside
hyper	above or excessive
hypo	below or deficient
kerat/o	hard or cornea
ocul/o	pertaining to the eye
ophthalm/o	eye
phot/o	light
thromb/o	platelet
retina	nerve tissue layer of eye
-a	word ending
-ectomy	removal
-itis	inflammation
-pathy	disease
-penia	deficiency
-phobia	excessive fear
-plasty	surgical repair
-scopy	examination
-tropia	condition of turning

1. disease of the retina ______
2. type of squint when the eye looks downward ______
3. inflammation of the membrane lining the inner eyelid and the eyeball ______
4. excision of a lesion on the eyelid ______
5. light beam test that detects refractive errors ______
6. operation to correct defect in eyelids ______
7. visualizes the optic nerve for color and shape ______
8. mucous membrane lining the inner surface of the eye ______
9. inflammation of the eyelid ______
10. corneal transplant ______
11. outside the eye ______
12. deficiency of platelet cells (decreased platelets) ______

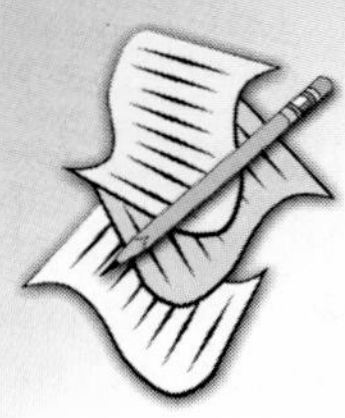

EXERCISE 5.6

Proofreading Review

Read the following partial report and look for errors in punctuation, spelling, plural vs. singular word forms, run-on sentences, and subject-verb agreement. Circle the errors; then key the report with the errors corrected.

1. **OBJECTIVE:** On examination visual aquity at distance was 20/20 in both eyes. The interocular pressure was 20 in both eyes. Motility was strait, with full versions and the pupils was normal. External exam revealed fat pertrusion on the lateral aspect of the upper and lower lids on both eye. There was a firmness on the right eye. The contacts were centered will, with good movement, slit lamp exam revealed a white conjunctiva, with a clear cornia. The lenses had some cortical changes. Dilated funduscopic exam revealed a normal cup-to-disc ratio, with a normal macule, blood vessels, and peripheral retina.

2. I found him to have papilodema as well as retinale hemorrhages. He occasionally notes some transient visual bluring when he suddenly goes from sitting to standing and occasional vertical deplopia.

Building Transcription Skills

The Consultation Letter/Report

The consultation letter (Figure 5.2) is a report that a patient's primary or attending physician requests of a specialist. Dictated in either letter or report form, this document provides an opinion on a particular problem or diagnosis. The specialist dictates the letter/report and addresses it to the primary physician.

Required Headings/Content JCAHO guidelines require no special headings in consultation letters; the format varies among institutions. The content includes sections similar to a history and physical, including date of consultation, reason for consultation, present history, past history, physical and laboratory evaluation, and the consultant's impression and recommendations. At the end of the dictation, physicians often add a phrase such as *Thank you for referring this patient to me.*

Turnaround Time For emergency room situations, specialists' consultations are available within approximately 30 minutes; initial consultation through two-way voice communication is acceptable. Consultations should be dictated within 24 hours from the time the request is received by the physician, and the report should be transcribed and on the chart within the next 24 hours. This guideline varies among institutions.

Preparing to Transcribe

To prepare for transcribing dictation, review the tables of common ophthalmology terms, drugs, and abbreviations presented in the Building Language Skills section of this chapter. Then, study the format and organization of the model document shown in Figure 5.4, and key the model document. Proofread the document by comparing it with the printed version. Categorize the types of errors you made, and document them on a copy of the Performance Comparison chart provided in Chapter 1. A template of this chart is included on the IRC that accompanies this text.

Patient Studies

Transcribe, edit, and correct each report in the following patient studies. Consult reference books for words or formatting rules that are unfamiliar.

As you work on the transcription assignment for this chapter, fill in the Performance Comparison chart that you started when you keyed the model document. For at least three of the reports, categorize and document the types of errors you made. Answer the document analysis questions on the bottom of the chart. With continuous practice and assessment, the quality of your work will improve.

After you have produced a final version of each transcribed report, complete the Performance Report cover sheet, attach it to the top of the transcripts, and submit them to your instructor for evaluation.

To prepare for transcribing dictation, key the consultation letter shown in Figure 5.2. You will later key the identical report from dictation. Follow these guidelines:

- Study the format and organization of the document.
- Review the word list presented earlier in this chapter.
- Consult reference books for words or formatting rules that are unfamiliar.
- Proofread your final copy by comparing it to the printed version.

1" top and side margins → **left justification**

Wills Eye Hospital
5849 Garfield Drive
Fort Worth, TX 76555-1223

2 or more line spaces, depending on length of letter

November 29, XXXX

2 or more line spaces, depending on length of letter

Dr. Albert J. Eisner
Brookfield University Medical School
One University Place
Fort Worth, TX 76104-3223

ds

RE: Lawrence Johnson, Jr.

ds

Dear Al:

ds

We rechecked Lawrence Johnson under anesthesia on November 21. It has been 9 months since he completed his course of external beam radiation therapy as management of unilateral sporadic retinoblastoma in the left eye.

ds

On our exam today, our findings remain the same as on our prior exam in August. The tumor is completely regressed, and there is no evidence of viability. There are no new tumors in the left eye. The optic disc is healthy, and there are no signs of radiation retinopathy or papillopathy.

ds

The right eye is perfectly normal, with no evidence of retinoblastoma. Regarding the visual prognosis, because of the macular location of the regressed retinoblastoma, his visual prognosis is very guarded. We will try patching of the right eye in an attempt to stimulate any possible vision in the left eye.

ds

Thank you for allowing us to assist in his care.

ds

Very sincerely yours,

quadruple-space

Richard Sowers, MD

ds

RS/XX

FIGURE 5.2
Consultation Letter

Patient Study 5.A — Lawrence Johnson

Lawrence Johnson is an infant who was diagnosed with retinoblastoma by Dr. Richard Sowers at Wills Eye Hospital. He was referred to Dr. Albert J. Eisner at Brookfield University Medical School for followup care. Dr. Eisner sent Lawrence to Dr. Jorge Frieze, a specialist in radiation oncology, for radiotherapy.

REPORT 5.1 Consultation Letter

- Listen for these troublesome terms:
  enucleation
  unilateral sporadic retinoblastoma
- Measurements of tumors are done with metric terms, as in 15 by 15 by 5.9 mm. Transcribe "by" as x with one space before and after. The abbreviation for millimeters requires no period, and the abbreviation should be keyed only once, at the end of the measurement.

REPORT 5.2 Letter of Referral

- The word *followup* functions as a noun, an adjective, and a verb. Key the term as one word when used as a noun or adjective and as two words when used as a verb. A hyphenated construction (*follow-up*) is also acceptable for adjective uses, but one word is preferred. In this report, *followup* is used three times as a noun. See Chapter 3 for a more complete discussion of compound words.

REPORT 5.3 Consultation Letter

Patient Study 5.B — Ronald Jones

Ronald Jones is a 21-year-old male diagnosed with osteosarcoma. While hospitalized for administration of chemotherapy, he developed difficulty with his vision, and a specialist in ophthalmology, Dr. Regina Smyth, was called as a consultant to assist with this complication.

REPORT 5.4 Consultation Report

- Listen for these difficult terms:
  metastatic osteosarcoma
  scotoma
- Visual acuity results are dictated as two numbers ("twenty twenty") and transcribed as two numerals separated by a diagonal slash, as in 20/20.
- The word *re-examine* requires a hyphen since the prefix ends with the first letter of the following word, *examine.*

REPORT 5.5 Consultation Letter

Patient Study 5.C — Reling Quang

Reling Quang is a 47-year-old secretary who reports that she has been finding it more difficult to see her computer screen and that her eyes tire easily. She has never worn glasses, but thinks that it may be necessary now.

REPORT 5.6 Office Note

- When transcribing visual acuity test results, separate the abbreviation (for example, OD) and the numbers with a space but no comma. However, include a comma between the results for the right and left eyes, as in OD 20/20, OS 20/20.

Patient Study 5.D — Elizabeth Hammers

Elizabeth Hammers is a young woman who has been referred to an ophthalmologist for an opinion about her dimness of vision in the right eye. Although the problem has been present since birth, Elizabeth's primary physician wanted to ensure that no disease process was occurring in the eye.

REPORT 5.7 Consultation Letter

- Listen for these difficult terms:
  afferent
  amblyopic
  cup-to-disc ratio
  disc edema
  dot-and-blot hemorrhage
  fluorescein angiogram
  ischemia
  pupillary
  rubeosis

Patient Study 5.E — Glen Brian

Glen Brian is a child who has a disorder of the eye because of increased pressure within the brain. His pediatrician, Dr. Richard Golden, has referred him to Sanford Guterman, MD, Ophthalmologist, for treatment.

REPORT 5.8 Consultation Letter

- Listen for these difficult terms:
  bimedial rectus recession
  esotropia
  hydrocephalus
  oblique over-action
  strabismus

Patient Study 5.F

Christopher Barney

Christopher Barney is a young man who is diagnosed with acute myeloblastic leukemia. He is being evaluated by the ophthalmologist for followup for visual problems resulting from retinal hemorrhages.

REPORT 5.9 Consultation Letter

- Listen for these difficult terms:
  papilledema
  afferent pupillary defect
  irides (plural of iris)
  dot-to-blot
  vitreous heme

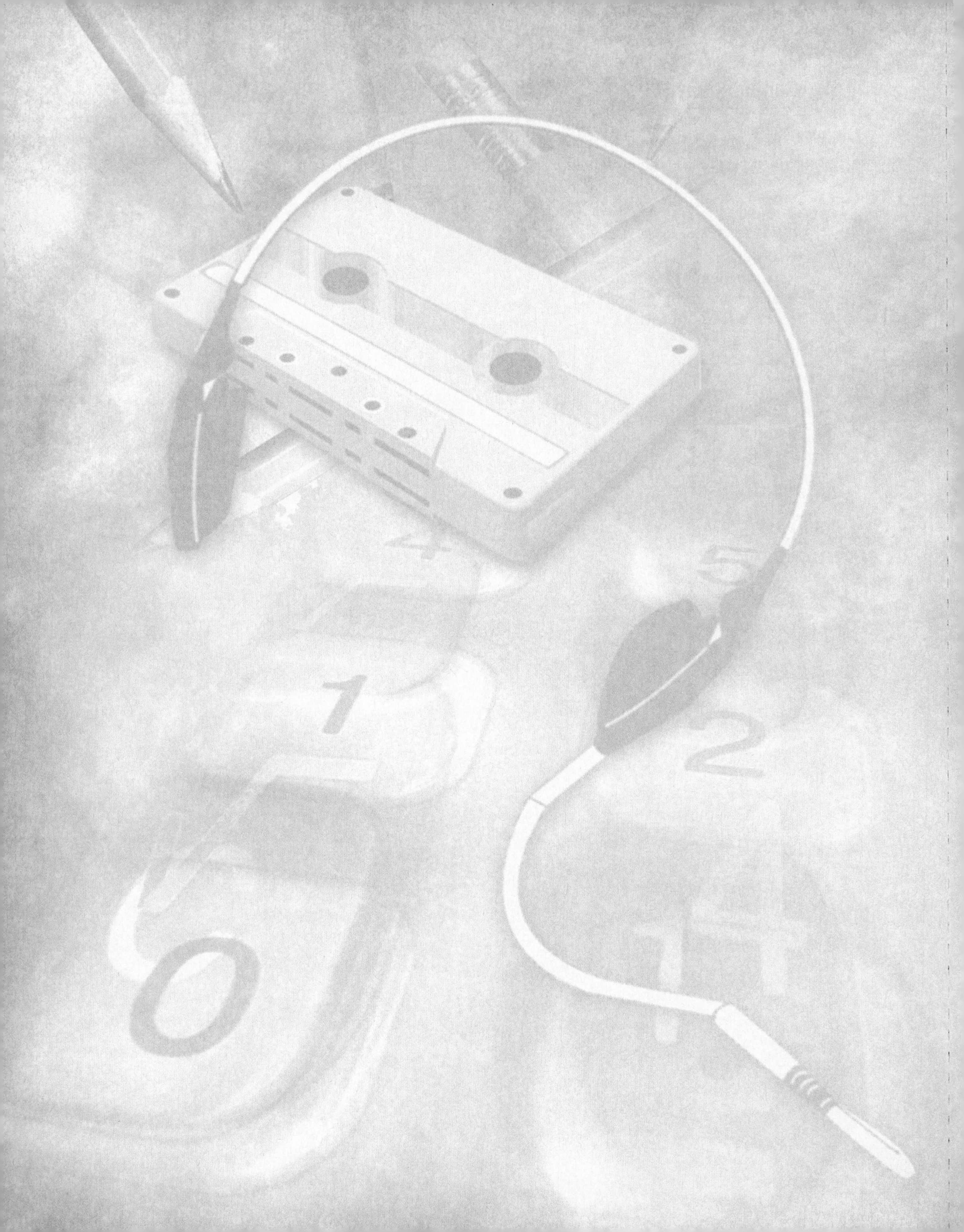

Using Medical References

Use the appropriate medical reference to locate the correct spelling and additional usage information for the words below. (If the reference is not available, use the glossary in this text.) Circle the correct spelling; then write a sentence using the word correctly.

1.	accomodation	accommodation	acommodation
2.	conjunctivi	conjunctiva	conjunktiva
3.	retinopathy	retanopathy	retinopathey
4.	glaucoma	glacoma	gloucoma
5.	phacoemulsification	phacoemulcifikation	phakoemulsiphication
6.	tosis	ptosis	phtosis
7.	nystagmis	nistagymus	nystagmus
8.	cattaract	catarachT	cataract
9.	pterygim	pterygium	terygium
10.	blepharitis	blepharytis	blefaritis

Making Expert Decisions

Circle the correct word from the choices in parentheses.

1. Examination noted the iris, ciliary body, and choroid to be inflamed; thus, the diagnosis of (conjunctivitis/uveitis) was considered.
2. A physician who specializes in the treatment of disorders of the eyes is called an (ophthalmologist/optometrist).
3. The (anterior/posterior) portion of the sclera becomes the cornea.
4. The (macula/macule) revealed a small, patchy lesion on the surface of the skin.
5. The condition whereby the eyes turn toward the nose is called (esotropia/exotropia); turning the eye toward the temple is called (esotropia/exotropia).
6. Examination of the optic nerve for color, shape, and vascularization was performed during (funduscopy/ophthalmoscopy).
7. The patient had yellow (sclerae or scleras/conjunctivae), so we ran liver function tests.
8. The (iris/pupil) regulates the size of the (iris/pupil).
9. The patient squinted downward, indicating (hypertropia/hypotropia).
10. A (cataract/corneal) transplant was done due to excessive scarring.

Transcribing Professional Documents

Transcribe the documents named Chapter 5 Assessment 1 and Assessment 2. Before you key, review the appropriate document formatting guidelines. Proofread your transcribed document and revise it until you think it is error-free.

Otorhinolaryngology

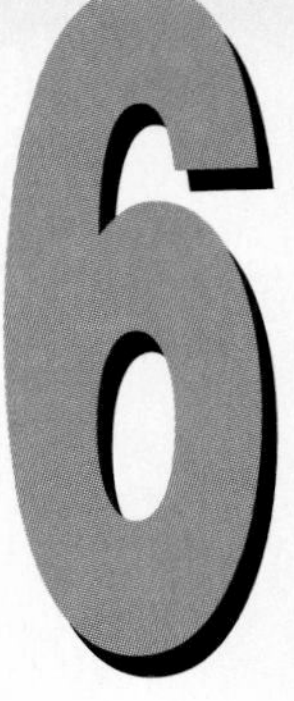

The ears, nose, and throat are important passageways into the body that can be affected by a variety of medical conditions. Otorhinolaryngology, from the Greek for ear *(oto),* nose *(rhis),* and larynx *(larynx),* is the medical specialty that deals with these passageways. Physicians who practice in this area are called otorhinolaryngologists or ENT specialists.

OBJECTIVES

- Use otorhinolaryngology terms correctly according to the context and purpose of the dictation.
- Select and use appropriate general and specialty reference materials.
- Key otorhinolaryngology documents of varying complexity and format.
- Transcribe authentic medical dictation requiring concentration and listening skill.
- Edit medical reports to conform with AAMT style guidelines.
- Proofread and correct transcripts to produce error-free documents.

Exploring Otorhinolaryngology (ENT)

The specialty of otorhinolaryngology is concerned with diseases of the ears, nose, and throat. Because many common illnesses affect the ears, nose, and throat, people frequently visit the doctor with complaints of symptoms affecting these areas. In addition, because the ears and nose are so visible and prominent, people often seek corrective treatment for deformities or malformations of these structures.

Structure and Function

The ear is the organ of hearing and equilibrium. It has three parts: the external, middle, and inner ear. Figure 6.1 shows the sections of the ear, consisting of the external auricle, or pinna, and the external ear canal. The auricle is designed to collect sound waves from the air and conduct them through the external ear canal into the middle ear. Figure 6.2 shows the structures of the inner ear.

When sound waves enter the ear canal, they strike against the tympanic membrane, or eardrum, which is located at the outer end of the middle ear (also called the tympanic cavity). From the tympanic membrane, the sound waves pass through bones called the ossicles. The ossicles include the malleus (hammer), the incus (anvil), and the stapes (stirrup). All of the parts of the ossicular chain (group of three ear bones) must be working properly for the sound-pressure ratio to be in balance and for hearing to be in the normal range.

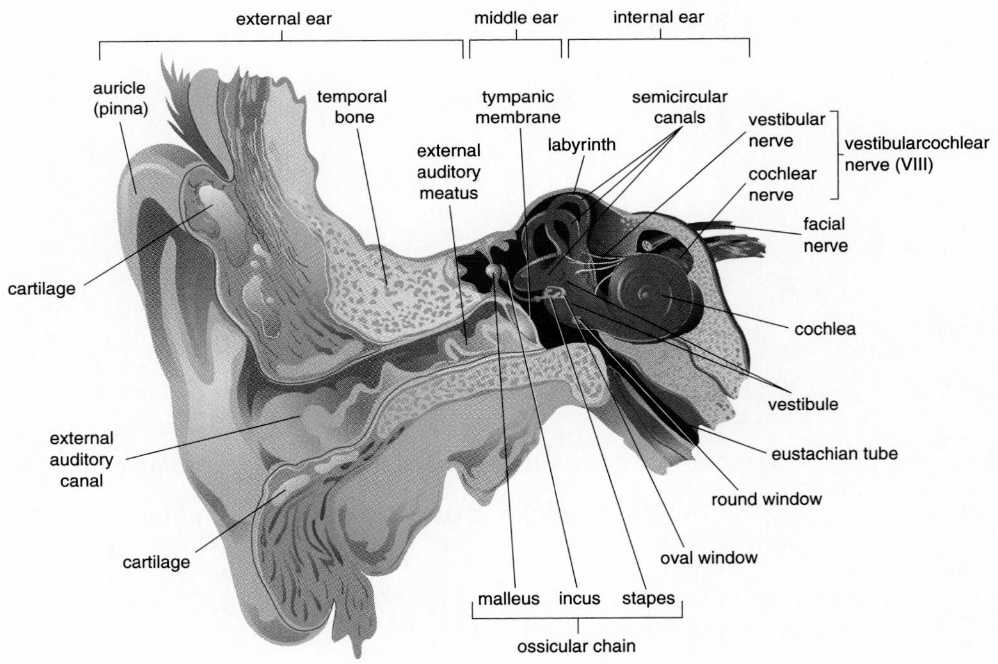

FIGURE 6.1
Divisions of the Ear: External, Middle, and Inner Ear

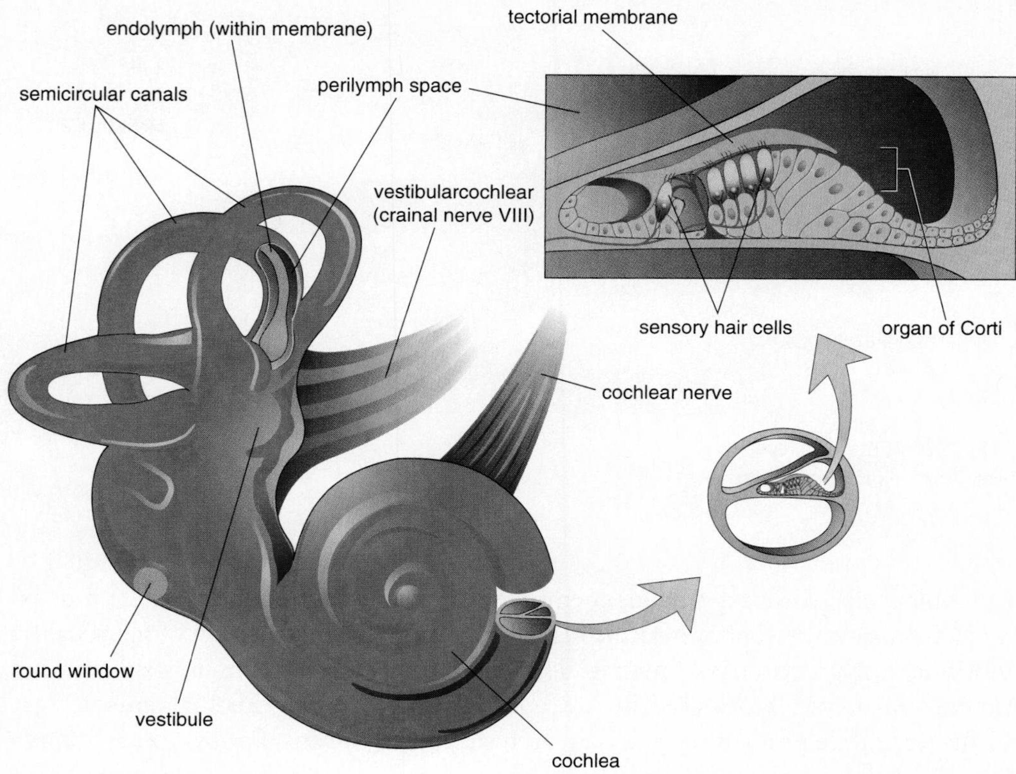

FIGURE 6.2
Structures of the Inner Ear

The structures of the inner ear, or labyrinth, include the cochlea, the vestibule, and the semicircular canals, as well as the auditory and vestibular receptors of the eighth cranial nerve (the vestibulocochlear nerve). The inner ear receives sound waves when the stapes gently pushes on the membrane of the oval window, or fenestra ovalis, forcing fluid to move within the cochlea. This moving fluid stimulates nerve endings on the hairs of Corti within the cochlea. The auditory nerve transmits the neural stimulation to the brain, where it is interpreted as sound.

Cerumen, or ear wax, is a normal byproduct of a healthy ear. It prevents foreign particles from entering the passageway. Cerumen is produced by glands in the middle ear.

The eustachian tube connects the middle ear with the nasal passages and larynx. This tube equalizes the pressure on the two sides of the eardrum.

The nose is an important structure with multiple functions. Besides being the organ of smell, the nose is the passageway for air into the sinuses and the respiratory tract. It assists with the production of sound during speech and is the disposal system for tears. In addition, the mucous membrane within the nose catches inhaled dust and germs and moistens and warms air as it enters the body.

A cartilage called the septum divides the nose into right and left nasal cavities. The lateral wall of the septum contains three bony structures: the inferior, middle, and superior turbinates, or conchae. The nasal cavities open into the paranasal sinuses—frontal, maxillary, ethmoid, and sphenoid sinuses (see Figure 6.3).

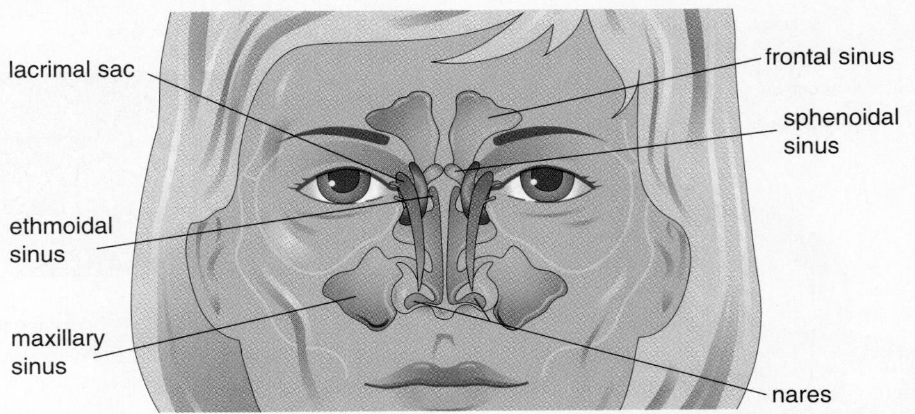

FIGURE 6.3
The Paranasal Sinuses

Goblet cells, within a mucous membrane covering, continuously secrete mucus. This mucus is moved back into the nasopharynx by the ciliary action of hairs, called vibrissae, within the nasal cavities. The nasal passages also contain sophisticated nervous tissue which detects odors and promotes sneezing to expel irritants.

Above and behind the tongue is an arch shaped by the anterior and posterior pillars, soft palate, and uvula. The tonsils, made of lymphoid tissue, form a protective ring in the mouth and back of the throat where they filter invasive particles from the nose and mouth. As the first line of defense against the outside environment, the tonsils often become infected. Figure 6.4 shows the three sets of tonsils: the palatine tonsils, located on each side of the throat; the pharyngeal tonsils, or adenoids, located in the posterior opening of the nasopharynx; and the lingual tonsils, located on both sides of the base of the tongue.

The larynx, or voice box, is a cartilaginous structure containing the pharynx and the trachea. The principal function of the larynx is vocalization. It contains the epiglottis, the glottis, and the thyroid and cricoid cartilage, as shown in Figure 6.5.

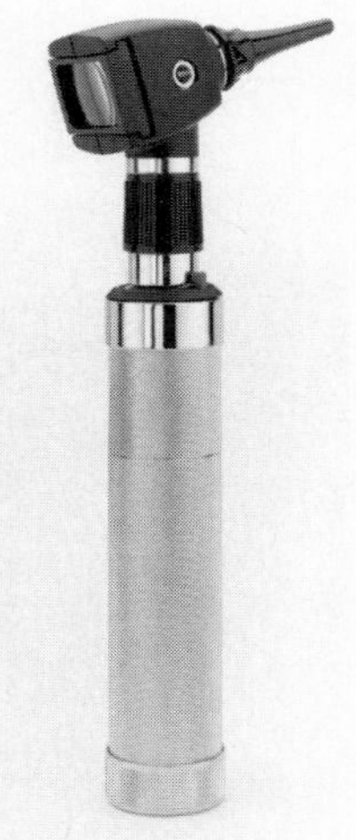

The otoscope's bright light allows the physician to examine the patient's ears, nose, or throat

Physical Assessment

The physician assesses the ears, nose, and throat through otoscopy, using an instrument called an otoscope. The otoscope is equipped with a bright light; it illuminates and magnifies internal areas.

During physical examination of the ear, the speculum is inserted into the external auditory meatus. The physician can see a portion of the tympanic membrane and important landmarks: the malleus, the annulus, and Wilde's triangle, which is a triangular area that under normal conditions reflects the otoscope's light. A normal tympanic membrane should be flat or concave and pearly gray in color. It should reflect a good cone of light.

The physician also observes the external areas of the ears, nose, and throat for abnormalities such as low-set ears (which may indicate genetic syndromes), malformations, or discharge.

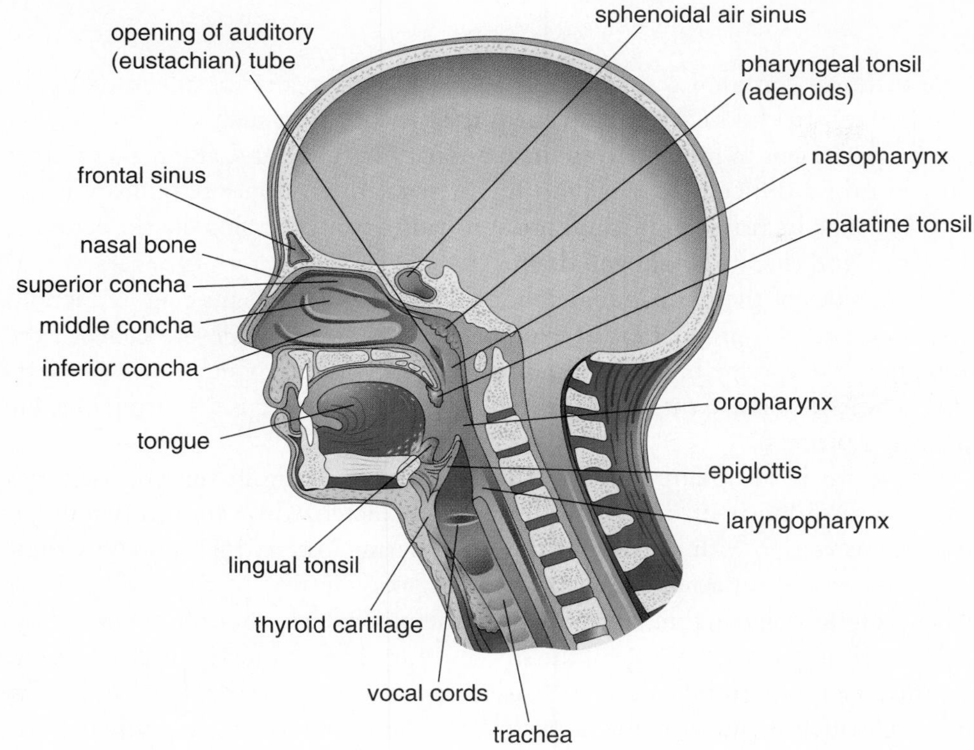

FIGURE 6.4
Sagittal View of the Head and Neck

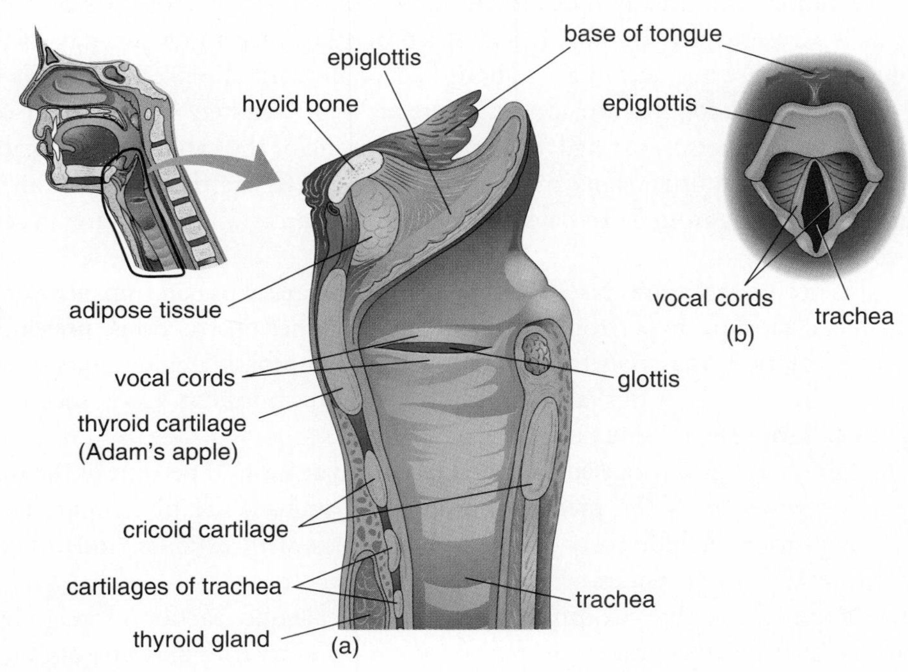

FIGURE 6.5
Structures within the Neck *(a) Sagittal view (b) Superior view*

Diseases and Conditions

One of the most common complaints of the ear is otitis media, an inflammation of the middle ear. In children, the eustachian tube is curved in such a manner that it is easy for pathogens to migrate from the nasopharynx. The curve also makes proper drainage of fluid difficult, especially in the presence of an upper respiratory infection (URI). The increase in fluid and pressure causes pain; occasionally the eardrum will rupture and then the fluid will drain.

Abnormalities of the tympanic membrane include injection, bulging, retraction, perforation, and the production of exudate. Ear diseases include otosclerosis, the hardening of the spongy bone surrounding the oval window, which results in hearing loss; cholesteatoma, a tumor in the middle ear; and presbycusis, hearing loss due to the aging process.

Labyrinthitis is an inflammation of the inner ear resulting in vertigo. Meniere's disease is a disturbance of the labyrinth that is characterized by various manifestations, such as vertigo with or without tinnitus, hearing loss, and nausea and vomiting. Balance may be affected because of the vertigo.

There can be congenital malformations of the nose which not only are unsightly, but also cause improper drainage of the sinuses, tears, and/or mucus. Malformations make the area prone to infections such as sinusitis. When chronic, this can lead to meningitis (inflammation of the surrounding brain tissue). The septum may be deviated or perforated.

Because the nose is often exposed to the sun's dangerous ultraviolet light, it is one of the most common sites of basal cell or squamous cell carcinomas, both malignant skin tumors.

The common cold usually refers to an upper respiratory infection (URI). Colds are actually viruses which are shed (transmitted to others) for about two days before symptoms appear. They account for about half of all work absences. Winter is the most common time for colds to appear. There are approximately 100 different cold viruses, but once a person has had a particular virus, he or she can no longer "catch" that cold again. The usual signs and symptoms of a URI are rhinitis, pharyngitis, and laryngitis lasting from 5–14 days. Coryza (acute rhinitis) is the term for an acute head cold.

Sinusitis occurs as a result of a URI in persons whose nasal passages are obstructed by a deviated septum, hypertrophied turbinates, or other obstructions, preventing fluids and infectious materials from draining. The symptoms include pressure and pain over the affected sinus areas, with or without purulent nasal secretions. Allergens can cause acute sinus infections.

Although pharyngitis is caused by a viral pathogen at least 70 percent of the time, group A *Streptococcus* is the most common cause of bacterial pharyngitis (strep throat). Symptoms include pain, fever, swollen tonsils with exudate, and enlarged and often tender lymph nodes.

Obstruction of the pharynx can occur from severe allergic reactions, foreign bodies, or epiglottitis, usually caused by *Haemophilus influenzae.* Epiglottitis can create a partial or complete airway obstruction, leading to a medical emergency. Other common conditions of the upper airway include sleep apnea syndrome, tonsillitis, and chronic cryptic tonsillitis.

Common Tests and Surgical Procedures

A patient's hearing at various sound frequencies can be assessed through audiometry, which measures nerve conduction. Other common hearing tests include the Rinne test and the Weber test.

Airway obstructions are cleared in an emergency by means of the Heimlich maneuver, designed to force food or other obstructions from the airway; severe obstructions may require an emergency tracheotomy to create an artificial airway.

Common ENT procedures include tonsillectomies and adenoidectomies, which may be performed in patients who have had recurrent bouts of tonsillitis that have caused enlarged tonsils and adenoids or in those who have hearing loss from frequent infections.

In cancers of the larynx, an ENT specialist may perform a laryngectomy, which can involve partial or complete removal of the organs of the larynx, depending upon the extent of the cancer involved.

ENT physicians also perform numerous constructive or reconstructive surgeries: otoplasty to correct an ear deformity, myringoplasty and tympanoplasty to reconstruct the eardrum, and myringotomy, most common in small children, to place a small tube into the eardrum in order to provide proper drainage of fluid from the middle ear.

Dacryocystorhinostomy is a surgical procedure for creating an opening into the nose for the drainage of tears. Rhinoplasty is the surgical restructuring of the nose, which can be performed for cosmetic reasons or for medical necessity—to improve breathing, for example.

Building Language Skills

The following tables list common otorhinolaryngology terms, drugs, and abbreviations. The list of terms and definitions includes the most difficult words contained in the dictated reports in this chapter. These words are identified in GREEN type. A list of common drugs is found in Appendix D.

Medical Terms and Pharmacologic Agents

adenitis
(ad-e-**nI**-tis) (n) inflammation of a lymph node or gland

adenoidectomy
(**ad**-e-noy-**dek**-tO-mee) (n) surgical removal of the adenoids from the nasopharynx

ala nasi
(**a**-la **nay**-sI) (adj) the outer flare of each nostril; alae nasi (**a**-lee) (pl)

allergen
(**al**-er-jen) (n) a substance that produces an allergic reaction

amphotericin
(**am**-fO-tear-a-sin) (n) a toxic antibiotic reserved for use in serious, potentially fatal infections of fungi and protozoa; amphotericin B

amplitude
(**am**-pli-tood) (n) the extent of a vibrating or alternating movement or wave from the average to the extreme; a louder sound has a greater amplitude

annulus
(**an**-yoo-lus) (n) a circular structure or opening

arytenoid
(ar-i-**tee**-noyd) (n) cartilage and muscles of the larynx

audiologic
(aw-dee-O-**loj**-ik) (adj) pertaining to hearing disorders or loss

audiometry
(aw-dee-**om**-e-tree) (n) test used to measure hearing (using an audiometer)

aural
(**aw**-ral) (adj) relating to the ear

auricle
(**aw**-ri-kl) (n) external ear; pinna

buccal
(**buk**-al) (adj) relating to the area inside the cheek

cavernous sinus thrombosis
(**kav**-er-nus **sI**-nus throm-**bO**-sis) (n) a group of symptoms caused by an obstruction in the cavernous intracranial sinus

cerumen
(se-**roo**-men) (n) earwax

cholesteatoma
(kO-les-tee-a-**tO**-ma) (n) a tumor-like mass of scaly epithelium and cholesterol in the middle ear

ciliary action
(**sil**-ee-ar-ee) (n) the lashing movement of a group of cilia, which can produce a current of movement in a fluid

cochlea
(**kok**-lee-a) (n) a spiral-shaped cavity in the internal ear

concha
(**kon**-ka) (n) a shell-shaped anatomical structure, such as the auricle of the ear; conchae (pl)

conductive deafness
(n) hearing impairment due to obstruction of sound waves; the sound waves are not passed on to the inner ear

coryza
(ko-**rI**-za) (n) acute rhinitis; acute head cold; inflammation of the mucous membrane of the nose with sneezing, tearing, and watery nasal discharge

cricoid cartilage
(**krI**-koyd) (n) a ring-shaped cartilage in the lower part of the larynx

culture
(**kul**-chur) (n) propagation of microorganisms in a solid or liquid medium

dacryocystorhinostomy
(**dak**-ree-O-**sis**-tO-rI-**nos**-tO-mee) (n) a surgical opening to provide drainage between the tear duct and the nasal mucosa

debride
(da-**breed**/dee-**brId**) (v) to remove unhealthy tissue and foreign material to prevent infection and permit healing

distress
(n) trouble; mental or physical suffering

dysphagia
(dis-**fay**-jee-a) (n) difficulty swallowing

en bloc
(ahn blok) (adj) as a whole, in one piece

epiglottis
(**ep**-I-**glot**-is) (n) flap of elastic cartilage at the back of the mouth that covers the opening to the windpipe during swallowing, thereby preventing choking.

epiglottitis
(ep-i-glot-**tI**-tis) (n) inflammation of the epiglottis, causing potentially fatal airway obstruction, especially in small children

epistaxis
(**ep**-i-**stak**-sis) (n) nosebleed

ethmoidal
(eth-**moy**-dal) (adj) relating to the ethmoid bone or ethmoid sinus

eustachian tube
(yoo-**stay**-shun/yoo-**stay**-kee-an) (n) a tube leading from the middle ear to the nasopharynx; thus air pressure is equalized on both sides of the tympanic membrane

excision
(ek-**si**-zhun) (n) cutting out; surgical removal of all or part of a lesion, structure, or organ

exudate
(**eks**-oo-dayt) (n) any fluid that has oozed out of a tissue, usually due to inflammation or injury

exudative
(**eks**-oo-dayt-iv) (adj) relating to exudate

fenestra ovalis
(fe-**nes**-tra O-**val**-is) (n) an oval opening between the middle ear and the vestibule; closed by the base of the stapes

fixation
(fik-**say**-shun) (n) process of securing a part, as by suturing

foramen
(fO-**ray**-men) (n) hole or opening, especially in a bone or membrane

gingival
(**jin**-ji-val) (adj) relating to the gums

glossopharyngeal neuralgia
(**glos**-O-fa-**rin**-jee-al noo-**ral**-jee-a) (n) a condition of sharp spasmic pain in the throat or palate

helix
(**hee**-liks) (n) the folded edge of the external ear

incus
(**ing**-kus) (n) the anvil-shaped bone in the middle ear

jugular
(**jug**-yoo-lar) (adj) relating to the throat or neck

labial
(**lay**-bee-al) (adj) relating to the lips

labyrinth
(**lab**-i-rinth) (n) an anatomical structure made up of a complex of cavities, such as the inner ear

labyrinthitis
(**lab**-i-rin-**thI**-tis) (n) inflammation of the inner ear (labyrinth) or ethmoidal labyrinth (nose)

lacrimation
(**lak**-ri-**may**-shun) (n) secretion of tears

laryngectomy
(**lar**-in-**jek**-tO-mee) (n) surgical removal of the larynx

laryngostomy
(**lar**-ing-**gos**-tO-mee) (n) surgically creating an opening into the larynx

larynx
(**lar**-ingks) (n) the voice box, located between the pharynx and the trachea

lucency
(**loo**-sen-see) (n) giving off light; being luminous or translucent

lymph
(limf) (n) fluid that bathes the tissues of the body and circulates through lymphatic vessels

malleus
(**mal**-ee-us) (n) the largest of the three inner ear bones; club-shaped; attached to the tympanic membrane

mandibular
(man-**dib**-yoo-lar) (adj) relating to the lower jaw

mastoiditis
(mas-toy-**dI**-tis) (n) inflammation of the mastoid process (part of the temporal bone behind the ear)

maxilla
(mak-**sil**-a) (n) the upper jaw

maxillary sinus
(**mak**-si-layr-ee **sI**-nus) (n) an air cavity in the body of the upper jaw bone; connects with the middle passage (meatus) of the nose

meatus
(mee-**ay**-tus) (n) a passage or channel, especially with an external opening

Meniere's disease
(mayn-**yairz**) (n) a disease of the inner ear with attacks of dizziness, nausea, ringing in the ear, and increasing deafness

meninges
(me-**nin**-jeez) (n) membranes covering the brain and spinal cord

meningitis
(men-in-**jI**-tis) (n) inflammation of the meninges

mucoperiosteum
(**myoo**-kO-per-ee-**os**-tee-um) (n) the mucous membrane covering the hard palate at the front of the roof of the mouth

mucosa
(myoo-**kO**-sa) (n) mucous membrane

myringitis
(mir-in-**jI**-tis) (n) inflammation of the tympanic membrane; tympanitis

myringoplasty
(mi-**ring**-gO-**plas**-tee) (n) surgical repair of the eardrum

myringotomy
(mir-ing-**got**-o-mee) (n) surgical incision into the tympanic membrane

nafcillin
(naf-**sill**-in) (n) an antibiotic; one of the varieties of penicillin

naris
(**nay**-ris) (n) nostril; nares (**nay**-rees) (pl)

neoadjuvant
(nee-O-**ad**-joo-vant) (adj) used in conjunction with other types of therapy

neuroblastoma
(**noor**-O-blas-**tO**-ma) (n) malignant (cancerous) tumor containing embryonic nerve cells

neuroectodermal
(**noo**-rO-ek-tO-**der**-mal) (adj) embryonic tissue that gives rise to nerve tissue

node
(nOd) (n) a small knot of tissue, distinct from surrounding tissue; a lymph node

orbital cellulitis
(**or**-bit-al sel-yoo-**lI**-tis) (n) inflammation of tissue around or behind the eye

organism
(**or**-ga-nizm) (n) a living plant, animal, or microorganism

orifice
(**or**-i-fis) (n) an opening

ossicles
(os-i-kls) (n) small bones, such as the auditory ossicles (the three bones of the inner ear)

ostectomy
(os-**tek**-tO-mee) (n) surgical removal of all or part of a bone

otalgia
(**Otal**-jeea) (n) earache

otitis externa
(O-**tI**-tis eks-**ter**-na) (n) inflammation of the external ear

otitis media
(O-**tI**-tis **mee**-dee-a) (n) inflammation of the middle ear

otorhinolaryngology
(**O**-tO-**rI**-nO-lar-in-**gol**-o-jee) (n) study of the ears, nose, and throat

otosclerosis
(**O**-tO-sklee-**rO**-sis) (n) a growth of sponge-like bone in the inner ear, eventually leading to deafness

otoscope
(**O**-tO-skOp) (n) an instrument for examining the eardrum

otoscopy
(O-**tos**-kO-pee) (n) visual examination of the ear with an otoscope

ototoxic
(O-to-**tok**-sic) (adj) harmful to the organs of hearing or auditory nerve

palpable
(**pal**-pa-bl) (adj) able to be identified by touch

palate
(**pal**-at) (n) the roof of one's mouth, composed of the hard palate (front) and the soft palate (back)

pathogen
(**path**-O-jen) (n) any microorganism or substance that can cause a disease

periauricular
(**per**-ee-aw-**rik**-yoo-lar) (adj) around the ear

pharyngitis
(far-in-jI-tis) (n) inflammation of the pharynx

pharynx
(**far**-ingks) (n) throat; passageway for air from nasal cavity to larynx, and food from mouth to esophagus

pinna
(**pin**-a) (n) the external ear; auricle; pinnae (**pin**-ee) (pl)

polyp
(**pol**-ip) (n) an outgrowth of tissue from a mucous membrane

presbycusis
(**prez**-bee-**koo**-sis) (n) the loss of hearing acuity due to aging

pterygoid plate
(**ter**-i-goyd) (n) wing-shaped bones at the back of the nasal cavity

purulent
(**pyoor**-u-lent) (adj) relating to, containing, or forming pus

resection
(ree-**sek**-shun) (n) surgical removal of a portion of a structure or organ

rhinitis
(rI-**nI**-tis) (n) inflammation of the mucous membrane of the nose

rhinoplasty
(**rI**-nO-plas-tee) (n) surgery to correct a defect in the nose or to change its shape

Rinne test
(**rin**-ne) (n) also Rinne's (**rin**-ez); a hearing test comparing perception of air and bone conduction in one ear with a tuning fork; normally air conduction is more acute

semicircular canals
(**sem**-ee-**sir**-kyoo-lar ka-**nals**) (n) three fluid-filled loops in the labyrinth of the inner ear, associated with the body's sense of balance

sensorineural deafness
(**sen**-sOr-i-**noor**-al) (n) hearing impairment due to nerve disturbance

septum
(**sep**-tum) (n) division between two cavities or two masses of tissue, such as the nasal septum; septa (pl)

serous
(**seer**-us) (adj) relating to or having a watery consistency

serous otitis media
(**seer**-us O-**tI**-tis **mee**-dee-a) (n) inflammation of the middle ear accompanied by production of a watery fluid (serum)

shotty
(**shot**-ee) (adj) resembling shot (hard pellets) to the touch; as shotty nodes

sinus
(**sI**-nus) (n) a passageway or hollow in a bone or other tissue

sinusitis
(sI-nu-**sI**-tis) (n) inflammation of the nasal sinuses, occurring as a result of an upper respiratory infection, an allergic response, or a defect of the nose

sleep apnea syndrome
(**ap**-nee-a) (n) breathing stops, briefly and periodically, due to partial upper airway obstruction during sleep

speculum
(**spek**-yoo-lum) (n) an instrument used for examining the interior of a cavity

sphenoidal sinus
(sfee-**noy**-dal) (n) one of two sinuses in the sphenoid bone opening to the nasal cavity

stapes
(**stay**-peez) (n) the smallest and innermost of the three auditory bones in the inner ear; stirrup

strep
(n) short form of Streptococcus, a genus of bacteria; many species cause disease in humans

submandibular
(sub-man-**dib**-yoo-lar) (adj) under the lower jaw

supratentorial
(**soo**-pra-ten-**tO**-ree-al) (adj) located above the tentorium, a tent-like structure

symphysis
(**sim**-fi-sis) (n) joint in which fibrocartilage firmly unites the bones

thyroid
(**thI**-royd) (n) a gland in the neck that secretes thyroid hormone

tinnitus
(ti-**nI**-tus) (n) noise, such as ringing, in the ears

tonsils
(**ton**-silz) (n) lymphoid tissue structures in the oropharynx

trachea
(**tray**-kee-a) (n) the windpipe

tracheostomy
(**tray**-kee-**os**-tO-mee) (n) a surgical opening into the trachea

tracheotomy
(**tray**-kee-**ot**-O-mee) (n) the surgical procedure in which a tracheostomy is created

tragus
(**tray**-gus) (n) the small projection of cartilage in front of the external opening to the ear canal

turbinate
(**ter**-bi-nayt) (n) one of several thin, spongy, bony plates within the walls of the nasal cavity

tympanic membrane
(tim-**pan**-ik) (n) eardrum

tympanometric
(**tim**-pa-nO-**met**-rik) (adj) pertaining to tympanometry, a procedure for evaluation of motility of eardrum and middle ear disorders

tympanoplasty
(**tim**-pa-nO-plas-tee) (n) surgical repair of the middle ear

umbo
(**um**-bO) (n) the inner surface of the tympanic membrane where it connects with the malleus in the middle ear

unremarkable
(adj) nothing unusual is noted

upper respiratory infection (URI)
(n) an infection of the upper respiratory tract such as the common cold, laryngitis, sinusitis, and tonsillitis

uvula
(**yoo**-vyoo-la) (n) small, fleshy mass hanging from the soft palate in the mouth

uvulitis
(yoo-vyoo-**lI**-tis) (n) inflammation of the uvula

uvulopalatopharyngoplasty
(**yoo**-vyoo-lO-**pal**-a-tO-fa-**rin**-gO-plas-tee) (n) UPPP for short; a surgical treatment for sleep apnea for patients who cannot tolerate or respond to medical therapies

vertigo
(**ver**-tigO) (n) dizziness

vestibulum
(ves-**tib**-yoo-lum) (n) the central cavity of the labyrinth in the inner ear, between the cochlea and the semicircular canals

vibrissae
(vI-**bris**-a) (n) nose hairs

Weber test
(**web**-er) (n) a hearing test performed with a tuning fork placed at points in the middle of the skull to determine where the vibration is heard (not where it is felt)

xerostomia
(zeer-O-**stO**-mee-a) (n) dryness of the mouth

Abbreviations

AC	air conduction
AD	right ear (auris dextra)
AOM	acute otitis media
AS	left ear (auris sinistra)
C&S	culture and sensitivity
dB	decibel
EAC	external ear canal
EENT	eye, ear, nose, throat
ENT	ear, nose, throat
PE tubes	pressure-equalizing tubes
SAR	seasonal allergic rhinitis
T&A	tonsillectomy and adenoidectomy
TM	tympanic membrane
TMJ	temporomandibular joint
UPPP	uvulopalatopharyngoplasty
URI	upper respiratory infection

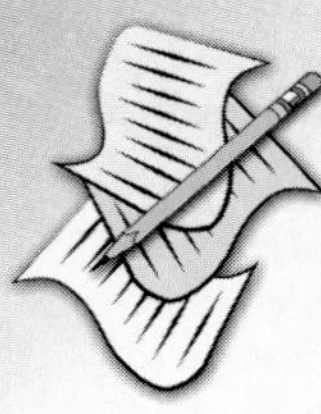

EXERCISE 6.1

Recognizing Look-Alikes and Sound-Alikes

Below is a list of frequently used words that look alike and/or sound alike. Study the meaning and pronunciation of each set of words, then read the following sentences carefully and circle the word in parentheses that correctly completes the meaning.

assistance	aiding, helping
assistants	individuals who give aid and support
aural	pertaining to the ear
oral	pertaining to the mouth
auricle	external ear
oracle	a wise person; a god-like person
dysphagia	difficulty swallowing
dysphasia	difficulty using language due to injury or disease
dysphonia	difficulty in speaking
dysphoria	depression
malleus	a structure in the inner ear
malleolus	a rounded bone on either side of the ankle
laryngitis	inflammation of the larynx
pharyngitis	inflammation of the pharynx
osteal	bony or bonelike
ostial	relating to an ostium (a small opening, e.g., eustachian tube)
passed	past tense of verb pass; to move, to accomplish
past	time that has gone by
serious	not joking
serous	resembling serum
shoddy	inferior or imitation goods
shotty	resembling shot to the touch
subtle	hard to detect
supple	limber
tendinitis or tendonitis	inflammation of a tendon
tinnitus	ringing in the ears

1. (Aural, Oral) examination revealed cerumen in the canal.
2. Examination of the mouth reveals no (aural, oral) lesions.
3. The patient complains of tenderness around the (auricle, oracle).
4. Examination of the neck revealed a few (shoddy, shotty) nodes.
5. I feel great. I (passed, past) my exam!
6. The patient thinks his (tendinitis, tinnitus) and headache symptoms may be associated with his high blood pressure.
7. Examination of the face revealed only (subtle, supple) changes in the pigmentation of the skin.
8. NECK: (Subtle, Supple) without masses.
9. We will be adding three new medical (assistance, assistants) to the staff this month.
10. Could you please give me some (assistance, assistants) in lifting this patient?

11. While the patient was making a (serious, serous) effort to get out of bed, we noticed the (serious, serous) drainage from his ear.
12. The eustachian tube is blocked, the eardrum is retracted, and the (malleolus, malleus) looks shorter and more horizontal.
13. The injury resulted from a rolling bowling ball, which caused a fractured (malleolus, malleus).
14. A sore throat with (dysphagia, dysphasia) made the child uncomfortable when eating solid foods.
15. The patient's (osteal, ostial) opening was about 1.2 centimeters.

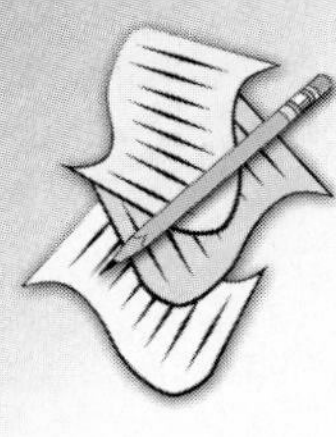

EXERCISE 6.2

Matching Sound and Spelling

The numbered list that follows shows the phonetic spelling of hard-to-spell words. Sound out the word, then write the correct spelling in the blank space provided. Each of the words can be found in the Glossary or in the drug list in Appendix D.

1. nee-O-**ad**-joo-vant ________________
2. **pyoor**-u-lent ________________
3. yoo-**stay**-shun ________________
4. **aw**-ri-kl ________________
5. fO-**ray**-men ________________
6. **per**-ee-aw-**rik**-yoo-lar ________________
7. **nay**-ris ________________
8. **ver**-ti-gO ________________
9. tim-**pan**-ik **mem**-brayn ________________
10. **sim**-fi-sis ________________
11. O-**tal**-jee-a ________________
12. **mal**-ee-us ________________
13. ti-**nI**-tus ________________
14. **loo**-sen-see ________________
15. ep-i-**stak**-sis ________________

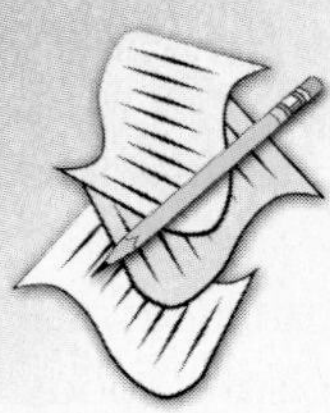

EXERCISE 6.3

Choosing Words from Context

When transcribing dictation, the medical transcriptionist frequently needs to consider the situation when determining the word that correctly completes the sentence. From the list below, select the term that meaningfully completes each of the following statements.

buccal	jugular	otitis
culture	laryngostomy	palpable
erythematous	mandibular	purulent
excision	mastoiditis	shotty
exudate	node	

1. Examination of the external ear showed a periauricular lymph _________ .
2. DIAGNOSIS: Upper respiratory infection, with acute bilateral __________ media.
3. The central line was changed from her right subclavian to her right internal __________.
4. Her throat is slightly red; however, no drainage or ___________ is noted.
5. The patient's throat _________ came back positive for strep.
6. The examining physician found a (an) ___________ mass in the abdomen.
7. The tympanic membrane on the right is ___________ and bulging.
8. The en bloc ____________ to remove the tumor left a large scar.
9. I instructed the patient to call us promptly if she develops any __________ drainage from the wound site.
10. Mr. Johnson had large open sores on his gingiva and ________ cavity on the right side of his mouth.

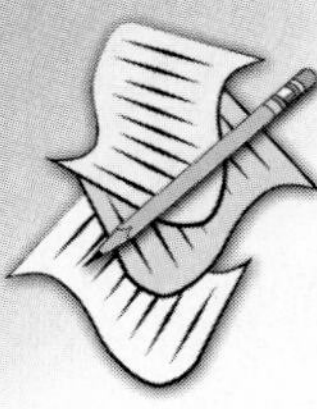

EXERCISE 6.4

Pairing Words and Meanings

From this list, locate the term that best matches each of the following definitions. Write the letter of the term in the space provided by each definition.

A.	gingival	F.	neuroblastoma	J.	tracheostomy
B.	labial	G.	otitis	K.	aural
C.	mandibular	H.	pathogen	L.	cerumen
D.	mastoiditis	I.	periauricular	M.	buccal
E.	myringotomy				

1. around the ear ____________________
2. inflammation of the ear ____________________
3. opening created surgically in the trachea ____________________
4. relating to the gums ____________________
5. relating to the lower jaw ____________________
6. substance capable of producing a disease ____________________
7. pertaining to the lips ____________________
8. infection of the mastoid bones ____________________
9. surgical incision into tympanic membrane ____________________
10. malignant tumor of nerve cells ____________________

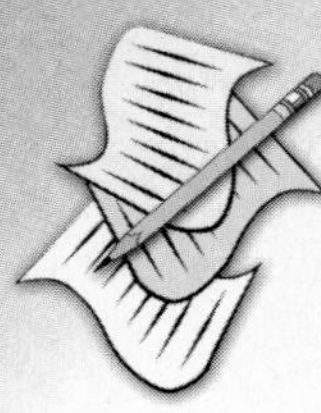

EXERCISE 6.5

Creating Terms from Word Forms

Combine prefixes, root words, and suffixes from this list to create medical words that fit the following definitions. Fill in the blanks with the words you construct.

a-	without, absence	-auricular	pertaining to the ear
dys-	difficult	-blastoma	malignant cell/tumor
ex-	out	-cision	to cut
laryng/o-	larynx	-ectomy	removal of body structure
neur/o-	nerve	-gen	to produce
or/o-	mouth	-itis	inflammation or infection
oste/o-	bone	-mandibular	lower jaw
oto-	ear	-pharyng/o	throat
peri-	around	-phonia	voice; sound
rhin-	nose	-stomy	artificial or surgical opening
sub-	beneath, under		

1. loss of voice ______
2. difficulty in speaking ______
3. cut out ______
4. surgical opening into the larynx ______
5. malignant tumor containing nerve cells ______
6. surgical excision of a bone ______
7. inflammation of the ear ______
8. middle of the throat, between roof of mouth and upper edge of epiglottis ______
9. surrounding the ear ______
10. inflammation of the nasal mucosa ______

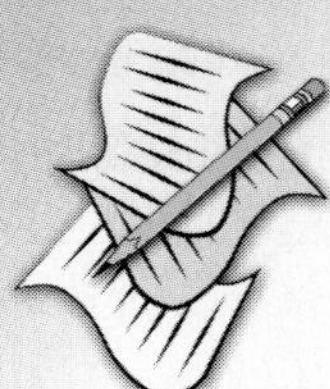

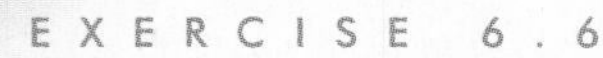

Proofreading Review

Read the following partial report and look for errors in format, usage, and spelling. Circle the errors, then key the report with the errors corrected.

CHIEF COMPLAINT: The patient Had been well until about four wks ago when he develloped a runy nose, sore throat, and pain in both ears. He was seen by his peditritian, who gave him an antibiotic for seven days. Two week later the ear pain has not resolved.

PAST MEDICAL HX: Noncontributory.

PHYSICAL EXAMINATION: L TM is injected with whitish exadate. Palpable shoddy L submandibalar lymph nodes and a 2 cm firm periaurcular lymph node. Physical exam is otherwise within normal limits.

Building Transcription Skills

The Operative Report

The operative report (Figure 6.6) is a narrative description of an operation or other invasive procedure. The surgeon or an assistant to the surgeon dictates the report. This type of document is often quite long and detailed. It is likely to be the most technically demanding report a medical transcriptionist will encounter.

Required Headings/Content Operative reports are variously structured but usually include the preoperative and postoperative diagnoses, the surgeon's name, the title and date of the procedure, the indications for surgery, the anesthesia, the surgical findings, the specimen removed, and the actual description of the surgery, called the procedure. The report usually contains a sponge count and an estimate of blood loss. It typically ends with the patient being taken to the recovery room.

Other headings in the operative report may include the assistant surgeon's name, the name of the anesthesiologist, type of incision, drains used, complications. The operative report may also include information on when an informed consent document was presented by the surgeon and signed by the patient.

Many hospitals break down the operative description into three sections: (1) positioning, prepping and draping, and opening the incision; (2) the internal operation; and (3) the closing.

Turnaround Time An operative report is dictated or written in the medical record immediately after surgery and ideally transcribed within six hours. This guideline applies to all surgical procedures done in hospitals, outpatient surgical centers, and clinics.

Preparing to Transcribe

To prepare for transcribing dictation, review the tables of common otorhinolaryngology terms, drugs, and abbreviations presented in the Building Language Skills section of this chapter. Then, study the format and organization of the model document shown in Figure 6.6, and key the model document. Proofread the document by comparing it with the printed version. Categorize the types of errors you made, and document them on a copy of the Performance Comparison chart provided in Chapter 1. A template of this chart is included on the IRC that accompanies this text.

Patient Studies

Transcribe, edit, and correct each report in the following patient studies. Consult reference books for words or formatting rules that are unfamiliar.

As you work on the transcription assignment for this chapter, fill in the Performance Comparison chart that you started when you keyed the model document. For at least three of the reports, categorize and document the types of errors you made. Answer the document analysis questions on the bottom of the chart. With continuous practice and assessment, the quality of your work will improve.

After you have produced a final version of each transcribed report, complete the Performance Report cover sheet, attach it to the top of the transcripts, and submit them to your instructor for evaluation.

1" top and side margins

Aligning information at tab settings is another acceptable format

NAME: Jane Henry
MEDICAL RECORD #: 7054922
DATE OF SURGERY: 8/18/XX
SURGEON: Jack Einhorn, MD
ASSISTANT: Neil Fischer, MD

ds

PREOPERATIVE DIAGNOSIS

No colon since entry for this heading begins on next line

Mandibular symphysis osteotomy. Open wound at floor of mouth and buccal mucosa.

ds

POSTOPERATIVE DIAGNOSIS

Mandibular symphysis osteotomy. Open wound at floor of mouth and buccal mucosa.

ds

PROCEDURE

left justification

Repair with internal fixation and repair of soft tissue defect.

ds

ANESTHESIA

General.

ds

OPERATIVE INDICATIONS

This is a youngster with a history of neuroblastoma whom I had first seen 6 months earlier. At that time, the lesion presented as a neck mass, which was biopsied. Subsequent studies showed extensive involvement of the right neck and right cranial base, namely extension into the jugular foramen. The patient received neoadjuvant chemotherapy and is slated for radical en bloc excision today.

ds

OPERATIVE PROCEDURE

Through the mandibular-splitting approach, a radical neck dissection with en bloc resection of the tumor from the cranial base around the jugular foramen was carried out without complication after tracheostomy had been performed. The right floor of the mouth incision, extending from the posterior middle third of the tongue up to the anterior floor of the mouth, was closed with interrupted sutures of Vicryl, with care being taken to maintain a watertight closure.

(continued) **Include this notation on multiple-page reports**

FIGURE 6.6
Operative Report

OPERATIVE REPORT
NAME: Jane Henry **Include a header on second and succeeding pages**
MEDICAL RECORD #: 7054922
DATE: 8/18/XX
Page 2

ds

The mandibular symphysis osteotomy was carried out through the socket of the extracted right mandibular central incisor halfway down the vertical height of the symphysis and then stair-stepped to the left and then down across the mandibular border. Care was taken to preserve both mental nerves bilaterally. The horizontal portion of the osteotomy had necessarily coursed through 2 tooth buds of the permanent dentition, and these were subsequently debrided. An anatomic approximation of the symphysis was carried out and held in place while a 2.0 compression plate made of titanium was applied to the lower rim of the symphysis. Good solid bony union was achieved. The mucosa, both labial and gingival, of the lower lip were then reapproximated with 5 interrupted sutures of Vicryl. The gingiva was then brought up to the tooth crowns and secured into the mucosa in the anterior floor of the mouth with sutures. These sutures encircled the teeth and created a nice watertight seal, with no exposure of the underlying mandible. The lip was then prepared, and the remainder of the neck closure was carried out by Dr. Fischer.

ds

ESTIMATED BLOOD LOSS
Negligible.

ds

COMPLICATIONS
None.

ds

SPECIMENS
None.

qs

____
Jack C. Einhorn, MD

ds

JCE/XX
D: 8/18/XX
T: 8/18/XX

FIGURE 6.6
Operative Report (Continued)

Patient Study 6.A — Mark Rankin

Pediatrician Marcus Green, MD, treats 5-year-old Mark Rankin for ear pain. When the antibiotic regimen is unsuccessful, Dr. Green refers Mark to Dr. Joseph Strong, otorhinolaryngologist, for consultation.

REPORT 6.1 Office Note

- CBC stands for complete blood count, a common laboratory test that measures levels of red blood cells, white blood cells, and platelets. The abbreviation for CBC and white blood cells, WBC, is frequently dictated letter-by-letter. The measurement unit, cubic millimeters, should be transcribed as mm with a superscript 3. Because not all equipment allows superscripts, the form *cu mm* is the preferred alternative.
- Use the abbreviations HGB for hemoglobin results and HCT for hematocrit.
- The shortened forms *polys, lymphs,* and *monos* can be transcribed as dictated.

REPORT 6.2 Office Note

- Listen for these difficult words:
  exudate (noun) and exudative (adjective)
  submandibular
  periauricular
  mastoiditis
  myringotomy

Patient Study 6.B — Yarvella Harves

Yarvella Harves is an 11-week-old girl who had been well until a few days ago. She had a neck mass that did not appear to be painful, but it had been growing steadily for several days. The baby was referred to the specialist from the pediatrician's office.

REPORT 6.3 Consultation Letter

- BUMC stands for Brookfield University Medical Center
- Nafcillin is the generic name of a penicillin antibiotic

Patient Study 6.C

Jane Henry

Jane Henry is a 2-year-old girl who was diagnosed with a neuroblastoma arising from the floor of the mouth and extending to the neck and lower base of the skull. She has been treated with chemotherapy and is now undergoing surgery to remove any residual tumor. Dr. Einhorn is an otorhinolaryngologist who is performing the surgery with the assistance of a plastic surgeon, Dr. Fischer.

REPORT 6.4 Operative Report

Patient Study 6.D

Julia Wang

Fifty-three-year-old Julia Wang is seeing the physician regarding a snoring problem that disrupts her sleep, leaving her feeling chronically tired. She also thinks she may have allergies or a sinus infection because of an annoying drainage into her throat.

REPORT 6.5 Office Note

- Vancenase Nasal Spray and Allegra are brand-name drugs.
- Listen for these terms:
  apnea
  somnolence

Patient Study 6.E — Cynthia Mancini

Cynthia Mancini is a 35-year-old woman who was in an automobile accident 5 years ago. At that time she had a fracture of the septum, causing a deviation. She presents to the surgeon for correction of the nasal obstruction.

REPORT 6.6 Operative Report

- Every operative report must contain a preoperative and postoperative diagnosis, the name of the procedure, the name of the surgeon, and a description of the procedure.
- In many operative reports, the preoperative and postoperative diagnoses are the same. Most hospitals require that the diagnosis be repeated, even if the dictator says "same." Do this efficiently by blocking and copying the item.
- Suture size is dictated as "four O" and should be transcribed as 4-0.

Patient Study 6.F — Rosa Valdez

Rosa Valdez is seeking relief for recurring headaches and dizziness, for which she has been treated in the past. This 30-year-old ad agency account manager leads a hectic work life and wants to resolve her medical problem before it worsens and requires her to miss work for an extended period.

REPORT 6.7 Office Note

- The abbreviation PO stands for *postoperative.* In other instances, this abbreviation can stand for *by mouth* (p.o.) from the Latin phrase *per os.*
- Listen for these drug names:
  Bactrim-DS
  Beconase
  Antivert

Case Study 6.G — Sara Vagts

Sara Vagts is a 44-year-old woman who has been seen by her primary physician for recurrent sinusitis. A consultation with the ENT specialist results in a recommendation for an ethmoidectomy and a different antibiotic.

REPORT 6.8 Office Note (Phone Call Note)

- Aspergillus is the genus name of a fungus. Aspergillosis is an infection caused by that fungus.
- Listen for these drug names:
  vancomycin
  amphotericin
  Tussionex

Patient Study 6.H — Irene Callahan

Irene Callahan is a 16-year-old with a diagnosis of a brain tumor. She was sent to the audiology clinic for evaluation of her hearing status prior to beginning chemotherapy which may potentially cause some hearing loss.

REPORT 6.9 Audiology Report

- Decibel(s) will be transcribed as dB. Hertz is transcribed as Hz.
- Minus 5 to 10 is transcribed as –5 to 10.

Using Medical References

Use the appropriate medical reference to locate the correct spelling and additional usage information for the words below. (If the reference is not available, use the Glossary in this text.) Circle the correct spelling, then write a sentence using the word correctly.

1.	cerumen	serumen	cerumun
2.	tinitus	tinnitus	tinnitis
3.	aretinoid	aretynoid	arytenoid
4.	labrinthitis	labyrinthitis	labirynthitis
5.	pharyngitis	pharingitis	pharingytis
6.	turbunate	turbinate	terbinate
7.	disphagia	dysphagea	dysphagia
8.	malleus	maleus	malleas
9.	buccal	buckal	bucchal
10.	epitaxsis	epistacsis	epistaxis

Making Expert Decisions

Circle the correct word from the choices in parentheses.

1. There was a large lesion in the (oral/aural) cavity on the buccal mucosa.
2. There were several (shoddy/shotty) nodes located in the neck.
3. Redness of the external ear canal was noted; (otits media/otitis externa) was diagnosed.
4. There was fluid in the middle ear and recurrent otitis media, so a (tympanoplasty/myringotomy) was performed with insertion of polyethylene tubes.
5. The (osteal/ostial) opening of the eustachian tube was blocked.
6. This (past/passed) year, the patient had PE tubes placed because of chronic infections.
7. It was felt that the patient had (vertigo/tinnitus) when she said she had a sensation of spinning, even when standing still.
8. A (Rinne/Weber) test was performed by placing a tuning fork on the center of the forehead, the vertex.
9. This was a 47-year-old male with basal cell carcinoma located on the right (naris/nares).
10. Using a Zeiss microscope, the physician examined the middle ear; the incus was malformed and fused to the head of the (malleus/malleolus).

Transcribing Professional Documents

Transcribe the document named Chapter 6 Assessment. Before you key, review the document formatting guidelines. Proofread your transcribed document and revise it until you think it is error-free.

7

Pulmonology

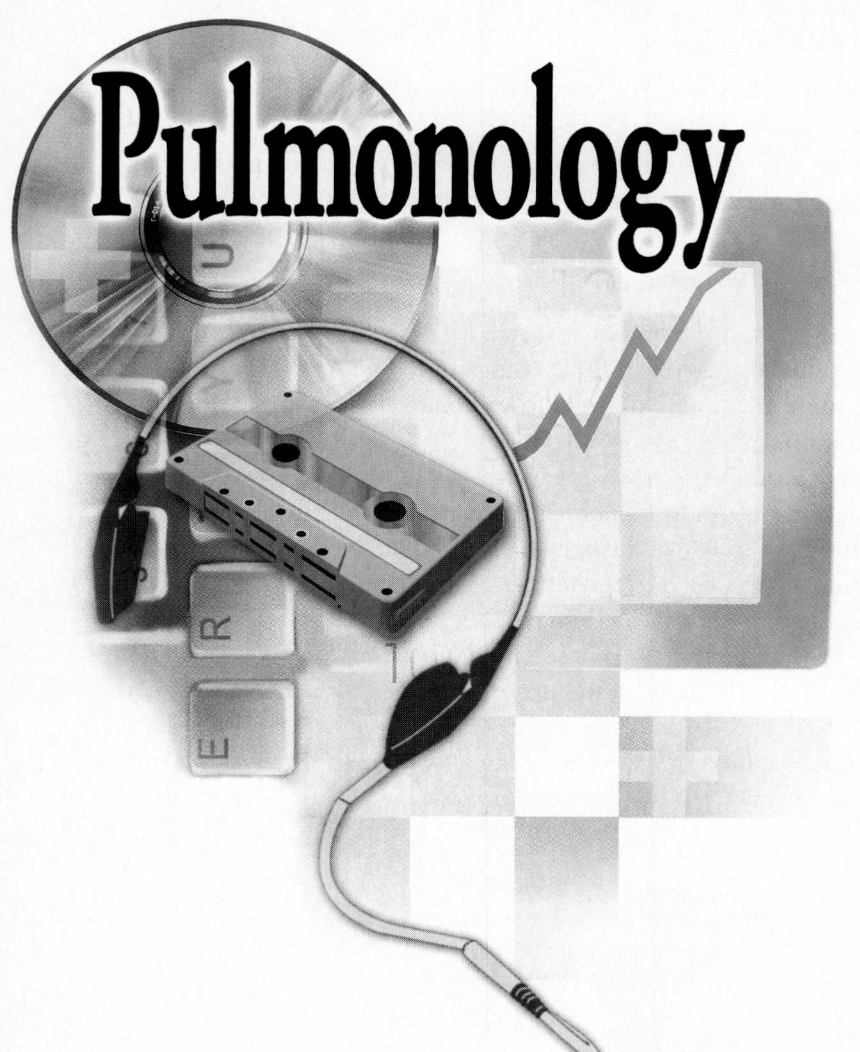

Pulmonology, from the Latin for lung *(pulmo)*, is the medical specialty that deals with the respiratory system. The respiratory system functions with the circulatory system to transport oxygen and carbon dioxide between the lungs and tissues of the body. The organs of the respiratory system include the nose, mouth, pharynx, larynx, epiglottis, trachea, lungs, bronchi, bronchioles, and alveoli. The physician who specializes in the respiratory tract is called a pulmonologist.

OBJECTIVES

- Use pulmonology terms correctly according to the context and purpose of the dictation.
- Select and use appropriate general and specialty reference materials.
- Key pulmonology documents of varying complexity and format.
- Transcribe authentic medical dictation requiring concentration and listening skill.
- Edit medical reports to conform with AAMT style guidelines.
- Proofread and correct transcripts to produce error-free documents.

Exploring Pulmonology

Our bodies need oxygen to function properly. The air we breathe, inhaled through the nose and mouth, contains oxygen. The respiratory system uses this oxygen and, in the processs, converts the gas to carbon dioxide. It then eliminates this waste gas from the body. Each step of the respiratory process is essential for good health.

Structure and Function

The central part of the respiratory system is located in the chest, or thorax, which contains the sternum, ribs, thoracic vertebrae, and lungs. The muscles of the respiratory tract are also important. These muscles transfer air by moving the ribs during inspiration and expiration.

Air enters the body through the nose or mouth, then passes through the pharynx and into the trachea, or windpipe. The air is warmed and filtered of noxious substances, and then passes into the tracheobronchial tree (Figure 7.1). This tree, so named because of its branching into the left and right bronchi, is further divided into bronchioles, which terminate into air sacs, called alveoli. Adjacent to the alveoli lie tiny capillary beds (Figure 7.2). These circulatory beds enable exchange of oxygen from the alveoli to the blood and carbon dioxide from the blood to the alveoli.

During the normal respiratory cycle there is an inspiratory phase that requires active muscle movement, and a passive expiratory phase. During inspiration the

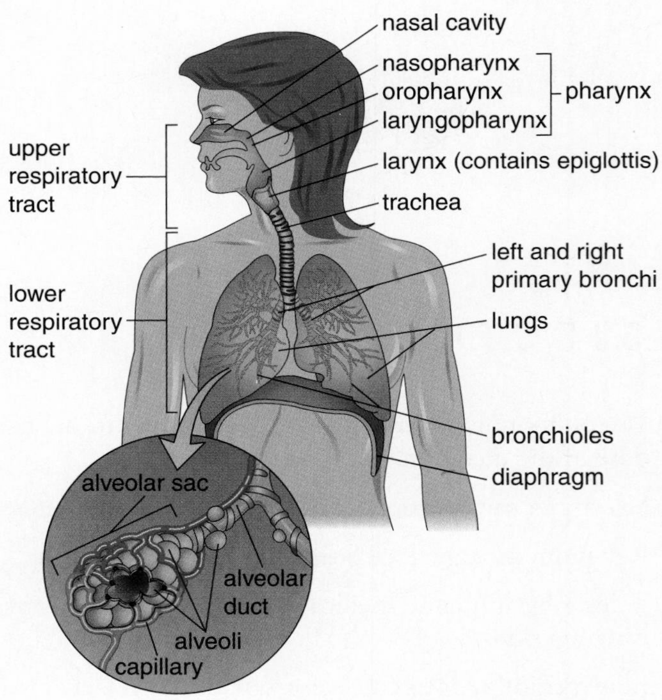

FIGURE 7.1
Respiratory System

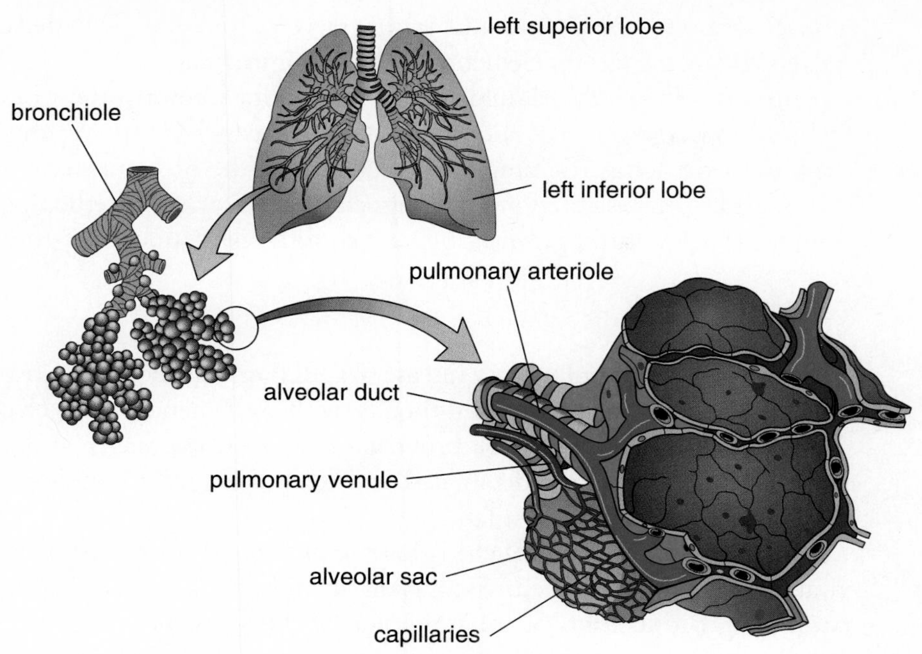

FIGURE 7.2
Capillary Beds in the Lungs

muscles between the ribs elevate the ribs, increasing the diameter of the chest. At the same time, the diaphragm drops to allow free entry of air. The recoiling of the thoracic cavity expels the air and causes the expiration to occur. In the normal adult, there is a 6–8 cm expansion during each of the 16–20 cycles per minute.

Respiration is divided into the external and internal processes. External respiration is the exchange of oxygen and carbon dioxide between the person and the environment. Internal respiration takes place on a cellular level, exchanging the oxygen carried on the red blood cells with the carbon dioxide in the tissues. After this dual exchange takes place, the lungs eliminate the carbon dioxide.

Physical Assessment

Assessment begins with visualization of the nose, observing for deviated septum or other abnormalities that would decrease the amount of air entry. Inspection of the chest includes counting the respirations, observing the movement of the chest during inspiration and expiration, and noting the

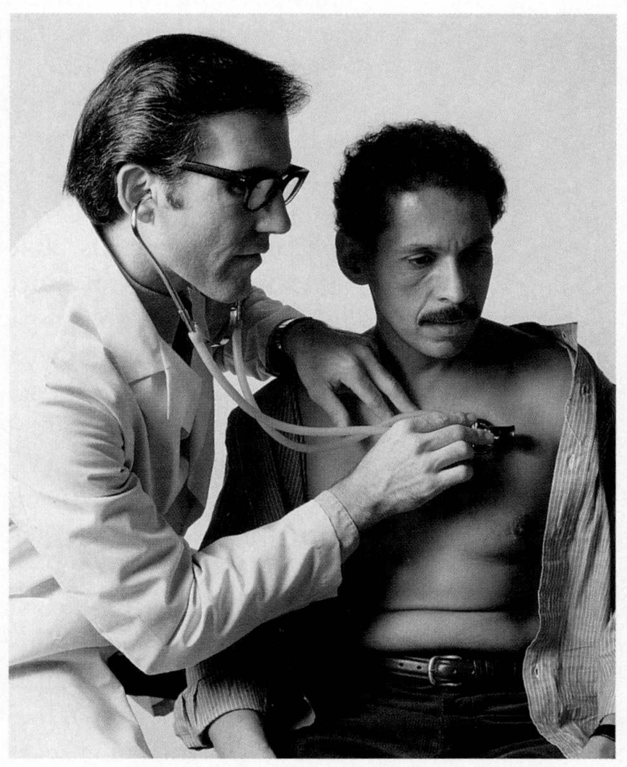

The physician listens to breath sounds with a stethoscope.

general shape of the thorax and symmetry of expansion. Posture, contour, and movement are important elements in proper air exchange.

Palpation of the back should include feeling for fremitus, the vibrations caused by breathing. A resonant sound should be produced when tapping on the chest over the area of the lungs. Tapping, or percussing, on the ribs and sternum produces a dull sound. On auscultation, the physician listens with a stethoscope for breath sounds as well as rattling, wheezing, and snoring-like sounds.

Diseases and Conditions

Chronic obstructive pulmonary disease (COPD) or chronic obstructive lung disease (COLD) occurs when there is difficulty with oxygenation. It is characterized by dyspnea and hyperplasia of the bronchial tissues. In late stages of this disease, the patient may become very debilitated and require oxygen to be delivered continuously via a nasal cannula or mask.

Inflammation of the bronchi is known as bronchitis. It is usually caused by a viral or bacterial pathogen. Symptoms include cough, usually productive, and chest pain. Bronchiolitis is inflammation of the bronchioles and is usually found only in children.

Emphysema results from chronic asthma, bronchitis, and/or smoking. It occurs when the alveoli lose their elasticity and air is trapped within. This constant expansion leads to the characteristic "barrel chest." During periods of difficult breathing, the patient must remain erect, either sitting up continuously or in an orthopneic position, leaning over a table with arms resting on the surface and extended over the head. This position allows for better air exchange.

Asthma is a common obstructive airway disease producing intermittent attacks that usually are reversible. It is characterized by a narrowing of the airways, resulting in dyspnea, cough, and wheezing in response to various stimuli. An asthma attack may be triggered by known or unknown allergens, or by exercise, an upper respiratory infection (URI), or emotions. Asthma is usually controlled with the use of pharmacologic agents, although severe asthma can lead to chronic lung problems.

Pneumonia is an inflammatory process affecting the tissue of the lung. It is usually caused by infectious organisms. The types of pneumonia are described by the causative agent: bacterial, viral, fungal, or parasitic. Other causes include chemical inhalations or aspirated foreign material. Manifestations may include cough, with or without sputum production; lethargy; fever; pain in the chest; changes in the respiratory rate; grunting; and nasal flaring. Assessment includes adventitious (abnormal) breath sounds; increased tactile fremitus; dullness on percussion; bronchovesicular breath sounds; egophony; and pectoriloquy. A diagnostic evaluation includes physical examination, chest x-ray, sputum culture if productive cough exists, and blood culture if bacteremia is a concern.

Respiratory distress syndrome (RDS) is a series of symptoms found most commonly in premature infants and small children. It is characterized by very rapid breathing, cyanosis, nasal flaring, grunting, and retractions of the muscles between the ribs. Premature infants are at risk because their immature lung tissue has not yet developed surfactant, the substance that the lungs require to expand. Without surfactant, the alveoli collapse and breathing is difficult.

Cystic fibrosis is a hereditary disorder affecting the lungs, pancreas, and digestive system. Thick, viscous mucus is produced, blocking the airway and trapping air in the lungs. Pancreatic enzymes are not produced, causing problems with digestion and fatty, frequent, foul-smelling stools. Presently, lifelong treatment with pancreatic enzyme replacement, respiratory or pulmonary toilet including postural drainage, and antibiotic therapy for frequent, associated pneumonia is necessary. The genetic abnormality causing this disease has been discovered and progress is being made to replace the aberrant gene in order to develop a cure for persons affected with cystic fibrosis.

Common Tests and Surgical Procedures

X-ray visualization of the chest is one of the most commonly used procedures to diagnose conditions such as pneumonia, tuberculosis, and abnormalities of the lungs and surrounding structures.

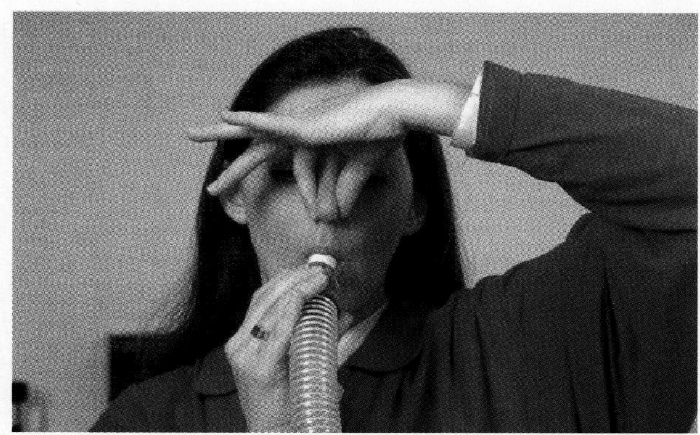

Patient pinches nose and mouth-breathes, allowing spirometer to measure and record airflow.

Pulmonary function tests are essential to diagnosing chronic obstructive pulmonary disease and other lung ailments. These breathing tests include measurement of lung volume and the distribution of gases along with diffusion studies. Spirometry measures the amount of air exchanged during each breath, and the results are compared with established results from healthy individuals.

Another common procedure is bronchoscopy. The examination is usually performed with a flexible bronchoscope that allows the physician to see even the small airways and to remove pieces of tissue for biopsy. The same type of instrument is used to view the trachea and esophagus for signs of disease and abnormalities.

Thoracentesis is a surgical procedure to remove fluid from the pleural cavity. Pneumonectomy, or pulmonectomy, is an excision of all lobes of a lung in a single operation.

Pulse oximetry uses a small, portable, non-invasive monitoring device that measures the saturation of oxygen in the hemoglobin.

Building Language Skills

The following tables list common pulmonology terms, drugs, and abbreviations. The list of terms and definitions includes the most difficult words contained in the dictated reports in this chapter. These words are identified in GREEN type. A list of common drugs is found in Appendix D.

Medical Terms and Pharmacologic Agents

abscess
(**ab**-ses) (n) a pus-filled cavity, usually because of a localized infection

aerosol
(**ayr**-O-sol) (n) a liquid or solution dispensed as a fine mist or a product dispensed from a pressurized container as a fine mist

afebrile
(ay-**feb**-ril) (adj) without fever

albuterol
(al-**byoo**-ter-ol) (n) bronchodilator available in oral and inhalent forms to be used in asthma, emphysema, and other lung conditions

alveolus
(al-**vee**-O-lus) (n) tiny chambers of the lungs where the exchange of oxygen and carbon dioxide takes place; alveoli (al-**vee**-O-lI) (pl)

anicteric
(an-ik-**ter**-ik) (adj) without jaundice or icterus (a yellowing of the skin and whites of the eyes)

anorexia
(an-O-**rek**-see-a) (n) loss of appetite

arytenoid
(ar-i-**tee**-noid) (adj) resembling a ladle or pitcher mouth; the muscle and cartilage of the larynx

asthma
(**az**-ma) (n) respiratory disorder with temporary narrowing of the airways, resulting in difficulty in breathing, coughing, gasping, wheezing

atelectasis
(at-e-**lek**-ta-sis) (n) condition in which lungs are unexpanded

atraumatic
(ay-traw-**mat**-ik) (adj) without injury or trauma

auscultation
(aws-kul-**tay**-shun) (n) act of listening through a stethoscope to sounds from within the body, including lungs, heart, and abdomen

bacteremia
(bak-te-**ree**-mee-a) (n) the presence of bacteria in the blood

bibasilar
(bI-**bays**-i-lar) (adj) occurring in both bases

bifurcation
(bI-fer-**kay**-shun) (n) forking into two branches

bleomycin
(blee-O-**mI**-sin) (n) antitumor agents

bolus
(**bO**-lus) (n) a mass of something such as masticated (chewed) food or substance that is ready to be swallowed; an amount of medication

brachial
(**bray**-kee-al) (adj) pertaining to the arm

bronchial
(**brong**-kee-al) (adj) relating to the bronchi

bronchiectasis
(brong-kee-**ek**-ta-sis) (n) persistent, abnormal widening of the bronchi, with an associated cough and spitting up of mucus

bronchiole
(**brong**-kee-Ol) (n) one of the smaller subdivisions of the bronchi

bronchitis
(brong-**kI**-tis) (n) inflammation of the bronchi

bronchovesicular
(**brong**-kO-ve-**sik**-yoo-lar) (adj) relating to the bronchioles and alveoli in the lungs

bronchus
(**brong**-kus) (n) the divisions of the trachea leading to the lungs; bronchi (**brong**-kI) (pl)

bulla
(**bul**-a) (n) large bleb in the skin that contains fluid; bullae (pl)

cannula
(**kan**-yoo-la) (n) a tube for insertion into a duct or cavity to allow the escape of fluid

cannulate
(**kan**-yoo-layt) (v) to introduce a cannula through a passageway

capillary
(kap-i-**layr**-ee) (n) tiny blood vessel connecting arterioles and venules

ceftazidime
(sef-**taz**-i-deem) (n) antibiotic used in the treatment of moderate to severe infections

cilium
(**sil**-ee-um) (n) a short hairlike extension of a cell surface, capable of lashlike movement, which aids in the movement of unicellular organisms and in the movement of fluids in higher organisms; eyelash; cilia (pl)

clavicular
(kla-**vik**-yoo-lar) (adj) pertains to the clavicle, or collarbone

clubbing
(**klub**-ing) (n) condition of the fingers and toes in which their ends become wide and thickened; often a sign of disease, especially heart or lung disease

conjunctival
(kon-junk-**tI**-val) (n) pertaining to the mucous membrane that lines eyelids and is reflected onto eyeball

consolidation
(kon-sol-i-**day**-shun (n) solidification into a firm, dense mass

cyanosis
(cI-a-**nO**-sis) (n) bluish discoloration of the skin and/or mucous membranes due to decreased amount of oxygen in the blood cells

cyanotic
(sI-a-**not**-ik) (adj) pertaining to cyanosis

cystic fibrosis
(**sis**-tik fI-**brO**-sis) (n) an inherited disease, in which the mucus-producing glands become clogged with thick mucus; digestion and respiration are affected

diffuse
(di-**fyoos**) (adj) spreading, scattered

distal
(**dis**-tal) (adj) away from the center, toward the far end of something

dorsal
(**dOr**-sal) (adj) relating to the back; posterior

dyspnea
(disp-**nee**-a) (n) shortness of breath; difficulty in breathing

edema
(e-**dee**-ma) (n) excessive accumulation of fluid in tissues, especially just under the skin or in a given cavity

effusion
(e-**fyoo**-zhun) (n) escape of fluid into a cavity or tissues; the fluid itself

egophony
(ee-**gof**-O-nee) (n) an abnormal voice sound, like the bleating of a goat

electrocautery
(ee-**lek**-trO-**caw**-ter-ee) (n) application of a needle or snare heated by an electric current to destroy tissue

electrolyte
(ee-**lek**-trO-lIt) (n) an ionized chemical capable of conducting an electric current; the body contains many different electrolytes in specific amounts to keep it functioning properly

endotracheal tube
(**en**-dO-**tray**-kee-al toob) (n) a catheter inserted through the mouth or nose into the trachea to maintain an open airway to deliver oxygen to permit suctioning of mucus or to prevent aspiration of foreign materials

epiglottis
(**ep**-I-**glot**-is) (n) flap of elastic cartilage at the back of the mouth that covers the opening to the windpipe during swallowing, thereby preventing choking.

epithelial
(ep-i-**thee**-lee-al (adj) composed of epithelium, cell layers covering the outside body surface as well as forming the lining of hollow organs and the passages of the respiratory, digestive, and urinary tracts

erythema
(er-i-**thee**-ma) (n) redness of the skin

esophagus
(ee-**sof**-a-gus) (n) the muscular canal that connects the pharynx and stomach

expectoration
(ek-spek-tO-**ray**-shun) (n) expelling by mouth; spitting

expiratory
(ek-**spI**-ra-**tO**-ree) (adj) relating to expiration, or breathing out air from the lungs

extraocular
(eks-tra-**ok**-yoo-lar) (adj) outside the eye

femoral
(**fem**-o-ral) (adj) relating to the thigh bone or femur

flaring
(**flayr**-ing) (adj) widening of an area, as the nostrils; a spreading area of redness around a lesion

fremitus
(**frem**-i-tus) (n) a vibration that can be felt by the hand on the chest

funduscopic
(fun-dus-**kop**-ik) (adj) pertaining to examinatiom of the fundus of the eye by an ophthalmoscope

fungal
(**fung**-gal) (adj) caused by fungus or pertaining to fungus

granulomas
(gran-yoo-**lO**-mas) (n) masses of nodular granulation tissues that cover lesions resulting from injury, infection, or inflammation

guttural
(**gut**-er-al) (adj) relating to the throat, or guttur

hemoptysis
(hee-**mop**-ti-sis) (n) expectoration of blood; spitting or coughing up blood

hemothorax
(hee-mO-**thOr**-aks) (n) blood in the chest cavity

hilar
(**hI**-lar) (adj) pertaining to a hilum, the part of an organ where the nerves and vessels enter and leave

histiocytes
(**his**-tee-O-sitz) (n) tissue cells

humeral
(**hyoo**-mer-al) (adj) near the shoulder or upper arm

hyperemia
(hI-per-**ee**-mee-a) (n) increased blood in part of the body, caused by inflammatory response or blockage of blood outflow

hyperplasia
(hI-per-**play**-see-a) (n) increase in the number of cells in a tissue or organ resulting in an increase in size (does not include tumor formation)

hyphae
(**hI**-fay) (n) cells forming the filaments of mold

infiltrate
(in-**fil**-trayt) (v) to pass into or through a substance or a space

inspiratory
(in-**spI**-ra-tO-ree) (adj) relating to inhalation, drawing air into the lungs

latissimus
(la-**tis**-i-mus) (n) denoting a broad anatomical structure, such as a muscle

linear
(**lin**-ee-ar) (adj) pertaining to or resembling a line

lobectomy
(lOb-**ek**-tO-mee) (n) the removal of a lobe from an organ or gland

lytic
(**lit**-ik) (adj) pertaining to lysis, a gradual subsidence of the symptoms of an acute disease

mediastinal
(mee-dee-as-**tI**-nal (adj) related to the mediastinum, a septum or cavity between two principal portions of an organ

metaphyseal
(met-a-**fiz**-ee-al) (adj) relating to a metaphysis

metaphysis
(me-**taf**-i-sis) (n) a conical section of bone between the epiphysis and diaphysis of long bones

metaplasia
(me-ta-**play**-zee-a) (n) conversion of a tissue into a form that is not normal for that tissue

metastasis
(me-**tas**-ta-sis) (n) the shifting of a disease from one part of the body to another, especially in cancer; metastases (pl)

multinucleated
(mul-ti-**noo**-klee-ay-ted) (adj) possessing several nuclei

nasopharynx
(**nay**-zO-**far**-ingks) (n) open chamber behind the nose and above the palate

nebulization
(**neb**-yoo-li-**zay**-shun) (n) production of fine particles, such as a spray or mist, from liquid

opacity
(O-**pas**-i-tee) (n) state of being opaque, impenetrable by visible light rays or by forms of radiant energy, such as x-rays

organomegaly
(**Or**-ga-nO-**meg**-a-lee) (n) abnormal enlargement of an organ, particularly an organ of the abdominal cavity, such as the liver or spleen

orthopnea
(Or-thop-**nee**-a) (n) difficulty in breathing when lying down

oximetry
(ok-**sim**-i-tree) (n) a method of measuring the amount of oxygen combined with the hemoglobin in a blood sample

pancrelipase
(pan-kree-**lip**-ase) (n) standardized preparation of enzymes with amylase and protease, obtained from the pancreas of hogs

parenchymal
(pa-**reng**-ki-mal) (adj) pertaining to the distinguishing or specific cells of a gland or organ contained in and supported by the connective tissue framework

parietal
(pa-**ree**-e-tal) (adj) pertaining to the inner walls of a body cavity

pathogen
(**path**-O-jen) (n) any microorganism or substance that can cause a disease

pathologic
(path-O-**loj**-ik) (adj) pertaining to pathology, the medical science concerned with all aspects of disease, especially with the structural and functional changes caused by disease

pectoriloquy
(pek-tO-**ril**-O-kwee) (n) voice sounds transmitted through the pulmonary structures, clearly audible on auscultation

pectus carinatum
(**pek**-tus kar-i-**nay**-tum) (n) forward protusion of the sternum; pigeon breast

pectus excavatum
(**pek**-tus eks-ka-**vay**-tum) (n) markedly sunken sternum; funnel breast

percussion
(per-**kush**-un) (n) a technique of physical examination in which the sound of fingers or a small tool tapping parts of the body is used to determine position and size of internal organs and to detect the presence of fluid

perihilar
(per-i-**hI**-lar) (adj) occurring near the hilum, the part of an organ where the nerves and vessels enter and leave

pharynx
(**far**-ingks) (n) throat; passageway for air from nasal cavity to larynx, and food from mouth to esophagus

pleura
(**ploor**-a) (n) membrane lining the chest cavity and covering the lungs

pleural
(**ploor**-al) (adj) relating to the pleura

pleurisy
(**ploor**-I-see) (n) inflammation of the pleura; pleuritis

pneumonia
(noo-**mO**-nee-a) (n) inflammation and congestion of the lung, usually due to infection by bacteria or viruses

pneumonitis
(noo-mO-**nI**-tis) (n) inflammation of the lungs

pneumothorax
(noo-mO-**thor**-aks) (n) abnormal presence of air or gas in the chest cavity

protuberant
(prO-**too**-ber-ant) (adj) pertaining to a part that is prominent beyond a surface, like a knob

Pseudomonas
(soo-dO-**mO**-nas) (n) a genus of bacteria commonly found in soil and water and which may cause infection

radiograph
(**ray**-dee-O-graf) (n) a negative image in photographic film made by exposure to x-rays or gamma rays that have passed through matter or tissue

rales
(rahls) (n) abnormal sounds, such as rattling or bubbling, heard on auscultation of the lungs

rectal
(**rek**-tal) (adj) relating to the rectum, the lower part of the large intestine

regimen
(**rej**-i-men) (n) plan of therapy, including drugs

respiration
(res-pi-**ray**-shun) (n) inhalation and exhalation; the exchange of gases—oxygen and carbon dioxide—between an organism and the environment

respiratory
(**res**-per-a-tOr-ee) (adj) relating to respiration

respiratory distress syndrome
(**res**-pi-ra-tOr-ee dis-**tres sin**-drOm) (n) acute lung disease, especially in premature newborn babies, caused by a lack of surfactant in the lung tissue

rhinorrhea
(rI-nO-**ree**-a) (n) a watery discharge from the nose

rhonchus
(**rong**-kus) (n) abnormal sound heard on auscultation of the chest, usually during expiration; rhonchi (pl)

sclera
(**skleer**-a) (n) a fibrous coat that covers approximately five-sixths of the outer tunic of the eye; sclerae (pl)

sclerotic
(skle-**rot**-ik) (adj) relating to sclerosis, or induration; in neuropathy, induration of nervous and other structures by a hyperplasia of the interstitial fibrous atructures

squamous
(**skway**-mus) (adj) scale-like

septum
(**sep**-tum) (n) division between two cavities or two masses of tissue, e.g., nasal septum; septa (pl)

sputum
(**spyoo**-tum) (n) spit; expectorated material

sternum
(**ster**-num) (n) the breast bone

supraglottic
(soo-pra-**glot**-ik) (adj) located above the glottis, the sound-producing apparatus of the larynx

tachycardia
(**tak**-I-**kar**-dee-a) (n) rapid heart rate

tachycardiac
(**tak**-e-**kar**-dee-ak) (adj) relating to or suffering from an abnormally rapid heart rate

tachypnea
(tak-ip-**nee**-a) (n) rapid rate of breathing

theophylline
(thee-**of**-i-lin) (n) a drug used in chronic obstructive lung disease

thoracotomy
(thOr-a-**kot**-O-mee) (n) surgical incision of the chest wall

thoracoscopy
(thOr-a-**kos**-kO-pee) (n) diagnostic examination of the pleural cavity with an endoscope

thorax
(**thor**-aks) (n) the chest

thyromegaly
(thI-rO-**meg**-a-lee) (n) enlargement of the thyroid gland

tibia
(**tib**-ee-a) (n) larger bone of the lower leg; shin bone

tibial
(**tib**-ee-al) (adj) relating to the tibia

tobramycin
(tO-bra-**mI**-sin) (n) an antibiotic drug

trachea
(**tray**-kee-a) (n) the windpipe

turbinates
(**ter**-bi-naytz) (n) three scroll-shaped bones that form the sidewall of the nasal cavity

turgor
(**ter**-gOr) (n) normal tension in a cell; swelling

tympanic membrane
(tim-**pan**-ik) (n) eardrum

vincristine
(vin-**kris**-teen) (n) an antineoplastic drug that disrupts cell division and is used to treat many cancers, especially those of the lymphatic system.

wheezing
(**hweez**-ing) (n) breathing with difficulty and with a whistling sound; can be heard aloud and/or on auscultation

Wright peak flow
(n) maximum flow of expired air as measured by the Wright flowmeter

Abbreviations

Abbreviation	Meaning
A&P	auscultation and percussion
ABG	arterial blood gas (gases)
AFB	acid-fast bacilli
AP	anterior posterior
ARDS	acute respiratory distress syndrome
BiPAP	bilevel positive airway pressure
BOOP	bronchiolitis obliterans with organizing pneumonia
CO_2	carbon dioxide
COLD	chronic obstructive lung disease
COPD	chronic obstructive pulmonary disease
CPAP	continuous positive airway pressure
CPR	cardiopulmonary resuscitation
CXR	chest x-ray
DNR	do not resuscitate
FEF	forced expiratory flow
FEF_{25-75}	forced midexpiratory flow during the middle half of the FVC
FEV	forced expiratory volume
FEV_1	forced expiratory volume in one second
FEV_3	forced expiratory volume in three seconds
FVC	forced vital capacity
FVL	flow volume loop
IPPB	intermittent positive pressure breathing
IS	incentive spirometry
MDI	metered dose inhaler
O_2	oxygen
PA	posterior anterior
PAP	positive airway pressure
PEEP	positive end expiratory pressure
PEF	peak expiratory flow
PND	paroxysmal nocturnal dyspnea
RDS	respiratory distress syndrome
SIDS	sudden infant death syndrome
SMR	submucosal resection
SOB	shortness of breath
TB	tuberculosis
URI	upper respiratory infection
VC	vital capacity

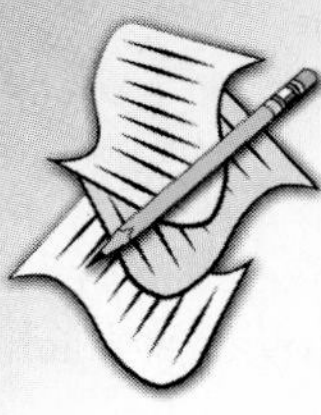

EXERCISE 7.1

Recognizing Look-Alikes and Sound-Alikes

Below is a list of frequently used words that look alike and/or sound alike. Study the meaning and pronunciation of each set of words, then read the following sentences carefully and circle the word in parentheses that correctly completes the meaning.

breath	(n) air taken into the lungs
breathe	(v) to take air into the lungs
coarse	rough; "coarse breath sounds"
course	progress or duration of time
dose	(n) a measure
doze	(v) to nap
expiratory	breathing out from the lungs
inspiratory	breathing into the lungs
loose	(adj) free from anything that restrains
lose	(v) to miss something
loss	(n) something that is missing
lost	(v) past tense of lose
lost	(adj) missing as in "a lost watch"
perfuse	to force blood or other fluid to flow; "toes are well perfused"
profuse	abundant; "the patient had profuse bleeding"
presence	(n) attendance; close proximity
presents	(n) gifts
presents	(v) manner in which the patient appears to the caregiver
afebrile	(adj) without fever
a febrile	(adj) with fever
viscous	(adj) sticky
viscus	(n) a hollow, multilayered, walled organ such as an organ of the digestive system or the heart
vicious	(adj) mean

1. The patient is to take three (doses, dozes) of the medication daily.
2. It was unfortunate that she (dosed, dozed) through the lecture.
3. The patient (presence, presents) for followup of his colitis.
4. On cardiac examination, I detected the (presence, presents) of a systolic murmur.
5. As the patient inhaled, I noted (expiratory, inspiratory) wheezing.
6. She is complaining of shortness of (breath, breathe) on exertion.
7. When she exercises, she feels like she cannot (breath, breathe) as easily.
8. We will have her complete her full (coarse, course) of antibiotics.
9. When she cut her finger, she noted (perfuse, profuse) bleeding.
10. The patient was directed to (loose, lose) 10 pounds by her next visit.

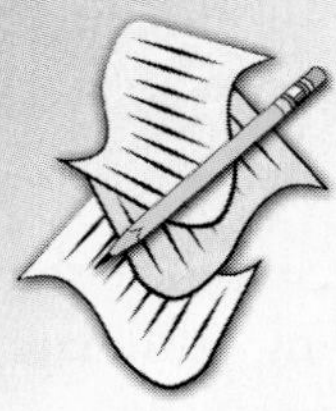

EXERCISE 7.2

Matching Sound and Spelling

The numbered list that follows shows the phonetic spelling of hard-to-spell words. Sound out the word, then write the correct spelling in the blank space provided. Each of the words can be found in the Glossary or in the drug list in Appendix D.

1. tak-i-**kar**-dee-a ______________________________
2. **ploor**-al ______________________________
3. an-ik-**ter**-ik ______________________________
4. thee-**of**-i-lin ______________________________
5. brong-kee-**ek**-ta-sis______________________________
6. noo-mO-**nI**-tis______________________________
7. **rong**-kus ______________________________
8. aws-kul-**tay**-shun ______________________________
9. tak-ip-**nee**-a ______________________________
10. thI-rO-**meg**-a-lee ______________________________
11. **nay**-zO-**far**-ingks______________________________
12. hee-**mop**-ti-sis ______________________________
13. di-**fyoos** ______________________________
14. **tray**-kee-a______________________________
15. **Or**-ga-nO-**meg**-a-lee ______________________________

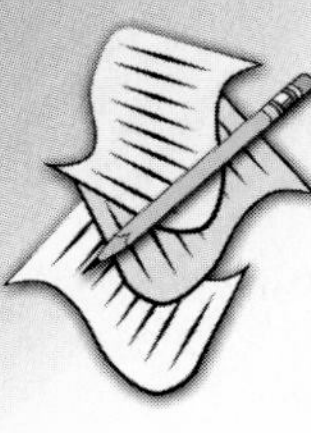

EXERCISE 7.3

Choosing Words from Context

When transcribing dictation, the medical transcriptionist frequently needs to consider the situation when determining the word that correctly completes the sentence. From the list below, select the term that meaningfully completes each of the following statements.

afebrile	respiratory distress	tachycardic
erythema	bolus	diffuse
alveoli	rhonchi	tachypneic
hemoptysis	cyanosis	effusion
auscultation	infiltrate	nebulizer
mediastinal	cyanotic	radiograph

1. Upon presentation to the emergency room, the patient was in severe _______________, making breathing painful.
2. On ___________ of the lungs, I heard rhonchi and rales.
3. Her fingernails were ________________, indicating that she needed oxygen.
4. Mrs. Smith is __________ today, with a temperature of 98.6° on exam.
5. The chest x-ray showed improvement in her pleural _________.
6. The patient has had two episodes of _________, when he noticed flecks of blood in his sputum.
7. Although she complains of rapid breathing, she is not _________ on exam.
8. On auscultation, there were ________ heard in the lower lung fields.
9. Jackie has developed a lot of chest congestion over the past 24 hours, with an increase in her wheezing. She has been using her _________ at home but no other medications
10. The patient is ______________, with a heart rate of 160.
11. The ____________ revealed a pleural effusion.
12. The CT scan showed a large ____________ mass in the center of the chest.
13. The color of the lips revealed ____________, an indication that there was an airway obstruction.
14. The chest x-ray revealed a left hilar ____________.
15. The medication was given very quickly by ____________ injection.

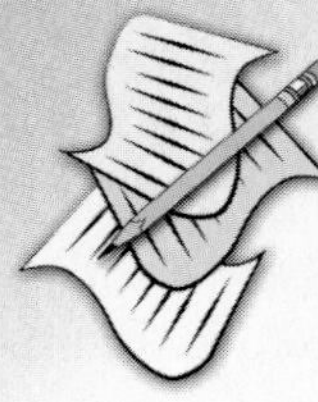

EXERCISE 7.4

Pairing Words and Meanings

From this list, locate the term that best matches each of the following definitions. Write the letter of the term in the space provided by each definition.

A. bronchiole	F. hyperemia	K. Ventolin
B. cystic fibrosis	G. pathogen	L. effusion
C. edema	H. Pseudomonas	M. hemothorax
D. epiglottis	I. theophylline	N. trachea
E. esophagus	J. tympanic membrane	

1. a drug resembling caffeine that dilates blood vessels ______
2. a genus of small, motile bacilli ______
3. a muscular canal that carries food from the mouth to the stomach ______
4. one of the smaller divisions of the bronchial tubes ______
5. a transparent membrane that separates the outer ear from the middle ear ______
6. abnormal collection of fluid in spaces between cells ______
7. a disease in which the passageways (including pancreatic and bile ducts, intestine, and bronchi) become clogged with thick mucus ______
8. cartilage at the back of the mouth cavity that covers the windpipe during swallowing ______
9. increased blood supply in part of the body ______
10. a microorganism that can produce disease ______

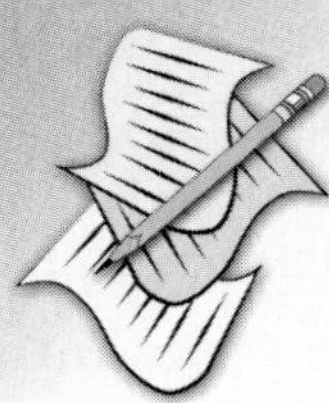

EXERCISE 7.5

Creating Terms from Word Forms

Combine prefixes, root words, and suffixes from this list to create medical words that fit the following definitions. Fill in the blanks with the words you construct.

bronch/o	airway	-capnia	carbon dioxide
hyper-	above or excessive	-cythemia	red blood cells
hypo-	below or deficient	-ectomy	removal of anatomical structure
oxa- or oxy- or oxo-	oxygen	-emia	blood condition
pneum/o or pneumon/o	air or lung	-ia	condition of
		-itis	inflammation or infection
pulmon/o	lung		
thyroid	gland	-plasia	formation; growth

1. excision of the thyroid ________________
2. reduction of oxygen supply to tissue ________________
3. excision of all pulmonary lobes from lung ________________
4. increase in number of cells, enlarging the organ ________________
5. excess of carbon dioxide ________________
6. underdevelopment of organ growth ________________
7. excess of red blood cells ________________
8. excision of entire lung ________________
9. deficiency of carbon dioxide ________________
10. inflammation of the mucosa of the bronchi ________________

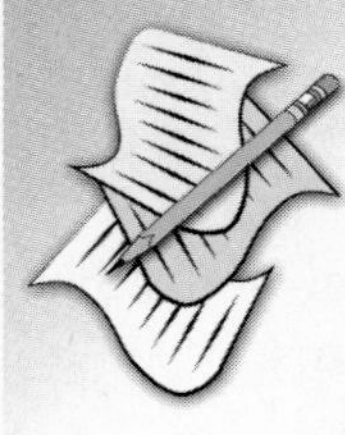

E X E R C I S E 7 . 6

Proofreading Review

Read the following partial medical report and look for errors in word use, spelling, the use of commas, pronoun and reference agreement, and subject and verb agreement. Also check for incomplete sentences. Circle the errors, then key the report with the errors corrected.

1. **PHYSICAL EXAMINATION:** Plus of 120, respertory rate of 30, temperature of 99° and weight 40.6 kg. She is a thin, pale, adolescence female in mild respiratory distress. Head is normocephalic and a traumatic. Pupil are equal, round and reaction to light. Extraocular movements are full. Sclera are anicteric. Conjunctavae is not injected. Nose is without discharge. No flareing. Her mouth have pink and moist mucosa with no lesions. Her lips are cyanotic. His face has a flush over the cheek bones. Her neck is supply, without palpable limph nodes.

2. Within the proxmal right humoral metaphysys ther is a mixed litic and sclerotic lesion. Since the previous exam this has worsened signifacantly.

Building Transcription Skills

The Discharge Summary

Sometimes called a dismissal summary or summary of hospitalization, the discharge summary (Figure 7.3) provides a review of the patient's hospitalization, including the reason for entering the hospital, the patient's medical history, and a description of the procedures and treatment performed during the stay.

Required Headings/Content Headings required by JCAHO include history, course in the hospital, instructions to the patient (disposition), and final diagnosis(es). Physicians may also add history of present illness, family history, social history, physical examination, laboratory data, x-ray findings, and condition on discharge.

The instructions for continuing care can include information on therapy, diet, activity, and medications prescribed for the patient at discharge.

Turnaround Time Medical records for discharged patients are to be completed within a time period specified by the hospital but not to exceed 30 days. Because subsequent medical care can proceed without the discharge summary, the turnaround time on this report is typically three to seven days, which is longer than for other, more critical chart reports.

1" top and side margins

Aligning name, dates, and record numbers is another acceptable format

left justification

PATIENT NAME: **tab** Jaheem Arnold
ADMISSION DATE: **tab** 2/13/XX
DISCHARGE DATE: **tab** 2/20/XX
MEDICAL RECORD #: **tab** 7013920

ds

ADMITTING DIAGNOSIS: Reactive airway disease.

ds

DISCHARGE DIAGNOSIS: Reactive airway disease.

ds

HISTORY OF PRESENT ILLNESS: The patient is a 19-month-old African-American male who had been well until 2 days prior to admission, when he developed a loose cough. Mother gave him an over-the-counter children's cough remedy several times each day. He was afebrile during this time. During the day, the child had increased difficulty breathing, and wheezing was noted in the late p.m., when the child was brought to the emergency room.

In the emergency room, the child was found to have a fever of 102°F rectally. He was found to be in respiratory distress and was given Ventolin nebulization and admitted.

ds

PHYSICAL EXAMINATION: Physical examination showed a patient sitting in bed with mild respiratory distress. He was alert. Respiratory rate was 40, heart rate was 115, temperature was 102.3°. Right tympanic membrane was slightly erythematous. There was slight nasal flaring. Throat was slightly injected. On auscultation, the lungs were found to have diffuse inspiratory and expiratory wheezes. The heart showed the presence of normal heart sounds with mild tachycardia.

ds

HOSPITAL COURSE: Reactive airway disease. The patient was admitted, started on theophylline, given a bolus of theophylline 1 mg/kg and subsequently put on a maintenance dose of theophylline. High-flow nebulization was also given p.o. every 2 hours.

With this management, the patient showed rapid improvement and his respiratory treatments were gradually spaced out so that, subsequently, the regimen was changed to oral medication of theophylline. Theophylline levels were monitored during the hospital course.

(continued)

FIGURE 7.3
Discharge Summary

DISCHARGE SUMMARY
PATIENT NAME: Jaheem Arnold
MEDICAL RECORD #: 7013920
DATE: 2/22/XX
Page 2

ds

DISPOSITION: The child was discharged after a 1 week hospitalization on theophylline therapy. Condition at time of discharge was improved. Mother was instructed to bring him to our office in 1 week.

qs

____
Mencer Alcott, MD

ds

MA/XX
D: 2/22/XX
T: 2/25/XX

FIGURE 7.3
Discharge Summary (Continued)

Preparing to Transcribe

To prepare for transcribing dictation, review the tables of common pulmonology terms, drugs, and abbreviations presented in the Building Language Skills section of this chapter. Then, study the format and organization of the model document shown in Figure 7.3, and key the model document. Proofread the document by comparing it with the printed version. Categorize the types of errors you made, and document them on a copy of the Performance Comparison chart provided in Chapter 1. A template of this chart is included on the IRC that accompanies this text.

Patient Studies

Transcribe, edit, and correct each report in the following patient studies. Consult reference books for words or formatting rules that are unfamiliar.

As you work on the transcription assignment for this chapter, fill in the Performance Comparison chart that you started when you keyed the model document. For at least three of the reports, categorize and document the types of errors you made. Answer the document analysis questions on the bottom of the chart. With continuous practice and assessment, the quality of your work will improve.

After you have produced a final version of each transcribed report, complete the Performance Report cover sheet, attach it to the top of the transcripts, and submit them to your instructor for evaluation.

Patient Study 7.A — Jaheem Arnold

Jaheem Arnold is a 19-month-old African-American male who came to the emergency room (ER) of the hospital at 10 p.m., with a history of cough for 2 days. He had begun wheezing and having increased difficulty breathing for 1 hour prior to coming to the ER.

REPORT 7.1 Discharge Summary

- When the dictator refers to nebulization given "pee oh," transcribe this abbreviation for *by mouth* as p.o.
- Listen for these drug names:
  Ventolin
  theophylline

Patient Study 7.B — Charles Ingrid

Charles Ingrid is a 4½-year-old male who was diagnosed with cystic fibrosis several months ago. He had a history of frequent colds, with large amounts of thick nasal discharge and thick respiratory sputum. His growth was slow, and his mother noticed that he had very sticky bowel movements. The diagnosis of cystic fibrosis was made after the pediatrician sent him for a sweat test that was positive for the disease. Charles is being admitted to the hospital because of a respiratory tract infection, which is common for persons with cystic fibrosis.

REPORT 7.2 Physical Examination Section of Discharge Summary

- PERRL and PERRLA are common abbreviations in the HEENT (head, eyes, ears, nose, and throat) examination. They stand for *pupils equal, round, reactive to light* or *pupils equal, round, reactive to light and accommodation.* This means that the pupils are equal in size and round in shape and that they constrict when a light is shined into the eyes. Accommodation refers to the changing shape of the lens in response to the patient focusing on an object across the room and then on an object a foot or two away.

REPORT 7.3 Consultation Letter

- Physicians sometimes use the words *regime* and *regimen* interchangeably in dictation. However, *regimen* is the word that is usually intended.
- A regime is a system of government or a social system.
- A regimen is a daily routine, as in a *medication regimen.*

Patient Study 7.C

Denise Sultan

Denise Sultan is a 17-year-old girl diagnosed 1 year ago with Hodgkin disease. She has been receiving chemotherapy for the past year. She was admitted to the hospital for difficulty breathing. She was diagnosed with pneumonia and had a complicated hospital course.

REPORT 7.4 Discharge Summary

- Blood gases are transcribed using the chemical abbreviations and numbers. The dictator may use the full term (for example, carbon dioxide) for some gases and may pronounce the letters of the abbreviation for others. In this report, the blood gases should be transcribed as pH of 7.5, pCO_2 of 31, pO_2 of 35, CO_2 of 24, and an O_2 saturation of 84.2.
- Listen for these shortened terms for blood cells in the CBC results:
  segs
  lymphs
  monos
  eos
  basos

Patient Study 7.D

Janis Miller

Janis Miller is a tour guide and part-time college student who has been feeling ill for about a week. She has had a runny nose and shortness of breath.

REPORT 7.5 Office Note

- Listen for these special terms:
  rhinorrhea
  Wright peak flow

Patient Study 7.E — Rhonda Bentz

A third-grader with chronic asthma, Rhonda Bentz is returning for a checkup following treatment for pneumonia.

REPORT 7.6 Office Note

- Listen for these pharmaceutical terms:
  albuterol inhaler with InspirEase
  Azmacort

Patient Study 7.F — Jordan White

Jordan White is an 11-year-old boy with Hurler's syndrome. Over the past months, he has been hospitalized several times with recurrent bronchitis. On this admission, he will undergo laryngoscopy and bronchoscopy to rule out tracheal granulomas.

REPORT 7.7 Operative Report

- Listen for these terms:
  arytenoids
  cannulate
  KTP laser

Patient Study 7.G

Thomas Kalamara

Thomas Kalamara is a 17-year-old young man who complained of severe pain on the right side and immediately collapsed. He was rushed to the emergency room. Chest x-ray revealed a collapse of his right lung. He is being taken to the OR for immediate surgery.

REPORT 7.8 Operative Report

- Listen for these difficult terms:
  pneumothorax
  pneumothoraces
  Surgiport
  apical
  bullous
  emphysematous bullae
  blebs
  latissimus
  2-0 Vicryl
  Scarpa's layer
  4-0 Monocryl

Patient Study 7.H

Rychena Karina

Rychena Karina is referred for a repeat chest x-ray by Dr. Ellinger. She has had recent surgery and has a pulse oximeter reading of 87% on room air.

REPORT 7.9 Radiology Report

- Listen for these difficult terms:
  metaphysis
  lytic
  sclerotic
  perihilar
  metastasis

Patient Study 7.I — Jeffrey Arron

Jeffrey has been diagnosed with a kidney tumor and is sent for CT scan to determine if there are metastases in the lungs. It is noted that there are some small pleural effusions.

REPORT 7.10 Radiology Report

- Listen for these difficult terms:
  postop (postoperative)
  atelectasis
  parenchymal

Using Medical References

Use the appropriate medical reference to locate the correct spelling and additional usage information for the words below. (If the reference is not available, use the Glossary in this text.) Circle the correct spelling, then write a sentence using the word correctly.

1. pneumothorax pneumothorix pneumothoracs
____

2. broncholes bronchiols bronchioles
____

3. abscess absess abcsess
____

4. theophyllin theophyline theophylline
____

5. pneumonitus pneumanitis pneumonitis
____

6. bronciectasis bronchiectasis bronchiectasus
____

7. thyromegaly thyromagely thyroidmegaly
____

8. bronchitis broncitis bronchitus
____

9. fibrous fibrus fibruos
____

10. diaphram diagphram diaphragm
____

Assessing Transcription Skills

Making Expert Decisions

Circle the correct word from the choices in parentheses.

1. (Expiratory/Inspiratory) wheezing was noted as the patient breathed out.
2. The patient had a ventilation (perfusion/profusion) scan to assess the pulmonary function.
3. The patient reports having difficulty breathing while lying down. She stated that she had 2-pillow (dyspnea/orthopnea).
4. Sounds heard on inspiration and expiration were normal, indicating (vascular/vesicular) breathing.
5. Lungs revealed good air entry and vesicular breathing. No rales or (coarse/course) rhonchi were heard.
6. Utilizing a stethoscope, the physician performed (auscultation/percussion) of the lung fields.
7. Air exchange takes place in the (alveoli/bronchi).
8. The patient stated that she could not (breath/breathe) through her nose.
9. Only the left lower lobe of the lung was removed during the (lobectomy/pneumonectomy).
10. During the hospital course, this (regime/regimen) was tried and deemed successful.

Transcribing Professional Documents

Transcribe the document named Chapter 7 Assessment. Before you key, review the document formatting guidelines. Proofread your transcribed document and revise it until you think it is error-free.

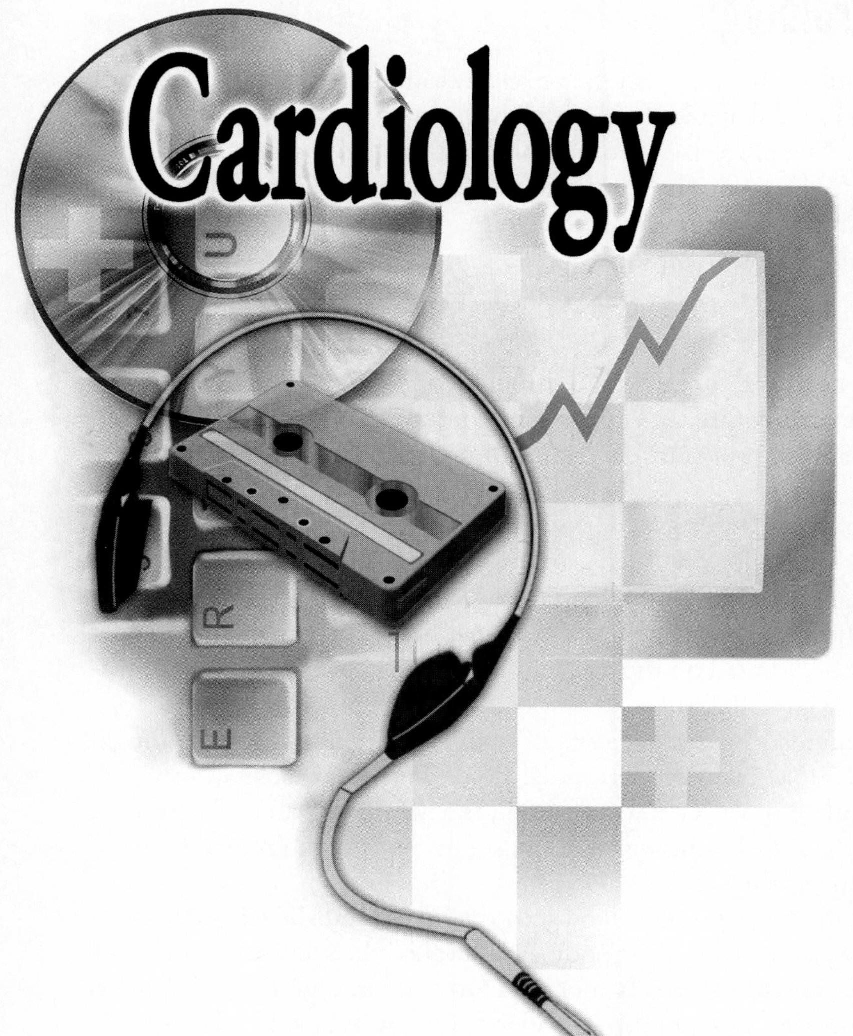

Cardiology is the study of the heart and the blood vessels that carry blood throughout the body. Cardiovascular diseases are the major cause of death in the United States and many other Western societies. Over the last few decades, however, advances in surgical techniques and knowledge about lifestyle and diet effects on the cardiovascular system have resulted in a significant decline in the death rate from heart disease. Medical transcriptionists working in cardiology are constantly challenged by the changing terminology for procedures, new drugs, and technology.

OBJECTIVES

- Use cardiology terms correctly according to the context and purpose of the dictation.
- Select and use appropriate general and specialty reference materials.
- Key cardiology documents of varying complexity and format.
- Transcribe authentic medical dictation requiring concentration and listening skill.
- Edit medical reports to conform with AAMT style guidelines.
- Proofread and correct transcripts to produce error-free documents.

Exploring Cardiology

Cardiology is the study of the heart and the vessels surrounding the heart. The heart is a muscular pump that circulates blood through the body via the pulmonary and systemic circulation. The physician who specializes in this field is the cardiologist. Subspecialists include interventional cardiologists, who assess the function of the heart through invasive and noninvasive procedures, and cardiovascular surgeons, who operate on the heart and its vessels.

Structure and Function

The function of the heart is to pump blood throughout the body. The blood vessels are arranged so that each contraction of the heart pumps blood through the pulmonary circulation and the systemic circulation simultaneously, although each has a distinct purpose.

The heart and great vessels are located between the lungs in the middle of the thoracic rib cage, which is called the mediastinum (Figure 8.1). The normal heart extends from the second to the fifth intercostal space and from the right sternal border to the left midclavicular line. The heart is shaped like a triangle with the wider portion, called the base, located on the top, and the point, or apex, pointing downward and to the left (Figure 8.2).

The heart is surrounded by several layers of tissue. The pericardium is a tough, fibrous protective sac that contains pericardial fluid. This fluid facilitates smooth movement of the heart muscle. The myocardium, the muscular wall of the heart, is the tissue that does the actual pumping. The endocardium is the thin membrane of tissue lining the inside of the heart.

The right side of the heart pumps blood into the lungs, and the left side simultaneously pumps blood throughout the body. A wall called the septum separates the two sides. Each side consists of two chambers: an atrium (anteroom), which holds the blood, and a ventricle, which pumps the blood. One-way valves at the entry to each chamber open only in response to pressure gradients in the blood, preventing backflow.

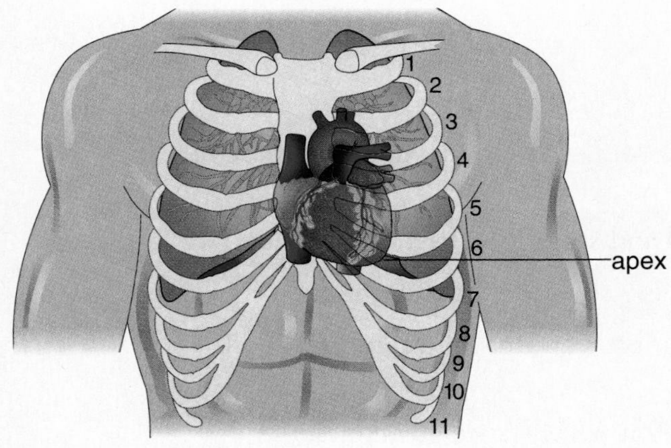

FIGURE 8.1
Position of the Heart in the Thoracic Cavity

The atrioventricular (AV) valves separate the atria and ventricles. The right AV valve is the tricuspid, and the left AV valve is the bicuspid, or mitral valve. The AV valves open during the heart's filling phase, or diastole. This allows the ventricles to fill with blood. During the systole phase, when the heart pumps blood out of the ventricles, the valves close to prevent regurgitation of blood back into the atria.

The semilunar (SL) valves are located between the ventricles and the arteries. The pulmonic valve is in the right side of the heart, and the aortic valve is in the left side. They open during systole to allow ejection of blood from the heart.

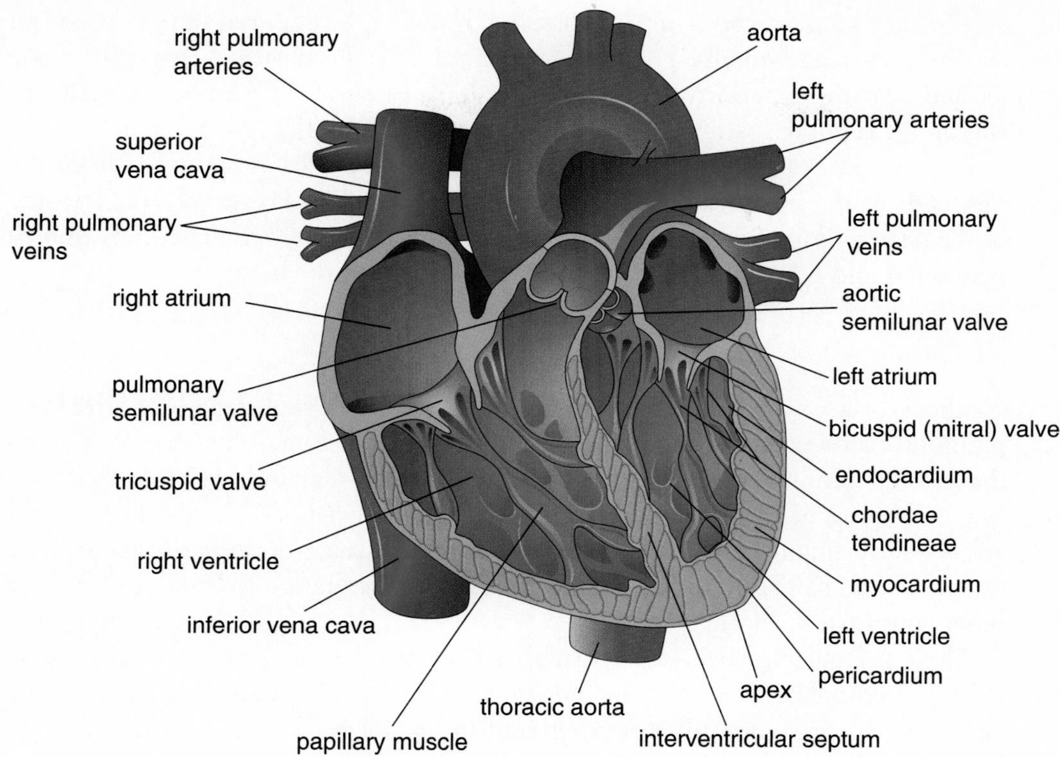

FIGURE 8.2
Internal Structures of the Heart

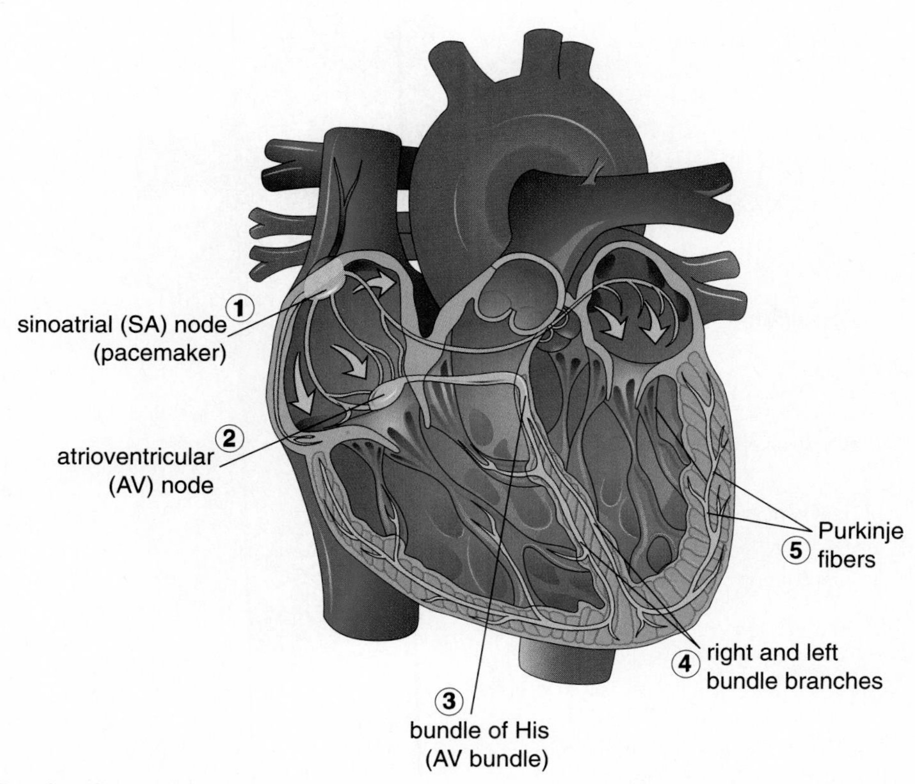

FIGURE 8.3
Electrical Current Flow in the Heart

The cardiac cycle, consisting of diastole and systole, is produced in response to an electrical current contained within specialized cells in the sinoatrial (SA) node located near the superior vena cava (Figure 8.3). Because the SA node has its own rhythm, it is known as the heart's "pacemaker."

During each cardiac cycle, unoxygenated red blood cells are pumped from the right side of the heart into the lungs for oxygenation. Simultaneously, the left side of the heart pumps oxygenated blood into the body (Figure 8.4). The heart pumps between 4 and 6 liters of blood per minute throughout the body.

Physical Assessment

Cardiovascular assessment begins by noting the patient's vital signs. Abnormal respirations, blood pressure, and pulse can indicate heart disease. A bluish color around the lips (circumoral cyanosis) and/or on the nail beds may indicate decreased oxygen. Clubbing of the fingers is a sign of chronic oxygen deficiency. The carotid artery and the jugular veins in the neck reflect the efficiency of cardiac function. The examiner uses palpation to feel for the pulses and auscultation to listen for bruits or other abnormal sounds.

The examiner may palpate the patient's chest for the point of maximal impulse (PMI). A complete assessment includes auscultation of the heart's sounds in all the "stations": aortic, pulmonic, tricuspid, and mitral valves. The rate and rhythm are noted. The start of systole, caused by the AV valves closing, is noted as S1 and serves

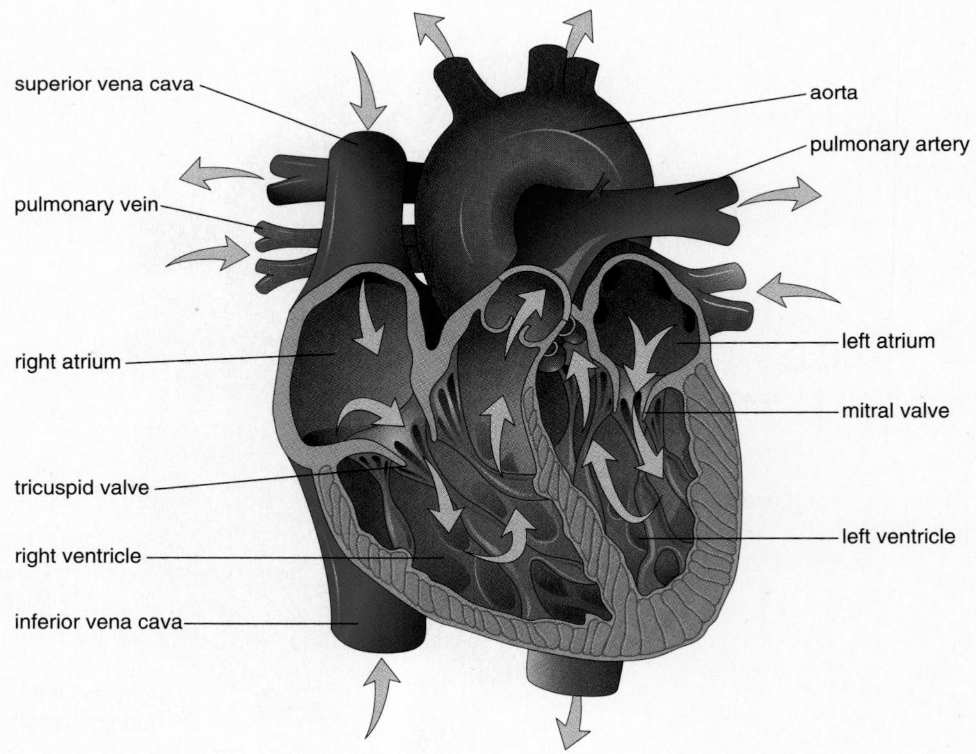

FIGURE 8.4
Blood Flow in the Heart

as the reference point for the other cardiac sounds. The S2 sound represents the closure of the semilunar valves.

The heart is examined with the patient in different positions to be sure that any murmurs or abnormal heart sounds are ascertained. The sound of a murmur is described by the intensity in terms of six grades. For example, the physician may dictate the phrase "a grade two over six systolic ejection murmur" (which is transcribed as 2/6 or, less commonly, using Roman numerals II/VI). The quality and location of the murmur may be described, and the physician may use words such as *gallop, whistle,* and *musical* to describe some abnormal heart sounds.

Diseases and Conditions

There are five main forms of heart disease: (1) hypertensive heart disease, in which the heart is overworked and gives way through exhaustion; (2) coronary artery occlusion, in which the heart muscle does not receive enough blood flow due to a blockage in narrowed coronary arteries; (3) rheumatic heart disease, which is caused by infection of the heart valves and which frequently leads to stenosis (narrowing of the valves); (4) bacterial endocarditis, in which the heart's action is damaged by inflammation; and (5) congenital heart disease, frequently caused by a malformation in the septum, or wall separating the right half of the heart from the left, and resulting in an intermingling of blood in the systemic and pulmonary circulations.

A condition in which damaged heart tissue interrupts the electrical currents is known as heart block. Another common condition in diseased hearts is atrial fibrillation in which the atria contract so rapidly that the ventricles pump inefficiently.

Heart disease can be treated by lifestyle changes (diet and exercise programs and smoking cessation), with drugs, and/or with surgical procedures.

Common Tests and Surgical Procedures

Evaluation of the heart includes a chest x-ray to determine size and position, an electrocardiogram (ECG) to record the conduction system (Figure 8.5), and an echocardiogram to record the anatomy and motion of the heart. Other tests include angiograms, arteriograms, and venograms. Cardiac catheterization provides a visualization of the coronary arteries. A small flexible tube (catheter) is threaded from an arterial access site toward the heart. Dye is injected and the resulting pictures are viewed to determine abnormalities.

Drug treatments include enzyme inhibitors, antianginals, antiarrhythmics, anticoagulants, antihypertensives, beta blockers, calcium channel blockers, cardiotonics, and hypolipidemics. Cardiac surgical procedures include coronary artery bypass surgery; embolectomy, thrombectomy, angioplasty or atherectomy to open or clear blocked arteries; valve replacement surgery; and pacemaker, internal defibrillator devices, and intravascular stent implantations.

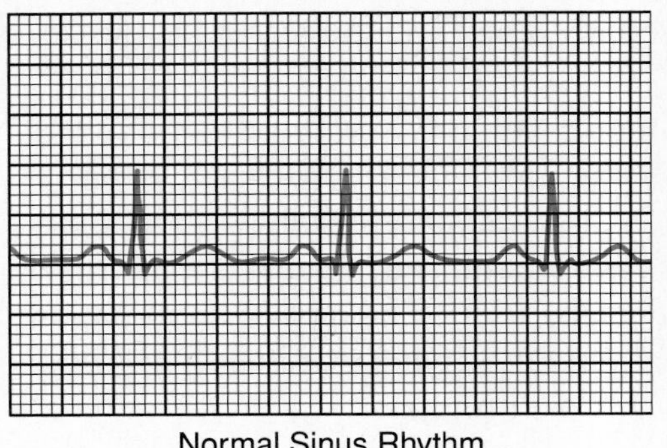

Normal Sinus Rhythm

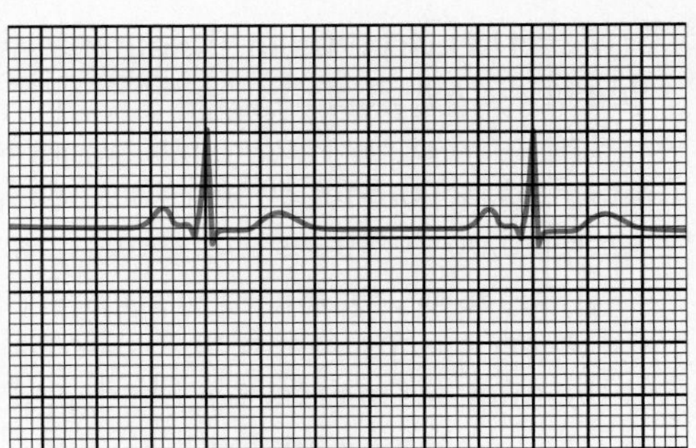

Sinus Bradycardia

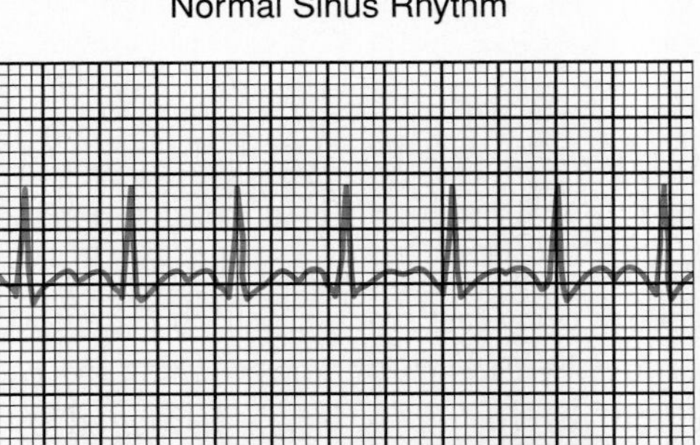

Sinus Tachycardia

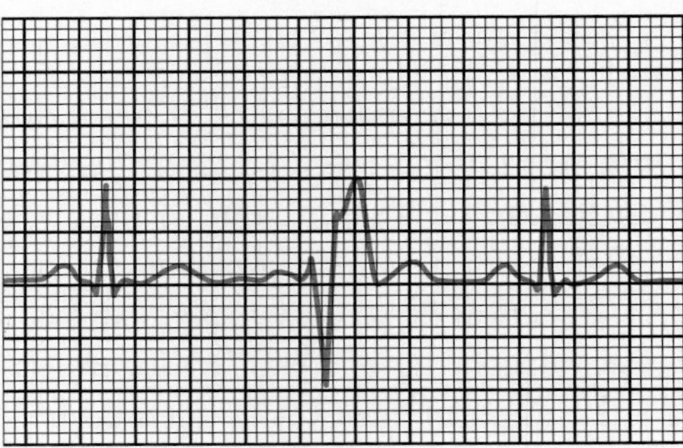

Premature Ventricular Contraction

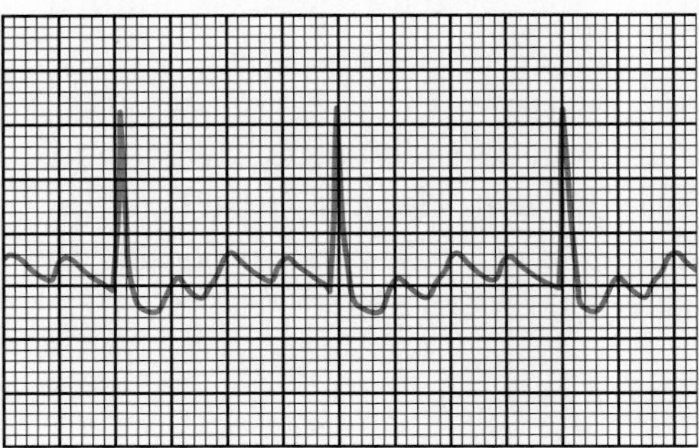

Atrial Flutter

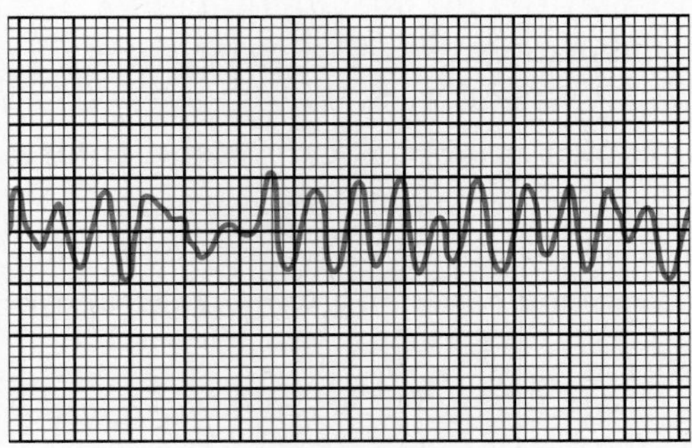

Ventricular Fibrillation

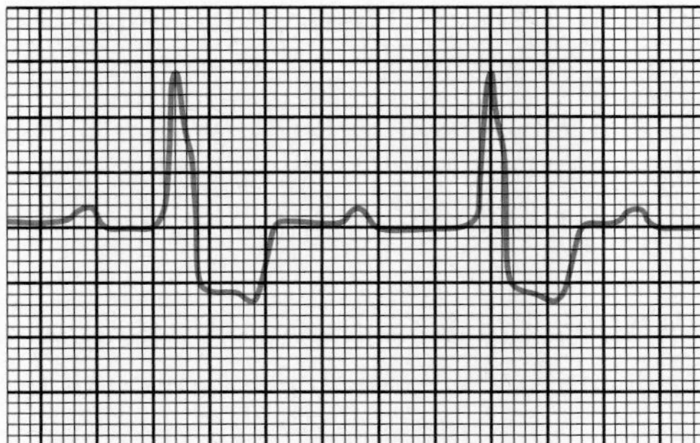

Atrioventricular Block

FIGURE 8.5
Heart Rhythms in ECG Tracings

Building Language Skills

The following tables list common cardiology terms, drugs, and abbreviations. The list of terms and definitions includes the most difficult words contained in the dictated reports in this chapter. These words are identified in GREEN type. A list of common drugs is found in Appendix D.

Medical Terms and Pharmacologic Agents

acyanotic
(ay-sI-a-**not**-ik) (adj) pertaining to the absence of cyanosis (slightly bluish, grayish, slatelike, or dark purple discoloration of the skin due to a reduction of oxygenated blood

ambulation
(am-byoo-**lay**-shun) (n) walking or moving about

anastomosis
(a-**nas**-tO-mO-sis) (n) a natural or surgical connection between two blood vessels, spaces, or organs

aneurysm
(**an**-yoo-rizm) (n) bulging out of an arterial wall due to a weakness in the wall

angina pectoris
(**an**-ji-na/an-**jI**-na **pek**-tO-ris) (n) an attack of intense chest pain; also known as stenocardia

angiography
(an-jee-**og**-ra-fee) (n) x-ray of blood vessels, usually after injecting a radiopaque substance

aorta
(ay-**Or**-ta) (n) the main artery leaving the heart

aortic root
(ay-**Or**-tik) (n) the opening of the aorta in the left ventricle of the heart

aortogram
(ay-**Or**-tO-gram) (n) x-ray of the aorta after injection of a radiopaque substance

arrhythmia
(a-**rith**-mee-a) (n) disturbance of normal rhythm; irregular heartbeat

arteriosclerosis
(ar-**teer**-ee-O-skler-**O**-sis) (n) hardening of the arteries

artery
(**ar**-ter-ee) (n) a vessel that carries blood away from the heart to other tissues throughout the body

ascending aorta
(n) the beginning section of the aorta, rising from the left ventricle of the heart to the arch

asymptomatic
(ay-simp-tO-**mat**-ik) (adj) without symptoms

atelectasis
(at-e-**lek**-ta-sis) (n) incomplete expansion of the lungs at birth or collapse of the adult lung

atherosclerosis
(**ath**-er-O-skler-**O**-sis) (n) buildup of fatty plaques inside arteries; a type of arteriosclerosis

atrial
(**ay**-tree-al) (adj) relating to the atrium

atrioventricular
(**ay**-tree-O-ven-**trik**-yoo-lar) (adj) relating to both the atria (upper chambers) and the ventricles (lower chambers) in the heart, or blood flow between them

atrioventricular groove
(n) a groove visible on the outside of the heart between the atria and the ventricles

atrium
(**ay**-tree-um) (n) one of the two upper chambers of the heart

attenuation
(a-ten-yoo-**ay**-shun) (n) process of weakening, such as the potency of a drug or the virulence of a disease-causing germ

auscultation
(aws-kul-**tay**-shun) (n) process of listening for sounds produced in some of the body cavities to detect abnormal conditions

autologous
(aw-**tol**-O-gus) (adj) indicating something that has its origin within an individual, especially a factor present in tissues or fluids

caliber
(**kal**-i-ber) (n) diameter of a tube or vessel, such as a blood vessel

capillary
(**kap**-i-layr-ee) (n) smallest type of blood vessels

cardiac tamponade
(**kar**-dee-ak tam-po-**nayd**) (n) compression of the venous return to the heart by fluid or blood in the pericardium

cardiomyopathy
(**kar**-dee-O-mI-**op**-a-thee) (n) disease of the heart muscle

catheter
(**kath**-e-ter) (n) a tube inserted into the body for removing or instilling fluids for diagnostic or therapeutic purposes

catheterization
(**kath**-e-ter-I-**zay**-shun) (n) the insertion of a catheter

circumflex
(**ser**-kum-fleks) (adj) bending around; describes anatomical structures that are shaped like an arc of a circle

collaterals
(ko-**lat**-er-als) (n) accompanying, as side by side; blood vessels that branch from larger vessels

compressible
(kom-**pres**-i-bl) (adj) pressed together; made more compact by or as by pressure

congestive heart failure
(CHF) (kon-**jes**-tiv) (n) condition in which the heart is unable to pump adequate blood to the tissues and organs, often due to myocardial infarction

coronary bypass surgery
(**kOr**-o-nayr-ee) (n) vein grafts or other surgical methods are used to carry blood from the aorta to branches of the coronary arteries in order to increase the flow beyond a local obstruction

coronary cusp
(n) one of the triangular parts of a heart valve

cyanosis
(cI-a-n**O**-sis) (n) bluish discoloration of the skin and/or mucous membranes due to decreased amount of oxygen in the blood cells

deep vein (or venous) thrombosis
(deep vayn throm-**bO**-sis) (n) a clump of various blood components in a blood vessel, forming an obstruction

defibrillator
(dee-**fib**-ri-lay-ter) (n) an agent, measure, or machine, e.g., an electric shock, that stops fibrillation of the ventricular muscle and restores the normal beat

diaphoresis
(**dI**-a-fO-**ree**-sis) (n) profuse perspiration or sweating

diaphragm
(**dI**-a-fram) (n) the muscle that separates the thoracic (chest) and abdominal cavities

digoxin
(di-**jok**-sin) (n) a heart stimulant

dilatation
(dil-a-**tay**-shun) (n) stretching or enlarging; dilation

distal
(**dis**tal) (adj) away from a center or point of reference; toward the far end of something

distally
(**dis**-ta-lee) (adv) occurring farthest from the center, from a medial line, or from the trunk

Doppler
(**dop**-ler) (n) a diagnostic instrument that emits an ultrasonic beam into the body

ductus arteriosus
(**duk**-tus ar-ter-ee-**O**-sus) (n) blood vessel in the fetus connecting the pulmonary artery directly to the ascending aorta, thus bypassing the pulmonary circulation

dysfunction
(dis-**funk**-shun) (n) abnormal or impaired function

echocardiogram
(ek-O-**kar**-dee-O-gram) (n) a sound-wave image of the heart's size, position, and motion

edema
(e-**dee**-ma) (n) abnormal accumulation of fluid in intercellular tissue

electrocardiogram
(ee-**lek**-trO-**kar**-dee-**O**-gram) (n) a graphic record of electrical waves within the heart

embolism
(**em**-bO-lizm) (n) blockage of a blood vessel by an abnormal object, such as a clot

endocarditis
(**en**-dO-kar-**dI**-tis) (n) inflammation of the endocardium and/or the heart valves

endocardium
(en-dO-**kar**-dee-um) (n) inner lining of the heart

exudates
(**eks**-oo-daytz) (n) accumulations of fluid in a cavity; matter that penetrates through vessel walls into adjoining tissues

femoral
(**fem**-o-ral) (adj) relating to the thigh artery or bone, the femur

femoralis
(fem-or-**awl**-is) (adj) pertaining to the femur, the longest and strongest bone in body, going from hip to knee

fibrinous
(**fI**-brin-us) (adj) pertaining to, of the nature of, or containing fibrin (a whitish filamentous protein)

foramen ovale
(fo-**ray**-men **O**-va-lay) (n) an oval opening through a bone or membrane; a hole normally found in the fetal heart that closes at birth

gestational age
(ges-**tay**-shun-al aj) (n) age of a fetus or newborn, usually expressed in weeks since the onset of the mother's last menstrual period

gross
(grOs) (adj) visible to the naked eye

hemodynamic
(**hee**-mO-dI-**nam**-ik) (adj) relating to the mechanics of blood circulation

hemostasis
(**hee**-mO-stay-sis/hee-**mos**-ta-sis) (n) stopping bleeding either naturally through blood coagulation, mechanically (as with surgical clamps), or chemically (with drugs)

hypokinesis
(**hI**-pO-ki-**nee**-sis) (n) decreased or slow motor reaction to stimulus

hypoperfusion
(**hI**-pO-per-**fyoo**-zhun) (n) lower-than-normal passage of a liquid through an organ or body part

infarction
(in-**fark**-shun) (n) formation of dead tissue as a result of diminished or stopped blood flow to the tissue area

inferior
(in-**fee**-ree-Or) (adj) lower; below; of lesser value

intimal
(**in**-ti-mal) (adj) relating to the innermost lining of a part, especially of a blood vessel; (n) intima

intravenous
(IV) (**in**-tra-**vee**-nus) (adj) within or by way of a vein

ischemia
(is-**kee**-mee-a) (n) decreased blood supply due to obstruction, such as narrowing of the blood vessels

lesion
(**lee**-zhun) (n) general term for any visible, circumscribed injury to the skin; such as, a wound, sore, rash, or mass

mammary
(**mam**-a-ree) (adj) relating to the breast

millicuries
(**mil**-i-**kyoo**-rees) (n) a unit of radioactivity, abbreviated mc

mitral
(**mI**-tral) (adj) relating to the bicuspid or mitral valve of the heart, between the atrium and the ventricle on the left side of the heart

murmur
(**mer**-mer) (n) abnormal heart sound

myocardial
(mI-O-**kar**-dee-al) (adj) relating to the myocardium, the heart muscle

obtuse
(ob-**toos**) (adj) dull or blunt; not pointed or acute

occlusion
(o-**kloo**-zhun) (n) blockage, such as coronary occlusion

orifice
(**or**-i-fis) (n) mouth, entrance, or outlet of any aperture

oscilloscope
(o-**sil**-O-scOp) (n) an instrument which displays electrical oscillations (waves) on a screen

oximetry
(ok-**sim**-e-tree) (n) measuring the amount of oxygen combined with the hemoglobin in a blood sample

pallor
(**pal**-or) (n) abnormal paleness of the skin; deficiency of color

palpitations
(pal-pi-**tay**-shuns) (n) stronger and more rapid heartbeats as felt by the patient; pounding or throbbing of the heart

parenteral
(pa-**ren**-ter-al) (adj) not through the digestive system, such as introduction of nutrients into the veins or under the skin

paroxysmal
(par-ok-**siz**-mal) (adj) relating to or recurring in paroxysms (sudden, severe attacks of symptoms or convulsions)

patent
(**pa**-tent) (adj) open; unblocked

pedal
(**ped**-al or **pE**dal) (adj) relating to the foot

pedicle
(**ped**-i-kl) (n) the stem that attaches a new growth

pedunculated
(pee-**dung**-Q-late-ed) (adj) possessing a stalk

perfusion
(per-**fyoo**-zhun) (n) passing of a fluid through spaces

pericardial
(per-i-**kar**-dee-al) (adj) surrounding the heart; relating to the pericardium

pericarditis
(per-i-kar-**dI**-tis) (n) an inflammatory disease of the pericardium (tough outer layer of the heart wall and lining of the pericardial sac that surrounds the heart)

pericardium
(per-i-**kar**-dee-um) (n) sac around the heart allowing movement without friction

peripheral vascular disease
(pe-**rif**-e-ral **vas**-kyoo-lar)(n) any disorder affecting the blood circulatory system, except the heart

phasic
(**fay**-sic) (adj) pertaining to a phase, a stage of development

phlebitis
(fle-**bI**-tis) (n) inflammation of a vein

phlebotomy
(fle-**bot**-O-mee) (n) incision into a vein for drawing blood

photon
(**fO**-ton) (n) a unit of radiant energy or light intensity

pleural
(**ploo**-ral) (adj) concerning the pleura (serous membrane that enfolds both lungs and is reflected upon the walls of the thorax and diaphragm

popliteal
(pop-**lit**-ee-al) (adj) concerning the posterior surface of the knee

precordial
(pree-**kor**-dee-al) (adj) pertaining to the precordium (region of the chest over the heart)

prolapse
(prO-**laps**) (n) dropping of an organ from its normal position, a sinking down

proximal
(**prok**-si-mal) (adj) nearest to a point of reference or center of the body

proximal
(**prok**-si-mal) (adj) nearest the point of attachment, center of the body, or point of reference

proximally
(**prok**-si-mal-lee) (adv) occurring nearest to the point of attachment, center of the body, or point of reference

radiopaque
(ray-dee-O-**payk**) (adj) opaque to x-rays or other radiation; an injection of a radiopaque dye or substance may be used to visualize areas of the body by x-ray

ramus
(**ray**-mus) (n) branch, especially of a nerve or blood vessel

reflux
(**ree**-fluks) (n) a return or backward flow

regurgitation
(ree-**ger**-ji-**tay**-shun) (n) a backward flowing, as a backflow of blood through a defective heart valve or the bringing up of gas or undigested food from the stomach

retrograde
(**ret**-rO-grayd) (adj) moving or going backward

rheumatic fever
(roo-**mat**-ik **fee**-ver) (n) fever following infection with *Streptococcus* bacteria; may affect the joints, skin, and heart

saphenous vein
(sa-**fee**-nus vayn) (n) either of two main veins in the leg that drain blood from the foot

scan
(n) scanning a tissue, organ, or system using a special apparatus that displays and records its image, such as computer tomography (CAT scan); the image so obtained

septal
(**sep**-tal) (adj) pertaining to a dividing partition

septum
(**sep**-tum) (n) a partition that separates a structure, as the two sides of the heart

sheath
(n) structure surrounding an organ, body part, or object

sinus rhythm
(**si**-nus **rith**-um) (n) normal cardiac rhythm

situs
(**sI**-tus) (n) a position

stenocardia
(sten-O-**kar**-dee-a) (n) an attack of intense chest pain; also called angina pectoris

stenosis
(ste-**nO**-sis) (n) narrowing or constriction of a passageway or opening, such as a blood vessel

sublingual
(sub-**ling**-gwahl) (adj) beneath the tongue

subxiphoid
(sub-**zif**-oyd) (adj) below a sword-shaped structure, as the xiphoid process, a structure beneath the lowest portion of the sternum

systolic
(sis-**tol**-ik) (adj) pertaining to systole, the part of the heart cycle in which the heart is in contraction

thermodilution
(**ther**-mO-di-**loo**-shun) (n) method of determining cardiac output; involves injecting a cold liquid into the bloodstream and measuring the temperature change downstream

thrombophlebitis
(**throm**-bO-fle-**bI**-tis) (n) inflammation of a vein with clot formation (thrombus)

thrombus
(**throm**-bus) (n) blood clot attached to the interior wall of a vein or artery

tibia
(tib-ee-a) (n) inner and thicker of the two bones of the human leg between the knee and the ankle

tibial
(tib-ee-al) (adj) pertaining to the tibia

transesophageal
(tranz-ee-sof-a-**jee**-al) (adj) pertaining to an abnormal opening between the trachea and esophagus

tomographic
(tO-**mog**-ra-feek) (adj) referring to an x-ray technique which displays an organ or tissue at a particular depth

vena cava
(**vee**-na **kav**-a) (n) one of the largest veins of the body; venae cavae (pl)

vascular
(**vas**-kyoo-lar) (adj) relating to the blood vessels

veno-occlusive
(**vee**-nO O-**kloo**-siv) (adj) concerning obstruction of veins

venous
(**vee**-nus) (adj) relating to a vein or veins

ventricle
(**ven**-tri-kl) (n) either of the two lower chambers of the heart

ventriculogram
(ven-**trik**-yoo-lO-gram) (n) an x-ray of the ventricles

ventriculography
(ven-trik-yoo-**log**-ra-fee) (n) x-ray visualization of heart ventricles after injection of a radiopaque substance

xiphoid
(**zif**-oyd) (adj) referring to the xiphoid process, the cartilage at the lower end of the sternum (breast bone); also spelled xyphoid

Abbreviations

ACG	angiocardiography
AICA	anterior inferior communicating artery
AS	aortic stenosis
ASD	atrial septal defect
ASHD	arteriosclerotic heart disease
BBB	bundle-branch block
CAD	coronary artery disease
CC	cardiac catheterization
CCU	coronary care unit
CF	circumflex (artery)
CHF	congestive heart failure
CPR	cardiopulmonary resuscitation
CV	cardiovascular
DVT	deep vein thrombosis
ECG or EKG	electrocardiogram
ICA	internal carotid artery
IMA	internal mammary artery
IV	intravenous
LAD	left anterior descending coronary artery
LCA	left coronary artery
LCF	left circumflex
LIMA	left internal mammary artery
LMCA	left main coronary artery
LPA	left pulmonary artery
MCL	midclavicular line
MI	myocardial infarction
MPA	main pulmonary artery
MS	mitral stenosis
MVP	mitral valve prolapse
OM	obtuse marginal [coronary artery]
PA	pulmonary artery
PAT	paroxysmal atrial tachycardia
PDA	posterior descending artery; patent ductus arteriosis
PICA	posterior inferior communicating artery
PMI	point of maximal impulse
PVC	premature ventricular contraction
RAO	right anterior oblique (view)
RCA	right coronary artery
RPA	right pulmonary artery
S-A	sinoatrial node
SFA	superficial femoral artery
VSD	ventricular septal defect

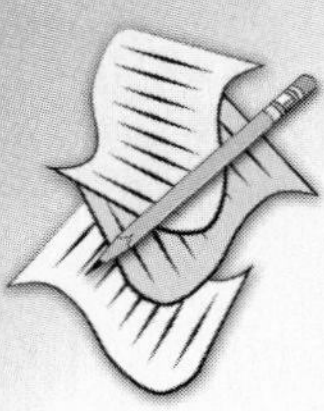

EXERCISE 8.1

Recognizing Look-Alikes and Sound-Alikes

Below is a list of frequently used words that look alike and/or sound alike. Study the meaning and pronunciation of each set of words, then read the following sentences carefully and circle the word in parentheses that correctly completes the meaning.

endocardial	within the heart
myocardial	relating to the heart muscle

pericardial	surrounding the heart
precordial	in front of the heart

inter-	between
intra-	within
infra-	below or under

nitrate	a salt of nitric acid; medication
nitrite	a salt of nitrous acid; found on urinalysis

palpation	examination by touching
palpitation	rapid or fluttering heartbeat

profuse	(adj) overabundant
perfuse	(v) to spread about

pulse	regular, rhythmic beat
plus	increased by or added to

pedal	(adj) relating to the foot
pedal	(n) a foot-operated mechanism
petal	(n) part of a flower

reinjected	injected again (as with a drug)
reinfected	infected again (as with an organism or pathogen)

recent	(adj) not long ago
resent	(v) to be annoyed at

1. The patient's (interocular, intraocular) pressure was within normal limits.
2. A (recent, resent) blood pressure check reveals the patient to be hypertensive.
3. The posterior tibial (pluses, pulses) were 2+/4+.
4. The patient had 1+ (pedal, petal) edema.
5. The patient was given an (infection, injection) of amoxicillin (intramuscularly, intermuscularly).
6. Her urine shows no white cells, trace leukocytes, and positive (nitrates, nitrites).
7. The patient has no tenderness to deep (palpation, palpitation).
8. She is complaining of (palpations, palpitations) after drinking several cups of coffee.
9. His night sweats are so (perfuse, profuse) that he regularly soaks his pajamas.
10. His previous surgeries resulted in (pericardial, precordial) adhesions.

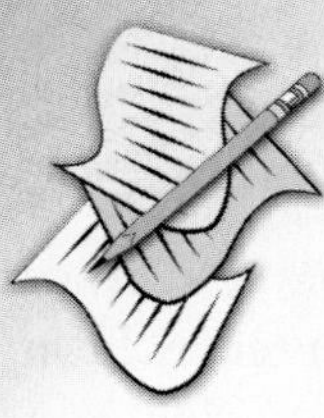

EXERCISE 8.2

Matching Sound and Spelling

The numbered list that follows shows the phonetic spelling of hard-to-spell words. Sound out the word, then write the correct spelling in the blank space provided. Each of the words can be found in the Glossary or in the drug list in Appendix D.

1. **zif**-oyd ______________________
2. a-**rith**-mee-a ______________________
3. a-**nas**-tO-mO-sis ______________________
4. ni-**fed**-i-peen ______________________
5. lIs-**in**-O-pril ______________________
6. lO-va-**stat**-in ______________________
7. **lee**-zhun ______________________
8. o-**kloo**-zhun ______________________
9. **an**-yoo-rizm ______________________
10. **vee**-nus ______________________
11. te-**ray**-zO-sin ______________________
12. pal-pi-**tay**-shuns ______________________
13. an-**jI**-na ______________________
14. ver-**ap**-a-mil ______________________
15. **cap**-tO-pril ______________________

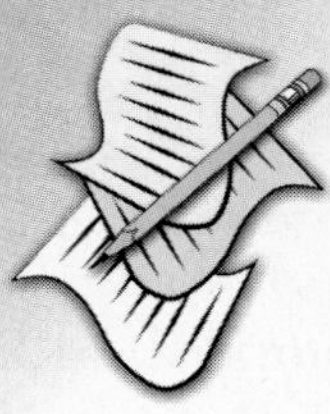

EXERCISE 8.3

Choosing Words from Context

When transcribing dictation, the medical transcriptionist frequently needs to consider the situation when determining the word that correctly completes the sentence. From the list below, select the term that meaningfully completes each of the following statements.

ambulating	diaphoresis	ischemia
arrhythmia	dilatation	oximetry
artery	hemodynamic	prolapse
attenuation	infarction	proximal
catheter	intravenous	ventricular

1. If the patient had an MI, it means he or she had a myocardial ____________________.
2. The patient is ______________________ well, with the use of a quad cane.
3. Due to dehydration, she will need ____________________________ fluids.
4. The blockage was not in a main ___________________.
5. While my father was in the hospital, he was monitored by pulse ____________________.
6. The patient's ECG showed left ______________________ dysfunction.
7. After the surgery, he needed a transfusion to return him to his usual ______________ state.
8. The patient's mitral valve __________________ meant she needed to take an antibiotic whenever she had dental work done.
9. A vaccine gives you an (a) __________________________________ of the disease.
10. He needed a Foley ____________________ inserted to collect the urine.

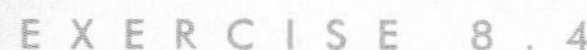
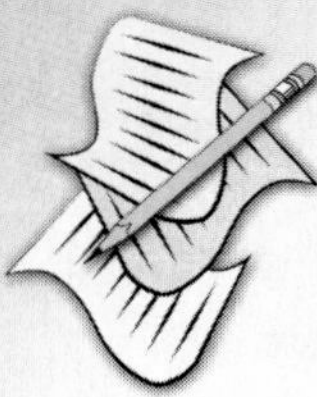

EXERCISE 8.4

Pairing Words and Meanings

From this list, locate the term that best matches each of the following definitions. Write the letter of the term in the space provided by each definition.

A. angiography	F. hypertension	J. ramus
B. aorta	G. ischemia	K. stenosis
C. atrium	H. myocardial	L. thermodilution
D. diaphoresis	I. pericardial	M. ventricle
E. hemostasis		

1. concerning the middle layer of the heart walls __________
2. branch of a nerve or blood vessel __________
3. method of cardiac output determination __________
4. study describing the blood vessels of the heart __________
5. main trunk of the arterial system __________
6. decreased blood supply to a given body part __________
7. abnormal narrowing of a passageway or opening __________
8. profuse sweating __________
9. either of the two upper chambers of the heart __________
10. cessation of bleeding __________

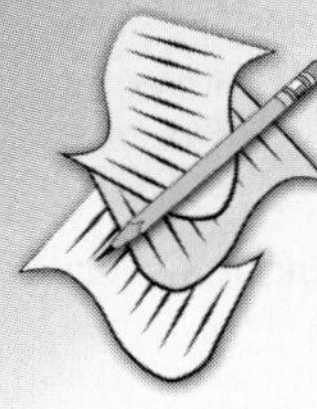

EXERCISE 8.5

Creating Terms from Word Forms

Combine prefixes, root words, and suffixes from this list to create medical words that fit the following definitions. Fill in the blanks with the words you construct.

a-	no, without	tachy-	swift, rapid
brady-	slow	cor	heart
cardio-	heart	-cardia/o	heart
circum-	around	-flect/-flex	bend
dia-	through, complete	-function	work, action, operation
dynamo-	relating to force, energy	-gram	letter, picture, printout
dys-	pain, improper, short	-lingual	tongue
electro-	current, conduction	-megaly	enlargement
hemo-	blood, bleeding	-pathy	disease
hem/o-	relating to blood	-pnea	breathing, breath
intra-	within	pre-	before
myo-	muscle	-stasis	stopping, halting
organ/o	organ	-stolic	sent, sending
peri-	around, near	-ventricular	front, ventricle
steno-	compressed	-xyph-oid	sword-shaped
sub-	beneath, under		

1. rapid heartbeat ____________________
2. under the tongue ____________________
3. a squeezing pain in the heart ____________________
4. the stopping of bleeding ____________________
5. around the heart ____________________
6. shortness of breath ____________________
7. sending through (blood into heart) ____________________
8. bent around ____________________
9. condition characterized by a slow heartbeat ____________________
10. complete picture ____________________
11. within the heart ____________________
12. beneath the lower end of the sternum (breastbone) ____________________
13. before (in front of) the heart ____________________
14. relating to the force of the blood going through the heart ____________________
15. a picture (recording) of the electrical activity of the heart ____________________

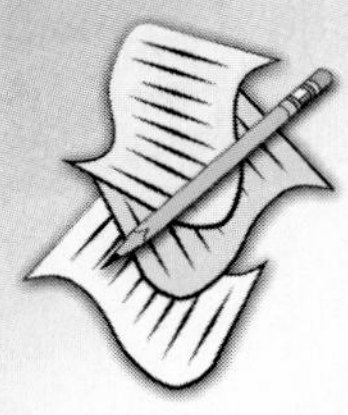

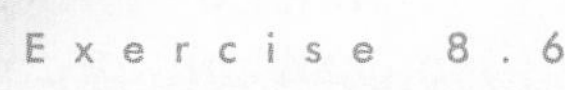

Exercise 8.6

Proofreading Review

Read the following report section and look for errors in spelling, punctuation, plural vs. singular word forms, subject-verb agreement, complete sentences, pronoun-reference agreement, capitalization, and special punctuation marks such as quotation marks. Circle the errors, then key the report with the errors corrected.

1. Left heart catheterization and coronary angiography was performed via Judkins Technique using the rite femoral artery. hemodynamic recordings was made in the ascending aorta at rest.

   blood samples for oximetry were obtained from the pulmonary artery and ascending aorta. Repeat hemodynamic recordings were made on pull-back. The catheter was then withdrawn and direct pressure was applied to the right femoral artery. Both good hemostasis and petal pluses were obtained. the patient tolerated the procedure well and left the laboratory in satisfactory condition.
2. The patent had no recurant chest pain throughout his admission her periferol adema improved somewhat but is still present.

Building Transcription Skills

The Radiology Report

The radiology report (Figure 8.6) is a description of the findings and interpretations of x-ray procedures. Dictated by a radiologist after reviewing the films or test results, the report can focus on bone and joint films, soft tissue films, or special studies of the internal organs. The major diagnostic procedures include roentgenograms (basic x-rays), CT scans (computerized tomography scans), MRI scans (magnetic resonance imaging scans), nuclear medicine procedures such as thyroid scans and bone scans with an injection or infusion of radioactive contrast, and fluoroscopic examinations.

Required Headings/Content Standard components include preliminary information, the type of examination performed and area of focus—for example, chest, skull—plus the contrast media used, and the findings or impressions.

Turnaround Time The usual turnaround time is 12 to 24 hours or even less. However, some hospitals make a voice report available as soon as the radiologist dictates the report.

Preparing to Transcribe

To prepare for transcribing dictation, review the tables of common cardiology terms, drugs, and abbreviations presented in the Building Language Skills section of this chapter. Then, study the format and organization of the model document shown in Figure 8.6, and key the model document. Proofread the document by comparing it with the printed version. Categorize the types of errors you made, and document them on a copy of the Performance Comparison chart provided in Chapter 1. A template of this chart is included on the IRC that accompanies this text.

Patient Studies

Transcribe, edit, and correct each report in the following patient studies. Consult reference books for words or formatting rules that are unfamiliar.

As you work on the transcription assignment for this chapter, fill in the Performance Comparison chart that you started when you keyed the model document. For at least three of the reports, categorize and document the types of errors you made. Answer the document analysis questions on the bottom of the chart. With continuous practice and assessment, the quality of your work will improve.

After you have produced a final version of each transcribed report, complete the Performance Report cover sheet, attach it to the top of the transcripts, and submit them to your instructor for evaluation.

Patient Study 8.A — Jim Andrews

The patient is a 63-year-old male who was admitted to the Intensive Care Unit with chest pain radiating down to the left hand, diaphoresis, and pallor. His physical examination, blood work, and ECG were within normal limits during a routine checkup 2 months ago.

REPORT 8.1 Office Note

REPORT 8.2 Radiology Report of Stress Thallium Scan

- Listen for these terms:
  thallium 201 chloride
  LAO 45 image
  SPECT studies

REPORT 8.3 Consultation Letter

1" top and side margins

DEPARTMENT OF RADIOLOGY

use left justification

PATIENT NAME:	Jim Andrews
MEDICAL RECORD #:	7093578
DATE:	1/12/XX
DOB:	12/23/XX
SEX:	Male
ROOM #:	804
REQUESTING PHYSICIAN:	Sondra Southward, MD

ds

STRESS THALLIUM SCAN WITH REINJECTION ← **test or x-ray name in all caps**

At the time of peak exercise, 4 mc of thallium-201 chloride was injected intravenously and exercise was continued for at least an additional minute. Single-photon emission computer tomographic study, as well as a planar LAO 45 image, was obtained immediately after exercise. The patient returned at least 3 hours later and was reinjected with 1 mc of thallium 201 chloride. Thirty minutes later, a single-photon emission computer tomographic exam was obtained. The SPECT studies were reconstructed with images obtained in the short, horizontal, long, and vertical long axes. Comparison was made with standard data base, as well as bull's eye plots. Images were evaluated on film, as well as on the computer console.

ds

Images reveal some mild fixed hypoperfusion of the inferior wall, compared with the rest of the myocardium. This is probable on the basis of diaphragmatic attenuation. Heart appears smaller on stress than it does on redistribution imaging. Findings consistent with normal response to exercise.

ds

Quantitative analysis reveals several inconsistent areas of hypoperfusion. The inferior wall is relatively unremarkable on these plots.

ds

IMPRESSION: NO EVIDENCE FOR STRESS-INDUCED ISCHEMIA.

qs

____

J. Kronin, MD

ds

JK:XX
D: 1/12/XX
T: 1/12/XX

FIGURE 8.6
Radiology Report

Patient Study 8.B

Chris Beltre

The patient is a 50-year-old male admitted for evaluation of coronary artery disease. His health history included a previous heart attack. During his last admission, the patient had severe chest pain and was diagnosed with acute anterior wall myocardial infarction. A cardiac catheterization showed severe left main coronary artery disease, and subsequent bypass surgery followed by a stress test showed persistent abnormalities at peak exercise. Cardiac catheterization was advised to evaluate the coronary disease and guide further therapy.

REPORT 8.4 Cardiac Catheterization Lab Report

Patient Study 8.C

Joshua Warren

Twenty-six-year-old Joshua Warren experienced mild chest pains while playing racquetball and subsequently was admitted to the emergency room. A treadmill stress test was ordered to determine the possibility of cardiovascular disease.

REPORT 8.5 Treadmill Stress Test

- Use figures for transcribing electrocardiographic chest leads and capital letters for waves and segments. The leads are V1 through V6 and aVL, aVR, and aVF. (It is also acceptable to transcribe the L, R, and F as subscript letters.) Waves include P, Q, R, S, T, and U and their combinations.

Patient Study 8.D

Baby Girl Smith

This female infant was born prematurely at approximately 24-1/2 weeks gestation. Cardiovascular surgeons will perform a ductus arteriosus ligation to stabilize the baby's heart function.

REPORT 8.6 Operative Report

Patient Study 8.E

Junice Monroe

Junice Monroe is a 65-year-old woman who presented with symptoms of congestive heart failure and lung collapse. A CT scan and an echocardiogram revealed a cardiac tumor, which surgeons will remove.

REPORT 8.7 Operative Report

- Listen for these difficult terms:
  atelectasis
  pedicle
  trilobulated
  Pacifico
  foramen ovale
  autologous
  pledgeted

Patient Study 8.F — Louis Frampton

This 65-year-old man has a history of atherosclerosis and suffered a heart attack 3 years ago. He presented to the ER with chest pain, profuse sweating, and shortness of breath, which his nitroglycerin tablets had failed to relieve.

REPORT 8.8 Discharge Summary

- Listen for these new laboratory and pharmaceutical terms:
  SMA-20
  BUN 21
  Isordil
  Slow-K
  Dalmane
  Lasix

Patient Study 8.G — Charles Bassinger

Charles Bassinger is a 16-year-old patient who is suffering from pain in his right leg. Although this may be due to his recent diagnosis of leukemia, Mr. Bassinger is sent for a B-mode Doppler study to rule out DVT.

REPORT 8.9 Doppler Study

- Spell out nonmetric units of measurement and omit comma between feet and inches.

Patient Study 8.H — Jennifer Malone

Jennifer Malone is a young lady who was diagnosed with a kidney tumor during childhood and was successfully treated using chemotherapy. However, as a result of the treatment, she has had a slight cardiac abnormality which is being followed by the New York Cardiology Associates. The following dictations describe Jennifer's condition over several years.

REPORT 8.10 Echocardiography Report

- Listen for these difficult terms:
  subxyphoid
  precordial
  situs solitus
  d-ventricular looping
  intracardiac
  milliseconds
  pedunculated
  SVC

REPORT 8.11 Letter

- Listen for these difficult terms:
  acyanotic
  thrill
  grade 2/6
  mid vibratory systolic murmur
  hemodynamic
  AV
  QRS
  ST-T
  +60°
  Vasotec

Using Medical References

Use the appropriate medical reference to locate the correct spelling and additional usage information for the words below. (If the reference is not available, use the Glossary in this text.) Circle the correct spelling, then write a sentence using the word correctly.

1.	benazepril	benazipril	benazaprel
2.	Cardezen	Cardizim	Cardizem
3.	Acupril	Accuprill	Accupril
4.	anurism	aneurysm	anurysm
5.	arrhythmia	arrythmea	arythmea
6.	parenteral	parentaral	parenterel
7.	paroxismal	paroxysmal	peroxsymal
8.	reumatic	rheumatic	rhuematic
9.	xiphioid	xipoid	xiphoid
10.	Coumidin	Coumadin	Cumadin

Making Expert Decisions

Circle the correct word from the choices in parentheses.

1. During the physical examination, the physician performed (auscultation/oscillation/oscitation/osculation) and percussion to hear the chest sounds.

2. Mr. Yoshida's blood pressure was 200/90, indicating (hypertensin/hypertension/hypotension).

3. Mrs. Lockhard's blood pressure was 90/60, indicating (hypertensin/hypertension/hypotension).

4. The cardiac catheterization showed that, although major vessels were obstructed, there was sufficient (canalization/cannulation/recanalization/rechannelization) that medical therapy, rather than bypass, could be tried.

5. After angioplasty, the patient's vessel restenosed, so a (canalization/cannulation/recanalization/rechannelization) was done.

6. (Canalization/Cannulation/Recanalization/Rechannelization) was done via the femoral artery with a JL4 guiding catheter.

7. There was diffuse inflammation of the (pericardial/pericardium/precordial/precordium) and congestive heart failure.

8. The patient complains of (pericardial/pericardium/precordial/precordium) chest pain.

9. An (osteal/ostial) lesion was noted near the takeoff of the posterior descending artery from the right coronary artery.

10. The ECG showed irregular rhythm, and the patient complained of (palpations/palpitations/papillations).

Transcribing Professional Documents

Transcribe the document named Chapter 8 Assessment. Before you key, review the document formatting guidelines. Proofread your transcribed document and revise it until you think it is error-free. This document is an echocardiogram report. The patient data portion can be transcribed like a table without lines.

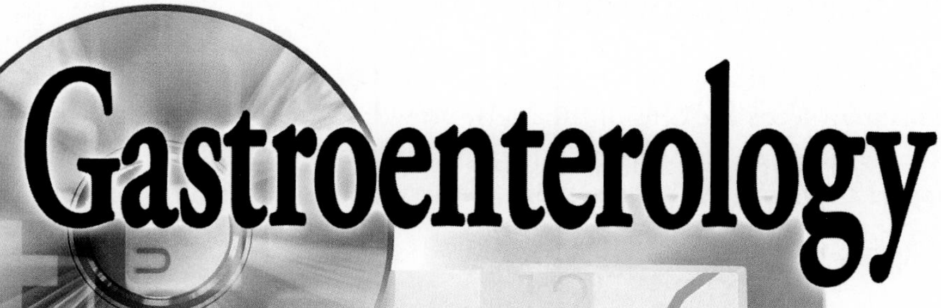

Gastroenterology

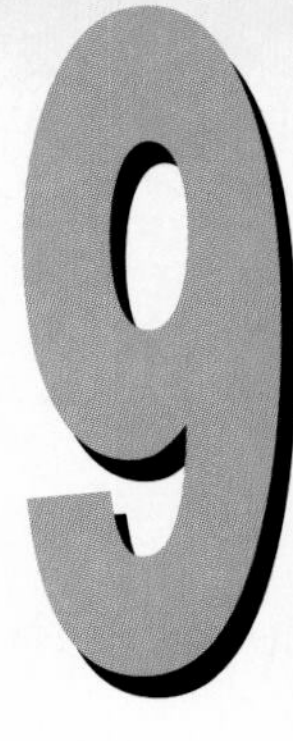

Gastroenterology is the study of the digestive tract, liver, and pancreas. The digestive tract, also called the alimentary canal or gastrointestinal (GI) tract, is similar to a tube with openings at both ends. It includes the mouth, pharynx, esophagus, stomach, and small and large intestines. It also incorporates accessory organs: the salivary glands, teeth, liver, gallbladder, pancreas, and appendix. The physician who specializes in the GI tract is called a gastroenterologist. A rectosigmoid specialist (proctologist) studies diseases of the lower end of the digestive tract.

OBJECTIVES

- Use gastroenterology terms correctly according to the context and purpose of the dictation.
- Select and use appropriate general and specialty reference materials.
- Key gastroenterology documents of varying complexity and format.
- Transcribe authentic medical dictation requiring concentration and listening skill.
- Edit medical reports to conform with AAMT style guidelines.
- Proofread and correct transcripts to produce error-free documents.

Exploring Gastroenterology

Digestion, absorption, and elimination are the processes of the gastrointestinal tract. This complex system feeds the cells of the body, providing energy for cellular functions. As with the other systems of the body, the digestive system involves several organs and interacts with other body systems to carry out its vital functions.

Structure and Function

The mouth is the first organ of digestion (Figure 9.1). Food enters the body through the mouth, and the teeth masticate, or chew, to break the food into small particles. The salivary glands (parotid, submaxillary, and sublingual) located in the mouth secrete digestive juices and salivary enzymes at the rate of about 1.5 liters per day.

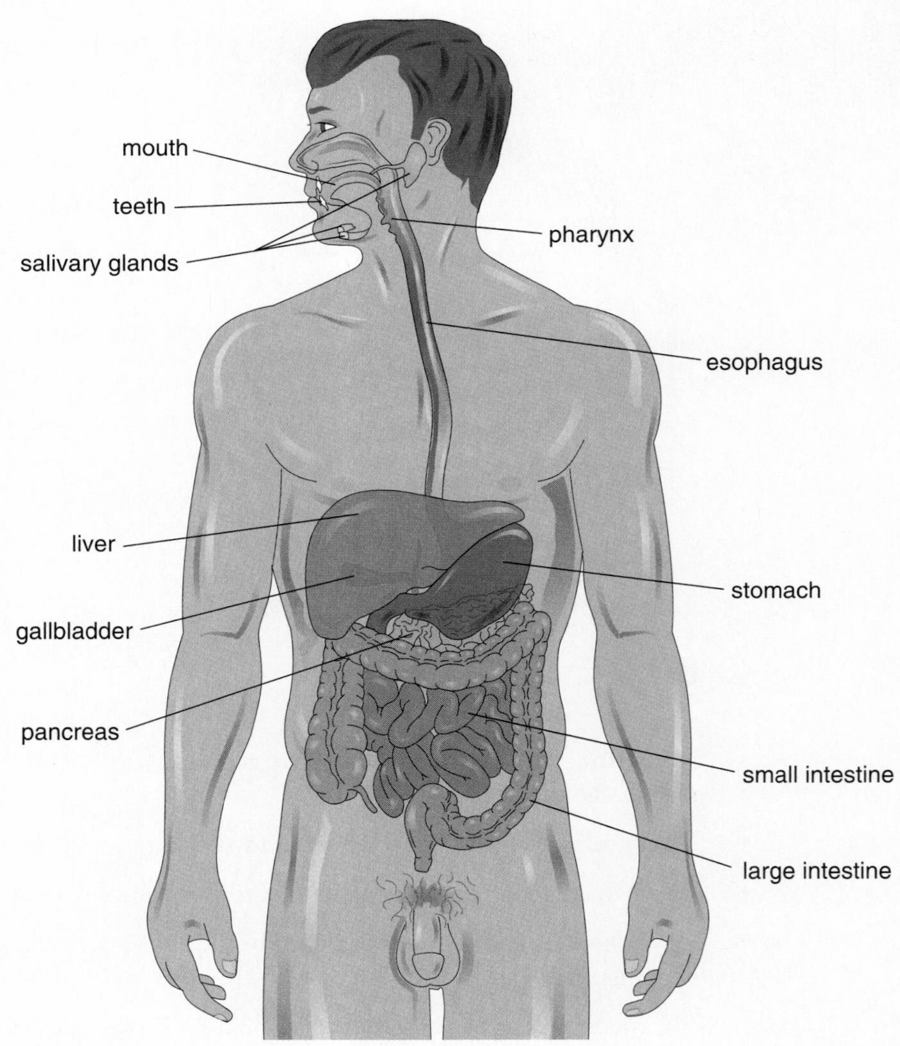

FIGURE 9.1
Organs of the Digestive System

These substances begin the digestion process. As the food is swallowed, it passes through the pharynx into the esophagus by an involuntary process that causes the epiglottis to cover the tracheal opening. This prevents the aspiration of food into the airways. Esophageal peristalsis, or rhythmic muscle movements, cause the food to move down the esophagus, passing the esophageal sphincter (or cardiac sphincter), and into the stomach. In order to prevent reflux into the esophagus, this sphincter closes tightly when the food enters the stomach.

In the stomach, hydrochloric acid is secreted by the gastric gland to further decompose the food particles. This highly acidic fluid is produced at the rate of about 2.5 liters per day. Pepsin is secreted to begin the digestion of proteins. Additionally, intrinsic factor is produced and aids in the absorption of vitamin B_{12} in the ileum.

The pyloric sphincter acts as a two-way valve moving small, digested particles toward the small intestine and preventing large particles from entering too soon to allow proper absorption of nutrients. In the small intestine (Figure 9.2), the duodenum continues the digestive processes. There are

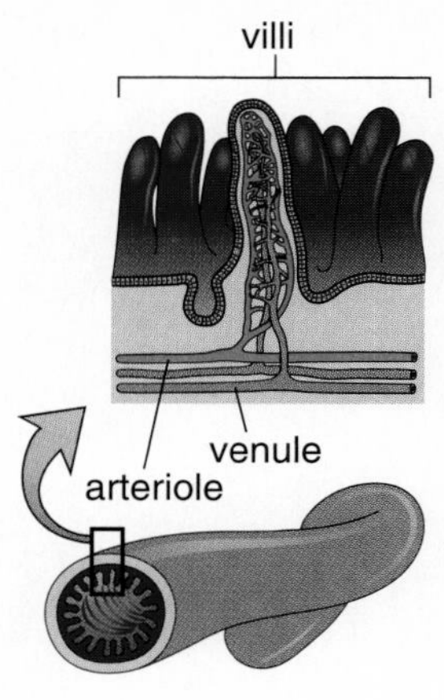

FIGURE 9.2
Cross Section of the Small Intestine

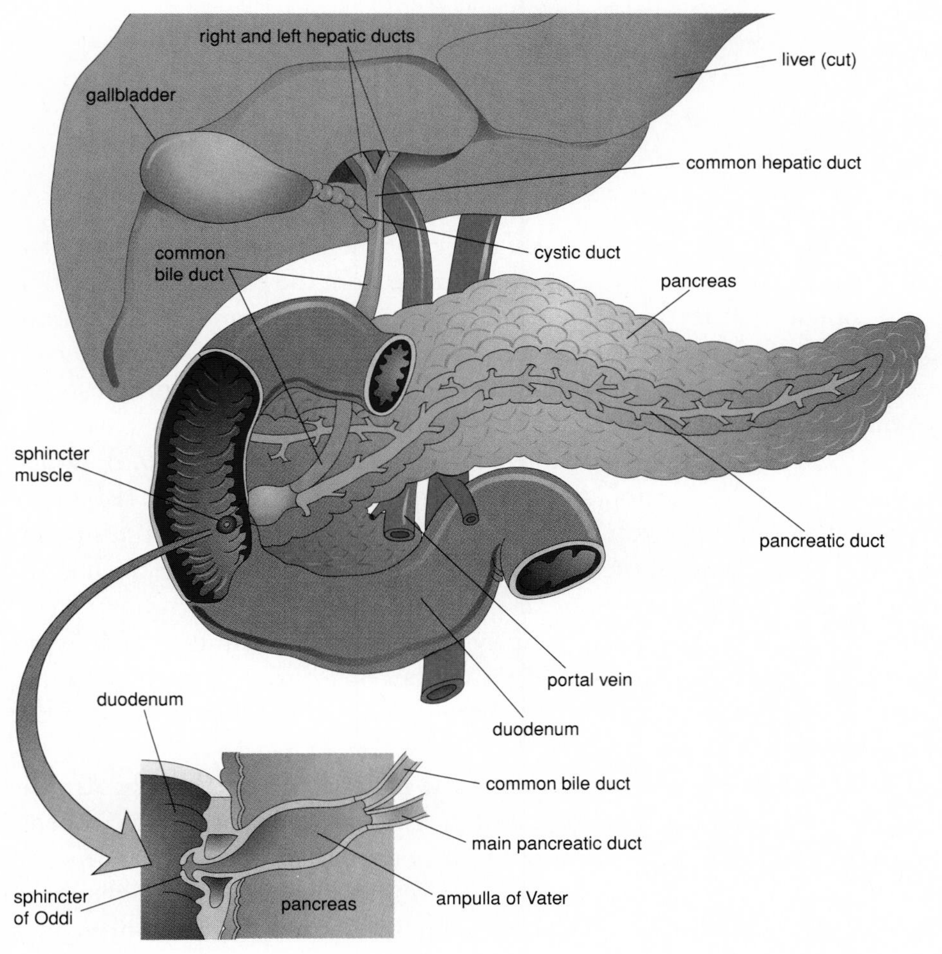

FIGURE 9.3
Gall Bladder and Bile Ducts

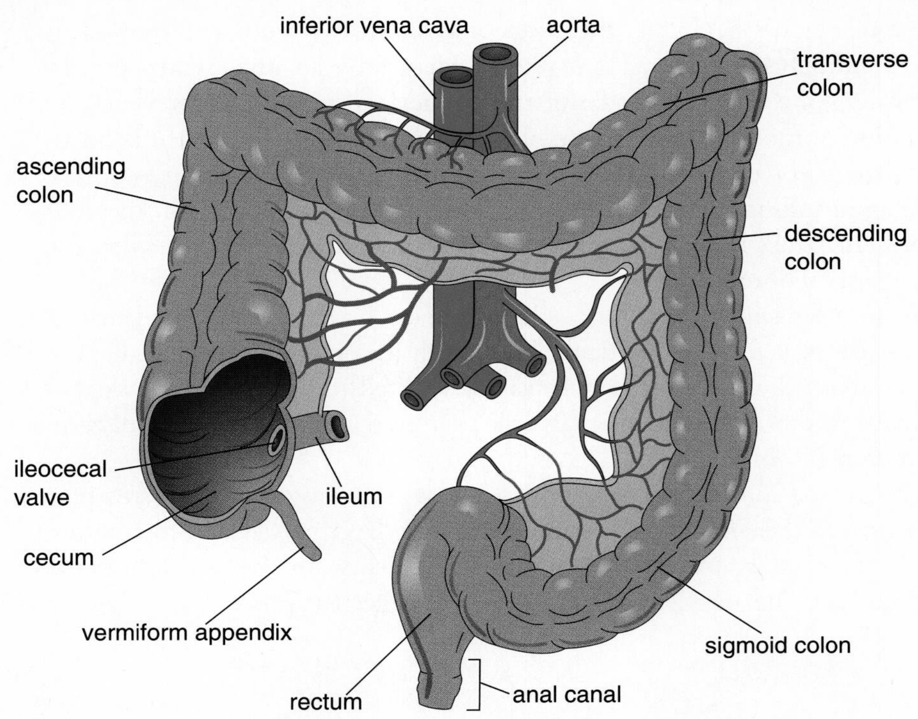

FIGURE 9.4
The Large Intestine

several hormones and other regulators that control the secretions of the digestive system. Alkaline digestive juices flow into the intestine from the pancreas and neutralize the acid contents. Other digestive enzymes produced in the pancreas continue to break down the food. Trypsin, amylase, and lipase assist in the digestion of proteins, starches, and fats respectively. The intestinal glands secrete mucus, which coats the lining of the intestine and protects it from erosion by the acidic juices.

Bile is secreted by the liver and stored in the gallbladder (Figure 9.3). When needed, the bile salts, cholesterol, and lecithin contained in the bile emulsify fatty substances into products that can be absorbed by the small intestine. At this point, peristalsis (the contractions of the intestine) causes the contents of the small intestine to be propelled into the colon, or large intestine (Figure 9.4).

Bacteria present in the large intestine play an important role in digestion, assisting with the absorption of bile salts and the further breakdown of waste products. *Escherichia coli,* or *E. coli,* is one of the most common bacteria that normally occur in the intestines.

The final step of digestion is moving the waste material out of the body. As peristalsis propels waste products through the small intestine, the ileocecal valve opens, allowing some contents to enter the colon. Once waste has moved past the ileocecal valve, the valve closes to prevent the products from moving back into the small intestine. As the waste fills the colon and reaches the rectum, the rectum expands until there is an urge to defecate. The movement of waste from the rectum and out of the body can take up to three days, a period that allows for the resorption of fluid and electrolytes.

Stool, or feces, contains undigested foodstuffs, bacteria, water, and inorganic matter. The characteristic brown color is produced as bile is broken down by bacteria within the intestine. The fecal odor is caused by chemicals produced during digestion. The gastrointestinal tract contains gas from swallowed air and the action of intestinal bacteria. Gas expelled through the mouth is called a *belch, burp,* or *eructation;* gas expelled from the anus is called *flatus.*

Physical Assessment

Obtaining an accurate, complete patient history is probably the most important technique for the examiner. The patient is asked to describe any problems, starting from the mouth and teeth, and ending with a description of bowel habits. Diet and eating habits can suggest routines that could lead to the improper functioning of the GI organs. The mouth is inspected for proper moisture, teeth alignment, and any deviations in the structures. Next, the examiner may auscultate the abdomen from the epigastric area down to the suprapubic area, using a stethoscope and dividing the abdomen into four sections called quadrants (see Figure 9.5). Each quadrant is examined since different sounds might be heard in different areas. The physician then percusses (taps) all four quadrants, listening for the different sounds from the gas-filled mid-abdomen versus the denser spleen and liver. Lastly, the examiner

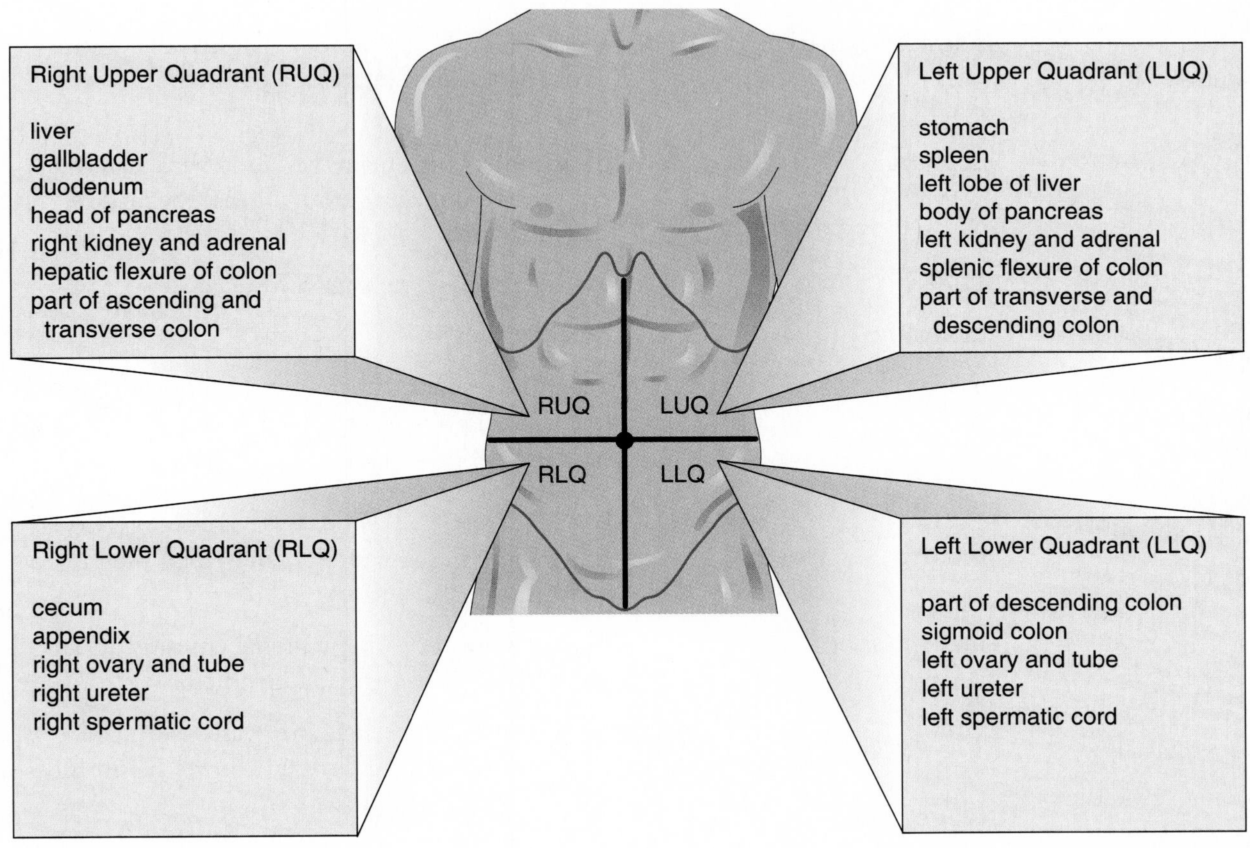

FIGURE 9.5
Divisions of the Abdomen

palpates the abdomen from the suprapubic area up to the ribs, watching the patient for signs of pain, tenderness, or rebound tenderness, and palpating for masses, adenopathy, or organomegaly. Although it is customary to perform palpation before auscultation with other systems of the body, this is reversed in the examination of the abdomen since palpation could change the sound and pattern of gas within the intestine, and this could have an influence on the results of the examination.

Diseases and Conditions

Because the GI tract encompasses so many organs and structures, the number of diseases affecting this region is extensive. Each area has its common maladies, as summarized in Table 9.1 and as illustrated in Figure 9.6.

Common Tests and Surgical Procedures

Many of the diagnostic procedures in gastroenterology center on the use of the endoscope and its variations. The endoscope is a flexible tube with fiberoptics,

TABLE 9.1 Areas of the Digestive Tract and Their Diseases

Area of GI Tract	Common Diseases
mouth and pharynx	candidiasis (thrush, moniliasis), herpetic stomatitis (Most illnesses are treated by the ENT specialist.)
esophagus	ulcers, infections, hiatal hernia, diverticula, cancer, gastroesophageal reflux disease, Schatzki's ring, strictures
stomach	gastric ulcers, tumors, gastritis, cancer
duodenum	cancer, ulcers
liver	hepatitis, syphilis, tuberculosis, fungal infections, leptospirosis, abscesses, tumors, parasites, cirrhosis, cancer
gallbladder	gallstones
pancreas	acute and chronic pancreatitis, benign pseudocysts, malignant tumors
small intestine	tumors, Crohn disease, regional enteritis, terminal ileitis, cancer, hernia, appendicitis
colon	cancer, polyps, diverticular disease, ulcerative colitis, Crohn disease, irritable bowel syndrome
rectum	hemorrhoids, cancer

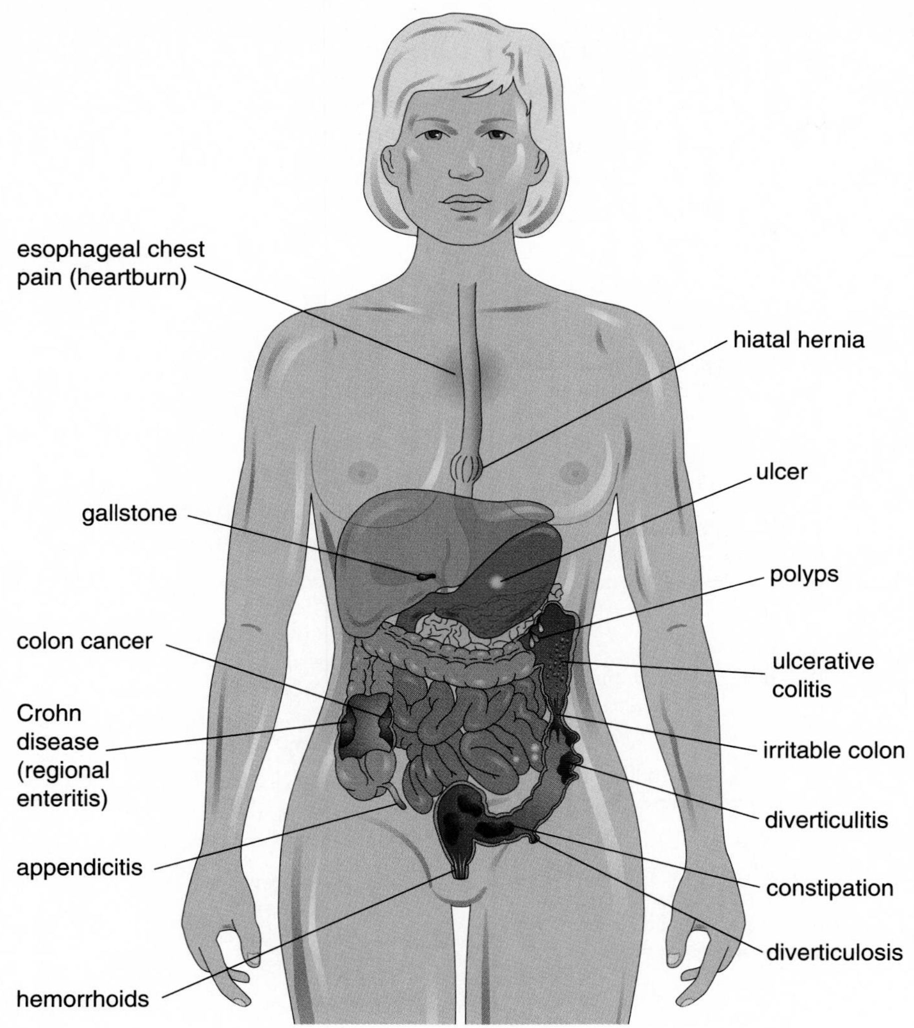

FIGURE 9.6
Common Diseases and Their Locations in the Digestive Tract

which allows the physician to look inside the esophagus, stomach, and other areas of the GI tract. Some of the common studies include gastroscopy (stomach), exploratory laparoscopy (intestinal tract), and colonoscopy and flexible sigmoidoscopy (colon). Other important tests include x-rays using barium (commonly called a GI series), computed tomography (CT scans), abdominal ultrasound, insertion of a PEG tube, and Whipple's operation (removal of all or part of the pancreas and duodenum). A hemorrhoidectomy is the surgical removal of hemorrhoids; an appendectomy is the surgical removal of the appendix.

Building Language Skills

The following tables list common gastroenterology terms, drugs, and abbreviations. The list of terms and definitions includes the most difficult words contained in the dictated reports in this chapter. These words are identified in GREEN type. A list of common drugs is found in Appendix D.

Medical Terms and Pharmacologic Agents

abdomen
(ab-**dO**-men/**ab**-dO-men) (n) that part of the body between the chest and the pelvis (the lower part of the trunk of the body)

adenocarcinoma
(ad-en-O-**kar**-si-n**O**-ma) (n) malignant tumor of epithelial cells arising from the glandular structures which are a part of most organs of the body

adenopathy
(ad-e-**nop**-a-thee) (n) swelling or enlargement of the lymph nodes

adipose
(**ad**-i-pOz) (adj) fatty

albumin
(al-**byoo**-min) (n) a type of simple protein, varieties of which are widely distributed throughout the tissues and fluids

alimentary canal
(al-i-**men**-ter-ee ka-**nal**) (n) gastrointestinal tract; tubelike structure through which food passes and is digested and absorbed

anesthesia
(**an**-es-**thee**-zee-a) (n) absence of sensation, especially pain; usually applied to the medical technique of reducing or eliminating a person's sensation of pain to enable surgery to be performed

anesthetic
(**an**-es-**thet**-ik) (n) the medications used to produce anesthesia

angiodysplasia
(**an**-jee-O-dis-**play**-zee-a) (n) degenerative stretching or enlarging of the blood vessels in an organ

anorexia
(an-O-**rek**-see-a) (n) diminished appetite; aversion to food

antiemetic
(**an**-ti-ee-**met**-ik) (n) pharmacologic agent used to decrease nausea and/or vomiting

aphagia
(a-**fay**-jee-a) (n) inability to swallow

aphthous stomatitis
(**af**-thus stO-ma-**tI**-tis) (n) small ulcers of the mucous membrane of the mouth

benign
(bee-**nIn**) (adj) describing a mild illness or a nonmalignant tumor

bile
(bIl) (n) a thick, yellow-green-brown fluid secreted by the liver

bilirubin
(bil-i-**roo**-bin) (n) a red bile pigment, formed from hemoglobin during normal and abnormal destruction of erythrocytes

biopsy
(**bI**-op-see) (n) removal of a small amount of tissue and/or fluid from the body for microscopic examination; the specimen obtained

bulimia
(boo-**lim**-ee-a) (n) a chronic disorder involving repeated and secretive bouts of binge eating followed by self-induced vomiting, use of laxatives, or vigorous exercise in order to prevent weight gain

cachexia
(ka-**kek**-see-a) (n) a general weight loss and wasting occurring in the course of a chronic disease or emotional disturbance

caliber
(**kal**-i-ber) (n) diameter of a tube or vessel; e.g., a blood vessel

carcinoma
(kar-si-**nO**-ma) (n) malignant growth of epithelial cells that occurs in the linings of the body parts and in glands

cauterization
(kaw-ter-i-**zay**-shun) (n) destroying tissue by burning for medical reasons

cecum
(**see**-kum) (n) any part ending in a cul-de-sac; specifically the closed, pocket-like beginning of the large intestine in the lower right part of the abdomen

cholangiography
(kO-lan-jee-**og**-ra-fee) (n) x-ray examination of the bile ducts

cholecystectomy
(**kO**-lee-sis-**tek**-tO-mee) (n) excision of the gallbladder

cholecystitis
(**kO**-lee-sis-tI-tis) (n) inflammation or irritation of gallbladder, usually caused by the presence of gallstones

choledocholithiasis
(kO-**led**-O-kO-lith-**I**-a-sis) (n) presence of calculi (stones) in the common bile duct

cholelithiasis
(**kO**-lee-lith-**I**-a-sis) (n) formation or presence of gallstones in the gallbladder which may not cause any symptoms or perhaps only vague abdominal discomfort and intolerance to certain foods

cirrhosis
(sir-**rO**-sis) (n) a chronic, degenerative disease of the liver

cirrhotic
(sir-**rot**-ik) (adj) affected with cirrhosis

colonic
(ko-**lon**-ic) (adj) pertaining to the colon

colostomy
(kO-**los**-to-mee) (n) surgical creation of an opening in the abdominal wall to allow material to pass from the bowel through that opening rather than through the anus

Crohn disease
(krOn) (n) chronic inflammatory condition affecting the colon and/or terminal part of the small intestine and producing frequent episodes of diarrhea, abdominal pain, nausea, fever, weakness, and weight loss

cryptitis
(crip-**tI**-tis) (n) inflammation of a crypt or follicle

cyst
(sist) (n) a bladder or an abnormal sac containing gas, fluid, or a semisolid material

cystic
(**sis**-tik) (adj) relating to a cyst

cystic duct
(n) the duct of the gallbladder which unites with the hepatic duct from the liver to form the common bile duct

dehydration
(dee-hI-**dray**-shun) (n) extreme loss of water from the body tissues

Demerol
(**dem**-err-all) (n) Brand name for meperidine, a narcotic analgesic

diathesis
(dI-a-**thee**-sis) (n) unusual predisposition to certain disease conditions

digital
(**dij**-i-tal) (adj) relating to or resembling a finger or toe

distention
(dis-**ten**-shun) (n) the state of being stretched out or inflated

diverticulosis
(**dI**-ver-tik-yoo-**lO**-sis) (n) presence of diverticula (pouches) in the intestinal tract

dyspepsia
(dis-**pep**-see-a) (n) imperfect digestion; epigastric discomfort

dysphagia
(dis-**fay**-jee-a) (n) difficulty swallowing

emetic
(e-**met**-ik) (n) pharmacologic agent used to induce vomiting and eliminate toxic substances

epiploic
(**ep**-i-**plO**-ik) (adj) relating to the omentum, a fold of peritoneum attached to the stomach and connecting it with the adjacent organs

epithelial
(ep-i-**thee**-lee-al) (adj) relating to or consisting of epithelium

epithelium
(ep-i-**thee**-lee-um) (n) cell layers covering the outside body surfaces as well as forming the lining of hollow organs (e.g., the bladder) and the passages of the respiratory, digestive, and urinary tracts

eructation
(ee-ruk-**tay**-shun) (n) belching

esophagus
(ee-**sof**-a-gus) (n) the muscular canal that connects the pharynx and stomach

extravasation
(eks-**trav**-a-**say**-shun) (n) a leakage of fluid (e.g., blood) to the tissues outside the vessel normally containing it, which may occur in injuries, burns, and allergic reactions

fissure
(**fish**-ur) (n) a deep furrow, cleft, or slit; e.g., in the liver, lungs, ligaments, brain, or teeth

fistula
(**fis**-tyoo-la) (n) abnormal opening or channel connecting two internal organs or leading from an internal organ to the outside. They are due to ulceration, a wound that does not heal, injury, or tumor

flatulence
(**flat**-yoo-lens) (n) presence of an excessive amount of gas in the stomach and intestines

flexure
(**flek**-sher) (n) a bend, as in an organ or structure

fungating
(**fung**-gayt-ing) (adj) growing rapidly like a fungus, applied to certain tumors

gallbladder
(**gawl-blad**-er) (n) pear-shaped organ that is located on the lower surface of the liver and is a reservoir for bile until discharged through the cystic duct

gastritis
(gas-**trI**-tis) (n) inflammation of the gastric (stomach) mucosa

gastroenteritis
(**gas**-trO-en-ter-**I**-tis) (n) inflammation of the gastric mucosa and intestine

Gastrografin
(Gas-tro-**graf**-in) (n) brand name for an oral contrast medium used for radiographic examination of the alimentary tract

gingiva
(**jin**-ji-va) (n) the gum; the tissue that attaches the teeth to the jaws

granuloma
gran-yoo-**lO**-ma) (n) a granular tumor or growth, usually of lymphoid and epitheloid cells

hematemesis
(hee-ma-**tem**-e-sis) (n) vomiting of blood

hematochezia
(**hee**-ma-tO-**kee**-zee-a) (n) passage of bloody stools

hematocrit
(**hee**-ma-tO-krit/**hem**-a-tO-krit) (n) centrifuge for separating solids from plasma in the blood; measure of the volume of red blood cells as a percentage of the total blood volume

hemorrhoid
(**hem**-a-royd) (n) varicose vein of anal opening

hemostasis
(**hee**-mO-stay-sis/hee-**mos**-ta-sis) (n) cessation of bleeding either naturally through the blood coagulation process, mechanically (with surgical clamps), or chemically (with drugs)

hemostatic
(**hee**-mO-**stat**-ik) (adj) relating to procedure, device, or substance that stops flow of blood

hepatitis
(hep-a-**tI**-tis) (n) acute or chronic inflammation of the liver

hepatoduodenal
(**hep**-at-O-doo-O-**dee**-nal) (adj) referring to the portion of the lesser omentum (fold of peritoneal tissue attaching and supporting the stomach and adjacent organs) between the liver and the duodenum

hernia
(**her**-nee-a) (n) protrusion of an organ or part of an organ or other structure through the muscle wall of the cavity that normally contains it

hiatal
(hI-**ay**-tal) (adj) pertaining to a hernia of part of the stomach into the opening in the diaphragm, through which the esophagus passes

homeostasis
(**hO**-mee-O-**stay**-sis) (n) equilibrium in the body with respect to various functions (e.g., temperature, heart rate) and to the chemical compositions of the fluids and tissues

hyperemesis
(hI-per-**em**-e-sis) (n) excessive vomiting

hyperemia
(hI-per-**ee**-mee-a) (n) increased blood in part of the body, caused by inflammatory response or blockage of blood outflow

hyperemic
(hI-per-**ee**-mik) (adj) showing hyperemia

ileostomy
(**il**-ee-**os**-tO-mee) (n) surgical formation of an opening of the ileum (distal portion of the small intestine) onto the abdominal wall through which feces pass

ileum
(**il**-ee-um) (n) the third portion of the small intestine, about 12 feet in length, extending from the junction with the jejunum to the ileocecal opening

ileitis
(il-ee-**I**-tis) (n) inflammation of the ileum (lower-three-fifths of the small intestines)

ileus
(**il**-ee-us) (n) obstruction of the intestines

ilium
(**il**-ee-um) (n) the broad, flaring portion of the hip bone

infraumbilical
(**in**-fra-um-**bil**-i-kal) (adj) below the umbilicus (navel)

intestine
(in-**tes**-tin) (n) the portion of the alimentary canal extending from the pyloric opening of the stomach to the anus (opening of the rectum)

intussusception
(**in**-tus-su-**sep**-shun) (n) taking up or receiving one part within another, especially the infolding of one segment of the intestine within another

lamina
(**lam**-i-na) (n) thin membrane or plate-like structure, such as the two parts of a vertebra that join to hold the spinous process of the vertebra over the spinal cord (pl laminae)

laminar
(**lam**-i-nar) (adj) relating to lamina

laparoscope
(**lap**-a-rO-skOp) (n) a device for observing the inside of an organ or cavity

lateral
(**lat**-er-al) (adj) relating to a side, away from the center plane; e.g., cheeks are lateral to the nose

leukocyte
(**loo**-kO-sIt) (n) white blood cell

leukoplakia
(loo-kO-**play**-kee-a) (n) a precancerous change in a mucous membrane, such as the mouth or tongue

ligament
(**lig**-a-ment) (n) band of fibrous connective tissue that binds joints together and connects bones and cartilage

lobe
(lOb) (n) rounded part of an organ, separated from other parts of the organ by connective tissue or fissures

lumen
(**loo**-men) (n) cavity, canal, or channel within an organ or tube; the space inside a structure

luminal
(**loo**-min-al) (adj) related to the lumen of a tubular structure, such as a blood vessel

lymph
(limf) (n) a thin fluid that bathes the tissues of the body, circulates through lymph vessels, is filtered in lymph nodes, and enters the blood stream through the thoracic duct

lymphatic
(lim-**fat**-ik) (adj) relating to lymph

lymphoid
(**lim**-foyd) (adj) resembling lymph or relating to the lymphatic system

lymphoma
(lim-**fO**-ma) (n) a general term for various types of tumors of the lymphatic system

malaise
(ma-**layz**) (n) a feeling of general discomfort or uneasiness, often the first indication of an infection or other disease

malignancy
(ma-**lig**-nan-see) (n) a cancer that is invasive and spreading

mastication
(mas-ti-**kay**-shun) (n) process of chewing food

melena
(me-**lee**-na) (n) passage of dark, tarry stool

mucosal
(myoo-**kO**-sal) (adj) concerning any mucous membrane

mucous
(**myoo**-kus) (adj) having the nature of or resembling mucus

mucus
(**myoo**-kus) (n) viscous (sticky, gummy) secretions of mucous membranes and glands

nausea
(**naw**-zee-a; **naw**-zha) (n) inclination to vomit

nauseous
(**naw**-zee-us; **naw**-shus) (adj) causing nausea or feeling nausea

nodular
(**nod**-yoo-lar) (adj) small, firm, and knotty

obstipation
(ob-sti-**pay**-shun) (n) severe constipation

opacification
(O-**pas**-i-fi-kay-shun) (n) clouding or loss of transparency, especially of the cornea or lens of the eye

organomegaly
(**Or**-ga-nO-**meg**-a-lee) (n) abnormal enlargement of an organ, particularly an organ of the abdominal cavity, such as the liver or spleen

palpable
(**pal**-pa-bl) (adj) perceivable by touch

palpation
(pal-**pay**-shun) (n) technique of examination in which the examiner feels the firmness, texture, size, shape, or location of body parts

pancreas
(**pan**-kree-as) (n) gland lying behind the stomach that produces and secretes insulin, glucagon, and digestive enzymes

parasite
(**par**-a-sIt) (n) an organism that lives on or in another and draws its nourishment therefrom

percutaneous
(per-kyoo-**tay**-nee-us) (adj) through the skin

perforation
(per-fO-**ray**-shun) (n) abnormal opening or hole in a hollow organ

pericolonic
(per-ee-ko-**lon**-ik) (adj) pertaining to the region around the colon

peristalsis
(per-i-**stal**-sis) (n) the movement of the intestine or other tubular structure, characterized by waves of alternate circular contraction and relaxation of the tube by which the contents are propelled onward

peritoneum
(per-i-tO-**nee**-um) (n) lining of the abdominal cavity

pharynx
(**far**-ingks) (n) throat; passageway for air from nasal cavity or larynx, and food from mouth to esophagus

pneumoperitoneum
(**noo**-mO-per-i-ton-**ee**-um) (n) condition in which air or gas is collected in the peritoneal cavity

polyp
(**pol**-ip) (n) a general descriptive term used with reference to any mass of tissue that bulges or projects outward or upward from the normal surface level

Prilosec
(**pry**-low-sec) (n) Brand name for omeprazole, a gastric acid secretion inhibitor

proximal
(**prok**-si-mal) (adj) nearest to a point of reference

pyrosis
(pI-**rO**-sis) (n) heartburn

reflux
(**ree**-fluks) (n) abnormal backflow, as sometimes occurs with fluids in the esophagus or other body parts

regurgitation
(ree-gur-ji-**tay**-shun) (n) the return of gas or small amounts of food from the stomach

salivary gland
(**sal**-i-vayr-ee) (n) a gland that secretes saliva into the mouth

sigmoid colon
(**sig**-moyd **kO**-lon) (n) that part of the colon extending from the end of the descending colon to the rectum

sigmoidoscopy
(**sig**-moy-**dos**-ko-pee) (n) the inspection of the rectum and colon via endoscope

sphincter
(**sfingk**-ter) (n) a muscle that encircles a duct, tube, or opening in such a way that its contraction constricts the opening

sterile
(**ster**-il) (adj) free from living microorganisms

subcuticular
(sub-kyoo-**tik**-yoo-lar) (adj) beneath the cuticle of epidermis

supine
(soo-**pIn**) (adj) lying on the back

suprapubic
(soo-pra-**pyoo**-bik) (adj) above the pubic arch

tachycardia
(**tak**-e-**kar**-dee-a) (n) an abnormally rapid heart rate

tachycardic
(**tak**-e-**kar**-dik) (adj) relating to or suffering from an abnormally rapid heart rate

tracheostomy
(tray-kee-**os**-tO-mee) (n) a surgically created opening into the trachea (windpipe)

transmural
(trans-**myoo**-ral) (adj) relating to the entire thickness of the wall of an organ

trocar
(**trO**-kar) (n) sharply pointed surgical instrument used for aspiration or removal of fluids from cavities

ulcerative colitis
(**ul**-ser-a-tiv kO-**lI**-tis) (n) a chronic disease characterized by ulcers in the colon and rectum

ultrasound
(**ul**-tra-sownd) (n) sound waves at very high frequencies used in the technique of obtaining images for diagnostic purposes

villi
(**vil**-I) (n) many tiny projections, occurring over the mucous membrane of the small intestine that accomplish the absorption of nutrients and fluids; villus (sing)

villous
(**vil**-us) (adj) relating to villi

Abbreviations

a.c.	before meals	H/O	history of
BaE or BE	barium enema	IVC	intravenous cholangiography
BCM	below costal margin	LLQ	left lower quadrant
BM	bowel movement (bone marrow in oncology)	LRQ	lower right quadrant
		LUQ	left upper quadrant
BX	biopsy	n.p.o.	nothing by mouth
EGD	esophagogastroduodenoscopy	p.c.	after meals
FBS	fasting blood sugar	p.p.	postprandial (after eating)
GB	gallbladder	PUD	peptic ulcer disease
GE	gastroesophageal	RLQ	right lower quadrant
GERD	gastroesophageal reflux disease	R/O	rule out
GI	gastrointestinal	RUQ	right upper quadrant
HAL	hyperalimentation	TPN	total parenteral nutrition
HCl	hydrochloric acid	UGI	upper gastrointestinal
H&E	hematoxylin and eosin (stains for specimens on microscopic slides)	ULQ	upper left quadrant
		URQ	upper right quadrant

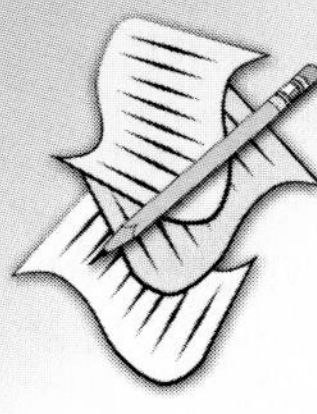

EXERCISE 9.1

Recognizing Look-Alikes and Sound-Alikes

Below is a list of frequently used words that look alike and/or sound alike. Study the meaning and pronunciation of each set of words, then read the following sentences carefully and circle the word in parentheses that correctly completes the meaning.

anesthesia	the loss of sensation of pain
anesthetic	the substance used to produce anesthesia
luminal	(adj) pertaining to a lumen (cavity or channel) within an organ or tube
Luminal	trade name for anticonvulsant and sedative phenobarbital
hemostasis	cessation of bleeding
hemostatic	pertaining to procedure, device, or substance that stops flow of blood
homeostasis	steady state in the internal environment of the body
dysphagia	difficulty swallowing
dysphasia	difficulty speaking
dyspnea	difficulty breathing

cite	(v) to quote or mention
sight	(n) vision, view
site	(n) location in the body
mucous	(adj) having the nature of or resembling mucus
mucus	(n) viscous (sticky, gummy) secretions of mucous membranes and glands
ileum	the last part of the small intestine, between the jejunum and the large intestine
ileus	obstruction of the intestines
ilium	superior portion of the hipbone
reflux	abnormal backflow of fluid
reflex	involuntary reaction or return

1. After adequate (anesthesia, anesthetic) was documented, the cyst was incised.
2. Local (anesthesia, anesthetic) consisting of 1% lidocaine with epinephrine was infiltrated into the chest region.
3. After sutures were placed, good (hemostasis, homeostasis) was documented.
4. Colonoscopy was normal to the terminal (ileum, ilium).
5. The patient is to call if he notices yellow or green (mucous, mucus).
6. The (mucous, mucus) membranes are injected, with clear rhinorrhea.
7. I (cited, sighted) to the patient several reasons for quitting smoking.
8. The excision (cite, site) showed good healing.
9. Due to her (dysphagia, dysphasia, dyspnea) she has had little food intake over the past 24 hours.
10. Due to an (ileum, ileus) the patient was placed on total parenteral nutrition.

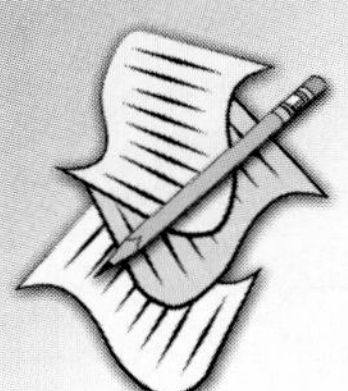

EXERCISE 9.2

Matching Sound and Spelling

The numbered list that follows shows the phonetic spelling of hard-to-spell words. Sound out the word, then write the correct spelling in the blank space provided. Each of the words can be found in the Glossary or in the drug list in Appendix D.

1. sir-**rO**-sis ______________________
2. a-**fay**-jee-a ______________________
3. ee-ruk-**tay**-shun ______________________
4. **pol**-ip______________________
5. al-**byoo**-min______________________
6. **af**-thus stO-ma-**tI**-tis ______________________
7. **in**-tus-su-**sep**-shun______________________
8. ma-**lee**-na______________________
9. **sfingk**-ter______________________
10. ka-**kek**-see-a______________________
11. me-**layz** ______________________
12. **flek**-sher______________________
13. hee-ma-**tem**-e-sis ______________________
14. bil-i-**roo**-bin______________________
15. **dI**-ver-tik-yoo-**lO**-sis ______________________
16. **il**-ee-um______________________

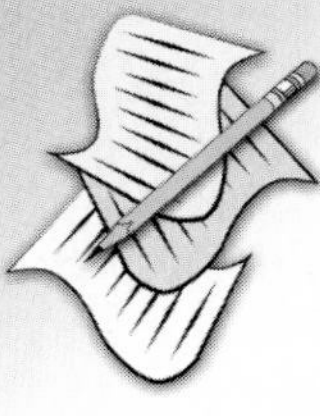

EXERCISE 9.3

Choosing Words from Context

When transcribing dictation, the medical transcriptionist frequently needs to consider the situation when determining the word that correctly completes the sentence. From the list below, select the term that meaningfully completes each of the following statements.

biopsy	palpable	hyperemesis
laparoscope	dehydration	hernia
cauterization	salivary glands	benign
malignancy	hyperemic	supine
Crohn disease	pyrosis	fistula

1. It was necessary to __________ the nodule to determine if it was malignant.
2. The homeless man was brought into the emergency room suffering from ______________. He was started on IV fluids.
3. They found Mrs. Arnold lying ____________ on her bed.
4. The patient had no __________ lymph nodes.
5. Mr. Johnson had a biopsy of the intestine which confirmed the diagnosis of __________________.
6. Her tonsils are enlarged and mildly _____________.
7. A ______________ was passed through the abdominal wall to examine the peritoneal cavity.
8. If it is suspected that you have a _________________, a biopsy may be performed.
9. __________________ was used during the procedure to prevent excess bleeding.
10. There was a swelling on the face, particularly about the cheeks, which led to the diagnosis of obstruction of the ______________________.
11. Joseph had a ______________________ between the trachea and esophagus.
12. During her pregnancy, Mrs. Andrews suffered from ______________________ when lying down.

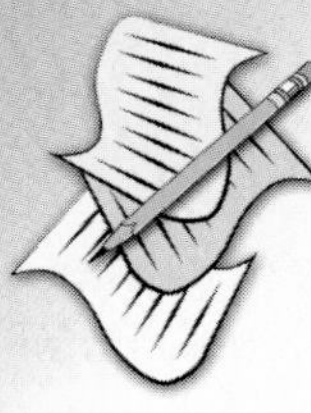

EXERCISE 9.4

Pairing Words and Meanings

From this list, locate the term that best matches each of the following definitions. Write the letter of the term in the space provided by each definition.

A. adenocarcinoma
B. adipose
C. cholecystectomy
D. cirrhosis
E. colostomy
F. epithelium
G. extravasation
H. lymph
I. pancreas
J. tachycardia
K. tracheostomy
L. lymphoma
M. gallbladder

1. cell layers that cover the outside body surfaces and line the hollow organs __________
2. a leakage of fluid from a vessel to the tissues outside it __________
3. an abnormally rapid heart rate __________
4. gland lying behind the stomach __________
5. surgical creation of an opening through the abdominal wall into the colon __________
6. excision of a gallbladder __________
7. a chronic disease of the liver __________
8. malignant tumor of a gland __________
9. fatty tissue __________
10. a thin fluid that bathes the tissues of the body and is filtered in nodes before entering the blood stream __________

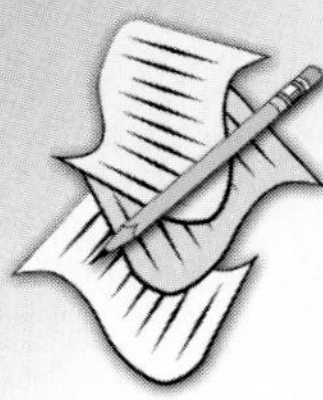

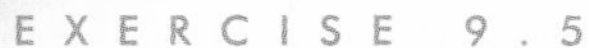

EXERCISE 9.5

Creating Terms from Word Forms

Combine prefixes, root words, and suffixes from this list to create medical words that fit the following definitions. Fill in the blanks with the words you construct.

aden/o	glands	per-	throughout, completely
carcin/o	cancer	stomat/o	mouth
chol/e	bile	cutaneous	skin
cyst/o	bladder	parotid	glands by the ear
dys-	poor or bad; painful	peptic	digestion
enter/o	small intestine	-blast	immature cell
epi-	upon	-emesis	vomiting
gastr/o	stomach, abdomen	-itis	inflammation
gloss/o	tongue	-oma	tumor
hemat/o	blood		
hepat/o	liver		

1. through the skin ______________________________
2. cancerous tumor ______________________________
3. inflammation of the gallbladder ______________________________
4. mumps (inflammation of the parotid gland) ______________________________
5. swelling, redness, and pain in the mouth ______________________________
6. malignant tumor in the glands ______________________________
7. inflammation of the tongue ______________________________
8. vomiting of blood ______________________________
9. imperfection of digestion ______________________________
10. maligant tumor in the liver ______________________________

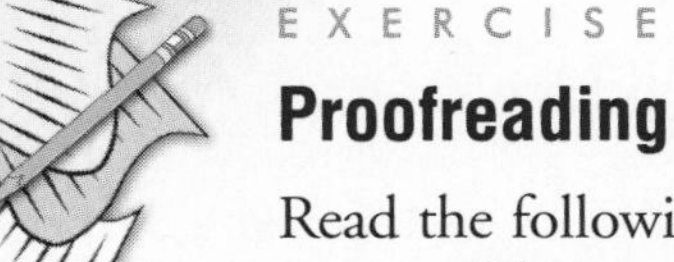

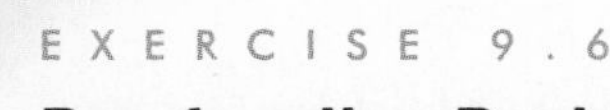

EXERCISE 9.6

Proofreading Review

Read the following reports and circle errors in format, usage, punctuation, capitalization, spelling, and mechanics. Then key the reports with the errors corrected.

1. **OPERATIVE PROCEDURE** The patient was placed on the operating table in the supine position. After satisfactory induction of general anesthesia, the abdomenal wall was prepared and drapped in the usual sterile fashion. Pneumoperitoneum was installed through a small infraumbilical excision and a Veress needle.

   Disection of the hepato-duodenal ligament was then commenced with identification of the cistic artery and the cystic duck.

   Earlier in the procedure a percutaneous liver biopsy was preformed to the right lobe of the liver, using a True-Cut needle under direct vision. No bleeding was found from this sight later in the operation.

   The abdomen was now copiously irritated through the lateral ports. The ports were now removed under direct vision.

2. **SPECIMEN:**
   A: ANTRUM B: GE JUNCTION

   CLINICAL DIAGNOSIS AND HISTORY:
   H/O DYSPEPSIA
   OPERATIVE PROCEDURE – EGD & BX

   PRE-OPERATIVE DIAGNOSIS:
   R/O PUD

   POST-OPERATIVE DIAGNOSIS:
   REFLUX ESOPHAGITIS, GASTRITIS

   GROSS DESCRIPTION:
   Specimen is received in 2 Parts. Part A is labelled Antrum and consists of 1 irregular piece of pink tan soft tissue measuring .4 x .3 x .3 cm. Entirly submitted in A1.

   Part B is labelled GE Junction and consistes of 2 irregular pieces of pink tan soft tissue, each piece measuring .3 x.3 x .2 cm. Entirely submitted in B1.

   FINAL DIAGNOSIS:

   PART A – ANTHRIUM BIOPSY:
   GASTRIC TISSUE WITH MILD CHRONIC INFLAMATION.
   NO HELICOBACTER ORGANISMS IDENTIFIED ON H&E.

   PART B – GE JUNCTION BIOPSY:
   MULTIPLE PORTIONS OF SQUAMOUS MUCOSA WITH MILD CHRONIC INFLAMMATION WITH RARE INTRAMUCOSAL EOSINOPHILS CONSISTENT WITH REFLUX ESOPHAGITIS ORIGIN.

Building Transcription Skills

The Pathology Report

The pathology report (Figure 9.7) is a diagnostic report describing the pathological or disease-related findings of a tissue sample taken during surgery, a biopsy, a special procedure, or an autopsy. Dictated by a pathologist, the report may also be called a biopsy report.

Required Headings/Content Although the wording of headings may vary among institutions, the following content categories are included in all pathology reports: name of specimen submitted, macroscopic (gross) findings, microscopic findings, remarks, and diagnosis(es). The central information in a pathology report includes the gross findings (the appearance of the specimen before it is prepared for microscopic study), the microscopic findings (cell- and blood-related), and the pathological diagnosis. Frequently, the gross descriptions of all the surgical specimens are dictated, transcribed, and given to the pathologist, who then dictates the microscopic descriptions. Once the microscopic descriptions are transcribed, the complete pathology reports are submitted to the pathologist for signature. Note that the pathology report is not the same as a laboratory report. The pathology report focuses on disease findings usually limited to tissue, while laboratory data usually concern body fluids.

Turnaround Time The expected turnaround time for a pathology report is generally 12–24 hours. However, in cases where a malignancy is suspected, the pathologist may render an opinion based on a frozen section of the specimen even before the patient is sutured, since more extensive surgery may be required.

Preparing to Transcribe

To prepare for transcribing dictation, review the tables of common gastroenterology terms, drugs, and abbreviations presented in the Building Language Skills section of this chapter. Then, study the format and organization of the model document shown in Figure 9.7, and key the model document. Proofread the document by comparing it with the printed version. Categorize the types of errors you made, and document them on a copy of the Performance Comparison chart provided in Chapter 1. A template of this chart is included on the IRC that accompanies this text.

Patient Studies

Transcribe, edit, and correct each report in the following patient studies. Consult reference books for words or formatting rules that are unfamiliar.

As you work on the transcription assignment for this chapter, fill in the Performance Comparison chart that you started when you keyed the model document. For at least three of the reports, categorize and document the types of errors

1" top and side margins → **use left justification**

PATIENT: Johnson, Sara
MR #: 7904532
SPECIMEN #: 30240
ROOM #: 931
SEX: Female
DATE OF BIRTH: 11/04/XX
PHYSICIAN: Binger, A
PROCEDURE: ABDOMINAL RESECTION
PROCEDURE DATE: 8/10/XX

ds

CLINICAL DIAGNOSIS: CARCINOMA OF RECTUM

ds

CLINICAL HISTORY: UNSTATED

ds

GROSS DESCRIPTION
The specimen is received in three portions.

ds

Portion one is stated to be "colon" and consists of a portion of large intestine, measuring 28.0-cm in length and 6.0-cm in greatest diameter. The serosal surface is reddish tan, smooth, and glistening with attached epiploic adipose tissue. The mucosal surface is tan-red, smooth, and glistening, with normal folds. At 0.5-cm from one surgical margin, there is a flat, fungating, ulcerated mass which occupies more than two-thirds of the circumference of the lumen and measures 6.5 x 3.5-cm in greatest diameter. Grossly, the tumor invades the serosal surface in the central portion. The surgical margin close to the tumor is inked. Representative sections of the tumor are submitted in three cassettes. Cassette A contains the surgical margin close to the tumor submitted in CM; surgical margin far from tumor submitted in FM; random sections in R, nodes close to tumor submitted in CN; nodes far from tumor submitted in FN.

ds

Portion two is stated to be "proximal ring" and consists of a ring of tan-pink soft tissue, measuring 1.5 x 1.4 x 0.5-cm, which has attached staples. The stapled portion of the specimen is removed, and the remainder of the specimen is submitted in cassette B.

ds

Portion three is stated to be "distal ring" and consists of a fragment of pinkish

(continued)

FIGURE 9.7
Pathology Report

PATHOLOGY REPORT
PATIENT: Johnson, Sara
MR #: 7904532
DATE: 8/10/XX
Page 2

tan, soft tissue, measuring 2.3 x 1.4 x 0.3-cm, and has some attached staples. The stapled portion is removed, and the remainder of the specimen is submitted in cassette C.

ds

DIAGNOSES (GROSS AND MICROSCOPIC)

A: Colon resection—infiltrating, moderately differentiated
indent adenocarcinoma with transmural invasion into pericolonic fat.
— No tumor seen in proximal and distal margins of resection.

ds

— Nine lymph nodes isolated, no tumor seen.

ds

— Based on the available histologic information, the tumor is classified as T3, N0, MX.

B: Proximal ring, segment—segment of large bowel with no evidence of malignancy.

C: Distal ring, segment—segment of large bowel with no evidence of malignancy.

qs

____

PATHOLOGIST: NURI BANO, MD

ds

NB/XX
D: 8/10/XX
T: 8/11/XX

FIGURE 9.7
Pathology Report (Continued)

you made. Answer the document analysis questions on the bottom of the chart. With continuous practice and assessment, the quality of your work will improve.

After you have produced a final version of each transcribed report, complete the Performance Report cover sheet, attach it to the top of the transcripts, and submit them to your instructor for evaluation.

Patient Study 9.A — James Welton

James Welton is a 34-year-old man who had eaten dinner and later complained of pain in his right side. He was nauseated and vomited several times during the evening and eventually was taken to the emergency room.

REPORT 9.1 Operative Report

- Listen for these special terms:
  Veress needle
  Tru-Cut needle

REPORT 9.2 Consultation Letter

- Listen for these special terms:
  Demerol
  D5W 0.45 NS (space between W and 0 and between 5 and N)

Patient Study 9.B — Sara Johnson

Sara Johnson is a 51-year-old woman who saw her physician after several weeks of intermittent constipation, abdominal distention, and bloody stools.

REPORT 9.3 Pathology Report

REPORT 9.4 Consultation Letter

- This report includes a tumor classification based on the TNM system described in the chapter overview. The classification should be transcribed as T3, N0, MX.

Patient Study 9.C — Jonathan Prince

Jonathan Prince is an 18-year-old young man who was diagnosed with Crohn disease one year prior to surgery. He had been doing well until last week when he began having intractable diarrhea, which required hospitalization for dehydration. He was given a presurgical barium enema and then sent to the operating room for a colostomy.

REPORT 9.5 X-Ray Report of Barium Enema

- Listen for the following new term:
  Gastrografin enema

REPORT 9.6 Pathology Report of Colostomy Procedure

- Transcribe the letter designations for specimen portions in capitals (A, B, etc.) and the labels in quotation marks, for example, "15-cm ileostomy."
- In the gross description section, treat each portion description as a separate paragraph.

Patient Study 9.D — David Dronen

David Dronen is a 52-year-old man who has been evaluated in the emergency room for severe abdominal pain.

REPORT 9.7 Flexible Sigmoidoscopy

Patient Study 9.E **Mary Gonzales**

Mary Gonzales is a 64-year-old woman with a long history of anemia. She was admitted to the hospital for tests to determine the cause of chest pain and dark, tarry stools.

REPORT 9.8 Discharge Summary

- Listen for these new words:
  guaiac-negative
  Prilosec
  Xanax

Patient Study 9.F **Jonathan Areade**

Jonathan Areade complained of sharp pain in the right upper quadrant. He went to the ER and on physical exam he was found to have jaundice and right upper quadrant tenderness.

REPORT 9.9 Pathology Report

Patient Study 9.G **Ronald Forest**

Ronald Forest is a 70-year-old gentleman who was found to have occult blood in his stool on routine examination. An abdominal CT scan revealed a mass in the colon.

REPORT 9.10 Pathology Report

Using Medical References

Use the appropriate medical reference to locate the correct spelling and additional usage information for the words below. (If the reference is not available, use the Glossary in this text.) Circle the correct spelling, then write a sentence using the word correctly.

1.	intusussception	intususception	intussusception
2.	guaiac	guiaic	guaic
3.	cachectic	cacechtic	cackhetic
4.	cirhossis	cirrhosis	cirhosis
5.	herniorhapy	herniorraphy	herniorrhaphy
6.	cholelithiasis	colelithiasis	cholelithisis
7.	diverticulae	diverticuli	diverticula
8.	hematochezia	hematachezia	hematocezia
9.	tenismus	tenesmus	tenesmis
10.	candydiasis	candidiosis	candidiasis

Making Expert Decisions

Circle the correct word from the choices in parentheses.

1. The patient had a hiatal hernia with esophageal (reflex/reflux).
2. The (mucous/mucus) membrane around the stomal opening was inflamed.
3. There was pain and tenderness in the area of the (carotid/parotid) gland.
4. The (acetic/acidic/ascitic) fluid was drained from the abdomen, which relieved a great deal of pressure.
5. Multiple (diverticula/diverticulum) were found along the wall of the colon.
6. Hyperactive bowel sounds were heard upon (auscultation/percussion) of the abdomen.
7. The patient had been suffering from inflammatory (bile/bowel) disease for two years now.
8. On endoscopic examination, the (ileum/ilium) was found to be normal.
9. Colonoscopic exam revealed a large tumor of the colonic mucosa and on pathological exam, this was found to be a (villi/villous/villus) adenoma.
10. The patient began to (retch/wretch) soon after eating dinner.

Transcribing Professional Documents

Transcribe the document named Chapter 9 Assessment. Before you key, review the appropriate report formatting guidelines. Proofread your transcribed document and revise it until you think it is error-free.

10

Obstetrics and Gynecology

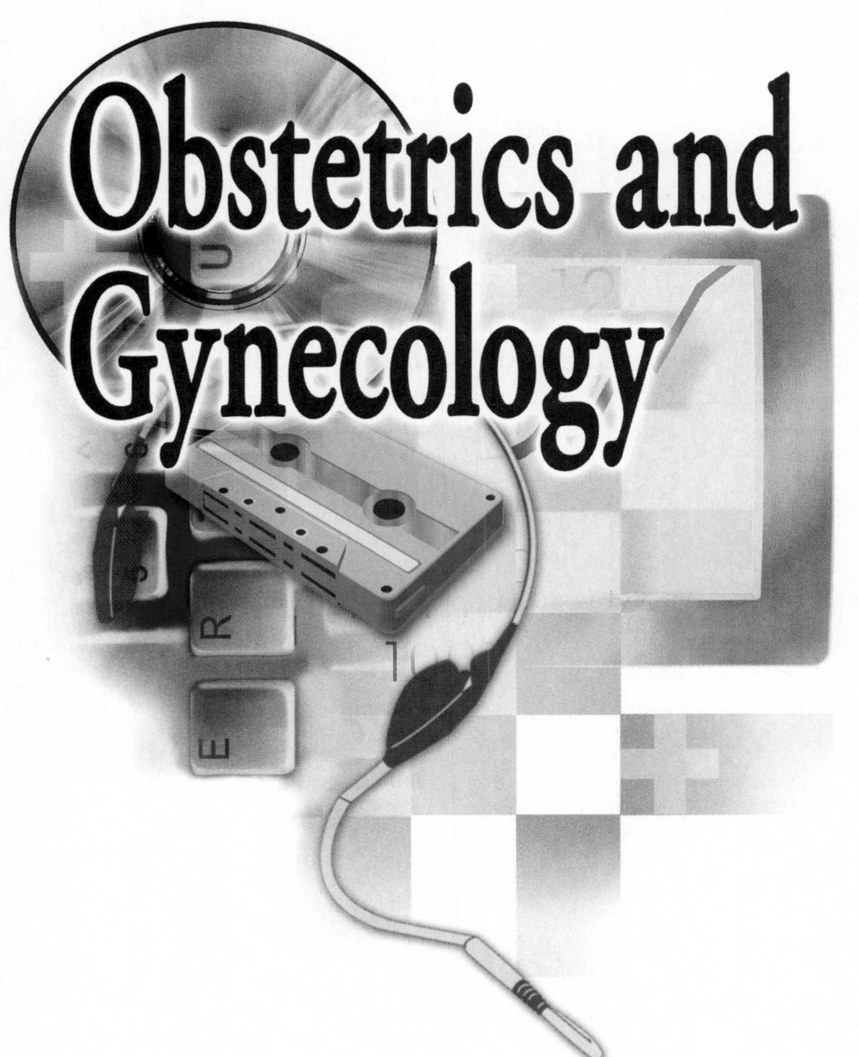

Obstetrics is the specialty concerned with the management of women's health during pregnancy, childbirth, and the three to six weeks following delivery. Gynecology is the study of the diseases of the female, particularly of the genital, urinary, and rectal organs. The practice of obstetrics and gynecology is usually done by the same physician, who is referred to as a gynecologist and/or obstetrician.

OBJECTIVES

- Use obstetrics and gynecology terms correctly according to the context and purpose of the dictation.
- Select and use appropriate general and specialty reference materials.
- Key obstetrics and gynecology documents of varying complexity and format.
- Transcribe authentic medical dictation requiring concentration and listening skill.
- Edit medical reports to conform with AAMT style guidelines.
- Proofread and correct transcripts to produce error-free documents.

Exploring Obstetrics and Gynecology

The joint specialty of obstetrics and gynecology has an acronym for its name: OB-GYN (pronounced letter by letter, O-B-G-Y-N, or as O-B-Gin). Recently, there have been separations in this specialty. There are physicians who only see patients during their prenatal, antenatal, and parturition periods. Other physicians deal only with high-risk pregnancies, that is, with women who have illnesses during pregnancy or who have fetuses that are considered at risk for problems in utero or at parturition. Other specialties include nurse-midwifery and fertility (usually for infertility). Some family and general practitioners also deliver babies, provide well-woman exams, and perform gynecologic/obstetric procedures.

Structure and Function

The female is born with a lifetime supply of eggs, or ova. These 30,000 to 40,000 eggs exist in an undeveloped form within the ovaries, which are almond-shaped glands located in the pelvic cavity on either side of the uterus (Figure 10.1). The uterus is a pear-shaped muscular organ that has a narrow neck called the cervix, a body or corpus, and the fundus, which is the uppermost part. The uterus is surrounded by the peritoneum and is held in the pelvic cavity by ligaments. The cor-

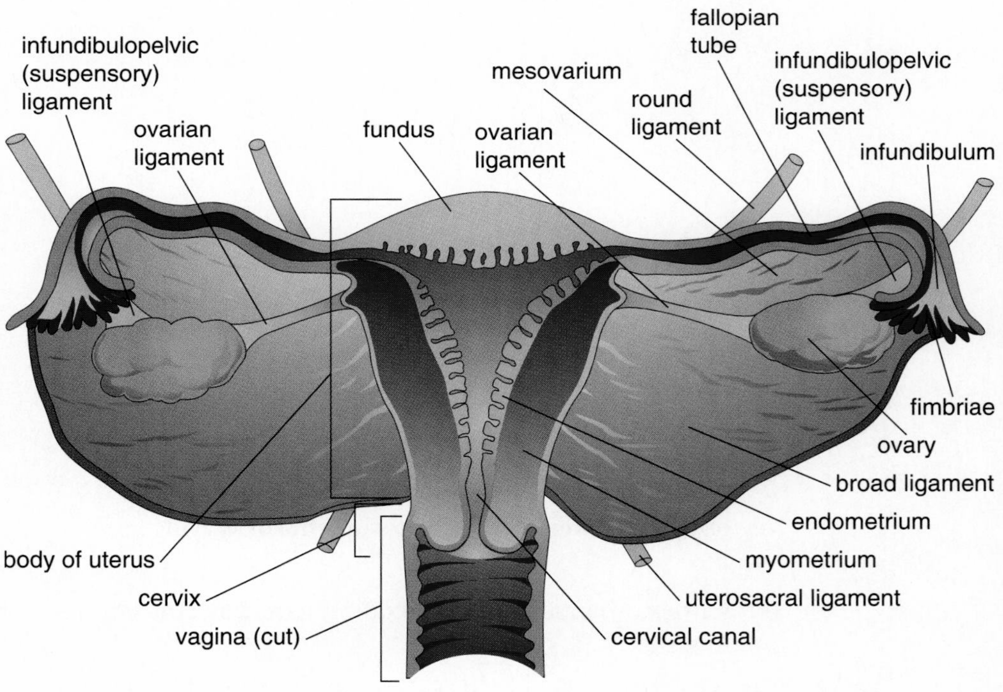

FIGURE 10.1
Internal Female Genitalia

nua is the upper lateral portion of the uterus from which the oviducts or fallopian tubes extend. The fallopian tubes are called the adnexa. The lumen of the fallopian tube is contiguous with the uterine cavity. At the distal end of each fallopian tube is the infundibulum, which is broad and funnel-like ending with an arm-like structure called the fimbria.

At puberty, hormones cause the ova to ripen and mature into a graafian follicle, a type of cyst that enlarges until it reaches the surface of the ovary. This is the beginning of the follicular phase of the menstrual cycle. The surface of the ovary ruptures, releasing an egg, or oocyte, into the pelvic cavity. The fimbriae sweep the oocyte into the fallopian tube.

The discharge of the oocyte from the ovary is referred to as ovulation, which may be accompanied by some pain, called mittelschmerz, in the lower groin area and some vaginal discharge. This is the luteal phase. If the oocyte is met by a spermatozoon, the male reproductive cell, conception takes place, usually occurring within the fallopian tubes. The cells of the graafian follicle become yellow and are referred to as the corpus luteum. The hormones secreted by the corpus luteum help prepare the uterus for the fertilized egg.

If conception does not occur, the ovum disintegrates and together with the upper layer of the endometrium of the uterus, is sloughed through the cervix and vagina. This blood flow is called menstruation and occurs approximately every 28 days during the reproductive life of the woman. Ovulation occurs about midway between menstrual periods.

The menstrual cycle occurs in response to the stimulation of hormones. The very first time menstruation occurs is known as menarche. Follicle-stimulating hormone (FSH) and luteinizing hormone (LH) are released by the pituitary gland located in the brain (see Chapter 13). Estrogen and progesterone are the hormones released by the follicle to prepare the uterus to receive the egg. This cycle continues until the woman reaches menopause, (average age is about 50 years). At this time the hormone production diminishes, causing atrophy of the genital organs, breast changes, loss in bone density, and vascular changes.

Physical Assessment

The physician begins the assessment of the female reproductive system by examining the external organs. The breasts are the first part of the assessment. Observation includes size, shape, deformities, markings (such as nevi), nipples, and areolar tissue (Figure 10.2). The breasts are then palpated for texture, masses, or abnormalities. The abdomen is examined as described in Chapter 9, Gastroenterology.

The external genitalia (Figure 10.3), or vulva, include the mon pubis, labia majora, labia minora, clitoris, vestibule of the vagina, the Skene or vestibular glands, and Bartholin glands. The physician inspects the genitalia, noting the urinary meatus, the anus, and the vulva.

Following the external inspection, the physician performs a digital examination of the organs, including a rectal exam with a stool swab for blood. A speculum (Figure 10.4) is usually inserted into the vagina to provide a wider opening for the visual exam of the cervix, fornices, and vaginal walls.

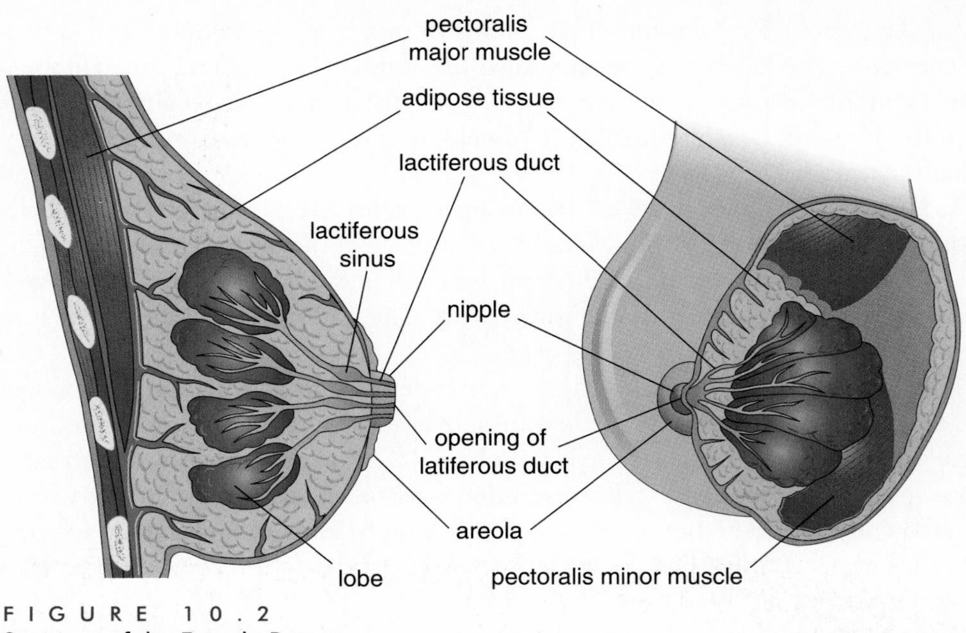

FIGURE 10.2
Structure of the Female Breast

Next, the physician completes a bimanual ("two hands") exam of the vagina and cervix, inserting one or two fingers of a gloved and lubricated hand into the vagina and placing the other hand on the patient's abdomen (Figure 10.5). This procedure allows the physician to assess the size, shape, and position of the uterus along with any masses or tenderness.

Diseases and Conditions

Along with cancers of the breast, uterus, ovaries, and cervix, common diseases of the female reproductive system include endometriosis, pelvic inflammatory disease, and sexually transmitted diseases.

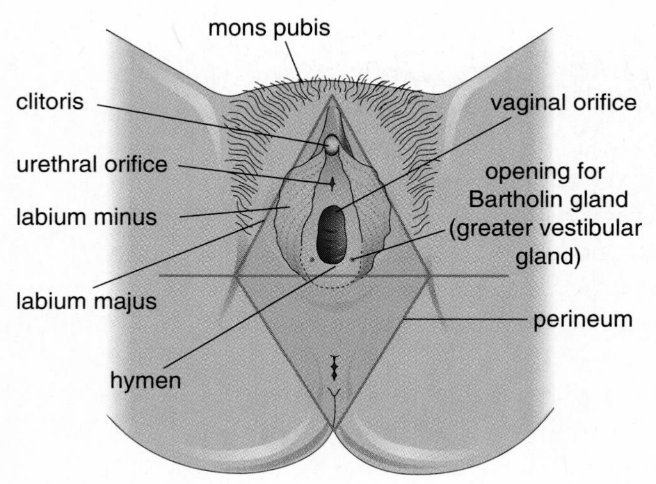

FIGURE 10.3
External Female Genitalia

Endometriosis is a benign condition in which there is aberrant uterine tissue growing outside the uterine wall. Symptoms associated with endometriosis include extreme menstrual pain, abnormal bleeding, infertility, and dyspareunia. Surgery and/or hormonal therapy to cause atrophy of the endometrium may be necessary to treat endometriosis.

Pelvic inflammatory disease (PID) is an inflammatory condition of the pelvic cavity that may be localized or spread throughout the reproductive organs. Also called acute salpingitis, the disease is usually caused by a bacterial agent such as gonococci or staphylococci and results in vaginal discharge, pain, and tenderness. PID is treated with the appropriate antibiotic therapy.

Human papillomavirus (HPV) is a sexually transmitted disease (STD) that is characterized by small growths on the genitalia. An increased risk of cervical cancer is associated with certain types of HPV; therefore, frequent Pap smears are indicated. Other STDs include gonorrhea, syphilis, Chlamydia, and herpes.

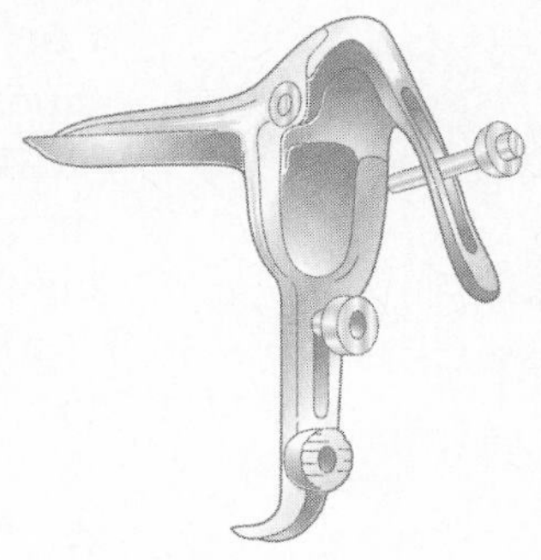

FIGURE 10.4
Vaginal Speculum

Common Tests and Surgical Procedures

The most common test performed during the gynecologic examination is the Papanicolaou (Pap) smear, which is a cytologic test that can detect cervical cancer.

The Bethesda System (TBS), a standardized system for reporting Pap smears is based on narrative reporting of descriptive diagnoses using clinically relevant cell findings. Physicians may incorporate within the narrative reporting a classification subsystem called the CIN system, which includes the following categories (CIN stands for cervical intraepithelial neoplasia, also called dysplasia, both of which are precancerous lesions):

- CIN-1: mild dysplasia
- CIN-2: moderate dysplasia
- CIN-3: severe dysplasia

Colposcopy is a procedure that is performed when there is an abnormal Pap smear. The colposcope is inserted into the cervix allowing visualization of the abnormal tissue. Biopsies are taken to provide more tissue for diagnosis. Cone biopsy is performed for the removal of premalignant cells. The patient has an excision of an inverted cone of tissue from the cervix.

Dilatation and curettage (D&C) is a surgical procedure performed to obtain endometrial or endocervical tissue for cytologic examination and to control abnormal uterine bleeding. The cervix is dilated and a curette is used to obtain uterine scrapings.

Hysterectomy is the surgical procedure to remove the cervix and uterus. A hysterectomy with removal of the fallopian tubes and ovaries is known as a total hysterectomy with bilateral salpingo-oophorectomy.

C-section (cesarean section) is the surgical delivery of a baby. This type of delivery accounts for approximately 20 to 25 percent of all deliveries and is carried out in

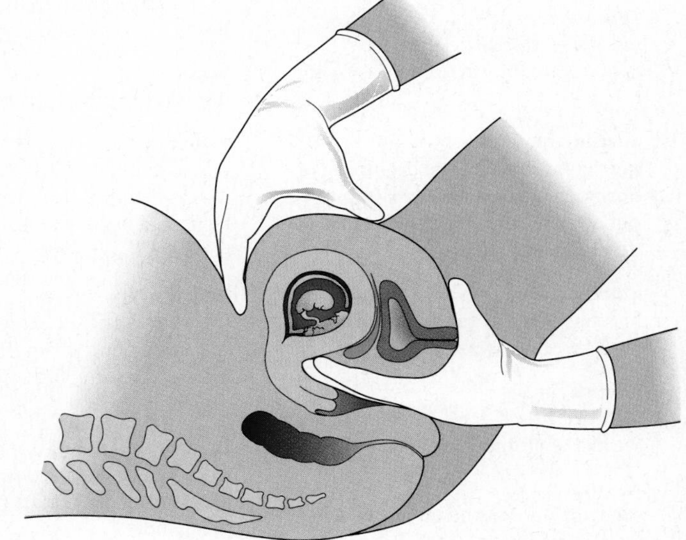

FIGURE 10.5
Bimanual Method of Palpating the Internal Genitalia

cases of ineffective labor, cephalopelvic disproportion, fetal distress, breech presentations, multiple births, and infections in the mother.

Mastectomy is the surgical removal of a breast, usually because of a cancerous tumor. The removal of only the tumor and minimal surrounding tissue is called a lumpectomy.

Mammogram is a radiographic image of the breast. It can detect abnormalities that cannot be palpated.

Building Language Skills

The following tables list common obstetrics and gynecology terms, drugs, and abbreviations. The list of terms and definitions includes the most difficult words contained in the dictated reports in this chapter. These words are identified in GREEN type. A list of common drugs is found in Appendix D.

Medical Terms and Pharmacologic Agents

adenocarcinoma
(**ad**-e-nO-kar-si-**nO**-ma) (n) a malignant adenoma arising from a glandular organ

adenopathy
(ad-e-**nop**-a-thee) (n) swelling or enlargement of any gland, especially the lymph nodes

adenosis
(ad-e-**nO**-sis) (n) any disease of a gland, especially of a lymphatic gland

adipose
(**ad**-i-pOz) (adj) containing fat

adnexal
(ad-**nek**-sal) (adj) relating to appendages or accessory parts of an organ

adrenarche
(**ad**-ren-ar-kee) (n) the beginning of hormonal activity that leads up to puberty and the associated sexual development

amenorrhea
(a-men-O-**ree**-a) (n) stoppage or absence of menses

amniocentesis
(**am**-nee-O-sen-**tee**-sis) (n) taking a sample of amniotic fluid

amnion
(**am**-nee-on) (n) the inner of the fetal membranes; a thin transparent sac that holds the fetus

anovulation
(an-ov-yoo-**lay**-shun) (n) absence of egg production or release from the ovary

anovulatory
(an-**ov**-yoo-la-tOr-ee) (adj) not accompanied by production of or discharge of an ovum (egg) or suppressing ovulation

anteflexion
(an-te-**flek**-shun) (n) the abnormal position of an organ that is bent forward over itself

Apgar score
(n) scoring system to assess newborn's physical condition

axilla
(**ak**-sil-a) (n) the armpit

axillary node
(**ak**-sil-ayr-ee nOd) (n) any of the lymph glands of the armpit that help to fight infection in the neck, chest, and arm area

biopsy
(**bI**-op-see) (n) the sampling of tissue and/or fluid from the body for microscopic study; the specimen obtained

Braxton Hicks sign
(n) irregular contractions of the uterus after the first trimester of pregnancy

breech presentation
(n) fetal position in which the feet or buttocks appear first in the birth canal

calcification
(**kal**-si-fi-**kay**-shun) (n) a hardening of tissue resulting from the formation of calcium salts within it

carcinoma
(kar-si-**nO**-ma) (n) a malignant growth of epithelial cells

cautery
(**kaw**-ter-ee) (n) a means of destroying tissue by electricity, freezing, heat, or corrosive chemicals

centimeter
(**sen**-ti-mee-ter) (n) unit of measurement; one hundredth of a meter; approximately 0.4 inches

cephalad
(**sef**-a-lad) (adv) toward the head

cerclage
(sair-**klazh**) (n) procedure to encircle tissues with a ligature, wire, or loop

cervical
(**ser**-vi-kal) (adj) relating to a neck, or cervix, especially the neck (cervix) of the uterus

cervix
(**ser**-viks) (n) the neck or part of an organ resembling a neck, such as the cervix of the uterus

chromosome
(**krO**-mO-sOm) (n) the structure in the cell nucleus that transmits genetic information; consists of a double strand of DNA in the form of a helix; there are normally 46 in humans

colostrum
(kO-**los**-trum) (n) the first milk secreted after childbirth

colposcopy
(kol-**pos**-ko-pee) (n) examination of the tissues of the vagina and cervix with a lighted instrument that magnifies the cells

condyloma
(kon-di-**lO**-ma) (n) warty growth in the genital area

cribriform
(**krib**-ri-fOrm) (adj) perforated with small holes of uniform size; (n) a polyporous structure

curettage
(**kyoo**-re-tahzh) (n) surgical scraping or cleaning, usually of the interior of a cavity or tract, for removal or sampling of tissue

cyanosis
(cI-a-**nO**-sis) (n) condition in which the skin and/or mucous membranes turn blue due to decreased amount of oxygen in the blood cells

decelerations
(dee-cel-er-**ay**-shunz) (n) decreases in speed or rate (of contractions)

dysgerminoma
(dis-jer-mi-**nO**-ma) (n) a rare cancerous ovarian tumor

dysmenorrhea
(dis-men-Or-**ee**-a) (n) painful menstruation

dyspareunia
(dis-pa-**roo**-nee-a) (n) painful sexual intercourse

ectopic pregnancy
(ek-**top**-ik) (n) pregnancy in which a fertilized ovum is implanted outside the uterus, often in a fallopian tube

edema
(e-**dee**-ma) (n) excessive accumulation of fluid in tissues, especially just under the skin or in a given cavity

emesis
(**em**-e-sis) (n) retching; throwing up

endocervical
(en-dO-**ser**-va-cal) (adj) pertaining to the lining of the canal of the cervix uteri

endometrium
(**en**-dO-**mee**-tree-um) (n) lining of the womb, composed of three layers and shed during menstruation

endometrial
(en-do-**mee**-tree-al) (adj) pertaining to the mucous membrane lining of the uterus

engorged
(en-**gOrjd**) (adj) filled to the limit of expansion

epidural
(ep-i-**doo**-ral) (adj) located over or under the dura

episiotomy
(e-peez-ee-**ot**-O-mee) (n) incision of perineum to facilitate delivery and prevent laceration (jagged tear)

epithelial
(ep-i-**thee**-lee-al) (adj) pertaining to or composed of epithelium, the layer of cells forming the epidermis of the skin and the surface layer of mucous and serous membranes

estradiol
(es-tra-**dI**-ol) (n) a hormone produced by the ovary; often used to treat menopausal symptoms

eversion
(ee-**vur**-zhun) (n) turning out or inside out

excrescence
(eks-**kres**-ens) (n) abnormal projection or outgrowth; such as a wart

fallopian tubes
(fa-**lO**-pee-an) (n) passageways from ovaries to uterus

fascia
(**fash**-ee-a) (n) fibrous connective tissue that supports and sheathes soft organs and muscles

fetal distress
(**fee**-tal) (n) life-threatening condition affecting the fetus

fibrosis
(fI-**brO**-sis) (n) a condition marked by thickening and scarring of connective tissue

fundus
(**fun**-dus) (n) the bottom or base of an organ; the part farthest from the opening; fundi (pl)

genital
(**jen**-i-tal) (adj) relating to reproduction or the organs of reproduction

genitalia
(jen-i-**tay**-lee-a) (n) male or female reproductive organs, especially the external ones

gestation
(jes-**tay**-shun) (n) the intrauterine development of an infant; pregnancy

gonorrhea
(gon-O-**ree**-a) a contagious disease usually affecting the genitourinary tract; transmitted chiefly by sexual intercourse

graafian follicle
(**graf**-ee-an) (n) a mature follicle on the ovary in which an oocyte matures and is released at ovulation

gravida
(**grav**-i-da) (n) a pregnant woman; may be used in combination with a number or prefix to indicate the number of pregnancies and their outcome

histiocytes
(**his**-tee-O-sitz) (n) cells present in loose connective tissues

homeostasis
(**hO**-mee-O-**stay**-sis/**hO**-mee-**os**-ta-sis) (n) equilibrium in the internal environment of the body, such as temperature and electrolyte balance

hypermenorrhea
(**hI**-per-men-O-**ree**-a) (n) lengthy or heavy menses; menorrhagia

hypomenorrhea
(**hI**-pO-men-O-**ree**-a) (n) decreased menses

hysterectomy
(his-ter-**ek**-tO-mee) (n) surgical removal of the uterus

immunohistochemistry
(**im**-yoo-nO-**his**-tO-**kem**-is-tree) (n) special techniques used on cells to identify certain characteristics, especially the presence of specific antigens

incised
(in-**sIzd**) (v) cut with a knife

Indocin
(in-**doe**-sin) (n) Brand name for indomethacin, an analgesic nonsteroidal anti-inflammatory drug

infundibulopelvic
(in-fun-**dib**-yoo-lO-**pel**-vik) (adj) relating to or located in the infundibulum (the end of the fallopian tube farthest from the uterus) and the pelvis

in situ
(in **sI**-too) (adj, adv) in position; at the original location, or site

intrauterine
(in-tra-**yoo**-ter-in) (adj) within the uterus

intraductal
(adj) inside a duct

introitus
(in-**trO**-i-tus) (n) an opening or entrance into a canal or cavity, such as the vagina

inversion
(in-**vur**-shun) (n) reversal of position, as upside down or inside out

knuckle
(**nuk**-l) (n) a finger joint; an abnormal kink or loop

laparotomy
(lap-a-**rot**-O-mee) (n) a surgical incision made into the abdominal wall

leiomyoma
(lI-O-mI-**O**-ma) (n) tumor in smooth muscle tissue

leukemia
(loo-**kee**-mee-a) (n) production of abnormal white blood cells; a type of cancer of the blood

lochia
(**lO**-kee-a) (n) vaginal discharge occurring after childbirth

loop
(n) a curve or bend forming a complete or almost complete oval or circle

loupe
(loop) (n) a magnifying lens

lumbar
(**lum**-bar) (adj) pertaining to the part of the back between the thorax and pelvis

lymphatic
(lim-**fat**-ik) (adj) relating to or resembling lymph or lymph nodes

lymphocyte
(**lim**-fO-sIt) (n) white blood cell that produces antibodies

lymphocytic
(lim-fO-**sit**-ik) (adj) relating to or characteristic of lymphocytes

mammogram
(**mam**-O-gram) (n) x-ray of the breast

meconium
(mee-**kO**-nee-um) (n) first bowel movement of a newborn, which are thick, sticky, greenish to black and composed of bile pigments and gland secretions

mediolateral
(**mee**-dee-O-**lat**-er-al) (adj) relating to the middle and side of a structure

menarche
(me-**nar**-kee) (n) the initial menstrual period

menometrorrhagia
(**men**-O-mee-trO-**rah**-jee-a) (n) excessive menstrual bleeding or bleeding between menstrual periods

menopause
(**men**-O-pawz) (n) the end of a woman's reproductive period of life and cessation of menses

menorrhagia
(men-O-**ray**-jee-a) (n) prolonged or heavy menses; hypermenorrhea

menorrhalgia
(men-O-**ral**-jee-a) (n) painful menstruation or pelvic pain accompanying menstruation

menses
(**men**-seez) (n) monthly flow of bloody fluid from the uterus

menstruation
(men-stroo-**ay**-shun) (n) the discharge of a bloody fluid from the uterus at regular intervals during the life of a woman from puberty to menopause

mesosalpinx
(**mez**-O-**sal**-pinks) (n) free end of the broad ligament which supports the fallopian tubes

metastatic
(met-a-**stat**-ic) (n) pertaining to metastasis (movement of cells, especially cancer cells, from one part of the body to another

metrorrhagia
(mee-trO-**rah**-jee-a) (n) bleeding from the uterus between menstrual periods

multipara
(mul-**tip**-a-ra) (n) a woman who has given birth to two or more children

necrosis
(ne-**crO**-sis) (n) dead areas of tissue or bone surrounded by healthy parts

nodule
(**nod**-yool) (n) a small mass, distinct from surrounding tissue

nuchal
(**noo**-kal) (adj) relating to the nape or back of the neck

nulligravida
(nul-i-**grav**-i-da) (n) a woman who has never been pregnant

occiput
(**ok**-si-put) (n) the back part of the skull

oligohydramnios
(**ol**-i-gO-hI-**dram**-nee-os) (n) abnormally small amount of amniotic fluid

oligomenorrhea
(**ol**-i-gO-men-O-**ree**-a) (n) infrequent or very light menstrual bleeding

omental
(O-**men**-tal) (adj) relating to the omentum

omentum
(O-**men**-tum) (n) fold of peritoneal tissue attaching to and supporting the stomach and intestines

oophorectomy
(O-of-Or-**ek**-tO-mee) (n) surgical removal of one or both ovaries

organomegaly
(**Or**-ga-nO-**meg**-a-lee) (n) abnormal enlargement of an organ, particularly an organ of the abdominal cavity, such as the liver or spleen

palpate
(**pal**-payt) (v) to examine by touch; to feel

para
(**par**-a) (n) a woman who has given birth to one or more children; the term may be used in combination with a number or prefix to indicate how many times a woman has given birth

pelvic
(**pel**-vik) (adj) relating to or located near the pelvis

pendulous
(**pen**-ju-lus) (adj) loosely hanging

perineum
(**per**-i-**nee**-um) (n) the external region between the urethral opening and the anus, including the skin and underlying tissues

peritoneal
(**per**-i-tO-**nee**-al) (adj) relating to the peritoneum

Pitocin
(**pit**-toe-sin) (n) Brand name for oxytocin, a synthetically produced, naturally-occurring hormone

peritoneum
(per-i-tO-**nee**-um) (n) lining of the abdominal cavity

polycystic
(pol-ee-**sis**-tik) (adj) having or consisting of many cysts

primipara
(prE-**mip**-ah-ra) (n) a woman who has had one pregnancy that produced a living infant

pyelogram
(**pI**-el-O-gram) (n) x-ray of the kidney and ureters; usually a radiopaque dye is injected into the patient to show the outline of the kidney and associated structures

rectovaginal
(**rek**-tO-**vaj**-i-nal) (adj) relating or located near the rectum and vagina

retraction
(ree-**trak**-shun) (n) the act of pulling back

sac
(sak) (n) pouch

sentinel node
(**sen**-ti-nal nOd) (n) an enlarged, supraclavicular lymph node infiltrated with cancer cells that have metastasized from an obscurely located primary cancer

sonometer
(**son**-O-mee-ter) (n) a bell-shaped instrument used to measure hearing

speculum
(**spek**-yoo-lum) (n) instrument for examination of canals

squamous
(**skway**-mus) (adj) covered with scale-like cells

supine
(soo-**pIn**) (adj) lying on the back

Tanner staging
(n) method of indicating the sexual development of a child or adolescent

thelarche
(thee-**lar**-kee) (n) the beginning of breast development in girls

thyroid
(**thI**-royd) (n) a gland in the neck that secretes thyroid hormone

thyromegaly
(thI-rO-**meg**-a-lee) (n) enlargement of the thyroid gland

transverse
(trans-**vers**) (adj) lying at right angles to the long axis of the body; crosswise

ureter
(**yoo**-re-ter) (n) the tube that carries urine from the kidney to the bladder

uterine
(**yoo**-ter-in/**yoo**-ter-In) (adj) relating to the uterus (the female reproductive organ where the fertilized egg develops before birth; the womb)

vertex
(**ver**-teks) (n) the crown or top of the head

vesicouterine
(**ves**-i-kO-**yoo**-ter-in) (adj) pertaining to the urinary bladder and uterus

vortex
(**vOr**-teks) (n) whirlpool; resembling a whirlpool

vulva
(**vul**-va) (n) external female genital organs; vulvae (pl)

vulvar
(**vul**-var) (adj) relating to the vulva

xeromammogram
(**zeer**-O-**mam**-o-gram) (n) type of x-ray of the breast

Abbreviations

AB, Ab	abortion
AIDS	acquired immune deficiency syndrome
BTL	bilateral tubal ligation (sterilization by cutting or cauterizing the fallopian tubes)
BBT	basal body temperature
BSO	bilateral salpingo-oophorectomy (removal of both ovaries and fallopian tubes)
CPD	cephalopelvic disproportion
CS, C-section	cesarean section
D&C	dilatation (or dilation) and curettage (instrumental expansion of the cervix and scraping of the uterine cavity)
DOB	date of birth
DUB	dysfunctional uterine bleeding
EDC	estimated date of confinement
FEKG	fetal electrocardiogram
FHR	fetal heart rate
FHT	fetal heart tones
FSH	follicle-stimulating hormone
FTND	full term normal delivery
FTNSVD	full term, normal spontaneous vaginal delivery
GC	gonorrhea
GYN	gynecology
HCG	human chorionic gonadotropin
HIV	human immunodeficiency virus
HRT	hormone replacement therapy
HSG	hysterosalpingography
IUD	intrauterine device
LH	luteinizing hormone
LMP	last menstrual period
NB	newborn
OB	obstetrics
PID	pelvic inflammatory disease
PMP	previous menstrual period
TAH	total abdominal hysterectomy
TAH/BSO	total abdominal hysterectomy with bilateral salpingo-oophorectomy
UC	uterine contractions
VH	vaginal hysterectomy
VBAC	vaginal birth after cesarean section

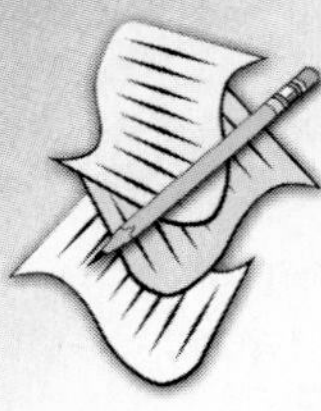

EXERCISE 10.1

Recognizing Look-Alikes and Sound Alikes

Below is a list of frequently used words that look alike and/or sound alike. Study the meaning and pronunciation of each set of words, then read the following sentences carefully and circle the word in parentheses that correctly completes the meaning.

thorough	complete, meticulous
through	nonstop, straight, finished, by way of

continual	regular or frequent
continuous	ceaseless; uninterrupted in time

menometrorrhagia	irregular or excessive bleeding during menses and between menses
menopause	cessation of reproductive period of life and cessation of menses for at least one year

menorrhagia	prolonged or heavy menses
menorrhalgia	painful menstruation or pelvic pain accompanying menstruation

perineum	external region between the urethral opening and the anus
peritoneum	lining of the abdominal cavity

elicit	(v) to bring out
illicit	(adj) illegal

decent	(adj) appropriate, conforming to acceptable behavior
descent	(n) downward movement, lowering

eminent	prominent, famous, standing out
imminent	about to occur

amenorrhea	absence of menses for three months or more
dysmenorrhea	painful menstruation
hypermenorrhea	prolonged or heavy menses
hypomenorrhea	diminished menses
oligomenorrhea	infrequent or scant menstrual bleeding

1. The patient denies use of (elicit, illicit) drugs.
2. Palpation of the area did not (elicit, illicit) pain.
3. She had a (continual, continuous) menstruation that lasted more than four weeks.
4. The patient seemed anxious to get (thorough, through) the physical examination.
5. The (decent, descent) of the laparoscope into the suprapubic area proceeded with minimal discomfort to the patient.
6. The patient states she has (amenorrhea, dysmenorrhea) with menses but Advil usually controls the pain.
7. Hypermenorrhea and (menorrhagia, menorrhalgia) mean the same thing.
8. Noting that the birth of the baby seemed (eminent, imminent), the nurse paged the obstetrician.
9. Dysmenorrhea and (menorrhagia, menorrhalgia) mean the same thing.
10. The end of one's reproductive life phase is called (menopause, menses).

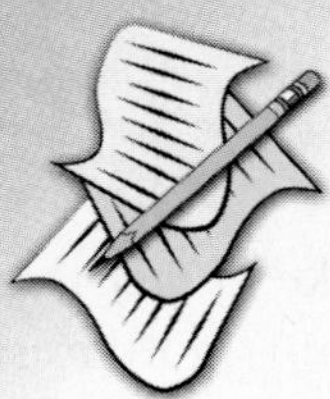

EXERCISE 10.2

Matching Sound and Spelling

The numbered list that follows shows the phonetic spelling of hard-to-spell words. Sound out the word, then write the correct spelling in the blank space provided. Each of the words can be found in the Glossary or in the drug list in Appendix D.

1. e-peez-ee-**ot**-O-mee ______________________
2. kol-**pos**-ko-pee ______________________
3. **krO**-mO-sOm ______________________
4. a-men-O-**ree**-a ______________________
5. kon-di-**lO**-ma ______________________
6. **graf**-ee-an ______________________
7. jes-**tay**-shun ______________________
8. his-ter-**ek**-tO-mee ______________________
9. **kyoo**-re-**tahzh** ______________________
10. in **sI**-too ______________________
11. mul-**tip**-a-ra ______________________
12. gon-O-**ree**-a ______________________
13. **men**-O-**rah**-jee-a ______________________
14. **ol**-i-gO-men-O-**ree**-a ______________________
15. **per**-i-**nee**-um ______________________

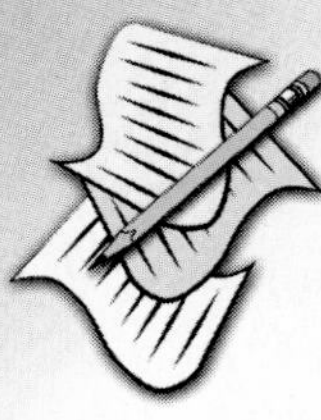

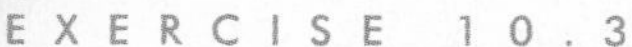

EXERCISE 10.3

Choosing Words from Context

When transcribing dictation, the medical transcriptionist frequently needs to consider the situation when determining the word that correctly completes the sentence. From the list below, select the term that meaningfully completes each statement.

carcinoma	menses	uterine
lymphocyte	gravida	para
dysmenorrhea	peritoneum	hypomenorrhea
mammogram	introitus	menopause
genital		

1. The ________________ showed she had a small, pea-sized mass in the right breast.
2. Mrs. Jones states she has severe cramping at the time of her _______________.
3. She has a condyloma on her external __________ area.
4. The ____________ is found at the entrance of the vagina.
5. Her blood count revealed an increased _____________ count, possibly indicating a viral infection.
6. The patient states that ibuprofen relieves the __________ during her menstrual periods.
7. The hysterectomy was performed after the biopsy revealed a _______________.
8. Mrs. Green is a (an) _______________2, para 1 and presents to the birthing center today in active labor.
9. The ________________contractions increased steadily until the baby was delivered.
10. After the tumor was removed from the abdominal wall, the _______________ was washed.

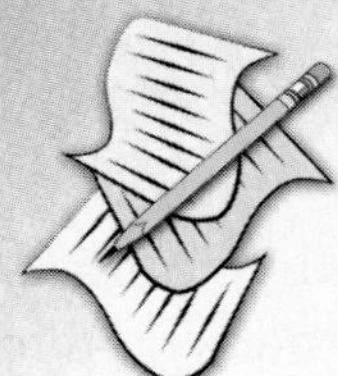

EXERCISE 10.4

Pairing Words and Meanings

From this list, locate the term that best matches each of the following definitions. Write the letter of the term in the space provided by each definition.

A. calcification
B. edema
C. menarche
D. nulligravida
E. oligomenorrhea
F. adrenarche
G. dysgerminoma
H. anovulation
I. menses
J. oophorectomy
K. dysmenorrhea
L. hysterectomy
M. amenorrhea

1. absence of egg release from an ovary __________
2. malignant neoplasm of an ovary __________
3. changes that occur at puberty __________
4. surgical removal of an ovary __________
5. a hardening of tissue from formation of calcium __________
6. painful menstruation __________
7. excessive amount of fluid in body tissues __________
8. first menstrual period __________
9. a woman who has never conceived a child __________
10. monthly flow of blood from the uterus __________

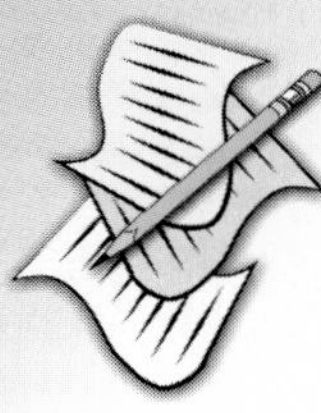

EXERCISE 10.5

Creating Terms from Word Forms

Combine prefixes, root words, and suffixes from this list to create medical words that fit the following definitions. Fill in the blanks with the words you construct.

a-	without; absence	son/o	sound waves
dys-	difficult, painful	thyr/o	thyroid
hepat/o	liver	germin	germinal tissue
lei/o	smooth	-algi/o	pain
mamm/o	breast	-ectomy	cutting out, removal
mast/o	breast	-gram	record
men/o	(month) mensus	-itis	inflammation
my/o	muscle	-megaly	enlargement
olig/o	little	-oma	tumor
oophor/o	ovary	-rrhagia	unusual or excessive flow (discharge)
organ/o	liver, spleen		
salping/o	tube	-rrhea	flow, discharge

1. removal of fallopian tubes ______
2. very large thyroid gland ______
3. inflammation of the ovary ______
4. menstruation ______
5. tumor of smooth muscle tissue ______
6. rare ovarian malignant tumor, that causes pain______
7. x-ray of breast ______
8. benign tumor in the uterus ______
9. removal of ovary ______
10. abnormally large liver______
11. removal of breast ______
12. ultrasound image/record ______
13. absence of menses ______
14. scanty menstrual flow______
15. excessive menstrual flow______
16. painful menstruation ______

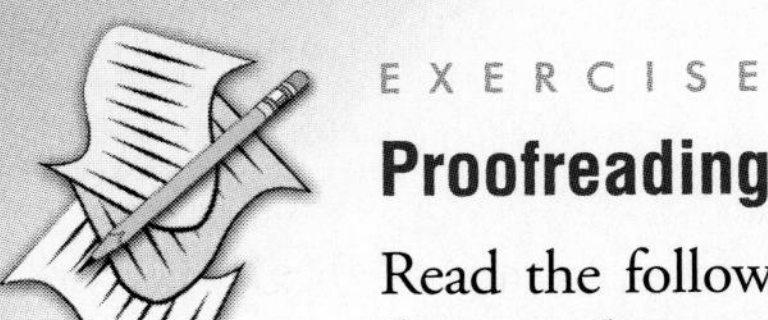

EXERCISE 10.6

Proofreading Review

Read the following report sections and circle errors in punctuation, spelling, plural forms, subject-verb agreement, incomplete sentences, and the placement of modifiers. Then key the report with the errors corrected.

Bilateral mammograms were preformed using film scream technique and compared with previous xeromammograms from June 1992 and February 1993. There appears to be a small and smoothly marginated oval shaped nodular in the upper quadrant of the right breast. Not as clearly visualised on the previous xeromammograms.

Increased density is again seen in the upper outer quadrants bilaterally, unchanged and consistent with fibroglandular tissue. Neither breasts demonstrates evidence of architectural distortion, clustered microcalcifications, skin thickening or retraction.

The patient was placed on the operating table in the supine position under satisfactory general endotracheal anesthesias. A #14 foley cathether was inserted. The abdomen was then prepped with betadine scrub and solution and was drapped in the usual sterile manner.

Building Transcription Skills

The Labor and Delivery Report

As its title suggests, the labor and delivery report (Figure 10.6) summarizes the procedures used in the delivery of a baby. Although most are brief reports, those describing a delivery that requires the physician's surgical intervention—for example, delivery by forceps—can be as extensive as an operative report.

Required Headings/Content Although no specific headings are required, the labor and delivery report includes headings similar to those in an operative report. Usually dictated are the preoperative and postoperative diagnoses, the title and date of the procedure, the indications for the procedure, and the actual description of the procedure.

Turnaround Time Generally, labor and delivery reports should be transcribed within 24 hours after dictation. However, this guideline varies among hospitals.

Preparing to Transcribe

To prepare for transcribing dictation, review the tables of common obstetrics and gynecology terms, drugs, and abbreviations presented in the Building Language Skills section of this chapter. Then, study the format and organization of the model document shown in Figure 10.6, and key the model document. Proofread the document by comparing it with the printed version. Categorize the types of errors you made, and document them on a copy of the Performance Comparison chart provided in Chapter 1. A template of this chart is included on the IRC that accompanies this text.

Patient Studies

Transcribe, edit, and correct each report in the following patient studies. Consult reference books for words or formatting rules that are unfamiliar.

As you work on the transcription assignment for this chapter, fill in the Performance Comparison chart that you started when you keyed the model document. For at least three of the reports, categorize and document the types of errors you made. Answer the document analysis questions on the bottom of the chart. With continuous practice and assessment, the quality of your work will improve.

After you have produced a final version of each transcribed report, complete the Performance Report cover sheet, attach it to the top of the transcripts, and submit them to your instructor for evaluation.

1" top and side margins → left justification

PATIENT NAME: Jung-Ah Wang
DATE: 10/21/XX

ds

PREOPERATIVE DIAGNOSIS: Arrest of Descent.

ds

POSTOPERATIVE DIAGNOSIS: Single viable female infant.

ds

OPERATION PERFORMED: Indicated low forceps delivery.

ds

INDICATIONS: This is a 33-year-old gravida 1, para 0 who pushed greater than 2 hours and then consented to epidural anesthesia. She pushed for 1 more hour and pushed the baby to +2 station and consented for assisted vaginal delivery.

ds

PROCEDURE: After adequate epidural anesthesia, the patient was placed in stirrups and was prepared and draped in the usual sterile fashion. The cervix was again examined and noted to be completely dilated, completely effaced. The pelvis was noted to be adequate. The estimated fetal weight was approximately 8 pounds. Position of the infant was noted to be right occiput posterior. The station was noted to be +2.

ds

The bladder was drained with a red Robinson catheter. Simpson forceps were then soaked in Betadine solution and the posterior blade was carefully placed, with the opposite hand protecting the vaginal side wall. The same procedure was repeated on the opposite site. Correct blade placement was then verified times 2. A midline episiotomy was then performed. With adequate maternal expulsive efforts, a viable female infant was delivered over a midline episiotomy. A vigorous cry was noted on the perineum. Inspection of the infant noted correct blade placement. The baby was bulb suctioned on the perineum and passed off to the awaiting pediatricians, who gave Apgar scores of 9 and 10. Weight of the infant was 3762 g. Cord pH was obtained; arterial 7.29, venous 7.33.

ds

The vagina was inspected for lacerations and there were none. The cervix and rectum were intact. The midline episiotomy was then reapproximated with 2-0

(continued)

FIGURE 10.6
Labor and Delivery Report

LABOR AND DELIVERY REPORT
PATIENT NAME: Jung-Ah Wang
DATE: 10/21/XX
Page 2
ds

Vicryl suture. The placenta was easily removed, followed by vigorous fundal massage, and intravenous Pitocin was given. Uterine tone was noted to be firm. There were no complications. After delivery of the infant at 0234, both mother and infant were doing well.

qs

____

Alexandra Mateo, MD
ds
AM:XX
D: 10/21/XX
T: 10/22/XX

FIGURE 10.6
Labor and Delivery Report (Continued)

Patient Study 10.A — Felicia Stallward

Felicia Stallward is a 25-year-old woman who had leukemia as a young child and presently complains of irregular menstruation. She is seen by the gynecologist.

REPORT 10.1 Consultation Letter

- Listen for these new abbreviations:
  TSH (thyroid-stimulating hormone)
  DHEAS (dehydroepiandrosterone sulfate)

Patient Study 10.B — Rosemary Barnes

Rosemary Barnes discovered a lump in her left breast when she was performing her monthly breast self-examination. She was seen in the gynecologist's office immediately. She was sent to the surgeon for examination and excision of the mass.

REPORT 10.2 Pathology Report

Patient Study 10.C — Irene Remona

Irene Remona is a 51-year-old woman who had a routine mammography as part of her annual checkup at the gynecologist. Her checkup was completely within normal limits. Her mammogram results follow.

REPORT 10.3 Radiology Report

Patient Study 10.D — Jung-Ah Wang

Jung-ah Wang is a 33-year-old woman who was admitted to the hospital to deliver her first child. She has had an unproductive labor and has agreed to an assisted vaginal delivery with forceps.

REPORT 10.4 Labor and Delivery Report

- Gravida refers to the number of times a woman has been pregnant. Para indicates the number of deliveries after the 20th week of gestation. A woman who has been pregnant five times (two term infants, one premature infant, one abortion, and one miscarriage) may be described in several different ways, all of which are acceptable:

  "The patient is gravida five, para three." (transcribed gravida 5, para 3)

  "The patient is G five, P three." (transcribed G5, P3)

  "The patient is gravida five, para three, aborta two." (transcribed gravida 5, para 3, aborta 2)

  "The patient is G five, P three, AB two [or A two]." (transcribed G5, P3, AB 2 [or A2])

  The physician may also use TPAL terminology, listing numbers in an order that correlates with the following designations: T = term infants, P = premature infants, A = abortions or miscarriages, L = living children

  Thus if the dictator says, "The patient is gravida five, para two one two three" or "obstetric history two one two three," you would key: The patient is gravida 5, para 2-1-2-3 or Obstetric history: 2-1-2-3.

- Some physicians use the military style for expressing time. For example, in this report, the dictator notes that the infant was delivered at "zero two thirty-four," which means 2:34 a.m., and which should be transcribed as 0234. See Chapter 3 for more information on transcribing time expressions.

Patient Study 10.E

Mary Ewing

Mary Ewing is an 18-year-old female who has experienced intermittent abdominal pain for several weeks. She was seen by her physician, and, at that time, there were no significant findings. Three weeks ago, she found that her waist had significantly increased in size. She also had continued abdominal pain and had some vomiting for the past several days. She returned to her physician who palpated a mass in the lower abdomen and referred her to the surgeon.

REPORT 10.5 Operative Report

Patient Study 10.F

Gena Martin

Gena Martin is a 21-year-old woman who was admitted to the hospital in labor with her first child. When tests indicated fetal distress, Gena agreed to undergo a cesarean section.

REPORT 10.6 Operative Report

- Listen for these new terms:
  DeLee suctioned
  vancomycin

Patient Study 10.G

Marta Valdez

Marta Valdez is a 22-year-old woman who is pregnant with twins. With her previous pregnancy, she developed cervical dilation at 20 weeks of gestation, which required cervical cerclage. Her obstetrician has recommended cervical cerclage with this pregnancy to prevent premature labor and delivery.

REPORT 10.7 Operative Report

- Physicians may use clock terminology to indicate areas on a circular surface. In this report, for example, the dictator describes the placement of a 5 mm Mersilene band at the "6 o'clock position" and the "2 o'clock" position of the cervix. Transcribe these expressions using figures and the word "o'clock" (6 o'clock and 2 o'clock).
- Listen for these terms:
  Unasyn
  Indocin
  Sims elevator
  amnion
  Trendelenburg position

Patient Study 10.H

Amy Bataglia

Amy Bataglia is a 21-year-old pregnant woman who was admitted to the hospital in labor. She has received her prenatal care in the medical center's OB clinic and is known to have a breech malpresentation with oligohydramnios. In consultation with her physician, she has agreed to a cesarean section.

REPORT 10.8 Operative Report

- Listen for these terms:
  Pfannenstiel incision
  Kocher clamp
  Metzenbaum scissors
  Mauriceau-Smellie-Veit maneuver

Patient Study 10.I — Marjorie Westenberg

This is the pathology report of a 68-year-old female who had an exploratory laparotomy with hysterectomy to remove a large pelvic mass.

REPORT 10.9 Pathology Report

- Listen for the following terms:
  Lap = laparotomy
  omentectomy
  multicystic
  multiloculated
  mucinous
  papillae
  omentum
  endomyometrium
  RPMI

Patient Study 10.J — Janine March

This pathology report is from a 31-year-old female who underwent a partial mastectomy, sentinel node biopsy with axillary node dissection.

REPORT 10.10 Pathology Report

- Listen for these terms:
  homogeneous
  fibrofatty
  subcapsular
  micrometastases
  in situ
  cribriform
  adenosis
  pan-cytokeratin

Using Medical References

Use the appropriate medical reference to locate the correct spelling and additional usage information for the words below. (If the reference is not available, use the Glossary in this text.) Circle the correct spelling; then write a sentence using the word correctly.

1.	colpscopy	colposcopy	colpuscopy
2.	adnexi	adnexa	adnexae
3.	falopian	faloppian	fallopian
4.	dilatation	dialatation	dilitation
5.	condyloma	chondyloma	condaloma
6.	oophorectomy	oopherectomy	ophorectomy
7.	ceaserean	caesarean	cesarean
8.	genetalia	gentalia	genitalia
9.	cytalogy	cytology	cytologey
10.	obsterics	obstetrics	obsetrics
11.	sists	cists	cysts
12.	ovaries	overies	ovares

Making Expert Decisions

Circle the correct word from the choices in parentheses.

1. After delivery, umbilical (chord/cord) blood samples were obtained and submitted for testing.
2. The baby was delivered from the (vertex/vortex) position after a lengthy labor period.
3. During the prenatal examination, it was determined that the baby was in a transverse (lay/lie).
4. There was one (loop/loupe) of (chord/cord) wrapped around the baby's neck.
5. The amniotic (sac/sack) was ruptured artificially when the patient was at 3 cm, revealing meconium-stained fluid.
6. During her pregnancy, the patient achieved a 20 pound (wait/weight) gain.
7. The (colposcope/culdoscope) was introduced through the posterior vaginal wall, and the rectovaginal pouch was visualized.
8. (Descent/Decent) of the baby's head into the birth canal was in progress.
9. Labor progressed rapidly, and it was felt delivery was (eminent/imminent).
10. The placental cord contained the normal (complement/compliment) of three vessels.

Transcribing Professional Documents

Transcribe the document named Chapter 10 Assessment. Before you key, review the report formatting guidelines. Proofread your transcribed document and revise it until you think it is error-free.

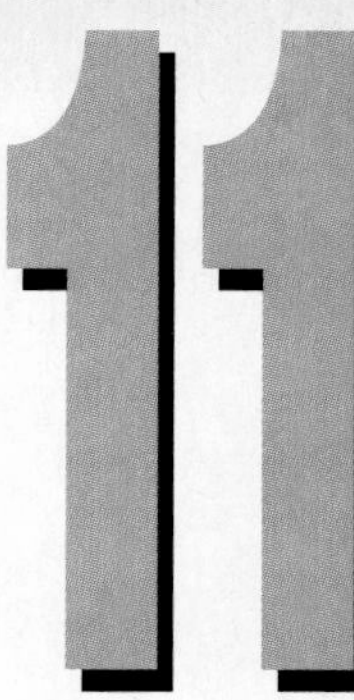

Urology and Nephrology

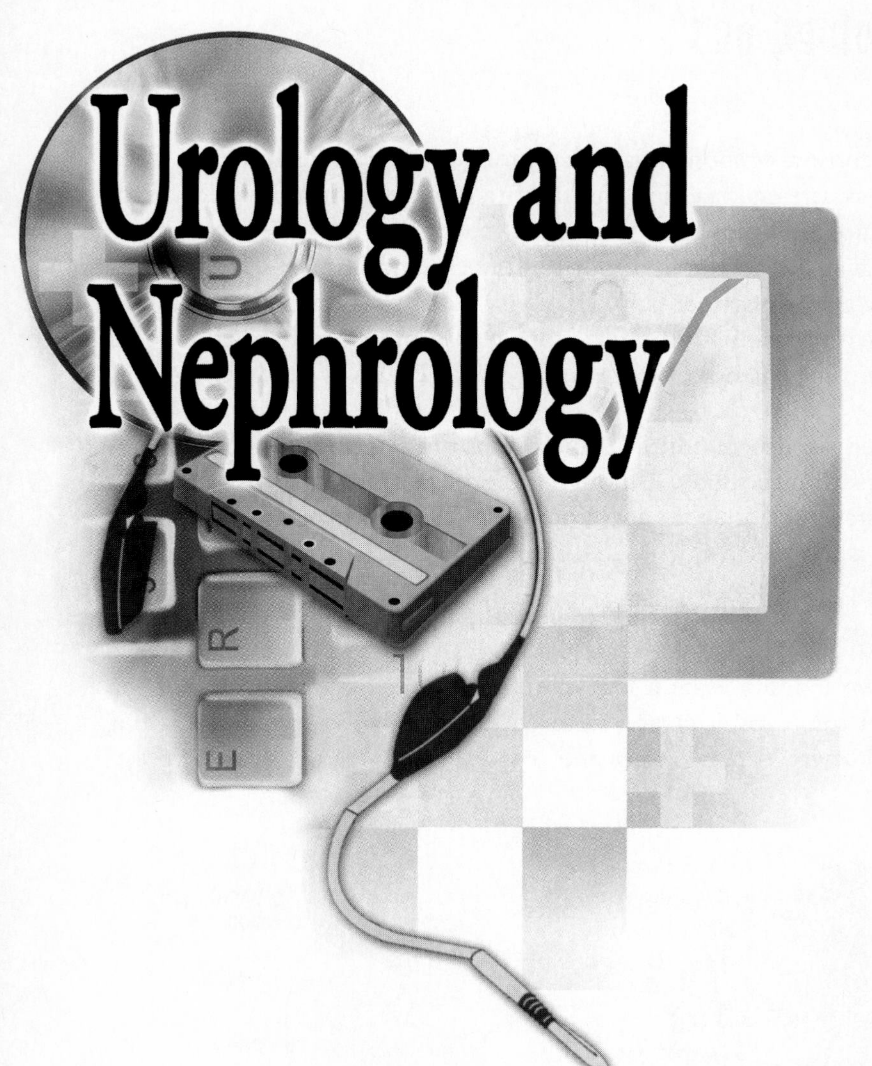

Urology is the study of the urinary tract in both sexes and the genital tract in the male. Nephrology is the science related to the structure and function of the kidney. Because the systems are interdependent, the specialties are often considered together in medical studies. The subspecialists concerned with the urinary system are the urologist and the nephrologist.

OBJECTIVES

- Use urology and nephrology terms correctly according to the context and purpose of the dictation.
- Select and use appropriate general and specialty reference materials.
- Key urology and nephrology documents of varying complexity and format.
- Transcribe authentic medical dictation requiring concentration and listening skill.
- Edit medical reports to conform with AAMT style guidelines.
- Proofread and correct transcripts to produce error-free documents.

Exploring Urology and Nephrology

The urinary system consists of those organs that produce urine and eliminate it from the body: the kidneys, ureters, bladder, and urethra (Figure 11.1). The body must have a proper balance of fluids and electrolytes to sustain life. Electrolytes are charged particles that make up the fluid portion of cells and intracellular, extracellular, and intravascular compartments. The urinary system regulates the fluid and electrolyte balance within the body by filtration, reabsorption, and secretion. The kidneys help maintain the balance by excreting about 1–2 liters of fluid per day and 6–8 grams of salt.

The urinary system is also responsible for transporting and excreting chemical and metabolic wastes from the body. Although there are other avenues by which the body eliminates wastes, such as sweat and stool, urine is the primary transporter of metabolic byproducts.

Structure and Function

The body houses two kidneys, each a few centimeters to the right and left of the thoracic vertebrae. A thin capsule surrounds each kidney to protect and separate it from the abdominal cavity. A renal artery and renal vein provide the blood supply.

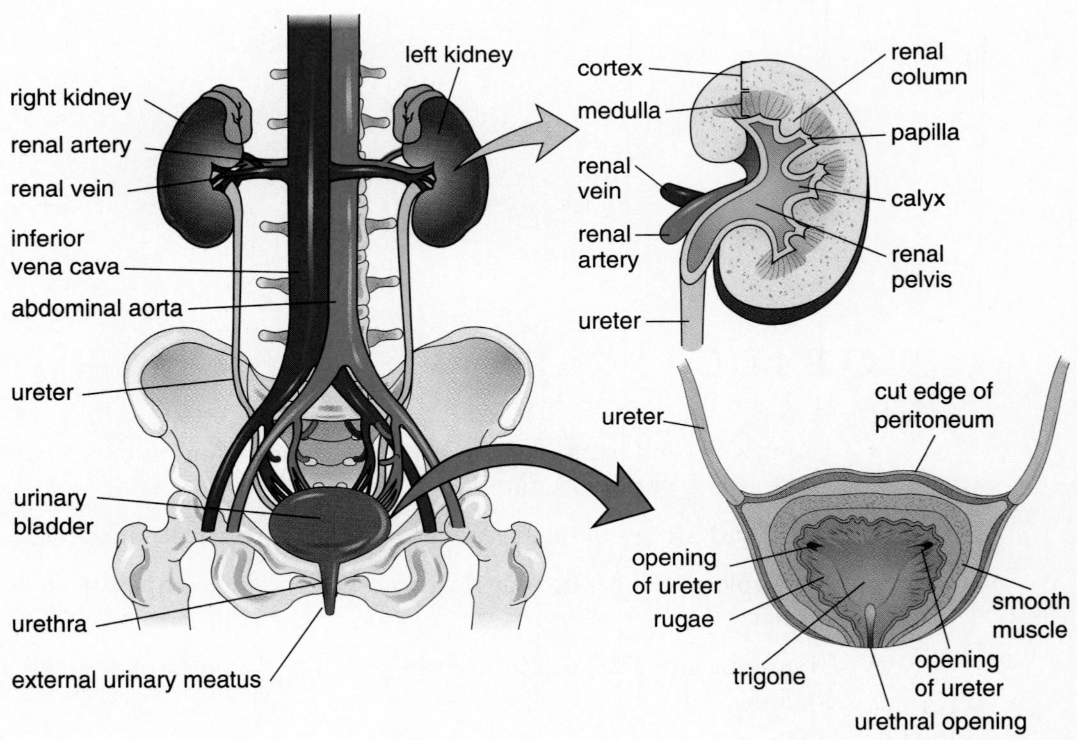

FIGURE 11.1
The Urinary System

The outer portion of the kidney is called the cortex; the inner portion is called the medulla. Within the kidney are approximately one million nephrons (Figure 11.2), which do the actual work of the kidney. Bowman's capsule surrounds the glomerulus, which contains capillaries composed of endothelial cells and basement membrane. The tubule is divided into four parts: a proximal convoluted tubule, the loop of Henle, a distal convoluted tubule, and a collecting tubule.

As blood flows through the glomerulus, fluid filters out through the walls of the glomerular capillary tufts. This filtrate is composed primarily of water and electrolytes. Some of the substances are selectively reabsorbed into the blood and the rest continue to travel through the tubule. The remaining fluid that reaches the kidney pelvis is urine.

From the renal pelvis, the urine travels through the ureters and into the bladder by peristaltic waves occurring about one to five times per minute. The bladder is lined with smooth muscle, which adapts to the slow filling and does not usually produce the sensation to void until there is approximately 200 to 300 ml of urine. The external urethral sphincter is a muscle that is under voluntary control, which is learned in early childhood. When there is a desire to urinate, the sphincter is relaxed. This allows the bladder muscles to contract and expel urine through the urethra and out the urinary meatus.

Men usually are seen by the urologist for problems with the urogenital system, which includes the male sexual organs. While male sexual dysfunction may be treated by the urologist, male infertility may be managed by infertility specialists. Figure 11.3 depicts the structures of the male urogenital anatomy.

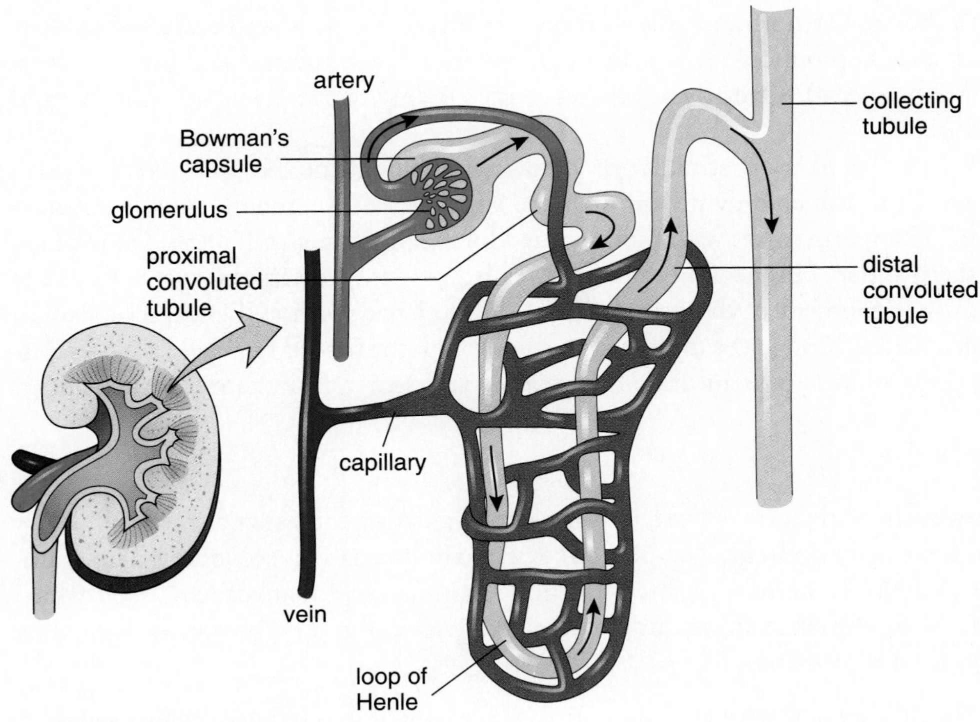

FIGURE 11.2
Structure of the Nephron

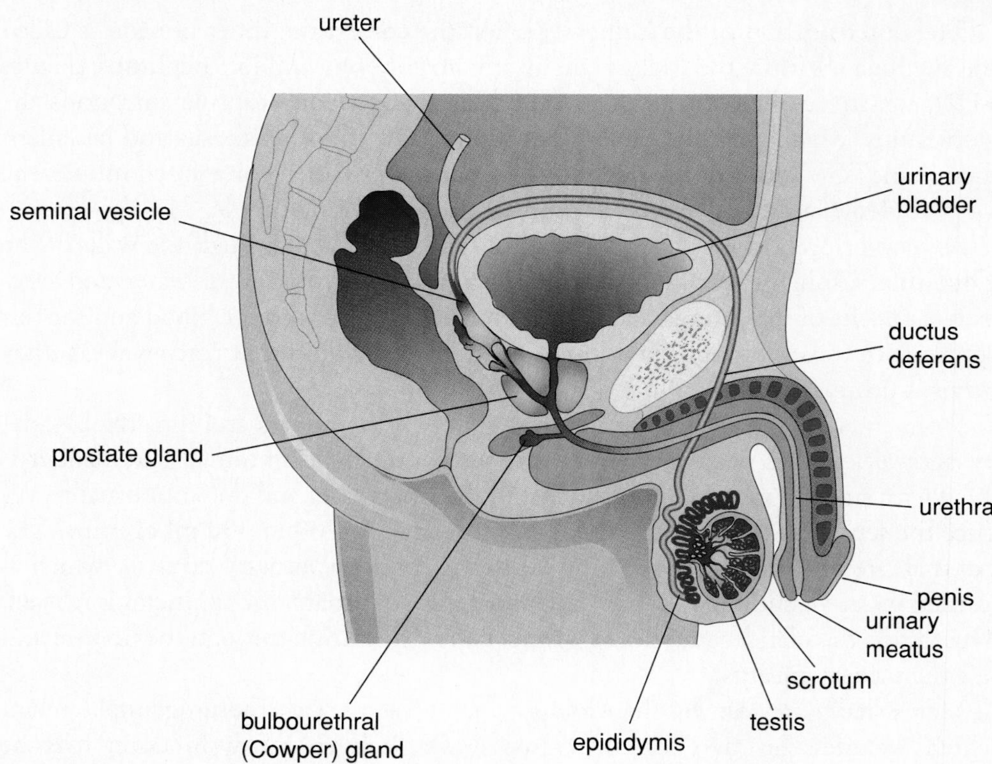

FIGURE 11.3
Male Urogenital System

The testes are contained in the scrotum. They are made of coils called seminiferous tubules. The hormone testosterone, responsible for male secondary sexual characteristics, is produced by the testes. The seminiferous tubules also produce spermatozoa (sperm). Over these tubules is the epididymis where sperm migrate and mature.

When the penis is stimulated, it fills with blood and becomes erect. Sperm travels from the epididymis through the vas deferens by smooth muscle contractions. The sperm mixes with fluid secreted by the prostate gland, located at the base of the bladder. This alkaline substance, called semen, protects the sperm from the acidic environment of the male urethra and the female vagina. During ejaculation, semen passes through the urethra. The sphincter at the base of the bladder closes during ejaculation to prevent urine from exiting and semen from entering the bladder.

Physical Assessment

Assessment of the urinary system is done by evaluating the patient's medical history and laboratory findings. The physical examination usually is secondary. The examiner asks about the color, odor, frequency, amount, and circumstances under which urine is produced. A urine sample obtained in one of the following ways provides important information:

- For urinalysis, the patient voids into a clean container. The specimen provides general characteristics of the urine and allows the physician to rule out problems.

- For clean-catch urine, the urinary meatus is cleaned with an antiseptic. The urine is collected midstream in a sterile container and then viewed through the microscope to determine the number and type of bacteria present. A clean-catch specimen is collected when the patient has complaints that suggest a urinary tract infection.
- For a catheterized specimen, a sterile, flexible tube, or catheter, is inserted through the meatus into the bladder. Urine is collected in a sterile receptacle for culture.

Diseases and Conditions

Diseases and pathology are described by the area of the urinary system involved. There are several diseases that affect the kidney and cause renal failure. Renal failure results in a decreased excretion of metabolic waste products, which can lead to serious and life-threatening complications. Decreased blood flow (prerenal), decreased urinary output (postrenal), or injury to the kidney (intrarenal) are causes of renal failure.

When there is a chronic dysfunction of the kidneys, the substances that are normally excreted accumulate in the body. This leads to uremic syndrome or uremia.

Nephrotic syndrome refers to a group of diseases of the glomerular apparatus that cause plasma proteins to spill into the urine.

Glomerulonephritis, an inflammation of the glomeruli, is often a result of a streptococcal infection. It is also associated with systemic lupus erythematosus (SLE), scleroderma, and other autoimmune disorders.

Kidney stones (nephroliths or nephrolithiases), cause a painful condition that occurs when urine salts are solidified and cannot be dissolved. When these salts, or stones, lodge in the urinary structures, painful spasms called renal colic occur. Urine may accumulate in the kidney, leading to hydronephrosis. If the stones cannot be passed, the physician may perform lithotripsy to break down the calculi.

Common Tests and Surgical Procedures

Urea is one of the end products of protein metabolism. Other components are creatinine, phosphates, sulfates, and uric acid. These substances can be measured in the blood, giving an indication of the functioning of the kidneys. A creatinine clearance is a measurement of the urine concentration of creatinine which indicates the glomerular filtration rate (GFR). The GFR is obtained by using a formula which measures the urine concentration in a volume of urine collected over a specific time and dividing that by the plasma concentration of the creatinine. This means that the patient must provide urine and blood samples to obtain the GFR result. A more exact method to determine the filtration rate is through a nuclear scan (nuclear GFR).

Blood urea nitrogen (BUN) is a blood test that measures the blood level of urea. In kidney disease, the BUN results will be elevated, indicating the kidneys' inability to excrete urea properly.

Orchidopexy is a surgical procedure performed to correct an undescended testicle. A vasectomy is a surgical procedure used as a method of birth control in which the vas deferens is bisected in order to prevent sperm from entering the semen.

Building Language Skills

The following tables list common urology and nephrology terms, drugs, and abbreviations. The list of terms and definitions includes the most difficult words contained in the dictated reports in this chapter. These words are identified in GREEN type. A list of common drugs is found in Appendix D.

Medical Terms and Pharmacologic Agents

auscultation
(aws-kul-**tay**-shun) (n) process of listening for sounds produced in some of the body cavities, especially chest and abdomen, in order to detect abnormal conditions

Bactrim
(**back**-trim) (n) brand name for co-trimoxazole, a sulfonamide antibiotic

biliary
(**bil**-ee-ayr-ee) (adj) relating to bile or the gallbladder and its ducts

biopsy
(**bI**-op-see) (n) the removal of tissue and/or fluid from the body for microscopic examination; the specimen obtained

bulbar
(**bul**-bar) (adj) bulb-shaped or relating to the medulla oblongata in the brain

calculus
(**kal**-kyoo-lus) (n) stone; a hard stone-like mass formed in the body; calculi (pl)

carotid
(ka-**rot**-id) (n) paired arteries (right and left) that arise from the aorta and provide the principal blood supply to the head and neck

catheter
(**kath**-e-ter) (n) a tube inserted into the body for removing or instilling fluids for diagnostic or therapeutic purposes

cerebrospinal
(**ser**-a-brO-**spI**-nal, se-**ree**-brO-**spI**-nal) (adj) referring to the brain and spinal cord

cystitis
(sis-**tI**-tis) (n) inflammation of the urinary bladder

cortex
(**kOr**-tex) (n) the outer layer of an organ, such as the kidney, as distinguished from the inner portion, or medulla

cystoscopy
(sis-**tos**-ko-pee) (n) examination of the inside of the urinary bladder with a lighted instrument inserted through the urethra

cystostomy
(sis-**tos**-tO-mee) (n) surgical creation of an opening in the bladder

dilation
(dI-**lay**-shun) (n) expansion of an organ or vessel

diltiazem
(dil-**tie**-a-zem) (n) a generic calcium channel blocker, used for hypertension

dysuria
(dis-**yoo**-ree-a) (n) difficult or painful urination

edema
(e-**dee**-ma) (n) excessive accumulation of fluid in tissues, especially just under the skin or in a given cavity

edematous
(e-**dem**-a-tus) (adj) having edema

electron
(ee-**lek**-tron) (n) a subatomic particle with a negative charge

encephalopathy
(en-sef-a-**lop**-a-thee) (n) any dysfunction of the brain

endocapillary
(**en**-dO-**cap**-layr-ee (n) within one of the tiny blood vessels

endoscope
(**en**-dO-skOp) (n) a lighted instrument for examining the inside of a body cavity or organ

enuresis
(en-yoo-**ree**-sis) (n) bed-wetting; involuntary urination, especially at night in bed

epididymis
(ep-i-**did**-i-mis) (n) one of a pair of long, coiled ducts in the scrotum; they carry and store spermatozoa between the testes and ductus deferens

epithelial
(ep-i-**thee**-lee-al) (adj) relating to or composed of epithelium

epithelium
(ep-i-**thee**-lee-um) (n) cell layers covering the outside body surfaces as well as forming the lining of hollow organs (such as the bladder) and the passages of the respiratory, digestive, and urinary tracts

extrahepatic
(eks-tra-he-**pat**-ik) (adj) unrelated to or located outside the liver

exudated
(eks-yoo-**day**-ted) (adj) pertaining to any fluid that has exuded out of a tissue or its capillaries

fascia
(**fash**-ee-a) (n) a thin layer of fibrous connective tissue that supports soft organs and covers structures such as muscles; fasciae (pl)

fetoprotein
(fee-tO-**prO**-teen) (n) antigen (substance or organism that produces an antibody) naturally present in the fetus and sometimes present in adults with certain cancers

fossa
(**fos**-a) (n) channel or shallow depression; fossae (pl)

fundus
(**fun**-dus) (n) the bottom or lowest parts of a sac or hollow organ; fundi (pl)

gastroesophageal
(**gas**-trO-ee-soph-a-**jee**-al) (adj) related to both stomach and esophagus

genital
(**jen**-i-tal) (adj) relating to reproduction or the organs of reproduction

genitalia
(**jen**-i-**tay**-lee-a) (n) the genitals; male or female reproductive organs, especially the external ones

glomerulus
(glO-**mayr**-yoo-lus) (n) a cluster of capillaries at the beginning of each nephron (the functional unit of the kidney); glomeruli (pl)

hematuria
(hee-ma-**too**-ree-a) (n) presence of blood in the urine

hemorrhagic
(hem-O-**raj**-ik) (adj) relating to or experiencing a hemorrhage

histology
(his-**tol**-O-jee) (n) a science of tissues, including their cellular composition and organization

hyperglycemic
(**hI**-per-glI-**see**-mic) (adj) pertaining to or characterized by hyperglycemia, an abnormally large concentration of glucose in the circulating blood

hyperplasia
(hI-per-**play**-see-a) (n) increase in size of a tissue or organ due to an increase in the number of cells (not including tumor formation)

hyperplastic
(hI-per-**plas**-tik) (adj) relating to hyperplasia

idiopathic
(**id**-ee-O-**path**-ik) (adj) of unknown cause; describes a disease for which no identifiable cause can be determined

idiopathy
(id-ee-**op**-a-thee) (n) any disease of unknown cause

inguinal
(**ing**-gwin-al) (adj) pertaining to the region of the groin

interstitial
(in-ter-**stish**-al) (adj) relating to or located in the space between tissues, such as interstitial fluid

intrahepatic
(**in**-tra-he-**pat**-ik) (adj) within the liver

kidneys
(**kid**-neez) (n) a pair of bean-shaped organs near the spinal column that filter blood and produce urine

levator
(le-**vay**-ter/le-**vay**-tOr) (n) muscle that lifts or raises the body part to which it is attached

lithotomy
(li-**thot**-O-mee) (n) surgical removal of a stone, especially from the urinary tract

lithotripsy
(**lith**-O-trip-see) (n) procedure using a laser to break apart stones (calculi)

lumen
(**loo**-men) (n) cavity, canal, or channel within an organ or tube; lumina or lumens (pl)

lymphadenitis
(lim-**fad**-e-**nI**-tis) (n) inflammation of one or more lymph nodes

lymphadenopathy
(lim-fad-e-**nop**-a-thee) (n) any disorder of lymph nodes or of the lymphatic system

meatus
(mee-**ay**-tus) (n) a passage or channel, especially with an external opening

microscopy
(mI-**kros**-kO-pee) (n) use of a microscope to magnify and examine objects

mitotic
(mI-**tot**-ik) (adj) pertaining to mitosis, a type of cell division in which a cell divides into two genetically identical daughter cells

mucosa
(myoo-**kO**-sa) (n) mucous membrane

neoplasm
(**nee**-O-plazm) (n) any abnormal growth of tissue, usually malignant; tumor

nephrectomy
(ne-**frek**-tO-mee) (n) surgical removal of a kidney

nephrolithiasis
(**nef**-rO-li-**thI**-a-sis) (n) presence of stones (calculi) in the kidney(s)

nephrolithotomy
(**nef**-rO-li-**thot**-O-mee) (n) surgical incision into a kidney to remove stones (calculi)

nephron
(**nef**-ron) (n) the functional unit of the kidney that filters the blood

nephrostomy
(ne-**fros**-tO-mee) (n) surgical creation of an opening in the kidney for drainage

nocturia
(nok-**too**-ree-a) (n) frequent urination during the night

nodular
(**nod**-yoo-lar) (adj) containing or resembling nodules; having small, firm, knotty masses

obturator
(**ob**-too-ray-tor) (n) device or body structure that closes up or covers an opening

orchidopexy
(Or-ki-**dop**-eks-ee) (n) surgical procedure in which an undescended testicle is sutured into place; also orchiopexy

orchiectomy
(Or-kee-**ek**-tO-mee) (n) surgical removal of one or both testes

orchiocele
(**Or**-kee-O-seel) (n) scrotal hernia; tumor of a testis

papilledema
(pa-pill-e-**dee**-ma) (n) edema and inflammation of the optic nerve at its point of entrance into the eyeball

pendulous
(**pen**-ju-lus) (adj) loosely hanging

perineum
(**per**-i-**nee**-um) (n) the external region between the vagina and the anus in women and between the scrotum and the anus in men

polydipsia
(pol-ee-dip-**see**-a) (n) excessive thirst

polyphagia
(pol-ee-**fay**-jee-a) (n) eating abnormally large amounts of food at a meal

polyuria
(pol-ee-**yoo**-ree-a) (n) excessive urinary output

prostate gland
(**pros**-tayt) (n) a gland located at the base of the bladder and surrounding the beginning of the urethra in the male

prostatic
(pros-**tat**-ik) (adj) relating to the prostate gland

proteinaceous
(**prO**-tee-**nay**-shus/**prO**-tee-i-**nay**-shus) (adj) relating to or resembling proteins

proteinuria
(prO-tee-**noo**-ree-a) (n) presence of abnormally large amounts of protein in the urine

proximal
(**prok**-si-mal) (adj) nearest to a point of reference or center of the body

renal
(**ree**-nal) (adj) related to the kidney

renal failure
(**ree**-nal) (n) inability of the kidneys to function

retinopathy
(re-ti-**nop**-a-thee) (n) any disorder of the retina

rhabdomyosarcoma
(**rab**-dO-**mI**-O-sar-**kO**-ma) (n) highly malignant tumor developing from striated muscle cells

sclerotic
(sklee-**rot**-ic) (adj) pertaining to or affected with sclerosis, a condition that shows hardness of tissue resulting from inflammation, mineral deposits, or other causes

sonography
(so-**nog**-ra-fi) (n) ultrasonography; use of high-frequency sound waves to produce an image of an organ or tissue

steroid
(**steer**-oyd) (n) any of a large number of similar chemical substances, either natural or synthetic; many are hormones; produced mainly in the adrenal cortex and gonads

stress incontinence
(stres in-**kon**-ti-nens) (n) inability to retain urine under tension, such as sneezing or coughing

suprapubic
(soo-pra-**pyoo**-bik) (adj) above the pubic bones

testicular
(tes-tik-yoo-lar) (adj) related to the testes, a pair of male gonads or sex glands that produce sperm and secretes androgens

thyromegaly
(thI-rO-**meg**-a-lee) (n) enlargement of the thyroid gland

transaminase
(trans-**am**-i-nays) (n) an enzyme that catalyzes transamination, the transfer of an animo group from one compound to another or the transposition of an animo group within a single compound

transperineal
(trans-per-i-**nee**-al) (adj) across or through the perineal region between the urethral opening and the anus, including the skin and underlying tissues

transurethral
(trans-yoo-**ree**-thral) (adj) through the urethra, such as a surgical procedure

trochanteric
(trO-kan-**ter**-ik) related to a trochanter, either of the two bony processes below the neck of the femur)

ureter
(yoo-**ree**-ter/**yoo**-ree-ter) (n) either of a pair of tubes that carry urine from the kidney to the urinary bladder

ureteral
(yoo-**ree**-te-ral) (adj) relating to the ureters

urethra
(yoo-**ree**-thra) (n) a tube that drains urine from the bladder to the outside

urethroscopy
(yoo-ree-**thros**-ko-pee) (n) an examination of the inside of the urethra with a urethroscope, a lighted instrument

vesical
(**ves**-i-kul) (adj) referring to the bladder or gallbladder

vesicle
(**ves**-i-kl) (n) blister; small, raised skin lesion containing clear fluid

viscera
(**vis**-er-a) (n) main internal organs within the trunk of the body, especially those in the abdominal cavity

visceral
(**vis**-er-al) (adj) relating to or located near the viscera

vasectomy
(va-**sek**-tO-mee) (n) excision of a portion of the vas deferens, in association with prostatectomy or to produce sterility

visceromegaly
(**vis**-er-O-**meg**-a-lee) (n) generalized enlargement of the abdominal organs

visualization
(**vich**-oo-al-I-**zay**-shun) (n) the act of viewing an object, especially the picture of a body structure as obtained by x-ray study

Abbreviations

AGN	acute glomerulonephritis
ATN	acute tubular necrosis
BPH	benign prostatic hypertrophy
BUN	blood urea nitrogen (lab test)
CVA	costovertebral angle
cysto	cystoscopy
ESWL	extracorporeal shock-wave lithotripsy
GFR	glomerular filtration rate
GU	genitourinary
I&O	intake and output
IVP	intravenous pyelogram
KUB	kidneys, ureters, bladder (x-ray)
PD	peritoneal dialysis
PE	physical exam
RP	retrograde pyelogram
SLE	systemic lupus erythematosus
TUR; TURP	transurethral resection of the prostate (prostatectomy)
UA; U/A	urinalysis
UTI	urinary tract infection
VDRL	Venereal Disease Research Laboratory (test for syphilis)

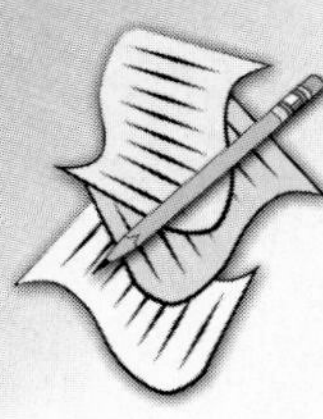

EXERCISE 11.1

Recognizing Look-Alikes and Sound-Alikes

Below is a list of frequently used words that look alike and/or sound alike. Study the meaning and pronunciation of each set of words, then read the following sentences carefully and circle the word in parentheses that correctly completes the meaning.

addition	counting, increase
edition	issue of a publication
dilatation	synonym of dilation
dilation	expansion of an organ or vessel
dilution	a substance that has been diluted (liquid has been added)
do	to perform
due	owing
farther	(adv) refers to physical distance
further	(adv) additional, extra, greater
further	(v) to advance, to help
father	(n) male parent
hole	opening
whole	total, complete
seen	noticed, viewed
scene	sight, background, display of emotion
states	(n) government units of land
states	(v) expresses, says
status	(n) rank, condition
to	toward, through
too	also, additionally
two	numerical unit, a pair

1. A tracheostomy establishes a (hole, whole) into the trachea.
2. Are you going to the medical conference with them (to, too, two)?
3. He lives (farther, further) from the hospital than I do.
4. If you have (farther, further) questions about the medical procedure, please call.
5. The ambulance arrived on the (scene, seen) within a few minutes.
6. The lesion was (to, too, two) small to be seen by the naked eye.
7. The patient is (states, status) post hysterectomy.
8. We went (to, too, two) the anatomy lecture yesterday.
9. With the (addition, edition) of hydrochlorothiazide, her blood pressure is now under good control.
10. The pupils were (dilated, diluted) on exam.

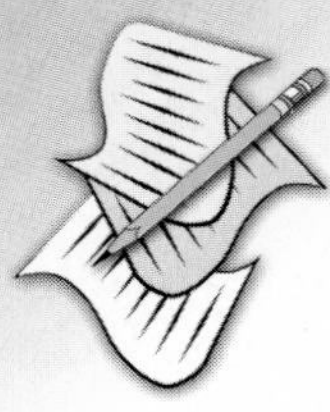

EXERCISE 11.2

Matching Sound and Spelling

The numbered list that follows shows the phonetic spelling of hard-to-spell words. Sound out the word, then write the correct spelling in the blank space provided. Each of the words can be found in the Glossary or in the drug list in Appendix D.

1. dis-**yoo**-ree-a ______________________________
2. pol-ee-**yoo**-ree-a ______________________________
3. lim-**fad**-e-**nI**-tis ______________________________
4. nok-**too**-ree-a ______________________________
5. **rab**-dO-**mI**-O-sar-**kO**-ma ______________________________
6. **prO**-tee-**noo**-ree-a ______________________________
7. **nef**-rO-li-**thot**-O-mee ______________________________
8. ep-i-**did**-i-mis ______________________________
9. Or-kee-**ek**-tO-mee ______________________________
10. **kal**-kyoo-lus ______________________________
11. **prO**-tee-**nay**-shus ______________________________
12. ep-i-**thee**-lee-um ______________________________
13. ne-**fros**-tO-mee ______________________________
14. **Or**-kee-O-seel ______________________________
15. **pros**-tayt ______________________________

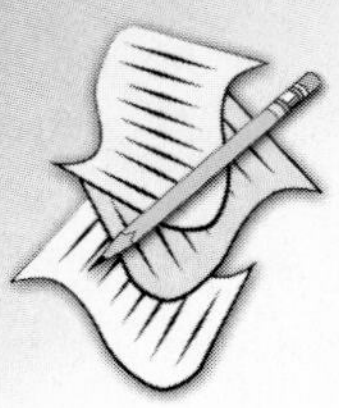

EXERCISE 11.3

Choosing Words from Context

When transcribing dictation, the medical transcriptionist frequently needs to consider the situation when determining the word that correctly completes the sentence. From the list below, select the term that meaningfully completes each statement.

catheter	genitalia	steroid
pendulous	renal failure	neoplasm
endoscope	hematuria	vesicle
proximal	meatus	urethra

1. When we saw Mr. Johnson in our office, his exam revealed a blood pressure of 210/100, ascites, and pitting pedal edema. He was admitted to the hospital immediately with the diagnosis of impending ____________________.
2. The __________ was inserted, and the urinary collection totaled only 50 cc in the first hour.
3. Breast exam revealed ______________ breasts, probably accounting for the patient's upper back pain.
4. The IV catheter was placed _______________ to the antecubital fossa.
5. There was an oozing ____________ on the abdomen where the incision had been made.
6. It was decided to place Mr. Arnold on ______________ therapy to decrease the allergic reaction.
7. After the Foley catheter was removed, the patient had a small amount of gross ________________, which cleared with the next void.
8. In our differential diagnosis, we considered an infectious process versus a (an) ___________.
9. Pelvic exam revealed normal female _______________.
10. During the procedure, the ____________ was repositioned several times to obtain different views.
11. The urinary catheter was inserted through the ____________ in order to obtain the specimen.
12. There was a blockage in the ____________, thus preventing urine from exiting the meatus.

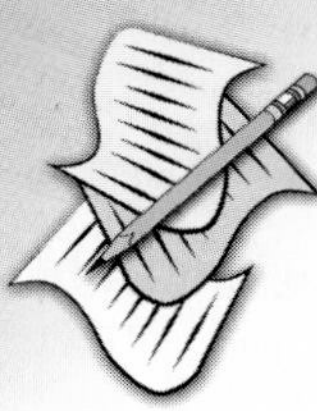

EXERCISE 11.4

Pairing Words and Meanings

From this list, locate the term that best matches each of the following definitions. Write the letter of the term in the space provided by each definition.

A.	edema	E.	perineum	H.	suprapubic
B.	epididymis	F.	proteinuria	I.	transurethral
C.	fascia	G.	sonography	J.	viscera
D.	idiopathic				

1. pertains to an operation performed through the urethra ________________
2. region between the urethral opening and the anus ________________
3. presence of large amounts of protein in the urine ________________
4. abnormal collection of fluid in spaces between cells ________________
5. fibrous connective tissue that supports soft organs ________________
6. a pair of long, tightly coiled ducts that carry sperm ________________
7. a disease for which no cause can be determined ________________
8. main internal organs within body cavities ________________
9. use of ultrasound to produce an image ________________
10. the area above the pubis ________________

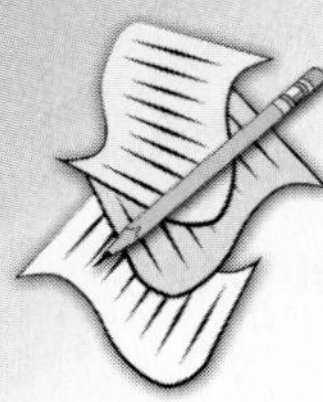

EXERCISE 11.5

Creating Terms from Word Forms

Combine prefixes, root words, and suffixes from this list to create medical words that fit the following definitions. Fill in the blanks with the words you construct.

aden/o	gland	ren/i (o)	pertaining to kidney
cyst/o	bladder or sac	ureter/o	ureter
dys-	painful	urethr/o	urethra
extra-	outside	ur/o	urine
hem/o (ato)	blood	noct	night
hepat/o	liver	-ectomy	removal, incision
hydr/o	water	-gram	recording; x-ray
intra-	inside	-ia/sis	condition of
lith/o	stone, calcification	-ic	pertaining to
lymph/o	clear, thin fluid	-itis	inflammation
meat/o	passageway	-lith	stone, calcification
nephr/o	kidney	-osis	condition of
orchi/o (do)	testicle	-pexy	repair
path/o	disease		

1. removal of the kidneys ______________________
2. difficult, painful urination______________________
3. related to the liver ______________________
4. blood in the urine ______________________
5. disease of the lymph glands______________________
6. urination during the night ______________________
7. excessive urea in the blood ______________________
8. removal of a testicle______________________
9. inflammation of the kidney______________________
10. outside of the liver ______________________
11. condition of having kidney stones ______________________
12. condition of having an obstruction preventing the flow of urine from the kidney __________
13. inflammation of the bladder ______________________
14. x-ray procedure to view the bladder ______________________

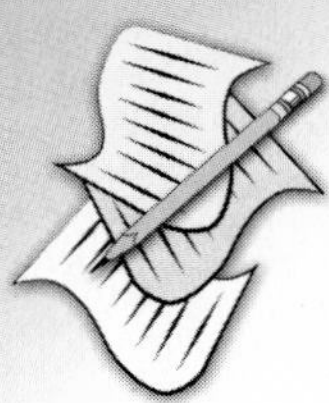

EXERCISE 11.6

Proofreading Review

Read the following partial report and look for errors in capitalization, word use, punctuation, spelling, meaning, and format. Key the report with the errors corrected.

S: 56-year-old middle eastern male who is seen in follow up for a elevated PSA, recent pylonephritis and microscopic hematuria. He has been referred to urology and will see them in 2 weeks. Today, he says he has occasional mild burning with urination but the disuria has overall improved. He denies any flake or abdominal pain, nausea or vomiting.

O: Routine laboratory was done at his last visit. His PSA was 14.3. He says that in the past his highest PSA was 6, and that was roughly six months ago. He had a transureteral resection of the prostrate in 1992. Other laboratories: A CBC showed a platelet count of 124,000. Hemoglobin 14.9. MCV 92. Chemistry profile within normal limits, including renal function.

A:
1. Resolved pyelonephritis.
2. Elevated PSA with a patient history of benign prostatic hypotrophy raises the question of possible prostate cancer.

P:
1. Will give another 7-day course of Bactrim to insure that the urinary track infection is resolved by the time of his Urology appointment in two weeks.
2. Patient is to call if he has any worsening of his symptoms.

Building Transcription Skills

The History and Physical

When a patient enters a healthcare system, the physician or examiner generates a comprehensive document called a history and physical (H&P) (Figure 11.4). This report focuses on the patient's medical and social history and the illness or complaint that prompted the person to seek medical attention. The primary purpose of the history and physical is to provide the information the physician needs to make a diagnosis and choose the appropriate care and treatment for the patient. The MT transcribes the H&P to provide a written documentation for the chart.

Required Headings/Content As the title of the report suggests, there are two main sections: (1) a complete history, including the current medical problem; and

PATIENT: Raymond Cheever
DATE: 7/10/XX
HOSPITAL NO: 93-22-17
PHYSICIAN: Harry Washington, MD
ds
CHIEF COMPLAINT: Severe pain in the left hip.
ds
HISTORY OF PRESENT ILLNESS: The patient is a 57-year-old white male who is admitted from the emergency department with hypertension, hyperglycemia, and greater trochanteric bursitis. The patient has been under treatment for greater trochanteric bursitis with Lortab and Naprosyn. He returns today because of increasing left hip pain. In the emergency room, he was noted to be significantly hypertensive and hyperglycemic. He is unaware of having a history of either.

ALLERGIES: No known allergies.

PRESENT MEDICATIONS
1. Lortab 7.5 mg q.d.
2. Naprosyn 375 mg q.d.

PAST MEDICAL HISTORY: Negative.

SURGICAL HISTORY: Tonsils and adenoids removed in early childhood.

SOCIAL HISTORY: The patient does not smoke at present. He stopped smoking 6 to 7 years ago; he smoked an average of a pack per day for many years. He denies ethanol use. He is married. He has 2 children who are alive and in good health. He works as a plant manager for a chemical company.

FAMILY HISTORY: His mother is alive and in good health. His father is deceased secondary to complications of black lung and asthma. He has 2 brothers and 1 sister. He thinks his sister has a history of hypertension.

REVIEW OF SYSTEMS: A full review of systems was negative. He states that his weight has been stable in the past year. He denies polyuria, polydipsia, or polyphagia.

(continued)

FIGURE 11.4
History and Physical

HISTORY AND PHYSICAL
PATIENT: Raymond Cheever
HOSPITAL NO.: 93-22-17
DATE: 7/10/XX
Page 2
ds
PHYSICAL EXAMINATION
GENERAL: Well-developed, well-nourished male in no acute distress.
ds
VITAL SIGNS: Blood pressure 200/104. Repeat, after rest and pain medication, was 170/96. The pulse was 72. Respiratory rate was 18 and labored. Patient refused to be weighed at this time because of pain.
HEENT: Pupils were somewhat constricted, but fundi were visualized minimally. No hypertensive retinopathy, exudates, hemorrhages, or papilledema were noted. Oral examination revealed no ulcerations, erosions, or masses.
NECK: Supple, without lymphadenopathy. The carotid upstrokes were brisk and equal bilaterally, without bruits. Thyroid nonpalpable.
CHEST: Chest was clear to auscultation in all fields.
CARDIOVASCULAR: Regular rate and rhythm, without murmurs, thrill, gallop, or click.
ABDOMEN: Abdomen nontender, nondistended, without masses, organomegaly, guarding, tenderness, or rebound.
EXTREMITIES: No clubbing, cyanosis, or edema. Peripheral pulses were intact, with good upstrokes. Palpation of the left hip did reveal tenderness, although the patient did report it was much improved after analgesia.

LABORATORY DATA: Review of the Chem-7 revealed a blood sugar of 201. His urinalysis revealed greater than 1000 glucose. CBC revealed a hemoglobin of 16.3 and hematocrit of 50. White count was 14.7. Platelets were 291,000. Differential was essentially within normal limits.

IMPRESSION
1. Marked hypertension.
2. Asymptomatic hyperglycemia with glycosuria.
3. Left greater trochanteric bursitis.

PLAN
1. Admit.
2. Orthopedic consultation.
3. Endocrinology consultation.
4. Cardiology consultation.

FIGURE 11.4
History and Physical (Continued)

HISTORY AND PHYSICAL
PATIENT: Raymond Cheever
HOSPITAL NO.: 93-22-17
DATE: 7/10/XX
Page 3

qs

____
Harry Washington, MD
ds
HW/XX
D: 07/10/XX
T: 07/11/XX

FIGURE 11.4
History and Physical (Continued)

(2) the results of the physical examination performed by the physician. For the entire report, the Joint Commission on the Accreditation of Healthcare Organizations (JCAHO) requires these headings: Chief Complaint, History of Present Illness, Review of Systems, Physical Examination, and Impression or Admitting Diagnosis(es). Individual hospitals and physicians, however, may expand the headings beyond these basic requirements. Medical transcriptionists need to be aware of the specific format the employer prefers.

History In the history section of the report, several variations or subheadings are possible, including details of present illness, past medical history, social history, surgical history, operations, habits, and risk factors. Despite the variety of subheadings, most physicians follow the same order when dictating the report, including more or less information, depending on the complexity of the patient's complaint.

Chief Complaint: The healthcare provider frequently documents the actual words used by the patient in describing the subjective data. This information may be called the Chief Complaint (CC) or History of Present Illness (HPI). Or, the physician may dictate both headings, using a brief summary statement for the Chief Complaint and a longer explanation under History of Present Illness. Also included may be objective data, organized through review of available clinical information, such as vital signs, measurements, laboratory tests, x-ray findings, and so on, which have been performed before admission and for which results are known.

Past History: This section begins by listing the patient's childhood illnesses and includes all past medical history with reference to diseases, illnesses, surgical procedures, accidents, medications, immunizations, and allergies (each topic is often indented as a subheading and keyed in capital letters). A history of pregnancies and deliveries is recorded for a female. Social history is another subheading that may be included. This subsection describes social habits such as alcohol use, smoking history, occupation, recreational interests, home environment, marital status, and sexual history. This information helps the interviewer develop an understanding of the patient as an individual and as a member of a family and a community.

Family History: Information on the health of the patient's parents, siblings, and grandparents may follow as a separate section. These data can point to the possibility of genetic traits or diseases.

Review of Systems: This section is a question-and-answer review of all the body systems conducted by the healthcare provider. The review is in cephalocaudal order—from head to foot.

- SKIN: Lesions, rashes, discolorations, itching, moles, eruptions
- HAIR: Texture, distribution, scalp problems
- HEENT: (Head, Ears, Eyes, Nose, Throat)
  Head: Headaches, dizziness
  Eyes: Visual problems, glaucoma, conjunctivitis, discharge, use of glasses
  Ears: Earaches, hearing loss, discharge, dizziness, fainting, ringing in the ears, pain

Nose: Discharges, sense of smell, colds, allergies, nosebleeds
Mouth and Throat: Condition of teeth, dental history, difficulty in swallowing, hoarseness, tonsillectomy

- NECK: Thyroid, movement of neck
- RESPIRATORY: Shortness of breath, cough with or without production of sputum or blood
- HEART: Increased heart rate, angina, or chest pain
- GASTROINTESTINAL: Appetite, indigestion, difficulty swallowing, vomiting, changes in weight, stool history, jaundice, gallbladder problems
- GENITOURINARY: Pain on urination, blood in urine, frequency, incontinence, urgency, sexually transmitted diseases
- GYNECOLOGIC: Menarche, menstrual history, discharges, contraceptive use, obstetric history, painful menses
- MUSCULOSKELETAL: Pain, stiffness, limitation of movement, fractures
- NEUROLOGICAL: Headaches, dizziness, fainting, pain, paralysis, difficulty walking, convulsions, emotional state

Physical A complete physical exam (PE) is usually performed after the history is recorded. This is arranged in cephalocaudal order, beginning with the visible areas of the body. Four basic procedures are included in the exam:

1) Inspection: looking at the body
2) Palpation: feeling various parts and organs
3) Percussion: listening to the sounds produced when a particular region is tapped using the hands or a small hammerlike tool
4) Auscultation: listening to body sounds

After noting general appearance, height, weight, age, race, nutritional state, and possibly emotional status (euphoric, lethargic, distracted, alert, oriented, agitated, flat affect), the physician dictates vital signs and then a description of findings on the rest of the body, similar to those described above in "Review of Systems."

A final section in the history and physical is the impression or diagnosis (may be called differential or admitting diagnosis), which lists many possibilities to explore or rule out. The plan of care is often dictated as a numbered list, written in order of most important to least, or as a random list. It will include recommendations for further studies and treatment and followup.

Turnaround Time The history and physical examination should be completed, dictated, and transcribed within the first 24 hours of admission as an inpatient. If a complete exam has been performed within 30 days before admission, such as in a physician's office, a copy of this report is placed in the patient's medical record and—in some hospitals—no new exam is required (provided no changes have occurred or provided changes that have occurred are noted in the medical record at the time of admission).

Preparing to Transcribe

To prepare for transcribing dictation, review the tables of common nephrology terms, drugs, and abbreviations presented in the Building Language Skills section of this chapter. Then, study the format and organization of the model document shown in Figure 11.4, and key the model document. Proofread the document by comparing it with the printed version. Categorize the types of errors you made, and document them on a copy of the Performance Comparison chart provided in Chapter 1. A template of this chart is included on the IRC that accompanies this text.

Patient Studies

Transcribe, edit, and correct each report in the following patient studies. Consult reference books for words or formatting rules that are unfamiliar.

As you work on the transcription assignment for this chapter, fill in the Performance Comparison chart that you started when you keyed the model document. For at least three of the reports, categorize and document the types of errors you made. Answer the document analysis questions on the bottom of the chart. With continuous practice and assessment, the quality of your work will improve.

After you have produced a final version of each transcribed report, complete the Performance Report cover sheet, attach it to the top of the transcripts, and submit them to your instructor for evaluation.

Patient Study 11.A — Alice Castanza

Alice Castanza is a 5-year-old child whose mother noticed that her pants were fitting tightly at the waist. When she was in the bathtub, her mother also noticed that her stomach appeared to be larger than usual. Alice had no complaints of pain, but her mother took her to the pediatrician, who was able to palpate an abdominal mass. She was sent for x-rays, lab work, and other tests. A surgical procedure was performed to remove a tumor and the right kidney to which it was attached. Alice was diagnosed with a Wilms' tumor, a malignant tumor of the kidney, treated by surgery and chemotherapy.

REPORT 11.1 Radiology Report

- Listen for these new words:
  echogenicity
  intrahepatic
  extrahepatic

Patient Study 11.B — Melissa Perlman

Melissa Perlman is a 3½-year-old child who was healthy until June of (last year) when she developed tonsillitis. The throat culture was negative for strep. In July, her mother noted that her diapers were not wet for 1 whole day and she was edematous. She was taken to the pediatrician and, after testing, was diagnosed with renal failure.

REPORT 11.2 Pathology Report

- Listen for these new words:
  hypercellularity
  PAS (physician will dictate individual letters)
  pseudocrescents
  proteinaceous
  glomerulosclerosis

Patient Study 11.C

Jonathan Blondell

Jonathan Blondell is a 35-year-old male who was having difficulty voiding for about 2 weeks. He saw his internist, who diagnosed a urinary tract infection. After treatment for several days, Jonathan continued to have pain on urination and blood in the urine. He was referred to the urologist for further evaluation.

REPORT 11.3 Operative Report

- Listen for these instrument names:
  Vim-Silverman needle
  #20-French 2-way tube
  #24-French 3-way catheter with 5-cc balloon

Patient Study 11.D

Raymond Cheever

Raymond Cheever is a 57-year-old male who is admitted from the emergency department with hypertension, hyperglycemia, and greater trochanteric bursitis. He came to the emergency department because of increasing left hip pain and was unaware of his hypertension and hyperglycemia.

REPORT 11.4 History and Physical

Patient Study 11.E — Dennis Chang

Dennis Chang is a 9-month-old male who was well until 2 weeks ago when his parents noticed that his left testicle was enlarged. The pediatrician referred the Changs to Dr. Roland Browne, a urologist, who scheduled a biopsy.

REPORT 11.5 Consultation Letter

- The results for the alpha fetoprotein test should be transcribed as 1652.5 (N: <9.0), and the beta subunit HCG should be transcribed using symbols and abbreviations, as follows: <2.0 IU/L.

Patient Study 11.F — William Booth

William Booth has an appointment for his annual physical. Since he lives in an out-state area and was once treated by this urologist for a prostate problem, he continues to have his annual checkup with the urologist.

REPORT 11.6 History and Physical

Patient Study 11.G

Marc Bario

Marc Bario is a 32-year-old male who was admitted through the emergency department with a history of 6 hours of acute ureteral colic on the right side. Subsequent testing revealed a large stone in his right ureter.

REPORT 11.7 History and Physical

- Listen for these special terms:
  ureterovesical junction
  JV distention

Patient Study 11.H

Sandra Davis

Sandra Davis is a 78-year-old woman who was recently hospitalized for a herpes infection. Two days after she was discharged, she was brought to the emergency room with a possible stroke and subsequently was admitted to the hospital for tests and treatment.

REPORT 11.8 Discharge Summary

- This report includes an exception to the hyphenation rule for the prefix *non.* If this prefix appears with a hyphenated compound adjective (insulin-dependent), add a hyphen after the prefix (non-insulin-dependent diabetes mellitus) to clarify meaning. Without a hyphen, the prefix appears to apply only to the word *insulin.* When the hyphen is included, the reader understands that non applies to the entire compound adjective *insulin-dependent.*
- Listen for these disease and drug terms:
  bilateral ureteral lithiasis
  clindamycin
  ceftazidime
  diltiazem-CD
  Nephro-Vite
  DSS

Patient Study 11.I — Rishera Subramanian

Rishera is a 24-month-old girl referred for evaluation and treatment of a left upper abdominal mass noted on recent examination consistent with a renal tumor.

REPORT 11.9 Operative Report

- Listen for these special terms:
  ballotable
  prepubertal
  electrocautery
  fascial
  tenotomy scissors
  Gerota's fascia
  Para-aorta
  contiguous
  splenocolic ligaments
  #2-0 PDS sutures
  PICU (may be dictated as Pick-U, or each letter may be said individually)

Using Medical References

Use the appropriate medical reference to locate the correct spelling and additional usage information for the words below. (If the reference is not available, use the Glossary in this text.) Circle the correct spelling; then write a sentence using the word correctly.

1.	epididymis	epidydimis	epididymus
2.	ideopathic	idiopathec	idiopathic
3.	rhabdomyosarcoma	rabdomyocarcoma	rhabdomysarcoma
4.	fulgeration	fulguration	folguration
5.	meatus	meaetos	meatis
6.	nephrolithiesis	nephrolithiasis	neprolithiasis
7.	glomerular	glamerular	glumerular
8.	dysuria	disuria	dysurea
9.	cystoscopy	cystascopy	cystoscapy
10.	orchectomy	orchictomy	orchiectomy

Making Expert Decisions

Circle the correct word from the choices in parentheses.

1. The bladder neck was inspected beginning distally after (ureteral/urethral) dilatation.
2. There was 3+ bacteria noted on microscopic exam and the patient was started on antibiotics after a specimen was obtained for (CNS/C&S)
3. A contracture of the (vesical/vesicle) neck was noted.
4. At the end of the cystoscopy, both ureters were seen to be (effluxing/reflexing/refluxing) clear urine from both sides.
5. (Testis/Testes) were descended bilaterally.
6. The main function of the urinary (track/tract) consists of production and elimination of urine.
7. The patient was started on a (regime/regimen/regiment) of diet, activity, and medication.
8. With the (addition/edition) of Bactrim-DS, the patient's UTI subsided.
9. Upon visualization, there were (to/too/two) patent ureters.
10. Examination revealed the (prostate/prostrate) to be normal in size and benign in consistency.

Transcribing Professional Documents

Transcribe the document named Chapter 11 Assessment. Before you key, review the appropriate report formatting guidelines. Proofread your transcribed document and revise it until you think it is error-free.

12

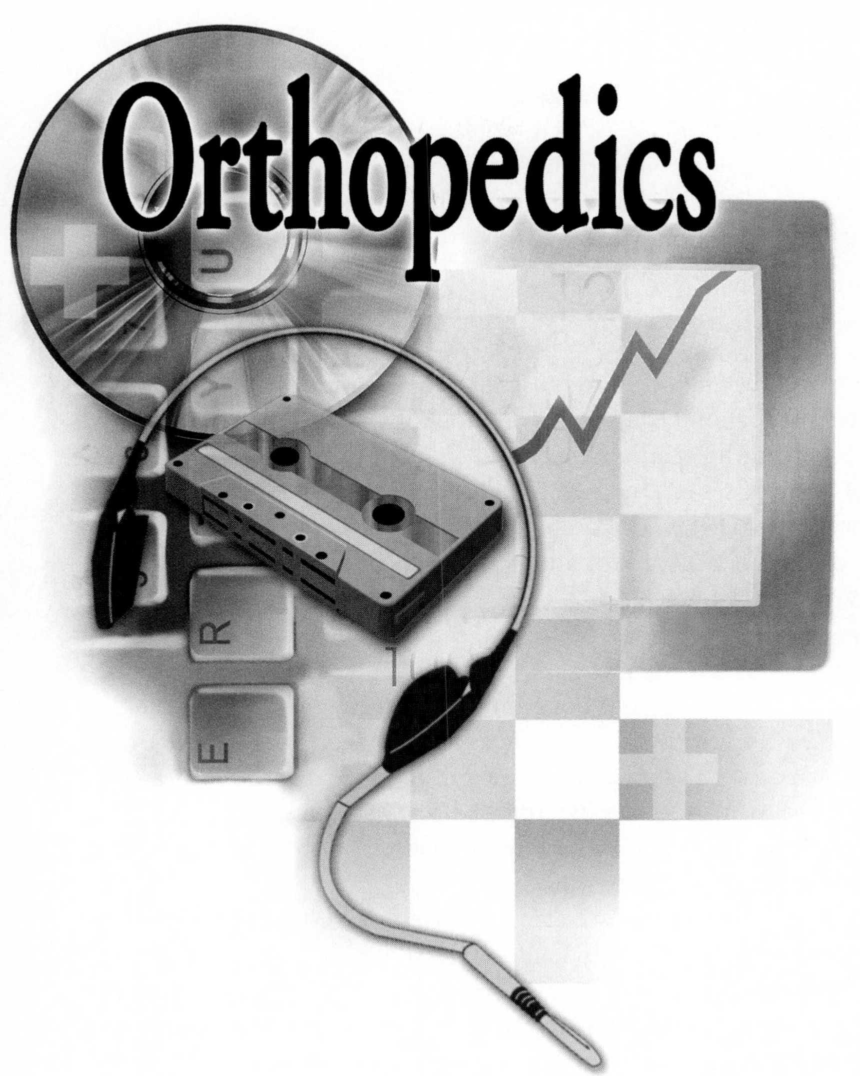

Orthopedics is the field of medicine concerned with diseases, injuries, and deformities of the musculoskeletal system, which includes the joints, muscles, and the fibrous connective tissue surrounding the bones and joints. Specialists in orthopedic medicine are orthopedists, who may also be skilled orthopedic surgeons. Due to the complexity of problems within the musculoskeletal system, orthopedic surgeons may further specialize in one anatomic area such as hip, knee, shoulder, foot, hand, or spine. The chiropractor is concerned with the relationship between the musculoskeletal system and health. Rheumatologists treat disease of the joints, connective tissues, collagen, and other structures of the body.

OBJECTIVES

- Use orthopedics terms correctly according to the context and purpose of the dictation.
- Select and use appropriate general and specialty reference materials.
- Key orthopedics documents of varying complexity and format.
- Transcribe authentic medical dictation requiring concentration and listening skill.
- Edit medical reports to conform with AAMT style guidelines.
- Proofread and correct transcripts to produce error-free documents.

Exploring Orthopedics

The musculoskeletal system (Figure 12.1) enables the body to move. It also provides support and protection for body organs. Within the bone is the bone marrow, which has the equally important responsibility of producing blood cells, a process called hematopoiesis. Bones are responsible for storing calcium and phosphorus. There are 206 named bones in the human body.

Structure and Function

Bone is the major tissue component of the musculoskeletal system. A complex type of calcified connective tissue, bone is made up of approximately 95 percent organic material and about 5 percent inorganic minerals.

The center of the bone is called the medullary cavity, which contains the bone marrow (Figure 12.2). The marrow looks like blood that has gritty and fatty particles in it. All bones of the body contain marrow. However, blood cells are formed mostly in the long, large, flat bones.

An extensive vascular system feeds the bones and moves blood cells in and out of the bone marrow (Figure 12.3). Osteocytes, the small living cells contained within the bone, are continually cycling through bone formation and bone destruction (via osteoblasts and osteoclasts, respectively). This cycle occurs throughout the life of a healthy individual in response to physical pressure and hormonal stimuli.

A periosteal layer of cells forms the covering of bone. This is a dense, fibrous membrane that contains the nerves, blood, and lymph vessels. The periosteum is the attachment point for muscles, ligaments, and tendons.

The long bones, like the humerus in the arm or the femur in the leg, are divided into the distal and proximal epiphyses (singular: epiphysis) on each end, and the diaphysis, the shaft or long section. The epiphyses are formed of spongy bone necessary to maintain growth, while the diaphysis is composed of compact bone that provides support. The articular cartilage on the end of the epiphyses provides the cushioning effect in the joints.

Flat bones provide protection for internal organs and wide surfaces for muscle attachment. The skull bones and sternum are flat bones. Short bones have a core of spongy or cancellous bone, surrounded by a layer of compact tissue. These bones are small and have an irregular shape, as in the wrists and phalanges. The irregular bones such as the vertebrae and bones of the ear do not fit into any one category.

Joints are the articulations that allow bones to move. There are three major classifications: diarthroses (Figure 12.4) are freely movable joints, amphiarthroses are slightly movable joints, and synarthroses are immovable joints. To allow free movement, synovial fluid is secreted into each joint cavity as a lubricant. Each joint capsule gains strength by the attachments of ligaments, made of fibrous bands of connective tissue.

Muscles (Figure 12.5) function to maintain posture, stabilize joints, provide movement, and generate heat. There are three types of muscle cells: skeletal, smooth, and cardiac. Each type has a different appearance under the microscope and has a particular function.

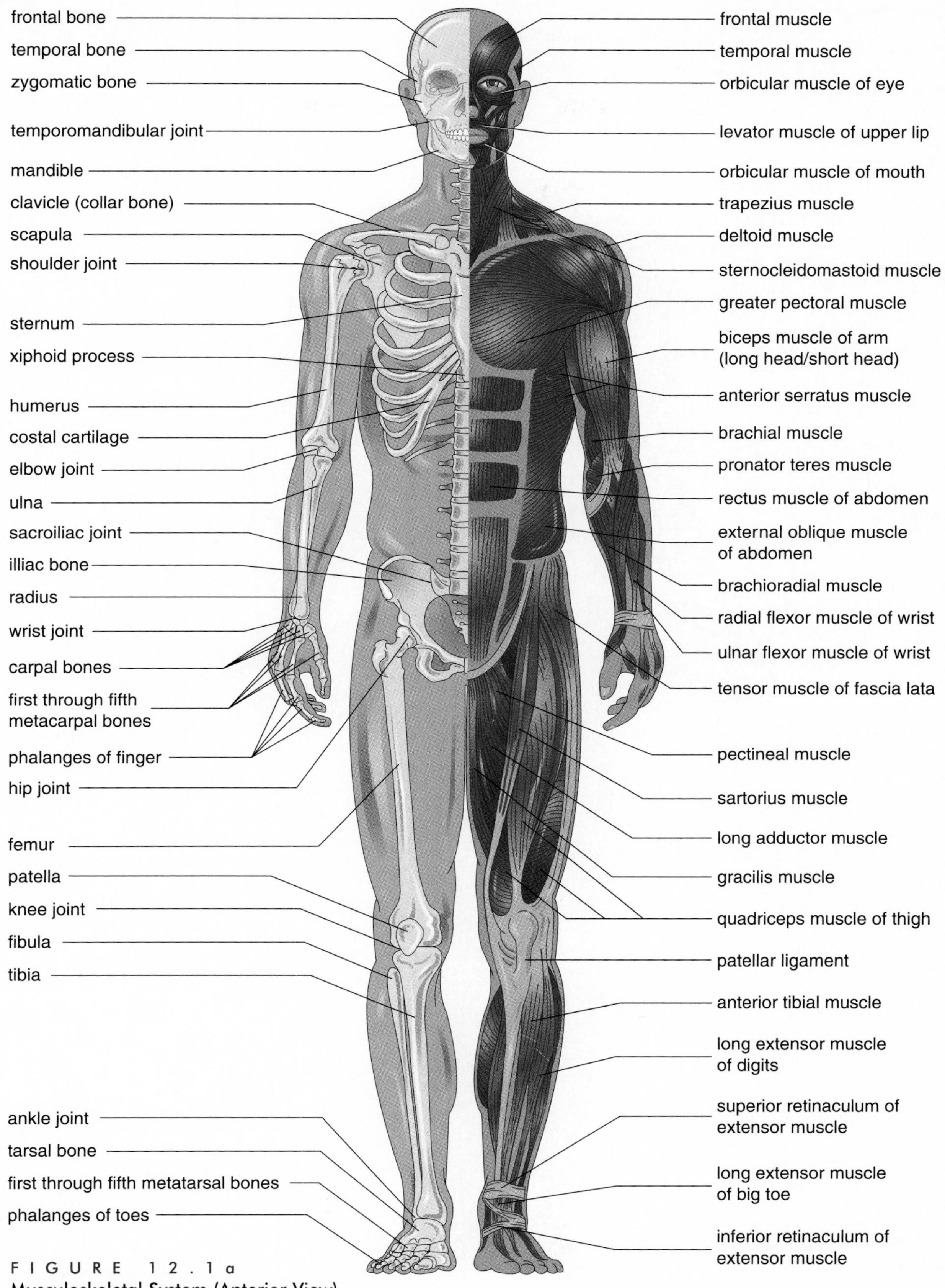
frontal bone
temporal bone
zygomatic bone
temporomandibular joint
mandible
clavicle (collar bone)
scapula
shoulder joint
sternum
xiphoid process
humerus
costal cartilage
elbow joint
ulna
sacroiliac joint
illiac bone
radius
wrist joint
carpal bones
first through fifth metacarpal bones
phalanges of finger
hip joint
femur
patella
knee joint
fibula
tibia
ankle joint
tarsal bone
first through fifth metatarsal bones
phalanges of toes
frontal muscle
temporal muscle
orbicular muscle of eye
levator muscle of upper lip
orbicular muscle of mouth
trapezius muscle
deltoid muscle
sternocleidomastoid muscle
greater pectoral muscle
biceps muscle of arm (long head/short head)
anterior serratus muscle
brachial muscle
pronator teres muscle
rectus muscle of abdomen
external oblique muscle of abdomen
brachioradial muscle
radial flexor muscle of wrist
ulnar flexor muscle of wrist
tensor muscle of fascia lata
pectineal muscle
sartorius muscle
long adductor muscle
gracilis muscle
quadriceps muscle of thigh
patellar ligament
anterior tibial muscle
long extensor muscle of digits
superior retinaculum of extensor muscle
long extensor muscle of big toe
inferior retinaculum of extensor muscle

FIGURE 12.1a
Musculoskeletal System (Anterior View)

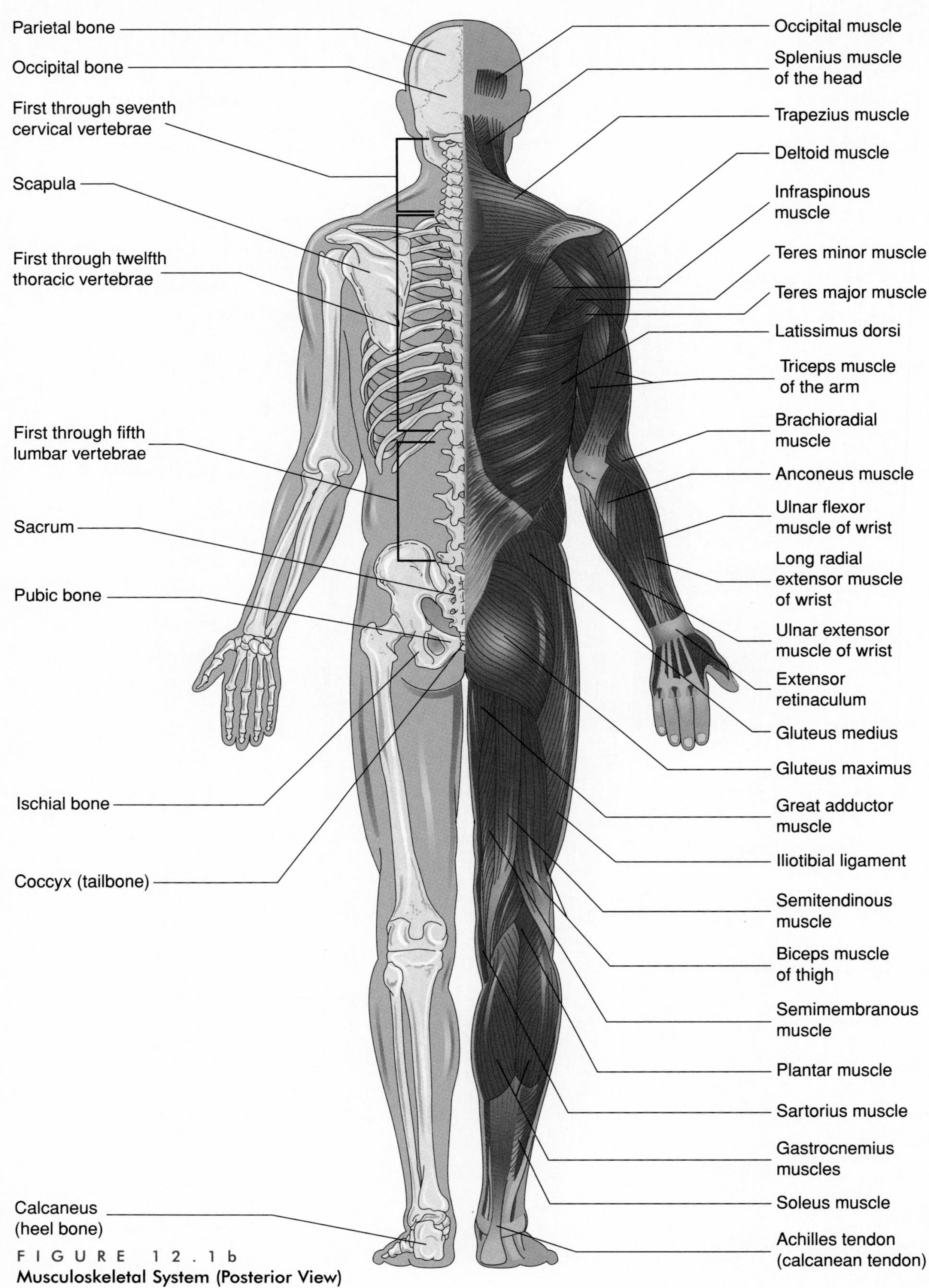
Parietal bone
Occipital bone
First through seventh cervical vertebrae
Scapula
First through twelfth thoracic vertebrae
First through fifth lumbar vertebrae
Sacrum
Pubic bone
Ischial bone
Coccyx (tailbone)
Calcaneus (heel bone)
Occipital muscle
Splenius muscle of the head
Trapezius muscle
Deltoid muscle
Infraspinous muscle
Teres minor muscle
Teres major muscle
Latissimus dorsi
Triceps muscle of the arm
Brachioradial muscle
Anconeus muscle
Ulnar flexor muscle of wrist
Long radial extensor muscle of wrist
Ulnar extensor muscle of wrist
Extensor retinaculum
Gluteus medius
Gluteus maximus
Great adductor muscle
Iliotibial ligament
Semitendinous muscle
Biceps muscle of thigh
Semimembranous muscle
Plantar muscle
Sartorius muscle
Gastrocnemius muscles
Soleus muscle
Achilles tendon (calcanean tendon)

FIGURE 12.1b
Musculoskeletal System (Posterior View)

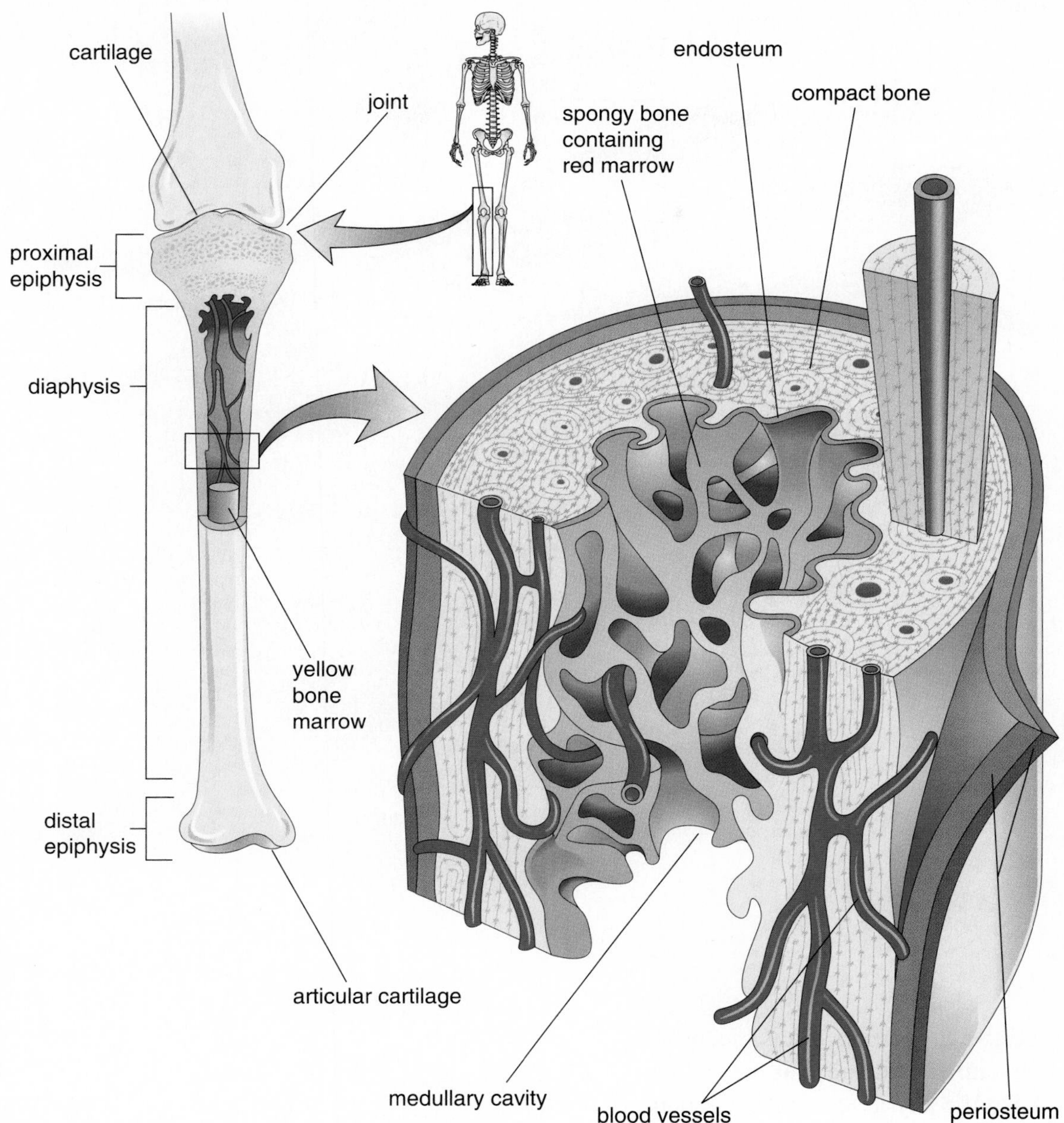

FIGURE 12.2
Structure of Long Bones

Skeletal muscle covers the skeleton. It is the only muscle type that is under our voluntary control. It is also called striated muscle because of its striped appearance. There are several parts of skeletal muscle as shown in Figure 12.3. Myofibrils actually do the work, or movement, in the skeletal muscle.

Smooth muscle lines the walls of the body's organs such as the stomach and small intestines. Cardiac muscle is involved with the heart's conduction system and the heartbeat. Both of these muscle groups are under involuntary control.

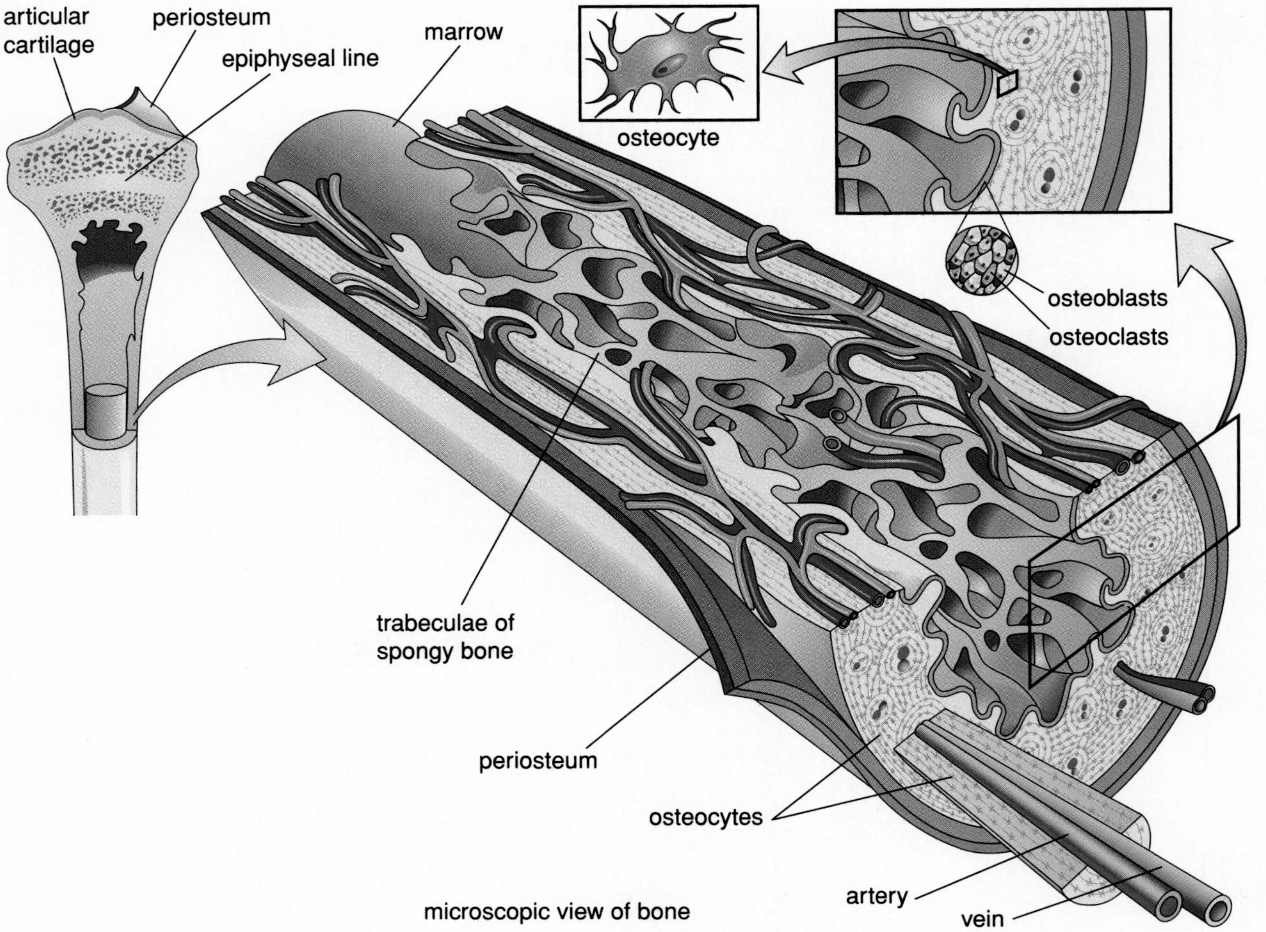

FIGURE 12.3
Microscopic View of Bone

Physical Assessment

The patient who sees the orthopedist is usually suffering from a fracture, an acute pain episode, or chronic pain. First, the physician assesses a patient's standing and walking movements. Noted at this time are posture, movement of the extremities, and any signs of pain (facial grimace is the giveaway). The orthopedist will ask about the history of the pain, the beginning of the pain, any precipitating events, and injuries. Information about activities, sports, sleeping habits, and lifestyle also will be noted in the medical record.

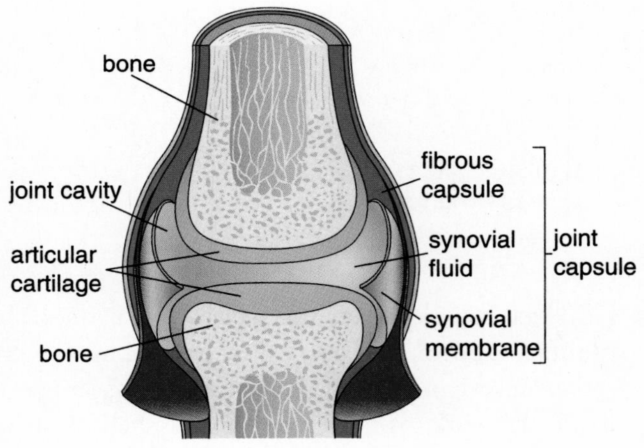

FIGURE 12.4
Diarthrotic (Synovial) Joint

The examination will include full range of motion activities and strength assessment for each

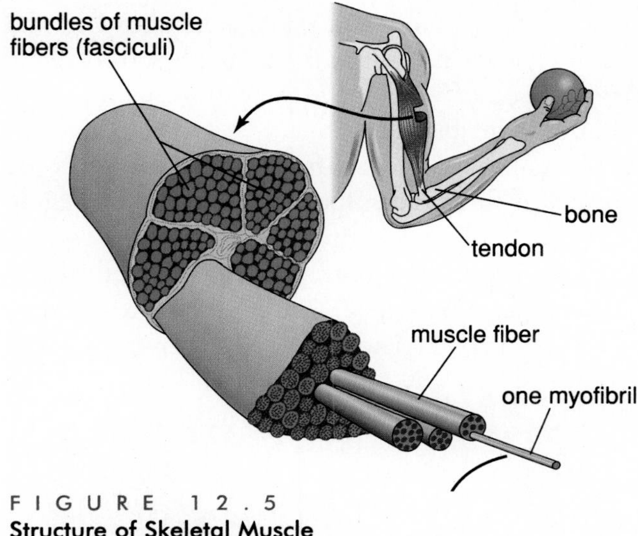

FIGURE 12.5
Structure of Skeletal Muscle

muscle group. Obvious malformations, such as scoliosis or kyphosis, will be noted. Asymmetry may be an indication of an abnormality. Because of the interrelationship of the nervous system with the musculoskeletal system, the physician will test reflexes, gait, and other areas.

Diseases, Conditions, and Injuries

For young people, a bone fracture may precipitate the first visit to the orthopedist. Inflammatory joint diseases or stress injuries are likely reasons for older adults to seek medical help from an orthopedist. Osteoarthritis, for example, is a degenerative disease characterized by pain, swelling, and a loss of flexibility in the area where cartilage is worn away. It affects mostly weight-bearing joints and is the main reason for total hip joint replacement surgery.

Another frequent disorder is herniated intervertebral discs (also spelled disks), which occur most often in patients between 20 and 45 years of age and more commonly in men. Some 90 percent of intervertebral herniations occur in one of two spinal interspaces, the areas experiencing the greatest amount of motion.

A common work-related orthopedic injury is carpal tunnel syndrome, which results from abnormal pressure on the median nerve passing through the wrist to the hand. Carpal tunnel syndrome is one of many repetitive stress injuries produced by years of continually repeated joint motions (for example, keyboarding).

Osteoporosis, or fragile bones, is a common disease in older women. Caused by the loss of bone mass, osteoporosis results in porous and brittle bones that break easily.

Common Tests and Surgical Procedures

Other than surgery to repair bone fractures, the most common procedures in orthopedics are probably x-rays and various kinds of computerized scans. Closed reduction refers to the repair of a fracture by manipulation, casting or cast application, and splinting. Open reduction is done when the area is surgically repaired. Arthrography produces a radiograph taken after injection of a radiopaque dye into a joint such as the knee or shoulder. The x-ray outlines the joint.

Arthrocentesis is a procedure to obtain synovial fluid for examination under the microscope. Usually this is performed if there is a suspected pathogen causing an infection.

Arthroscopy allows the physician to look inside a joint, most frequently the knee, using an instrument called an arthroscope. When there is an injury, an arthroscopic needle is inserted into the area. The area is viewed and a biopsy is taken if necessary.

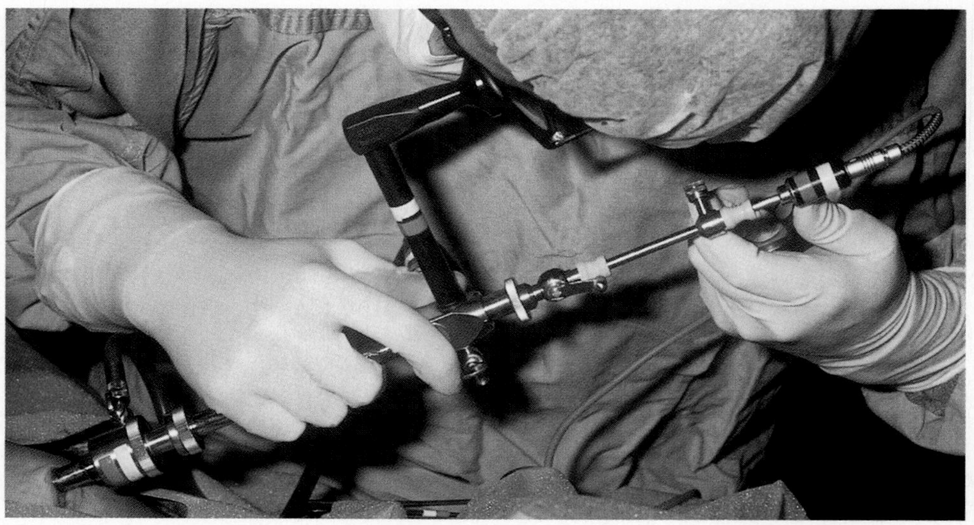

The arthroscope allows the visualization of the inside of a joint.

Building Language Skills

The following tables list common orthopedics terms, drugs, and abbreviations. The list of terms and definitions includes the most difficult words contained in the dictated reports in this chapter. These words are identified in GREEN type. A list of common drugs is found in Appendix D.

Medical Terms and Pharmacologic Agents

abduction
(ab-**duk**-shun) (n) movement of a leg or arm away from the middle of the body

adduction
(ad-**duk**-shun) (n) movement of a leg or arm toward the middle of the body

ankylosis
(**ang**-ki-**lO**-sis) (n) stiffening or rigidity of a joint either as a result of a disease process or from surgery

ankylotic
(ang-ki-**lot**-ik) (adj) relating to or having ankylosis

apophyseal
(a-pO-**fiz**-ee-al) (adj) relating to or having an apophysis

apophysis
(a-**pof**-i-sis) (n) a projection or outgrowth of a bone

arteritis
(**ar**-tur-**I**-tis) (n) inflammation of one or more arteries

arthralgia
(ar-**thral**-jee-a) (n) joint pain

arthritis
(ar-**thrI**-tis) (n) inflammation of one or more joints

arthroplasty
(**ar**-thrO-plas-tee) (n) surgical repair of a joint; creation of a new joint

articulation
(ar-tik-yoo-**lay**-shun) (n) the connecting of bones as a joint

asepsis
(a-**sep**-sis) (n) lack of germs; a state of sterility; methods used to create or maintain a sterile environment

aseptic
(a-**sep**-tik/ay-**sep**-tik) (adj) sterile; being without infection or contamination

calcaneus
(kal-**kay**-nee-us) (n) heel bone; calcanei (kal-**kay**-nee-I) (pl)

callous
(**kal**-us) (adj) pertaining to or resembling callus

callus
(**kal**-us) (n) thickened skin that develops at points of pressure or friction; the bony deposit which develops around the broken ends of bone during healing

carpal tunnel
(**kar**-pul **tun**-nul) (n) where the median nerve and flexor tendons pass through the wrist

cervical
(**ser**-vi-kal) (adj) relating to a neck or cervix

chondral
(**kon**-drul) (adj) relating to cartilage

chondritis
(kon-**drI**-tis) (n) inflammation of cartilage

chondromalacia
(**kon**-drO-ma-**lay**-shee-a) (n) softening of cartilage

claudication
(klaw-di-**ka**-shun) (n) limping; painful cramps in calf of leg due to poor blood circulation

clavicle
(**klav**-i-kl) (n) clavicula; collar bone

clavicula
(kla-**vik**-yoo-la) (n) clavicle; collar bone

condyle
(**kon**-dil) (n) the rounded projecting end of a bone where ligaments are attached

Coumadin
(**coo**-mah-din) (n) Brand name for warfarin, an agent to prevent blood clots

crepitus
(**krep**-i-tus) (n) grating sound or vibration made by movement of fractured bones (bone fragments); crepitation

dactylomegaly
(dak-til-O-**meg**-a-lee) (n) abnormal enlargement of one or more fingers or toes

degenerative
(di-**jen**-er-a-tiv) (adj) relating to or causing deterioration or worsening of a condition

diaphysis
(dI-**af**-i-sis) (n) shaft of a long bone

distal
(**dis**-tal) (adj) farthest from the center from a medial line, or from the trunk

edema
(e-**dee**-ma) (n) excessive accumulation of fluid in tissues, especially just under the skin or in a given cavity

edematous
(e-**dem**-a-tus) (adj) having edema

epiphyseal
(ep-i-**fiz**-ee-al) (adj) relating to an epiphysis

epiphysis
(e-**pif**-i-sis) (n) end of a long bone, separated by cartilage from the shaft until the bone stops growing when the shaft and end are joined

eversion
(ee-**vur**-zhun) (n) turning out or inside out

exacerbation
(eg-zas-er-**bay**-shun) (n) aggravation of symptoms or increase in the severity of a disease

facial
(**fay**-shul) (adj) relating to the face

fascia
(**fash**-ee-a) (n) fibrous connective tissue that supports soft organs and encloses structures such as muscles; fasciae (pl)

fascial
(**fash**-ee-al) (adj) relating to fascia

femoral
(**fem**-o-ral) (adj) relating to the thigh bone or femur

flexion
(**flek**-shun) (n) the act of bending or the condition of being bent, in contrast to extending

foramina
(for-**ray**-mi-na) (n) apertures or perforations through a bone or a membrane structure; plural of foramen

foramen
(fO-**ray**-men) (n) hole or opening, especially in a bone or membrane

fracture
(**frak**-chur) (v) to break; (n) a broken bone

girdle
(**ger**-dl) (n) a zone or belt

hemarthrosis
(**hee**-mar-**thrO**-sis/**hem**-ar-**thrO**-sis) (n) accumulation of blood in a joint

hematoma
(hee-ma-**tO**-ma) (n) a tumor or swelling that contains blood

hemodynamic
(**hee**-mO-dI-**nam**-ik) (adj) relating to the physical aspects of the blood circulation

hemostasis
(**hee**-mO-**stay**-sis) (n) arrest of bleeding or of circulation

hepatic
(he-**pat**-ik) (adj) pertaining to the liver

humeral
(hyoo-mer-al) (adj) pertaining to the humerus, the upper bone of arm extending from the elbow to the shoulder joint where it articulates with the scapula

humerus
(**hyoo**-mer-us) (n) the long bone of the upper arm

ischium
(**is**-kee-um/**ish**-ee-um) (n) bone upon which body rests when sitting; fuses with the ilium and pubis to form the pelvis; ischia (**is**-kee-a) (pl)

kyphosis
(kI-**fO**-sis) (n) abnormal curving of the spine causing a hunchback

lipping
(**lip**-ing) (n) excessive growth in a liplike shape at the edge of a bone

lordosis
(lOr-**dO**-sis) (n) abnormal curving of the spine causing a swayback

malleolus
(ma-**lee**-O-lus) (n) either of the two bumplike projections on each side of the ankle; malleoli (pl)

metatarsal
(**met**-a-**tar**-sal) (adj) relating to a metatarsus; (n) a metatarsal bone

metatarsus
(**met**-a-**tar**-sus) (n) any of the five long bones of the foot between the ankle and the toes

necrosis
(ne-**krO**-sis) (n) death of some or all of the cells in a tissue

necrotic
(ne-**krot**-ik) (adj) relating to or undergoing necrosis

neural
(**noo**-ral) (adj) relating to nerves or the nervous system

odontoid process
(O-**don**-toyd **pros**-es) (n) the toothlike projection from the upper surface of the second cervical vertebra on which the head rotates

osseous
(**os**-ee-us) (adj) bony; resembling bone; osteal

osteal
(**os**-tee-ul) (adj) bony; resembling bone; osseous

ostealgia
(os-tee-**al**-jee-a) (n) pain in a bone

osteophyte
(**os**-tee-O-fIt) (n) a bony outgrowth; projection or bone spur

osteoporosis
(os-tee-O-pO-**rO**-sis) (n) abnormal loss of bone tissue, causing fragile bones that fracture easily

ostial
(**os**-tee-ul) (adj) relating to any opening (ostium)

parietal
(pa-**rI**-e-tal) (adj) relating to the walls of a body cavity

plantar
(**plan**-tar) (adj) relating to the undersurface (sole) of the foot

prosthesis
(pros-**thee**-sis) (n) artificial replacement for a diseased or missing part of the body, such as artificial limbs; prostheses (pl)

proximal
(**prok**-si-mal) (adj) nearest the point of attachment, center of the body, or point of reference

radiograph
(**ray**-dee-O-graf) (n) an image produced through exposure to x-rays

residual
(re-**zid**-yoo-al) (adj) related to a residue which is left behind

rheumatoid
(**roo**-ma-toyd) (adj) resembling rheumatism, with pain, inflammation, and deformity of the joints

rigidity
(ri-**jid**-i-tee) (n) stiffness; inflexibility

scapula
(**skap**-yoo-la) (n) a large, triangular, flattened bone lying over the ribs

sclerosis
(sklee-**rO**-sis) (n) hardening or induration of an organ or tissue, especially that due to excessive growth of fibrous tissue

scoliosis
(skO-lee-**O**-sis) (n) abnormal curvature of the spine to one side

sphincter
(**sfingk**-ter) (n) circular muscle constricting an orifice

spinous
(**spI**-nus) (adj) pertaining to or resembling a spine, a short, sharp process of bone

splenic
(**splen**-ik) (adj) referring to the spleen

spondylitis
(spon-di-**lI**-tis) (n) inflammation of one or more vertebrae

sprain
(n) injury to a joint by overstretching the ligaments; (v) to injure a joint and sometimes the nearby ligaments or tendons

sternocleidomastoid
(**ster**-nO-**klI**-dO-**mas**-toyd) (n) one of two muscles arising from the sternum and the inner part of the clavicle

strain
(n) injury, usually to muscle, caused by overstretching or overuse; (v) to injure muscles by overstretching or overuse

synovial fluid
(si-**nO**-vee-al **floo**-id) (n) protective lubricating fluid around joints

tibia
(**tib**-ee-a) (n) the larger bone of the lower leg; shin bone

transverse
(trans-**vers**) (adj) at right angles to the long axis of the body or an organ; crosswise; side to side

trochanter
(trO-**kan**-ter) (n) one of the projections at the upper end of the femur (thigh bone)

vertebral
(ver-**tee**-bral) (adj) relating to a vertebra or the vertebrae

Vistaril
(**viss**-ta-rill) (n) Brand name for hydroxyzine, used for the treatment of anxiety and nausea

Abbreviations

AE	above the elbow (amputation)
AK	above the knee (amputation)
AP	anterioposterior
AROM	active range of motion
BE	below the elbow (amputation)
BK	below the knee (amputation)
C1, etc.	cervical vertebrae
CDH	congenital dislocation of the hip
DIP joint	distal interphalangeal joint
DJD	degenerative joint disease
DOS	date of service
EMG	electromyography
FROJM	full range of joint motion
fx	fracture
HD	hip disarticulation
HNP	herniated nucleus pulposus (disc)
HP	hemipelvectomy
ID	internal development (ortho)
IS	intracostal space
KD	knee disarticulation
L1, etc.	lumbar vertebrae
MCP joint	metacarpophalangeal joint
OA	osteoarthritis
ortho	orthopedics
PIP joint	proximal interphalangeal joint
PROM	passive range of motion
ROJM	range of joint motion
S1, etc.	sacral vertebrae
SD	shoulder disarticulation
T1, etc.	thoracic vertebrae
TENS	transcutaneous electric nerve stimulation
THA	total hip arthroplasty

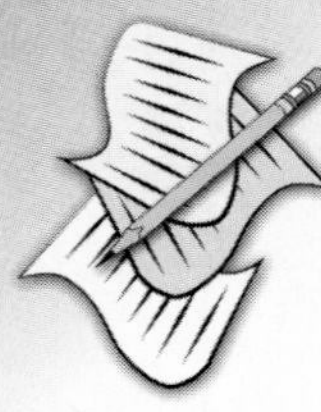

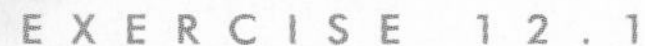
EXERCISE 12.1

Recognizing Look-Alikes and Sound-Alikes

Below is a list of frequently used words that look alike and/or sound alike. Study the meaning and pronunciation of each set of words, then read the following sentences carefully and circle the word in parentheses that correctly completes the meaning.

affect	(n) emotional or psychological disposition
affect	(v) to influence or alter
affective	(adj) pertaining to emotions
effect	(n) result
effect	(v) to bring about, accomplish
effective	(adj) producing the desired result

accept	(v) to take
except	(prep) other than; with exclusion of
except	(v) to leave out

weak	(adj) feeble, delicate
week	(n) a period of seven successive days

checkup	(n) an examination of the health of an individual
check up	(v) to investigate

ostial	(adj) relating to an orifice
osteal	(adj) bony

sprain	(v) to injure a joint
sprain	(n) traumatic injury to a joint
strain	(v) to injure a muscle
strain	(n) injury to a muscle

off	(adj) gone, absent
off	(adv) apart, away, below
of	(prep) indicating possession or origin

1. She complains of feeling (weak, week) and tired.
2. She has had flu symptoms for approximately one (weak, week).
3. The medication (affected, effected) her bladder control.
4. As steroids were gradually tapered (of, off, off of), the patient's strength returned.
5. The new medication was (affective, effective) in reducing inflammation.
6. The patient acknowledged the instruction and (accepted, excepted) the plan.
7. Mr. Braccia's pain was diagnosed as originating in the (osteal, ostial) tissue of the hip.
8. The patient displayed a flat (affect, effect).
9. During her gymnastics class, the patient jumped off the balance beam and (sprained, strained) her ankle.
10. The skin exam was unremarkable (accept, except) for a small lesion on the left cheek.

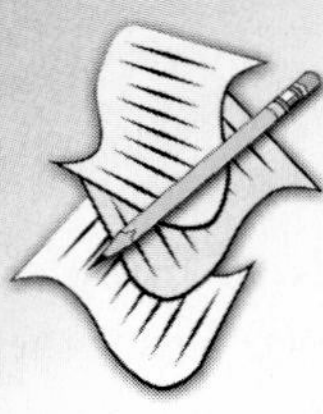

EXERCISE 12.2

Matching Sound and Spelling

The numbered list that follows shows the phonetic spelling of hard-to-spell words. Sound out the word, then write the correct spelling in the blank space provided. Each of the words can be found in the Glossary or in the drug list in Appendix D.

1. **os**-ee-us ______________________
2. **kon**-drO-ma-**lay**-shee-a ______________________
3. kal-**kay**-nee-us ______________________
4. **krep**-i-tus ______________________
5. trO-**kan**-ter ______________________
6. ang-ki-**lO**-sis ______________________
7. kI-**fO**-sis ______________________
8. kla-**vik**-yoo-la ______________________
9. dI-**af**-i-sis ______________________
10. kon-**drI**-tis ______________________
11. pa-**rI**-e-tal ______________________
12. **os**-tee-O-fIt ______________________
13. **is**-kee-um/**is**-shee-um ______________________
14. skO-lee-**O**-sis ______________________
15. **hyoo**-mer-us ______________________
16. **dak**-til-O-**meg**-a-lee ______________________
17. ang-ki-**lot**-ik ______________________
18. spon-di-**lI**-tis ______________________
19. **roo**-ma-toyd ______________________
20. os-tee-**al**-jee-a ______________________

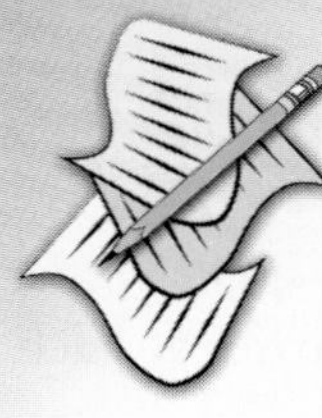

EXERCISE 12.3

Choosing Words from Context

When transcribing dictation, the medical transcriptionist frequently needs to consider the situation when determining the word that correctly completes the sentence. From the list below, select the term that meaningfully completes each of the following statements.

aseptic	chondritis	edematous
neural	degenerative	residual
kyphosis	radiograph	necrosis
cervical	crepitus	tibia
prosthesis	hemostasis	

1. It was necessary for Mr. Jones to have a(n) ____________ after the amputation.
2. The _______________ of the chest showed pneumonia.
3. Although there was considerable necrosis of the tumor after the chemotherapy, there was some ______________ tumor.
4. The boy suffered a fractured ___________ after he fell off his bicycle.
5. The legs were _____________ because the woman was in heart failure.
6. The pain was in the _____________ region of the back.
7. When he opened the sterile package, he used a(n) ________ technique.
8. He had ______________ of the thoracic spine, which caused pain when he stood too long.
9. The pathology report showed ________ tissue taken from the brain.
10. After the radiation treatments, there was considerable _________ at the tumor site.
11. A clamp was applied in order to assure _________ during the surgery.
12. Dr. Jones heard the _________ as the fractured bones rubbed when Jane attempted to walk.

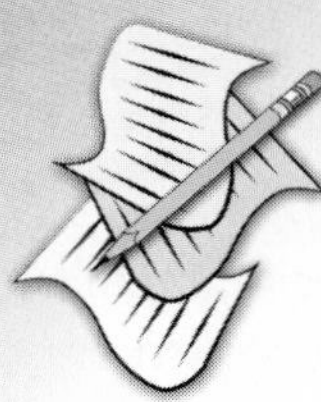

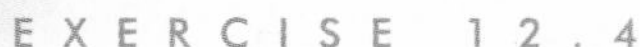

EXERCISE 12.4

Pairing Words and Meanings

From this list, locate the term that best matches each of the following definitions. Write the letter of the term in the space provided by each definition.

A.	apophysis	E.	fascia	I.	osteoporosis
B.	epiphysis	F.	malleolus	J.	synovial sarcoma
C.	femoral	G.	metatarsus	K.	proximal
D.	foramen	H.	odontoid process	L.	distal

1. a bone of the foot ____________________
2. a malignant tumor ____________________
3. loss of bone tissue ____________________
4. a small projection or outgrowth on a bone ____________________
5. toothlike projection that serves as pivot point when head turns ____________________
6. end portion of a long bone ____________________
7. a hole or opening in a bone or membrane ____________________
8. fibrous, connective tissue that supports small organs ____________________
9. a bumplike projection on the ankle bone ____________________
10. pertaining to the thigh bone ____________________
11. nearest to the center of the body ____________________
12. farthest from the center of the trunk ____________________

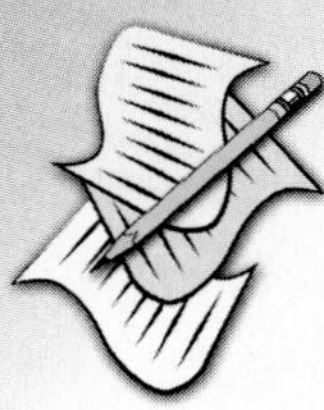

EXERCISE 12.5

Creating Terms from Word Forms

In the following exercise, combine prefixes, root words, and suffixes to create medical words that fit the definitions below. Fill in the blanks with the words you construct.

ankyl/o-	crooked, fusion, stiffness	necro/o-	death
		oste/o-	bone
arthr/o-	joint	por/o-	cavity, passage
articul/o-	joint	spondyl/o-	vertebra
chondr/o-	cartilage	tend/o-; tendin/o-	tendon
dia-	through	-physis	bone portion; growth
epi-	on, in addition to		
kyph/o-	humped	-phyte	outgrowth
lord/o-	bent	tarsus	instep of foot
meta-	after, beyond	-arthria	condition involving the ability to articulate
muscul/o	muscle		
myel/o	bone marrow or spinal cord	-itis	inflammation
my/o-	muscle	-osis	condition

1. abnormal loss of bone tissue______________________________
2. end of long bone, secondary bone ______________________________
3. inflammation of vertebra ______________________________
4. tissue death ______________________________
5. convexity of spine; sway back______________________________
6. inflammation of bone and marrow ______________________________
7. bone between ankle and toes ______________________________
8. inflammation of spinal cord______________________________
9. shaft of long bone ______________________________
10. hunchback, curved spine ______________________________
11. growth zone of long bone ______________________________
12. bony outgrowth______________________________
13. condition of crooked, stiff bones ______________________________
14. inflammation of the joint______________________________

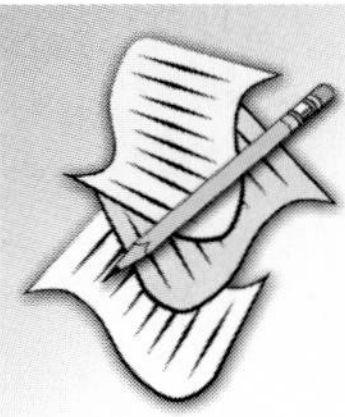

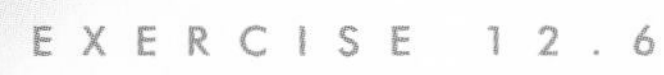

EXERCISE 12.6

Proofreading Review

Read the following report and look for errors in punctuation, plural vs. singular word forms, subject-verb agreement, complete sentences, and the use of numbers. Circle the errors, then key the document with the errors corrected.

DATE OF ADMISSION: August 5/XX

Jonathan is states post rite baloney amputation for synoviale sarcoma he is without complaints and is ambulating with his below knee prosthesis quiet well. His abdomen is soft and non-tender. there are no mass. The incisor is well heeled. The right thigh skin graph sight is clean. Their is no palpable mass and there is no open wound. If he experiences pain, he is to take one Vicodin p.o. q four to six hours.

Building Transcription Skills

The Emergency Room Note

Because emergency room cases can range from simple injuries to life-threatening traumas, ER reports (Figure 12.6) can likewise vary from short chart notes to lengthy, complex reports. The latter may include the results of laboratory studies, x-ray films, and ECGs, along with operative procedures and the results from detailed physical examinations. Common procedures in the emergency room include endotracheal intubation, insertion of chest tubes and nasogastric tubes, catheterization of the bladder, placement of central venous catheters, and suturing of wounds.

Transcribing emergency room reports presents challenges usually not encountered with other medical specialties. For example, sometimes a dictation may be incomplete or interrupted because the physician may have been handling several complex cases, including some that were life-threatening. This factor may also lead to inconsistencies in the dictation, which should be pointed out to the physician for correction.

Required Headings/Content JCAHO mandates no specific headings. However, reports typically include chief complaint, history of present illness, primary physician, physical examination, diagnosis, treatment plan, and condition at discharge. JCAHO does require ER physicians to record the patient's time of arrival, time seen by the physician, and the time of discharge or transfer. Sometimes the physician dictates these times; otherwise, the information is included in another part of the medical record.

Turnaround Time Rapid turnaround is required for ER reports since frequently the patient is admitted to the hospital and the information is vital for continued treatment. The ideal turnaround time is one to two hours, although critical cases may require that transcription is completed within an hour of dictation.

1" margins
left justification

PATIENT: Alex Cavara
MR#: 510-879-21
DATE SEEN: 9/5/XX

HISTORY: This 27-year-old Hispanic male was admitted today following a motor vehicle accident.

The patient was the unrestrained driver of a vehicle which struck a tree at approximately 40 miles per hour. The patient had a momentary loss of consciousness and appeared confused at the scene. He complained of immediate head and neck pain. Paramedics transported the victim in full spine precautions.

PHYSICAL EXAMINATION: On examination the patient noted pain in the right arm with left lateral flexion-rotation-compression maneuvers to the neck. There was profound hematoma along the course of the sternocleidomastoid muscle. Cervical flexion-extension maneuvers were limited. There was gross crepitus on palpation of the spinous processes of C5, C6, and C7.

Double-space between sections and between paragraphs within sections

The patient had a 5 x 8-cm hematoma of the left forehead and several small facial lacerations. The pupils were slow to respond but equal and round. The teeth were not broken. There were no intraoral lacerations. Pharynx was clear.

The lungs were clear to auscultation, and the heart showed regular rate and rhythm and no murmurs. The abdomen was mildly tender diffusely, but without signs of splenic or hepatic trauma.

There was an obvious spiral oblique fracture of the right humeral shaft with marked malangulation and shortening. Distal pulses were intact and the fingers were warm and well perfused.

IMPRESSION: Major polytrauma and major skeletal injuries secondary to motor vehicle accident.

TREATMENT PLAN: The patient will be admitted to the orthopedic surgical unit and taken immediately to surgery for internal fixation of his fractures. His hemodynamic status will be carefully monitored over the next few hours. Chest x-ray and labs will be followed serially.

(continued)

FIGURE 12.6
Emergency Department Report

EMERGENCY DEPARTMENT REPORT
PATIENT: Alex Cavara
MR#: 510-879-21
DATE: 9/5/XX
Page 2

CONDITION ON DISCHARGE: The patient is hemodynamically stable at the present time.

____
Jill McKensie, MD

JM/XX
D: 9/5/XX
T: 9/5/XX

FIGURE 12.6
Emergency Department Report (Continued)

Preparing to Transcribe

To prepare for transcribing dictation, review the tables of common orthopedics terms, drugs, and abbreviations presented in the Building Language Skills section of this chapter. Then, study the format and organization of the model document shown in Figure 12.6, and key the model document. Proofread the document by comparing it with the printed version. Categorize the types of errors you made, and document them on a copy of the Performance Comparison chart provided in Chapter 1. A template of this chart is included on the IRC that accompanies this text.

Patient Studies

Transcribe, edit, and correct each report in the following patient studies. Consult reference books for words or formatting rules that are unfamiliar.

As you work on the transcription assignment for this chapter, fill in the Performance Comparison chart that you started when you keyed the model document. For at least three of the reports, categorize and document the types of errors you made. Answer the document analysis questions on the bottom of the chart. With continuous practice and assessment, the quality of your work will improve.

After you have produced a final version of each transcribed report, complete the Performance Report cover sheet, attach it to the top of the transcripts, and submit them to your instructor for evaluation.

Patient Study 12.A — Roberta Flagner

Roberta Flagner is a 51-year-old woman who was complaining of back pain, particularly around the upper spine, radiating toward the left arm from the shoulder blade. She went to see her physician, Joseph White, MD, who referred her to an orthopedist, Samuel Larchmont, MD.

REPORT 12.1 Radiology Report

- To find the name of a joint, muscle, ligament, tendon, or bone, look first under the noun (joint, muscle, ligament, and so on). This also applies to surgical terms as there are many specialized names for the screws, nails, plates, and wires used to repair fractures.

REPORT 12.2 Consultation Letter

Patient Study 12.B

Steve Gatlin

Steve Gatlin is a 28-year-old man who cut his left index finger with a carving knife and came to the emergency room for treatment.

REPORT 12.3 Emergency Room Note

Patient Study 12.C

Arlene Elvin

Mrs. Arlene Elvin was walking through the Brookfield Natural History Museum when she tripped on a slanted floor board and twisted her foot. She felt immediate pain and was assisted by her husband and the security guard to a seat. The museum nurse brought a wheelchair, and ice was applied. Mrs. Elvin was taken to the Brookfield Emergency Room where she was diagnosed with a fracture of the foot.

REPORT 12.4 Radiology Report

REPORT 12.5 Discharge Summary

- Listen for a reference to another physician, Dr. Levendowski.

Patient Study 12.D — Alex Cavara

Alex Cavara is a 27-year-old man who was brought to the emergency room by ambulance following a car accident in which he ran into a tree while driving approximately 40 miles per hour. He suffered a momentary loss of consciousness and complained of immediate head and neck pain.

REPORT 12.6 Emergency Room Note

- The term *flexion-rotation-compression maneuvers* requires hyphens, as shown.
- Listen for these new terms:
  sternocleidomastoid muscle
  malangulation

Patient Study 12.E — Ivy Haines

Ivy Haines is a 72-year-old woman with a history of chronic, progressive left hip pain for the past 25 years. She has been admitted to the hospital for left total hip arthroplasty.

REPORT 12.7 History and Physical

Patient Study 12.F — Jane Stanley

Jan Stanley is a 36-year-old woman with a history of juvenile rheumatoid arthritis. In 1990 she had a bilateral total knee replacement with good results. In the past few years, however, she has experienced increasing left hip pain and was recently admitted to the hospital for a left total hip replacement.

REPORT 12.8 Discharge Summary

Using Medical References

Use the appropriate medical reference to locate the correct spelling and additional usage information for the words below. (If the reference is not available, use the Glossary in this text.) Circle the correct spelling, then write a sentence using the word correctly.

1.	acetabulem	acetabulum	ascetabulum
2.	humerous	humeres	humerus
3.	hematopoiesis	hematapoiesis	hematopoisis
4.	perosteum	periosteum	periostium
5.	epiphysis	epiphisys	epiphises
6.	hemearthrosis	hemarthrosus	hemarthosis
7.	calcaneus	calcaneas	calcuneas
8.	trocanter	trochanter	trochantor
9.	ischium	ishium	ischeum
10.	chondromalacia	condromalacia	chondromalace
11.	girdle	girdel	gridle
12.	flection	flexion	flecktion

Making Expert Decisions

Circle the correct word from the choices in parentheses.

1. Sterilization was (affected/effected) using Hibiclens followed by an alcoholic wash of the area.

2. There was a hard (callus/calus) noted on her heel.

3. The new equipment will be able to determine (osteal/ostial) density in women at risk for osteoporosis.

4. The patient was taken to the operating suite where an (open deduction/open reduction) and internal fixation were performed.

5. A preliminary (plain/plane) film of the abdomen revealed distended loops of bowel.

6. The patient had hypertension and arthritis and was taking nonsteroidal anti-inflammatory medication for the (later/latter).

7. The slip and fall was (humerus/humorous) when it happened, but upon discovery of a fractured (humerus/humorous), my friend apologized for laughing.

8. The doctor said he thought some ligamentous fibers were ruptured, but he thought my (sprain/strain) would heal nicely.

9. The physician's assistant had the patient (abduct/adduct) his foot by pushing against the assistant's hands, thereby testing for muscle strength.

10. The patient had a stroke last year with a residual of left (facial/fascial) weakness.

11. In order to prevent contractures in the comatose patient, the nurse provided (AROM/PROM).

12. During physical therapy John was able to perform (AROM/PROM) himself.

Transcribing Professional Documents

Transcribe the document named Chapter 12 Assessment. Before you key, review the document formatting guidelines. Proofread your transcribed document and revise it until you think it is error-free.

13

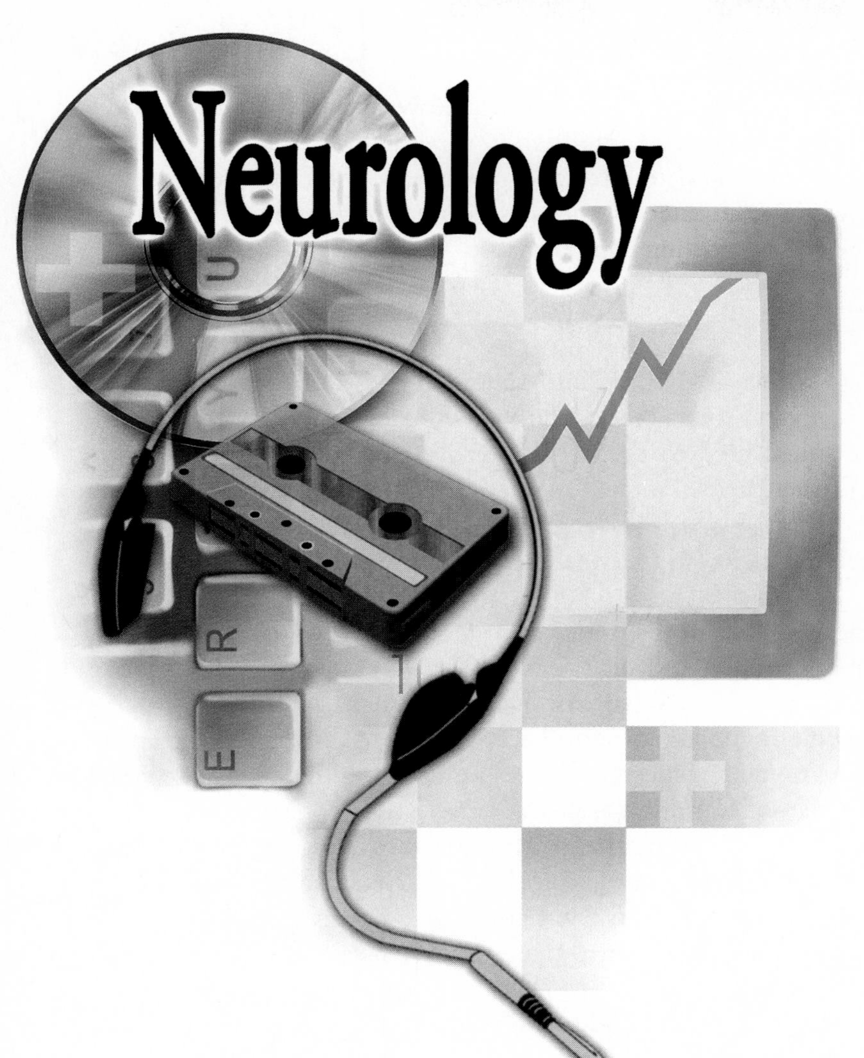

Neurology is the study of the nervous system—the body's communication network. The nervous system serves to conduct the impulses and signals that drive all bodily functions. The organs of the nervous system consist of the brain, the spinal cord, and nerves. The physician who treats diseases of the nervous system is the neurologist. A neurosurgeon performs surgery on organs of the nervous system.

OBJECTIVES

- Use neurology terms correctly according to the context and purpose of the dictation.
- Select and use appropriate general and specialty reference materials.
- Key neurology documents of varying complexity and format.
- Transcribe authentic medical dictation requiring concentration and listening skill.
- Edit medical reports to conform with AAMT style guidelines.
- Proofread and correct transcripts to produce error-free documents.

Exploring Neurology

The nervous system is probably the most complicated system in the human body. Think of it as the body's Internet, an information superhighway that activates and controls all bodily functions, and receives and processes stimuli from the outside world. The most powerful computers in the world cannot match the complexity of the human brain and the supporting components of the nervous system.

Structure and Function

The human nervous system is divided into the central nervous system (CNS), which includes the brain and spinal cord, and the peripheral nervous system (PNS), which connects the spinal cord to the nerve, sensory, and muscle fibers (Figure 13.1). The PNS is further divided into the somatic nervous system (SNS) and the autonomic nervous system (ANS). The somatic nervous system is under the voluntary control of the individual. It innervates nerves that control voluntary muscle movement.

The autonomic nervous system (Figure 13.2) produces the involuntary actions of the body such as the heartbeat and digestion. There are two subdivisions of the ANS: the sympathetic and parasympathetic nervous systems, which function as opposites. The hormones norepinephrine and acetylcholine, also opposites, mediate these responses. Most notably these two are responsible for the "fight or flight" response. At the first sign of fear, the sympathetic nerve fibers prepare the body to fight and move quickly by increasing the heart rate, constricting peripheral blood vessels to move more blood to the heart and skeletal muscles, dilating the pupils for better vision, slowing down peristalsis, and increasing energy production. The parasympathetic nervous system, by contrast, includes the nerves that function during quiet, nonstressful times.

The brain sends feedback to the endocrine system, which responds with the appropriate hormones. This combined system is known as the neuroendocrine system. The cerebrum (Figure 13.3) is the portion of the brain that generates thought through the cerebral cortex, which is the gray matter. Folds, or gyri, on the surface of the brain increase the amount of gray matter that can fit inside the skull. The brain is divided into two functional sides, the left and right hemispheres. The left brain, which controls muscles on the right side of the body, is involved with reasoning and language, as required for science and math. The right brain, which controls the muscles on the left side of the body, is responsible for imagination, insight, and artistic and musical abilities.

The cerebellum is located below the posterior portion of the cerebrum. It consists of the right and left cerebral hemispheres. The hemispheres are further divided by the brain's fissures, or crevices, called sulci. The brain stem is the continuation of the cervical segment of the spinal cord, which consists of bundles of nerve fibers and nuclei. Figure 13.4 shows the sections of the brain and the functions they control. Figure 13.5 is a sagittal section of the brain that shows structures involved in endocrine and sensory function.

The neuron (Figure 13.6) is the basic structural cell of the nervous system. Another class of cells called the neuroglia are supporting cells. The parts of a neuron

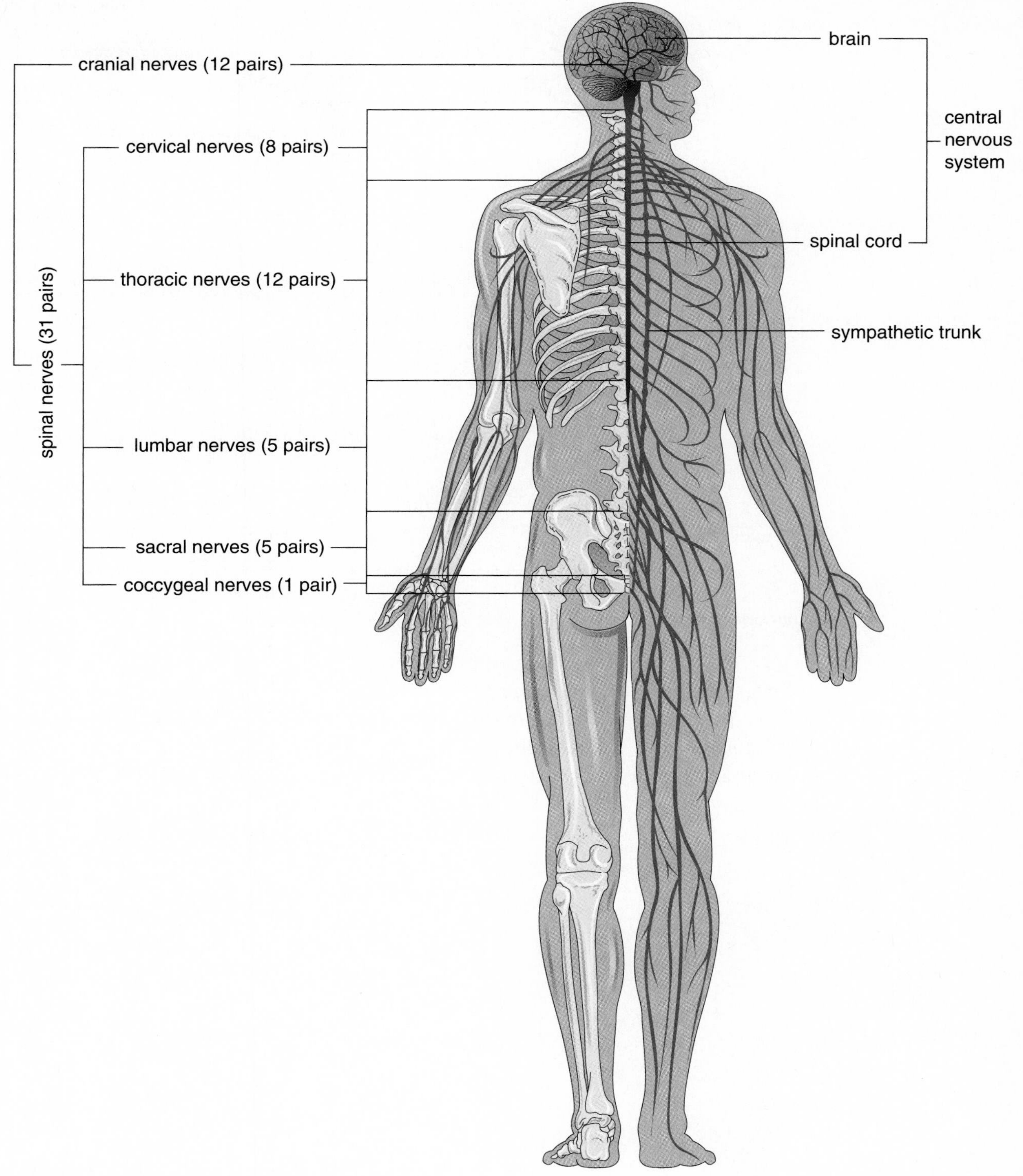

FIGURE 13.1
Structures of the Nervous System

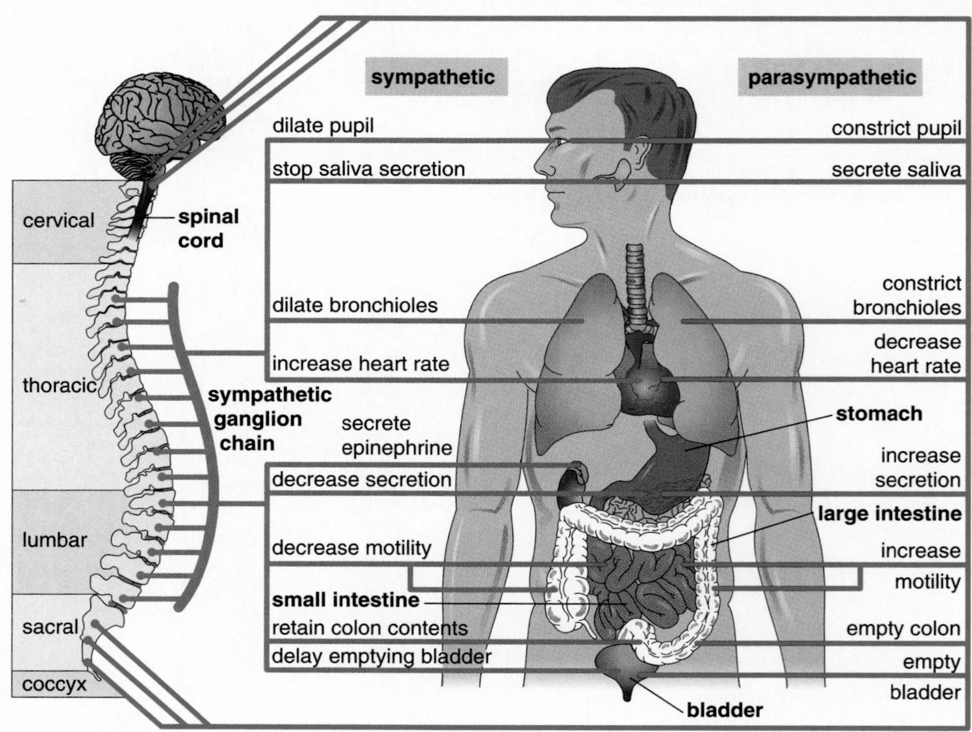

FIGURE 13.2
Autonomic Nervous System

include the soma (body), dendrites (branches leading toward the center of the soma), and an axon (a branch leading away from the soma). The soma contains the DNA for the cell. The dendrite is a tree-like area that receives signals from other neurons and sensory cells. The axon transmits signals away from the cell body and passes these signals to other neurons. Many of the axons are surrounded by a myelin sheath that protects the axon and accelerates impulses through it.

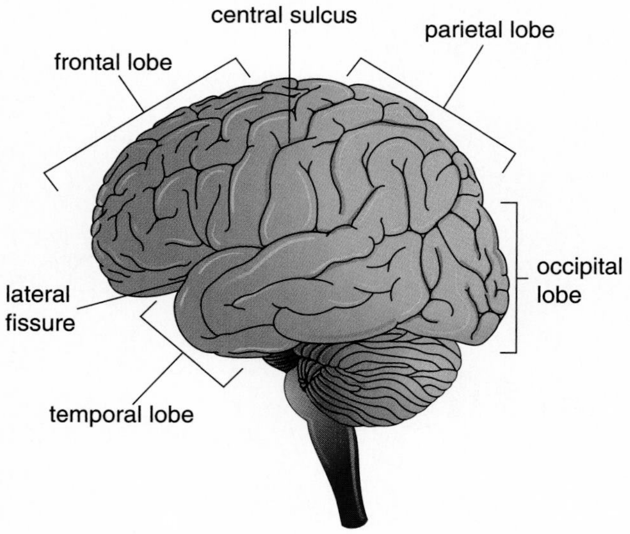

Communication between two neurons occurs when an electrical signal is converted into a chemical signal. This signal crosses a synapse, a minuscule space, where a neurotransmitter (a chemical) permits transmission at nearly unfathomable speed.

FIGURE 13.3
The Cerebrum

Physical Assessment

Neurologic diseases have presenting symptoms ranging from paralysis, numbness, shaking, and weakness to gait disturbances, recurring headaches, seizures, and passing out. Using both direct and indirect methods, the physician tests cerebral and cerebellar function, cranial nerves, motor and sensory systems, and reflexes.

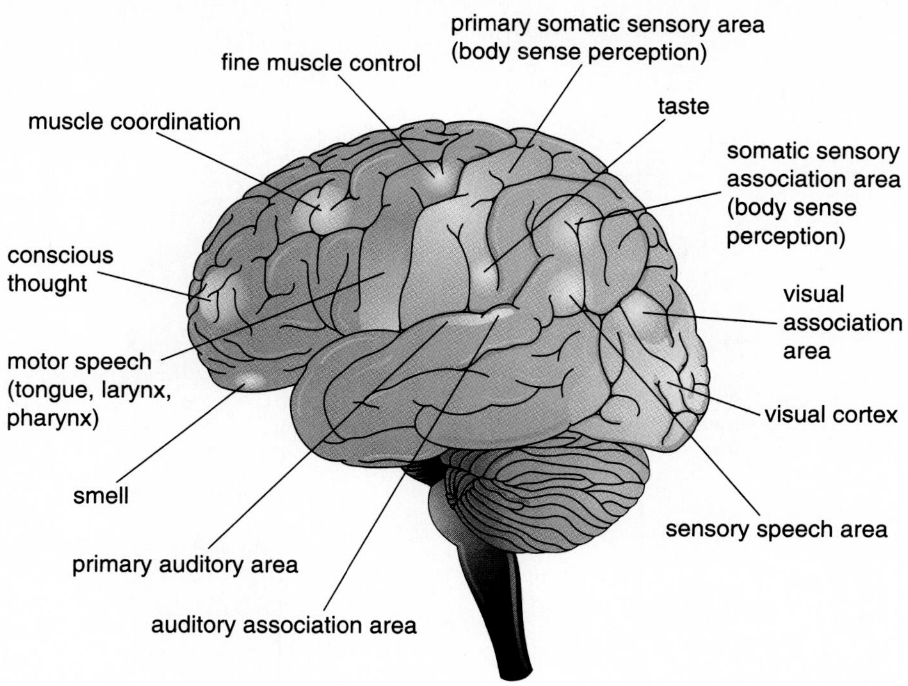

FIGURE 13.4
Functional Areas of the Cerebral Cortex

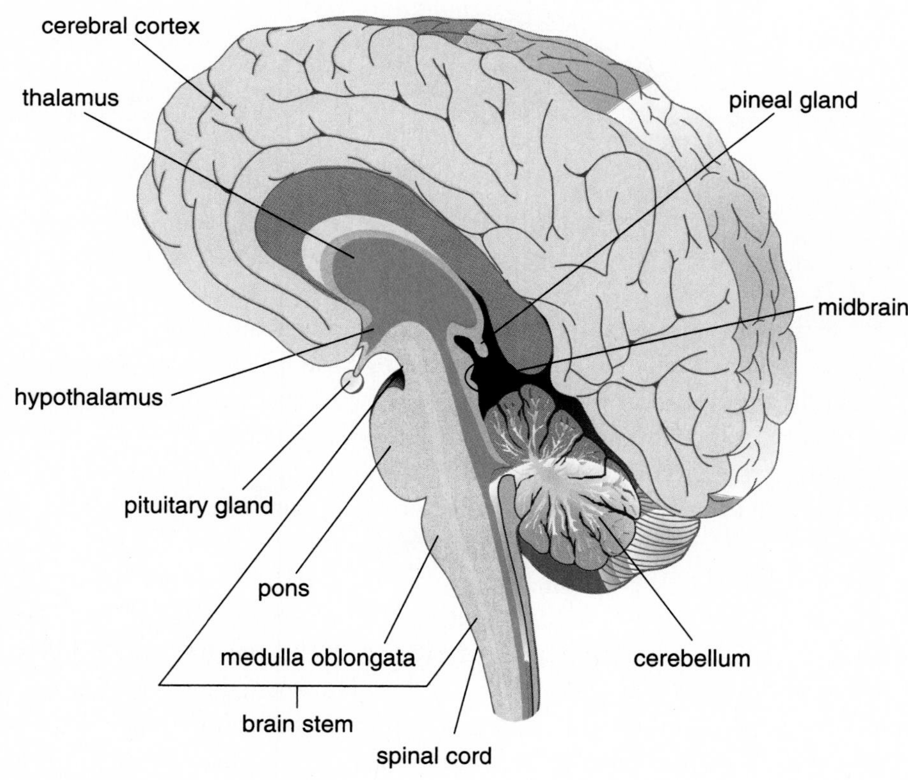

FIGURE 13.5
Sagittal Section of the Brain

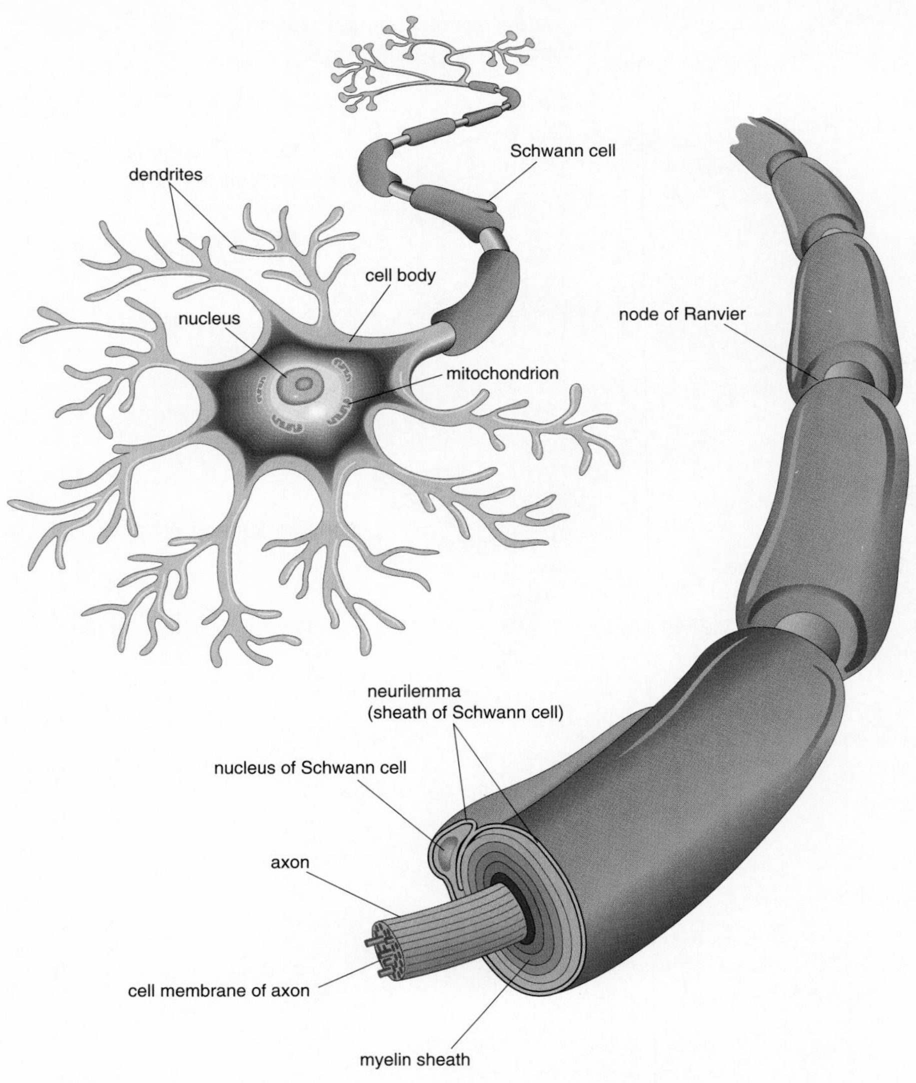

FIGURE 13.6
Neuron (Nerve Cell)

First, if the patient has use of all of the senses, can answer questions accurately, can coordinate muscle movements, and is oriented to time (time of day, date, season, year), person (identification of self, family, and friends), and place (location, city, and state), there is appropriate cerebral and cerebellar function.

Motor and sensory deficits are another level of the assessment. Weakness, paralysis, or atrophy of muscles are indicators of motor nerve impairment. Sensory nerves are tested by feel (touch and gentle pinpricks), temperature (heat, cold), vibration perception in a few areas, and position (limb position). The reflexes are examined by tapping a hammer over the tendons and watching for the contraction of the appropriate muscle. Reflexes tested include the biceps, triceps, patellar, and Achilles tendon. Another important reflex is the plantar reflex. The normal response is plantar flexion of all the toes; an abnormal response is known as Babinski's sign and consists of dorsiflexion of the great toe and spreading of the other toes. Results of the tendon reflex assessment are recorded as shown in Table 13.1.

TABLE 13.1 Tendon Reflex Assessment

Test Result	Meaning
0	no response
1+	diminished response
2+	normal response
3+	more brisk than average response
4+	hyperactive response (hyperreflexia)

The patient's state of consciousness is assessed in a range from alert to comatose. The affect, or mood, is described using words such as hyperactive, euphoric, hostile, agitated, or flat. A general assessment of intellect involves asking the patient to perform simple mathematical calculations, define familiar vocabulary, and describe recent, intermediate, and remote, or past, events (a test of memory).

A patient's behavior is evaluated by assessing the state of dress, appropriateness of language, gestures, facial expressions, and attentiveness to the examiner. Speech is an important part of the neurologic examination. It shows coordination of thought and muscle movements and function of the cranial nerves.

The cerebellum is the center for balance and muscle coordination. There are several tests that the physician uses to assess this function. Balance is tested by observing gait. If there is any abnormality, a cerebellar disorder is suggested. The Romberg is a test for sensory equilibrium. A positive Romberg test means the patient loses balance with eyes closed and feet together.

The finger-to-nose test assesses coordination by checking for "past-pointing" in which the patient brings the fingertip beyond the nose. The physician will test for muscle strength and range of motion and observe for involuntary body movements such as tics, twitches, and tremors.

Diseases and Conditions

Cerebrovascular disease accounts for the majority of patients treated by neurologists. This group of diseases includes cerebral arteriosclerosis, cerebral atherosclerosis, aneurysm, thrombosis, and embolism. Another major disease is a cerebrovascular accident (CVA), commonly known as a stroke. All these disorders are caused by mild to severe interruption of blood flow to the brain.

Seizures can occur at any age and involve different muscles and areas of the body. An aura, or particular smell or feeling, may occur before the seizure. This is known as the preictal phase—allowing the individual to anticipate a seizure. During the actual seizure, the ictal phase, the person may or may not lose consciousness or bowel and bladder control. Following the seizure, the postictal phase occurs and is characterized by tiredness and/or sleep.

Attention deficit hyperactivity disorder (ADHD) is usually diagnosed in early childhood. It is characterized by such symptoms as underachievement in school, hyperactivity with short attention span, obsessive-compulsive behaviors, and tics.

Parkinsonism usually begins in middle age. It is a defect of the extrapyramidal tract, especially in the basal ganglia. Classic motor disturbances include flat facial expression, stooping posture, balance and walking disturbances, excessive salivation, speech difficulties, and immobility.

Peripheral neuropathy is a disease category encompassing diseases of the peripheral nerves. In the United States the primary cause of peripheral neuropathy is diabetes mellitus. Worldwide, a common cause is leprosy.

Brain tumors, both malignant and benign, are another frequent neurologic affliction. Cancerous tumors either destroy or compress brain tissue and vary in aggressiveness. The most common brain tumors are tumors that have spread from another area, usually the breast or lung. Spinal cord tumors may be benign or malignant and occur one-tenth as frequently as brain tumors.

Degenerative disc disease is another common ailment treated by neurologists. Herniated discs may cause pressure on a nerve, resulting in arm, trunk, or leg pain.

Alzheimer disease results from structural changes in the brain, the exact cause of which is unknown. Patients experience a gradual loss of cognitive function that ends with total disability and death.

Common Tests and Surgical Procedures

Many procedures and studies give insight into the nervous system without requiring surgery or invasive techniques. Magnetic resonance imaging (MRI) is used extensively to visualize the brain or spinal cord. A contrast medium, usually gadolinium, is used to enhance or outline the structures. The computerized axial tomography (CT or CAT) scan provides section views of structures. Positron emission tomography (PET) is an imaging technology that uses a thin x-ray beam and an injection of a radioactive isotope to visualize the brain. Single photon emission computed tomography (SPECT) uses an injection of a radioactive sugar substance that is metabolized by the brain cells. The brain is then scanned for any abnormalities.

Myelography produces an x-ray picture of the spinal cord after injection of a radiopaque dye. This procedure has been largely replaced by newer, less invasive tests.

Electroencephalography (EEG) produces a graphic recording of the electrical activities of the brain, similar to an electrocardiogram (ECG) for the heart. Electrodes are placed on the scalp to detect and record brain impulses. This test assists in the diagnosis of epilepsy.

Cerebral angiography provides visualization of the vascular system using a radiopaque dye introduced through the carotid or vertebral artery. This technique has virtually been replaced by scans noted above.

Lumbar puncture (LP), or spinal tap, is performed by inserting a small gauge needle between the vertebrae into the spinal canal. This test is used to measure the pressure within the spinal canal and to withdraw cerebrospinal fluid (CSF) for examination under the microscope. Medications can be injected directly into the CSF through the needle.

Stereotactic surgery is a method of locating a precise area of the brain using a three-dimensional measurement. This operation is performed by a highly skilled neurosurgeon. Laminectomy can be performed by a neurosurgeon or an orthopedic surgeon. It involves excision of a portion of the vertebral body to relieve pressure on spinal nerves.

Trephination is performed by making a burr hole into the skull to decrease intracranial pressure.

Building Language Skills

The following tables list common neurology terms, drugs, and abbreviations. The list of terms and definitions includes the most difficult words contained in the dictated reports in this chapter. These words are identified in GREEN type. A list of common drugs is found in Appendix D.

Medical Terms and Pharmacologic Agents

abduction
(ab-**duk**-shun) (n) the lateral movement of a limb away from the median plane of the body

adenopathy
(a-den-**op**-a-thee) (n) swelling and morbid change in lymph nodes

agnosia
(ag-**nO**-see-a) (n) unable to perceive or recognize sensory stimuli

agraphia
(a-**graf**-ee-a) (n) impairment of the ability to write

akinesis
(ay-ki-**nee**-sis/ay-kI-**nee**-sis) (n) absence or loss of the power of voluntary motion; partial or incomplete paralysis

amnesia
(am-**nee**-zee-a) (n) a disturbance of long-term memory; total or partial inability to recall past experiences

angiography
(an-jee-**og**-ra-fee) (n) an x-ray taken after a radiopaque dye is given to visualize the vessels

aphasia
(a-**fay**-zee-a) (n) difficulty with using and understanding words

aphonia
(a-**fO**-nee-a) (n) loss of the voice as a result of disease or injury

arachnoid
(a-**rak**-noyd) (n) the middle of the three membranes covering the brain; it is a delicate fibrous membrane, resembling a cobweb

astereognosis
(a-**steer**-ee-og-**nO**-sis) (n) loss of the ability to judge the form of an object by touch

asymmetry
(ay-**sim**-e-tree) (n) lack of symmetry of parts or organs on opposite sides of body

ataxia
(a-**tak**-see-a) (n) muscular incoordination

atrophy
(**at**-rO-fee) (n) a decrease in size of a part or organ; a wasting away of tissue as a result of disuse, radiation therapy, surgery, disease

aura
(**aw**-ra) (n) a sensation, as of light or warmth, that may precede an attack of migraine or a seizure

auscultation
(aws-kul-**tay**-shun) (n) act of listening through a stethoscope to body sounds, including lungs, heart, and abdomen

axial
(**ak**-see-al) (adj) situated in or relating to an axis

Babinski reflex
(bab-**in**-skeez **ree**-fleks) (n) an extension or moving of the big toe upward or toward the head, with the other toes fanned out and extended when the sole of the foot is stimulated

Brudzinski sign
(n) in meningitis, if a leg is passively flexed, a similar movement occurs in the other leg; if the neck is passively flexed, the legs also flex

bruit
(**broo**-ee/broot) (n) an adventitious sound of venous or arterial origin heard on auscultation

causalgia
(kaw-**zal**-jee-a) (n) persistent severe burning sensation of the skin, usually following injury of a sensory nerve

central nervous system (CNS)
(n) portion of the nervous system consisting of the brain and spinal cord

cephalalgia
(**sef**-al-**al**-jee-a) (n) headache

cerebellar
(ser-e-**bel**-ar) (adj) relating to the cerebellum, the part of the brain concerned with the coordination and control of voluntary muscular activity

cerebrospinal
(**ser**-e-brO-spI-nal/se-**ree**-brO-spI-nal) (adj) relating to the brain and spinal cord

cerebrovascular
(**ser**-e-brO-**vas**-kyoo-lar) (adj) relating to the blood vessels of the brain, especially to pathological changes

Chvostek sign
(**khvosh**-teks) (n) an abnormal spasm of facial muscles when the facial nerve is tapped lightly

clonus
(**klO**-nus) (n) abnormal condition in which a skeletal muscle alternately contracts and relaxes

concussion
(kon-**kush**-un) (n) an injury of a soft structure, as the brain, resulting from a blow or violent shaking

corneal
(**kor**-nee-al) (adj) the clear, transparent, anterior portion of the fibrous coat of the eye composing about one-sixth of its surface

coronal
(ka-**rO**-nal) (adj) pertaining to a corona, a structure resembling a crown

cortex
(**kOr**-teks) (n) an outer part of an organ, such as the brain

cortical
(**kOr**-ti-kal) (adj) relating to a cortex

craniotomy
(cray-nee-**ot**-O-mee) (n) surgical opening into the skull, performed to control bleeding, remove tumors, relieve pressure inside the cranium, or insert electrodes for diagnosis

cranium
(**kray**-nee-um) (n) the bony skull that holds the brain

cyanosis
(sI-a-**nO**-sis) (n) bluish discoloration of the skin and mucous membranes, occurring when the oxygen in the blood is sharply diminished, as in carbon monoxide poisoning

decompression
(**dee**-kom-presh-un) (n) removal of bone to relieve pressure

dementia
(dee-**men**-shee-a) (n) a general mental deterioration due to organic or psychological factors

Dexedrine
(**dex**-a-dreen) (n) brand name for dextroamphetamine, a CNS stimulant

diffuse
(di-**fyoos**) (adj) spreading, scattered

Dilantin
(dill-**ann**-tin) (n) brand name for phenytoin, used for the prevention and management of seizures

diplopia
(di-**plO**-pee-a) (n) double vision

dorsum
(**dOr**-sum) (n) the back or posterior surface of a part

dural
(**doo**-ral) (adj) pertaining to the dura mater, the outer membrane covering the spinal cord and brain

dura mater
(**doo**-ra **may**-ter/**mah**-ter) (n) the outermost of the three membranes surrounding the brain and spinal cord; it is tough and fibrous

dyslexia
(dys-**lek**-see-a) (n) impairment of ability to read in which letters and words are reversed

echolalia
(ek-O-**lay**-lee-a) (n) involuntary repetition of a word or sentence just spoken by another person

electrophoresis
(ee-lek-trO-fO-**ree**-sis) (n) the movement of charged suspended particles through a liquid medium in response to changes in an electric field; for example, a hemoglobin electrophoresis measures the types of hemoglobin in the blood

encephalopathy
(en-**sef**-a-**lop**-a-thee) (n) disease or dysfunction of the brain

encopresis
(en-cO-**pree**-sis) (n) inability to control bowel movements, fecal incontinence

epilepsy
(**ep**-i-**lep**-see) (n) convulsive disorder

epileptiform
(ep-i-**lep**-ti-fOrm) (adj) having the form of epilepsy

erythema
(er-i-**thee**-ma) (n) abnormal redness of the skin resulting from dilation of the capillaries, as occurs in sunburn

exotropia
(ek-sO-**trO**-pee-a) (n) outward turning of one eye relative to the other

extensor
(eks-**ten**-ser, eks-**ten**-sOr) (n) muscle that, when flexed, causes extension of a joint or straightening of an arm or leg

extraocular
(eks-tra-**ok**-yoo-lar) (adj) outside the eye

fissures
(**fish**-urz) (n) deep grooves in the brain

flexor
(**flek**-ser, **flek**-sOr) (n) muscle that bends a joint

fundus
(**fun**-dus) (n) that part of the interior of the eyeball exposed to view through the ophthalmoscope; fundi (p1)

funduscopic
(fun-dus-**skop**-ik) (adj) the examination of the ocular fundus with an ophthalmoscope

gadolinium
(gad-O-**lin**-ee-um) (n) a rare earth metallic element

ganglion
(**gang**-glee-on) (n) a group of nerve cell bodies located in the peripheral nervous system

Glasgow coma scale
(**glas**-gO/**glaz**-gO) (n) a clinical scale to assess impaired consciousness; assessment includes motor responsiveness, verbal performance, and eye opening

glove-stocking anesthesia
(**an**-es-**thee**-see-a) (n) glove or gauntlet anesthesia is loss of sensation in the hand; stocking anesthesia is loss of sensation in the area covered by a stocking

hematocrit
(**hee**-ma-tO-krit, **hem**-a-tO-krit) (n) a measure of the packed cell volume of red cells

hemifocal
(hem-i-**fO**-kal) (adj) refers to half of the body; usually a type of seizure

hemiparesis
(hem-ee-pa-**ree**-sis, hem-ee-**par**-e-sis) (n) muscular weakness of one half of the body

hemoglobin
(hee-mO-**glO**-bin) (n) the iron-containing pigment of the red blood cells

hepatosplenomegaly
(**hep**-a-tO-**meg**-a-lee, hee-**pat**-O-**meg**-a-lee) (n) enlargement of both liver and spleen

hippocampus
(hip-O-**kam**-pus) (n) structure within the brain

hydrocephalus
(hI-drO-**sef**-a-lus) (n) an excessive accumulation of fluid in the brain

hyperreflexia
(**hI**-pur-re-**flek**-see-a) (n) condition in which deep tendon reflexes are abnormally strong

hypometabolism
(**hI**-pO-me-**tab**-O-lizm) (n) lowered metabolism

ichthyosis
(ik-thee-**O**-sis) (n) condition in which the skin is dry and scaly, resembling fish skin

ictal
(**ik**-tal) (adj) referring to the onset of a seizure

icteric
(ik-**ter**-ik) pertaining to jaundice

interictal
(in-ter-**ik**-tal) (adj) between seizures

ischemia
(is-**kee**-mee-a) (n) decreased blood supply due to obstruction, such as narrowing of the blood vessels

lethargy
(**leth**-ar-jee) (n) state of sluggishness, stupor, unresponsiveness

lobectomy
(lO-**bek**-tO-mee) (n) surgical procedure in which a lobe is removed (thyroid, brain, liver, and lungs are divided into lobes)

lymphadenopathy
(**lim**-phad-e-**nop**-a-thee) (n) disease of the lymph nodes

medulla oblongata
(me-**dool**-a ob-long-**gah**-ta) (n) the lowest part of the brain, connecting to the spinal cord; contains the cardiac, vasomotor, and respiratory centers of the brain

meninges
(me-**nin**-jeez) (n) membranes covering the brain and spinal cord

meningitis
(men-in-**jI**-tis) (n) inflammation of the membranes of the brain or spinal cord

meningocele
(me-**ning**-gO-seel) (n) protrusion of the brain or spinal cord through a defect in the skull or spinal column

mesial
(**mee**-zee-al; **mes**-ee-al) (adj) situated toward the midline of the body or the central part of an organ or tissue (also called medial)

myasthenia gravis
(mI-as-**thee**-nee-a **grav**-is) (n) a chronic progressive muscular weakness, beginning usually in the face and throat, due to a defect in the conduction of nerve impulses

nausea
(**naw**-zee-a, **naw**-zha) (n) an inclination to vomit

neoplastic
(nee-O-**plas**-tik) (adj) pertaining to the nature of new, abnormal tissue formation; usually refers to cancer

neuralgia
(noo-**ral**-jee-a) (n) pain of a severe, throbbing, or stabbing character along the course of a nerve

neurapraxia
(noor-a-**prak**-see-a) (n) loss of conduction in a nerve without structural degeneration

neurasthenia
(noor-as-**thee**-nee-a) (n) a condition, commonly accompanying or following depression, characterized by fatigue believed to be brought on by psychological factors

neurilemma
(noor-i-**lem**-a) (n) a cell that enfolds one or more axons of the peripheral nervous system

neuron
(**noor**-on) (n) nerve cell; the morphological and functional unit of the nervous system, consisting of the nerve cell body, the dendrites, and the axon

neuropathy
(noo-**rop**-a-thee) (n) disorder affecting the cranial or spinal nerves

nuchal
(**noo**-kal) (adj) pertaining to the neck, or nucha (nape of neck)

nystagmus
(nis-**tag**-mus) (n) involuntary, rhythmic oscillation of the eyeballs

palsy
(**pawl**-zee) (n) an abnormal condition characterized by partial paralysis

parietal
(pa-**rI**-e-tal) (adj) relating to the inner walls of a body cavity; a section (lobe) of the brain

peripheral nervous system
(per-**if**-er-al) (n) portion of nervous system that connects the CNS to other body parts

petit mal
(pe-**tee** mahl) (n) a type of seizure characterized by a brief blackout of consciousness with minor rhythmic movements, seen especially in children

phonation
(fO-**nay**-shun) (n) process of uttering vocal sounds

pia mater
(**pI**-a **may**-ter/**pee**-a **mah**-ter) (n) the innermost of the three membranes surrounding the brain and spinal cord; it carries a rich supply of blood vessels

pineal gland
(**pin**-ee-al) (n) small, cone-shaped gland in the brain thought to secrete melatonin

pituitary gland
(pi-**too**-i-tayr-ee) (n) gland suspended from the base of the hypothalamus

plantar
(**plan**-tar) (adj) relating to the undersurface (sole) of the foot; a reflex

plexus
(**plek**-sus) (n) a network of intersecting nerves and blood vessels or of lymphatic vessels

postictal
(pOst-**ik**-tal) (adj) relating to the period following a seizure

pronator
(**prO**-nay-ter, **prO**-nay-tOr) (n) muscle that moves a part into the prone position

proprioception
(**prO**-pree-O-**sep**-shun) (n) sensation due to receiving stimuli from muscles, tendons, or other internal tissues which provides a sense of movement and position of the body

proton
(**prO**-ton) (n) a positively charged particle that is a fundamental component of the nucleus of all atoms; used in radiotherapy

psychosomatic
(**sI**-kO-sO-mat-ik) (adj) relating to the influence of the mind upon the functions of the body

quadriceps
(**kwah**-dri-seps) (adj) four-headed, as a quadriceps muscle; one of the extensor muscles of the legs

quadriparesis
(kwod-ri-pa-**ree**-sis) (n) paralysis of both arms and both legs

radiculopathy
(ra-**dik**-yoo-**lop**-a-thee) (n) disease of the spinal nerve roots

refractory
(ree-frak-tO-ree) (adj) obstinate, stubborn; resistant to ordinary treatment

reticulocyte
(re-**tik**-yoo-lO-sIt) (n) a red blood cell containing a network of granules representing an immature stage in development

retina
(**ret**-i-na) (n) a 10-layered, delicate nervous tissue membrane of the eye that receives images of external objects and transmits visual impulses through the optic nerve to the brain

sagittal
(**saj**-i-tal) (adj) relating to a line from front to back in the middle of an organ or the body

sciatica
(sI-**at**-i-ka) (n) pain in the lower back and hip radiating down the back of the thigh into the leg, usually due to herniated lumbar disk

sclera
(**skleer**-a) (n) a tough white fibrous tissue that covers the so-called white of the eye

shunt
(shunt) (v) to turn away from; to divert

sickle cell anemia
(**sik**-l sel a-**nee**-mee-a) (n) hereditary blood disease in which abnormal hemoglobin causes red blood cells to become sickle-shaped, fragile and nonfunctional, leading to many acute and chronic complications

sphenoidal
(sfee-**noy**-dal) (adj) concerning the sphenoid bone

subdural hematoma
(sub-**doo**-ral hee-ma-**tO**-ma/hem-a-**tO**-ma) (n) an accumulation of blood under the dura mater surrounding the brain

syncopal
(**sin**-kO-pal) (adj) relating to fainting

syncope
(**sin**-ko-pee) (n) fainting

temporal
(**tem**-po-ral) (adj) pertaining to the temple of the head or the corresponding lobe of the brain

thecal
(**thee**-kal) (adj) referring to a covering or enclosure

thrombosis
(throm-**bO**-sis) (n) condition in which a blood clot forms within a blood vessel

uvula
(**yoo**-vyoo-la) (n) small, fleshy mass hanging from the soft palate in the mouth

ventricle
(**ven**-tri-kl) (n) either of the two lower chambers of the heart; areas of the brain that produce and drain cerebrospinal fluid (CSF)

Abbreviations

ADHD	attention deficit hyperactivity disorder	HNP	herniated nucleus pulposus
ALS	amyotrophic lateral sclerosis	LP	lumbar puncture
ANS	autonomic nervous system	MRI	magnetic resonance imaging
CAT or CT	computerized axial tomography	MS	multiple sclerosis
CNS	central nervous system	PD	Parkinson disease
CP	cerebral palsy	PET	positron emission tomography
CSF	cerebrospinal fluid	PNS	peripheral nervous system
CVA	cerebrovascular accident	SNS	somatic nervous system
DTR	deep tendon reflexes	SPECT	single photon emission computed tomography
EEG	electroencephalogram or electroencephalography	TIA	transient ischemic attack

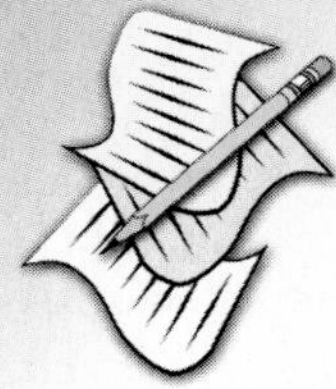

EXERCISE 13.1

Recognizing Look-Alikes and Sound-Alikes

Below is a list of frequently used words that look alike and/or sound alike. Study the meaning and pronunciation of each set of words, then read the following sentences carefully and circle the word in parentheses that correctly completes the meaning.

workup	(n) an intensive diagnostic study
work up	(v) to produce by mental or physical work
clinch	(v) confirm, ensure
clench	(n) fist, vise
clench	(v) clasp, clutch
conscience	(n) the sense of right and wrong
conscious	(adj) aware
pair	(n) two, couple
pare	(v) peel, scrape
pear	(n) fruit
radicle	(n) a nerve or vessel branch that joins others to form larger vessels or nerves
radical	(adj) aimed at the origin of a disease or condition; complete, as in surgical excision
there	(adv) in that place
their	(possessive pronoun) belonging to
they're	(contraction) they are
crisis	(n, sing) turning point
crises	(n, pl) turning points
hemifacial	half of the face
hemifocal	refers to half of the body; usually a type of seizure
recession	the withdrawal of a part from its normal position
resection	the cutting out of a portion of an organ
regression	a return to an earlier condition
repression	restraint
remission	partial or total disappearance of a disease

1. Because he did not take good care of his teeth, he now has (recession, regression, repression) of the gums.
2. He is suffering jaw pain because of frequent teeth (clenching, clinching).
3. Within two hours of surgery, the patient became (conscience, conscious).
4. I used a (pair, pare, pear) of tweezers to remove the splinter.
5. The surgeon had to (pair, pare, pear) the nerve from the bone.
6. She is suffering from situational depression precipitated by several (crisis, crises) in her life.
7. After experiencing severe trauma to the lower spine, the patient underwent (radical, radicle) surgery.
8. (Their, There, They're) children are both in college now.
9. The patient frequently suffered (hemifacial, hemifocal) seizures.
10. We are thankful his leukemia is now in (regression, remission, repression).

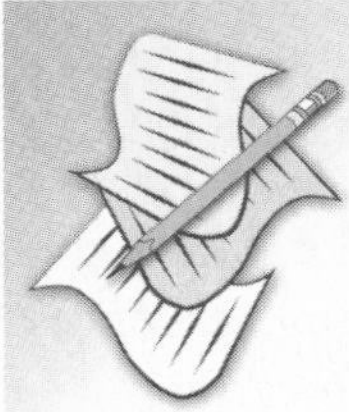

EXERCISE 13.2

Matching Sound and Spelling

The numbered list that follows shows the phonetic spelling of hard-to-spell words. Sound out the word, then write the correct spelling in the blank space provided. Each of the words can be found in the Glossary or in the drug list in Appendix D.

1. **sin**-ko-pee ______________________
2. ra-**dik**-yoo-**lop**-a-thee______________________
3. **naw**-zee-a/**naw**-zha ______________________
4. **noor**-on ______________________
5. me-**nin**-jeez ______________________
6. noor-as-**thee**-nee-a ______________________
7. a-**fay**-zee-a ______________________
8. noo-**ral**-jee-a ______________________
9. pe-**tee** mahl ______________________
10. **sI**-kO-sO-**mat**-ik ______________________
11. me-**ning**-gO-seel ______________________
12. pi-**too**-i-tayr-ee______________________
13. **ser**-e-brO-**spI**-nal/se-**ree**-brO-**spI**-nal______________________
14. a-**tak**-see-a ______________________

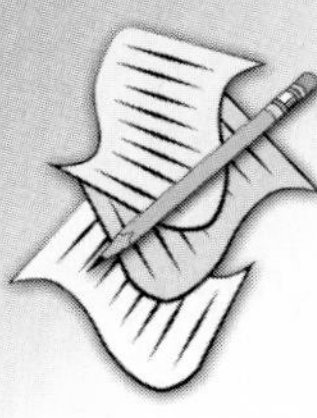

EXERCISE 13.3

Choosing Words from Context

When transcribing dictation, the medical transcriptionist frequently needs to consider the situation when determining the word that correctly completes the sentence. From the list below, select the term that meaningfully completes each of the following statements.

atrophy	cerebrovascular	plantar
hemiparesis	parietal	funduscopic
cerebellar examination	cranium	ventricle
postictal	interictal	clonus

1. The brain is found within the ____________________.
2. There was marked ______________________ after the stroke.
3. The ____________________ section of the brain was affected by the cerebrovascular accident.
4. The neurologic exam was normal, including ___________ flexion, a negative Babinski sign.
5. Increased intracranial pressure can be visualized by ____________ examination with the ophthalmoscope.
6. ______________________________ is best performed by having the patient walk down the hallway to see if there is any ataxia.
7. The radiation therapy caused a small amount of______________ of the parietal area of the brain.
8. Between seizures, the woman had a (an) ____________________ period where she slept for a few minutes.
9. There was a blockage of the right _______________ in the brain caused by a cystic lesion, most likely benign.
10. The 72-year-old man had a (an) ____________________ accident which caused him to have left-sided hemiparesis.
11. The patient had marked ____________________ of the left arm as an effect of the cerebral palsy.
12. The ____________________ phase of his seizures is always determined by his deep sleep.

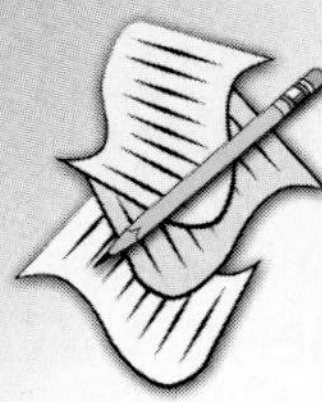

EXERCISE 13.4

Pairing Words and Meanings

From this list, locate the term that best matches each of the following definitions. Write the letter of the term in the space provided by each definition.

A. adenopathy
B. cerebrovascular
C. cyanosis
D. epileptiform
E. hemifocal palsy
F. icteric
G. retina
H. sagittal
I. thrombosis
J. uvula

1. an abnormal condition characterized by paralysis, aphasia, or amnesia ____________
2. the plane from front to back in the middle of an organ or body ____________
3. small structure hanging from soft palate in mouth ____________
4. formation of a blood clot within a blood vessel ____________
5. enlarged lymph nodes ____________
6. bluish discoloration of skin resulting from diminished supply of oxygen in blood ____________
7. having the form of epilepsy ____________
8. pertaining to jaundice ____________
9. pertaining to blood vessels of brain ____________
10. membrane of the eye that receives images and transmits visual impulses through the optic nerve to the brain ____________

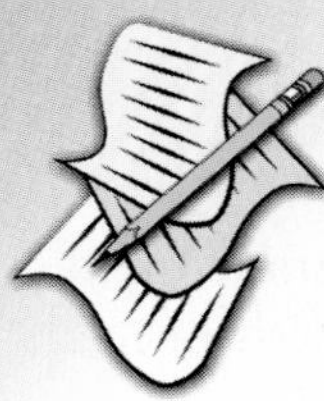

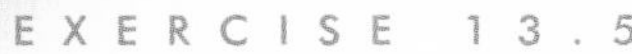

EXERCISE 13.5

Creating Terms from Word Forms

Combine prefixes, root words, and suffixes from this list to create medical words that fit the following definitions. Fill in the blanks with the words you construct.

cephal/o	head	ventricul/o	ventricle
cerebell/o	cerebellum	ictal	onset, as in a stroke or seizure
cerebr/o	cerebrum	neur/o	nerve
crani/o	cranium	path/o	disease
encephal/o	brain	somi	body, body of a cell
hemi-	half, slight	somni-	sleep
inter-	between	-itis	inflammation
mening/o	membrane	-lepsy	seizure
myel/o	spinal cord	-otomy	incision
para-	beside, abnormal; alongside	-paresis	minor paralysis
poly-	two or more, many	-plegia	paralysis
post-	after		

1. partial paralysis ________________
2. inflammation of brain tissue ________________
3. a sleep disorder ________________
4. paralysis of the lower extremities ________________
5. between seizures ________________
6. inflammation of the membrane(s) of the brain or spinal cord ________________
7. inflammation of large number of nerves ________________
8. following a seizure ________________
9. paralysis on one side ________________
10. inflammation of spinal cord ________________
11. cutting into the brain ________________
12. incision into the ventricle of the brain ________________

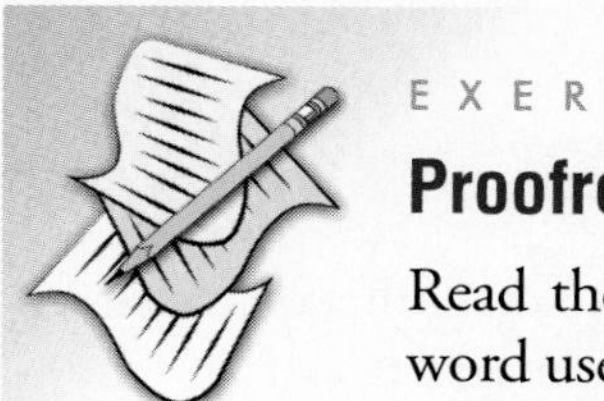

EXERCISE 13.6

Proofreading Review

Read the following emergency department note and look for errors in punctuation, word use, capitalization, spelling, and abbreviations. Then key the report with all errors corrected.

DOB: 3/29/56

ADMISSION DIAGNOSIS: LOC, drug OD.

HPI: The patient is a 40 y.o. female who was found blue in the face and unconscious by family this a.m. This occurred approximately 10 to 15 minutes after she had injected a line of heroin IV. Reportedly her son started CPR and she gasped for breath. Fire department arrived and administered Narcan.

The patient now complains of headache. She reports that she has not used heroin for several months. The family reports that she does heroin 4-5 x/week.

PMH: Seizure disorder, epilepsy since childhood. IVDA x 10 yrs.

MEDICATIONS: Percocet for migraine HAs, Dilantin, and Phenobarbital.

ALLERGIES: NKDA.

PHYSICAL EXAMINATION: A WDWN Caucasian female in NAD, awake, alert, oriented. HEENT: PERRLA; EOMI. Speech clear, respirations unlabored. Lungs clear to P&A. Heart: RRR. She follows instructions appropriately and moves all extremities. DTRs are symmetric.

ER COURSE: The patient was examined as above. She will be observed for another hour, and if she maintains her present level of consciousness, plan to DC to home with appropriate instructions.

ASSESSMENT: Heroin overdose.

PLAN: The patient is to be referred to the mental health unit for addiction counseling. She should continue with her Dilantin and Phenobarb and follow-up with her family M.D.

Building Transcription Skills

The Neuropsychological Evaluation

Neuropsychological evaluations or reports (Figure 13.7) contain information on patients seen in a clinic or hospital setting. A psychologist or neurologist dictates the report. The purpose of the report is to document a patient's history, mental status, assessment, and previous treatment to assist with planning care and treatment. The language on these reports includes terms related to neuropsychological development, human behavior, and treatment.

Required Headings/Content Typically, the information is provided in narrative format. Content includes a history of the present illness followed by the findings of both physical and neurologic examinations. The dictator may omit report headings. Sometimes, only neurologic information is included, along with the results of specific developmental and neurologic tests.

Turnaround Time If the patient is admitted to a hospital, the report is usually dictated and transcribed within the first 24 hours of admission. In clinic settings, the report may be dictated and transcribed within 48 hours.

Preparing to Transcribe

To prepare for transcribing dictation, review the tables of common neurology terms, drugs, and abbreviations presented in the Building Language Skills section of this chapter. Then, study the format and organization of the model document shown in Figure 13.7, and key the model document. Proofread the document by comparing it with the printed version. Categorize the types of errors you made, and document them on a copy of the Performance Comparison chart provided in Chapter 1. A template of this chart is included on the IRC that accompanies this text.

Patient Studies

Transcribe, edit, and correct each report in the following patient studies. Consult reference books for words or formatting rules that are unfamiliar.

As you work on the transcription assignment for this chapter, fill in the Performance Comparison chart that you started when you keyed the model document. For at least three of the reports, categorize and document the types of errors you made. Answer the document analysis questions on the bottom of the chart. With continuous practice and assessment, the quality of your work will improve.

After you have produced a final version of each transcribed report, complete the Performance Report cover sheet, attach it to the top of the transcripts, and submit them to your instructor for evaluation.

1" margins and left justification

RE: Rightman, Aaron
DOB: 8/30/XX
DOV: 7/10/XX

double-space

Aaron Rightman, age 7 years 10 months, was seen for a pediatric neurologic assessment on July 10. The parents were the informants. The reason for this visit was for a "second opinion." Aaron has been diagnosed as having a learning disability with an attention deficit disorder.

At 2 years of age it was noted that Aaron had articulation difficulties and delayed expressive language. He was given speech therapy. At 3 years of age he was placed in a preschool program for the handicapped. He had no problems socially and began to do well. At that time the school recommended that he attend a regular nursery school. Aaron was enrolled in the synagogue nursery school at the age of 4. He soon developed encopresis. The parents characterized Aaron's school experiences as being "a disaster." He began to exhibit poor attention, anger, and hostility. When he reached the age of 5, he was placed in a day school, which was also attended by his friends from nursery school. By this time he was "already viewed as a bad child by the other children."

Aaron recently completed second grade at the day school. There he received tutoring on a one-to-one basis. He was also seen by a learning disability expert twice a week. He had speech and language therapy one-half hour per week. He is still reading below grade level.

In March, Aaron had a neurobehavioral evaluation. It was noted that Aaron was "functioning within the High Average range perceptually and in the Very Superior range verbally." However, there was a 22-point disparity between his verbal and nonverbal abilities. He did best when he "was able to communicate verbally." His cognitive strengths included "word fluency and word knowledge, practical knowledge, common sense, and paper/pencil skills. Cognitive weaknesses included shifting of mental set, visual discrimination, visual searching, nonverbal deductive reasoning, and analysis/synthesis." The evaluators thought that Aaron did have an attention deficit hyperactive disorder syndrome and they noticed that he was a child with "poor phonological awareness, was unable to process certain sounds quickly enough, and encountered problems holding language sounds in short-term memory and manipulating them in active working memory. It is hard for him to break

(continued)

FIGURE 13.7
Neuropsychological Evaluation

NEUROPSYCHOLOGICAL EVALUATION
RE: Rightman, Aaron
DATE: 7/11/XX
Page 2

words down into their component sounds and reblend them or try to substitute a new sound for an existing one in a word."

Family history reveals that the father has reading problems. A paternal uncle has ADD. A paternal cousin is in a special education class and is said to have a learning disability and ADD. The mother's cousin has ADD. There is no family history of tics or obsessive-compulsive habits. There are 3 siblings—a 12-year-old and a 4-year-old are doing well. Daniel, who is 10, has mild learning difficulties and ADHD symptoms.

Aaron entered the examining room while his parents waited outside. He appeared to be anxious about the exam since there were 3 other observers in the room with me. Initially, he was very subdued and almost sad. However, he answered questions appropriately and showed no evidence of an activity disturbance. He is poorly oriented to left and right on himself and in space. When he copied geometric forms, he exhibited visual/motor integration difficulties, putting "ears" on the diamond figure. When he was given the Boder test for dyslexia, he had marked trouble spelling words which are in his sight vocabulary. From the screening test, he seemed to me to have a combination of dyseidetic-dysphonetic difficulties.

His height of 130 cm was in the 80th percentile; his weight of 26.6 kg was in the 60th percentile, and his head circumference of 52 cm was in the 50th percentile.

Head and neck were benign. Lungs were clear to percussion and auscultation. Heart—regular sinus rhythm, no murmurs. Abdomen—soft and nontender, liver and spleen not palpable. Genitalia—testes in scrotal sac. Tanner 1. Skin revealed mild ichthyosis over the dorsum of his legs. Skeletal was negative. There were no dysmorphic features.

On neurologic exam, Aaron's head was of normal shape. He had a single whorl on the right. He tracked well. He did have difficulty with rapidly moving his tongue from side to side. He could not isolate the tongue movement from movement of his jaw. The remainder of the cranial nerves were normal. Visual fields by confrontation were normal. Vision and hearing

(continued)

FIGURE 13.7
Neuropsychological Evaluation (Continued)

NEUROPSYCHOLOGICAL EVALUATION
RE: Rightman, Aaron
DATE: 7/11/XX
Page 3

were grossly normal. The tone of his muscles was normal. Fine and gross coordination was normal. Deep tendon reflexes were physiologic. Plantars were flexor. There was no clonus. He had some immature overflow phenomenon and a slightly positive Prechtl sign. He is right-handed. He held a pencil well.

In summary, Aaron has many symptoms of minimal cerebral dysfunction, which is probably on a genetic basis. These symptoms include: (1) a learning disability, primarily involving reading, which grossly appears to be the dyseidetic-dyskinetic type, (2) an attention deficit hyperactivity disorder, which is responding well to Dexedrine, (3) a vocal tic, which may be a precursor to developing Tourette syndrome, and (4) immature motor signs, as noted on the Prechtl, and overflow phenomenon. I think that Aaron's regression 6 months ago may reflect overt depression, which may still be present.

Therapeutically speaking, I think the parents are doing everything possible to help this young man. There is no question that he belongs in a psychotherapeutic relationship. I am assuming that the tricyclic antidepressant is being given for his depressive symptoms. (The parents think that this is helping.) The Dexedrine is effective for the ADHD symptoms. Personally, if his weight loss continues, I would suggest not using the sustained release form but, rather, giving him a dose in the morning, at noon, and at 4 p.m., and this should be given before meals.

I told the parents that they should not put too much stress on Aaron's academic learning, but look for activities where he might be successful, which would make him feel good about himself.

I also told them that I would discuss Aaron's case with Dr. Balla, a research educator who is utilizing a specific therapy for children who have problems with auditory processing. I promised to send the reports of the neuropsychological evaluation and my reports to Dr. Balla to see if she would be interested in seeing Aaron.

qs

____

Lawrence Trent, MD
Professor of Pediatrics

(continued)

FIGURE 13.7
Neuropsychological Evaluation (Continued)

NEUROPSYCHOLOGICAL EVALUATION
RE: Rightman, Aaron
DATE: 7/11/XX
Page 4
ds
LTT/XX
ds
C: Dr. L. Balla
ds
D: 7/11/XX
T: 7/12/XX

FIGURE 13.7
Neuropsychological Evaluation (Continued)

Patient Study 13.A — Brian Brendon

Brian Brendon is a 31-year-old gentleman who was diagnosed with a pineal region tumor 1 year prior to this visit. He had suffered dizzy spells, difficulty walking, and headaches for a month prior to his diagnosis. He was referred to Dr. Stone, who placed a ventricular shunt in the right ventricle to relieve the increased pressure caused by the tumor. He was then treated with chemotherapy and cranial irradiation. He is having an MRI of the brain as a follow-up study at the completion of his therapy.

REPORT 13.1 MRI Brain Scan

Patient Study 13.B — Michelle Kuvell

Michelle Kuvell is a 7-year-old girl diagnosed with a brain tumor arising in the brainstem. She has been treated with radiation therapy and chemotherapy. She is visiting the neurologist for continuing followup in the office.

REPORT 13.2 Consultation Letter

- The radiation therapy dosages should be transcribed as 120 cGy and 6480 Gy.

Patient Study 13.C — Michael Wright

Michael Wright is a 40-year-old male with a history of complex partial seizures for the past 23 years. Although he is taking Dilantin and Mysoline, his seizures have occurred more frequently in recent months. He was admitted to the hospital for evaluation and subsequently underwent a left anterior temporal lobectomy.

REPORT 13.3 Discharge Summary

- Listen for these terms and drug names:
  semiology
  Vicodin
  Decadron taper

Patient Study 13.D — Aaron Rightman

Seven-year-old Aaron Rightman has been diagnosed previously as having a learning disability with an attention deficit disorder. His parents have requested an evaluation and a second opinion by Dr. Lawrence Trent.

REPORT 13.4 Neuropsychological Evaluation

- Listen for these abbreviations and terms:
  ADD (attention deficit disorder)
  ADHD (attention deficit hyperactivity disorder)
  Boder test
  dyseidetic-dysphonetic difficulties
  encopresis
  whorl
  clonus
  Prechtl sign
  Tourette syndrome

Patient Study 13.E — Joseph Drinkowski

Joe Drinkowski is a 21-year-old man who has been experiencing episodes of involuntary contractions of his right arm followed by involuntary "shaking" of his legs. There are no other symptoms of seizures.

REPORT 13.5 History and Physical

- Listen for these terms:
  pronator drift
  proprioception

Patient Study 13.F — Tanisha Wilder

Tanisha Wilder is a 14-year-old child who has a history of sickle cell anemia. She has had multiple admissions for sickle cell crises and other complications related to sickle cell. She was admitted to the hospital with a history of confusion, lethargy, and inability to speak clearly.

REPORT 13.6 Discharge Summary

- Listen for these terms and drug names:
  Pen Vee-K
  Hib and Pneumovax vaccine
  reticulocyte
- Note that a primary physician name is supplied in the patient information section, but another physician has dictated the report.

Patient Study 13.G — Bryan Charles

Bryan Charles is a 5-year-old boy who has been diagnosed with a recurring primary brain sarcoma. He has had chemotherapy, a bone marrow transplant, and radiation therapy following surgery. His parents brought him to the Institute for the Study of Child Development for a neuropsychological evaluation.

REPORT 13.7 Neuropsychological Evaluation

- Test results for the Stanford-Binet Intelligence Scale should be transcribed in columnar form. List the subtests in the first column, the SAS (Standard Age Score) in the second column, and the percentile rank in the third column. The test includes four subtests (verbal reasoning, abstract/visual reasoning, quantitative reasoning, and short-term memory) and a composite score. Each subtest is further divided into parts, the names of which should be indented.

Using Medical References

Use the appropriate medical reference to locate the correct spelling and additional usage information for the words below. (If the reference is not available, use the glossary in this text.) Circle the correct spelling, then write a sentence using the word correctly.

1.	neurapathy	nueropathy	neuropathy
2.	neuropraxia	neuroproxia	neurapraxia
3.	hyereflexia	hyperreflexia	hyperefflexia
4.	neurilemma	neurolemma	neuralemma
5.	nuron	neuron	nueron
6.	sciatica	scyatica	sciattica
7.	Babinsky	Babinskey	Babinski
8.	meninges	meningies	menenges
9.	proprioception	propriaception	proprioseption
10.	quadraparesis	quadreparesis	quadriparesis
11.	nuchle	mukel	nuchal
12.	assymetry	asymmetry	asimetry

Assessing Transcription Skills

Making Expert Decisions

Circle the correct word from the choices in parentheses.

1. The patient fell asleep for 15 minutes after the seizure, when he was in a (an) (ictal/interictal/postictal) state.
2. The patient was alert and (conscience/conscious) at the time of my examination.
3. At discharge, the physicians recommended nursing home placement, but the family said (their/they/they're) willing to provide care for the patient.
4. The skin graft healed, but the plastic surgeon wants to (pair/pare/pear) down the surface after the swelling goes down.
5. The smallest branch of a nerve is called a (radical/radicle).
6. The dura mater is on top (of/off) the arachnoid.
7. "I was never more embarrassed," said the transcriptionist in training, "than when I transcribed (fecal/thecal) sac, rather than (fecal/thecal) sac, on the pathology report."
8. The thumb and fingers had good (apposition/opposition) when placed tip to tip.
9. An (excision/incision) was made into the subcutaneous tissue.
10. The patient stopped taking her medications and started to (recess/regress/repress), going back to a time when she felt safe and secure.

Transcribing Professional Documents

Transcribe the document named Chapter 13 Assessment. Before you key, review the appropriate document formatting guidelines. Proofread your transcribed document and revise it until you think it is error-free.

Hematology-Oncology 14

Hematology is the field of medicine devoted to diagnosing and treating diseases of the blood and blood-forming tissues. Oncology is the study and treatment of all kinds of cancers. Since many blood-related diseases are malignancies and since the blood is one of the means by which many cancers spread, the subspecialties of hematology and oncology are often combined in one practice. The physician who specializes in these areas is called a hematologist-oncologist.

OBJECTIVES

- Use hematology-oncology terms correctly according to the context and purpose of the dictation.
- Select and use appropriate general and specialty reference materials.
- Key hematology-oncology documents of varying complexity and format.
- Transcribe authentic medical dictation requiring concentration and listening skill.
- Edit medical reports to conform with AAMT style guidelines.
- Proofread and correct transcripts to produce error-free documents.

Exploring Hematology-Oncology

The word *hematology* is derived from the Greek word *haima,* for blood. The term cancer was first used by the Greek physician Hippocrates as a metaphor for the spreading tendency of the disease. He compared metastases to the tentacles of a crab. Cancer is Latin for "crab." Cancer is indeed frightening because of the destruction it causes within the body. Though life-threatening, many adult cancers and approximately 80 percent of pediatric cancers are curable today.

Structure and Function

Blood cells are produced in the bone marrow in a process called hematopoiesis. Bone marrow is found in the center of bones, particularly flat bones. Hematopoiesis begins with a pluripotential stem cell which is capable of becoming any type of blood cell. The types of blood cells and the phases of differentiation that they pass through as they mature are illustrated in Figure 14.1.

Blood has many components (Figure 14.2). The major kinds of blood cells are white blood cells, red blood cells, and platelets. These cells are suspended in the plasma portion of blood, which also contains proteins, such as albumin, immunoglobulins, and fibrinogen. Blood cells provide a vehicle for the transport of nutrients, gases, hormones, electrolytes, and cellular waste products. Table 14.1 lists blood cells by their type and function.

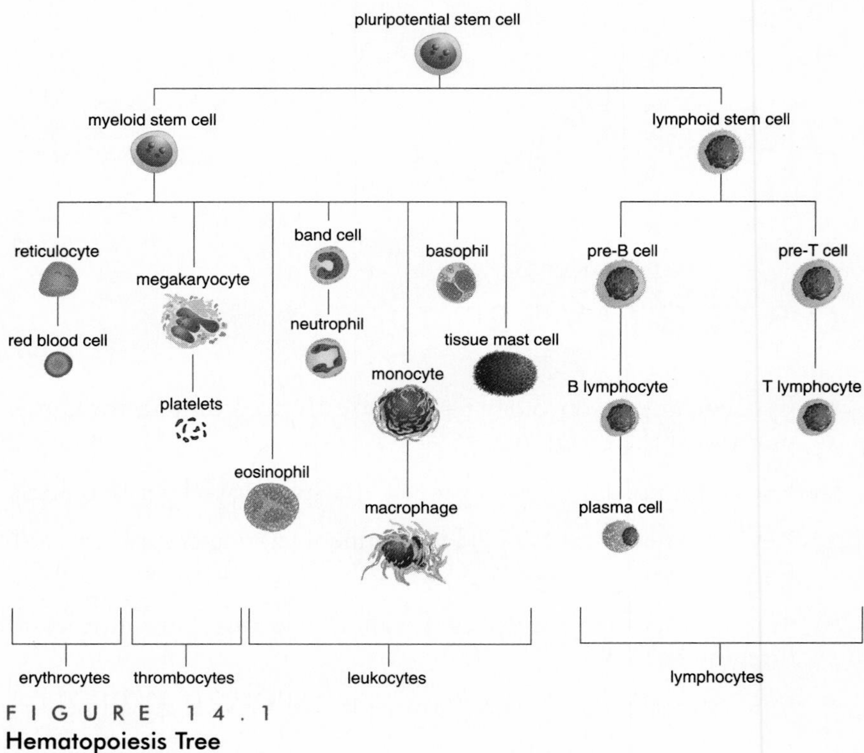

FIGURE 14.1
Hematopoiesis Tree

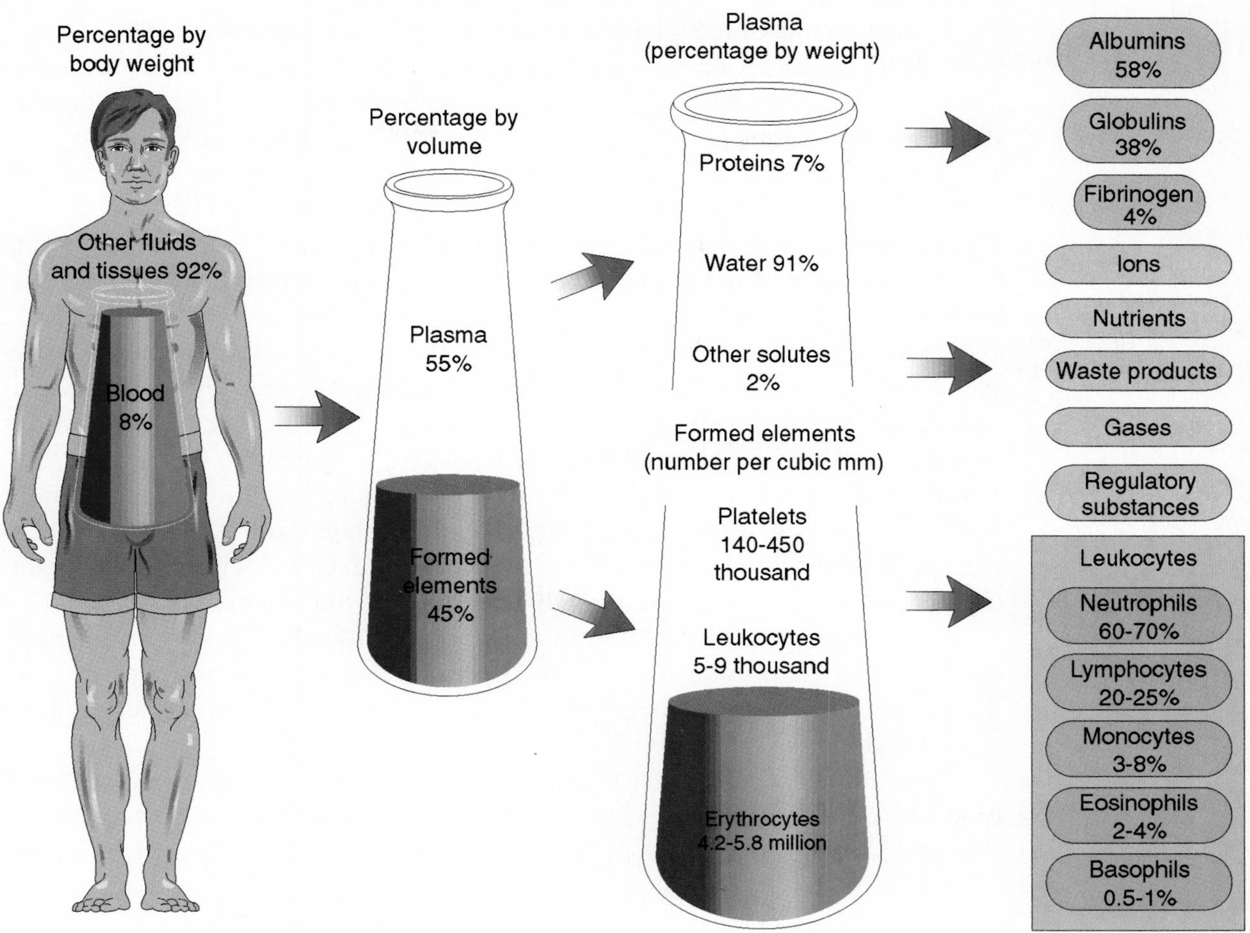

FIGURE 14.2
Components of Blood

TABLE 14.1 Types of Blood Cells

Cell Type	Function
red blood cells (RBCs)	carry oxygen to cells
white blood cells (WBCs)	fight invading substances such as bacteria and viruses
neutrophils	set up immune defenses
eosinophils	defend against parasites and allergic responses
basophils	involved in inflammatory response
lymphocytes	produce antibodies (B) create cellular immunity (T)
monocytes	set up immune defenses
platelets	promote blood clotting after injury

The membranes of red blood cells contain a variety of antigens, called agglutinogens, that have become attached in a process called agglutination. The presence or absence of these antigens is a major factor in blood typing. Blood typing is done to determine the specific blood type the person has inherited from both parents.

There are four major blood types: A, B, AB, and O. Individuals whose red cells carry only one antigen, A, are considered type A; those whose red cells carry antigen B are categorized as type B; and individuals carrying neither antigen are called group O. A small group of people have type AB blood, which means their red cells have both the A and B antigens.

Red blood cells may also carry Rh antigens (D, C, E, e, and c). People who carry the D antigen are called Rh-positive. Those who do not are called Rh-negative. This designation is added to the blood type. Thus, a person with type O blood who is found to be Rh-negative would be classified as type O negative.

One method of blood typing is the slide test (Figure 14.3), in which a drop or two of the patient's blood is placed on each end of a slide. Anti-A serum is added to one end and anti-B to the other. If antigen is present in either of the samples, agglutination will occur, and the results will determine the blood type.

If a person is given a blood transfusion of an incompatible blood type, a dangerous hemolytic transfusion reaction could occur. Table 14.2 lists the occurrence of the various blood types in the population, the agglutinins present in each, and the type(s) of donor blood needed for safe (compatible) transfusions.

Plasma protein factors in the blood work to provide the delicate balance between proper blood clotting and anticlotting. Along a pathway known as a clotting cascade (Figure 14.4), they make important contributions to hemostasis (proper balance of

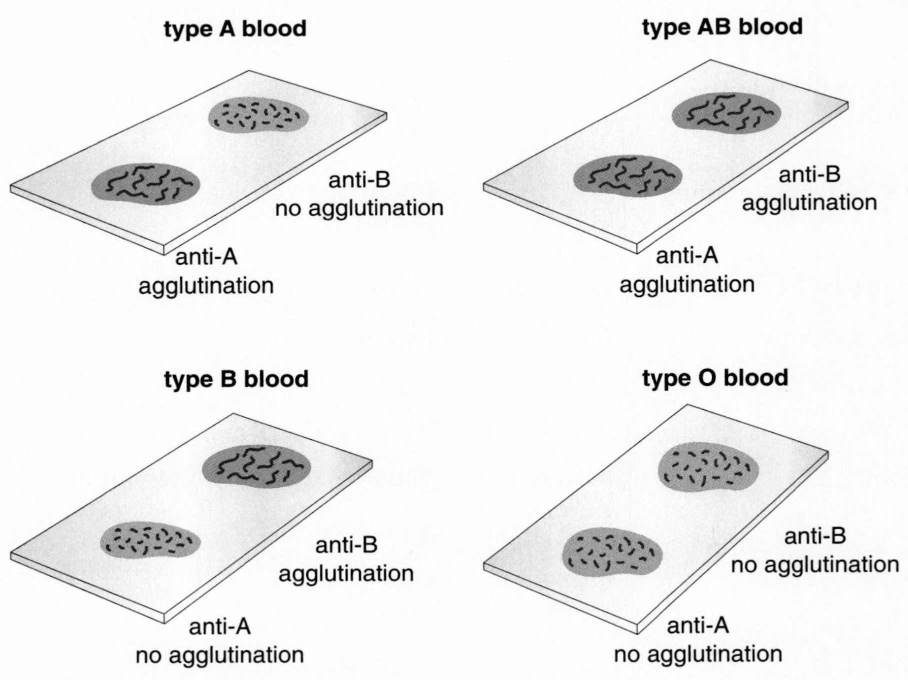

FIGURE 14.3
Blood Typing Based on the Principle of Agglutination

TABLE 14.2 Blood Types and Transfusions

Blood Type	Agglutinins in Plasma	Frequency of Occurrence	Safe Transfusions (may receive)
type A	anti-B	40%	types A, O
type B	anti-A	10%	types B, O
type AB	none	4%	types A, B, AB, O (universal recipient)
type O (universal donor)	anti-A, anti-B	45%	type O
Rh positive	none	85%	should receive Rh-positive blood but may receive Rh-negative blood if necessary
Rh negative	anti-D	15%	may receive only Rh-negative blood

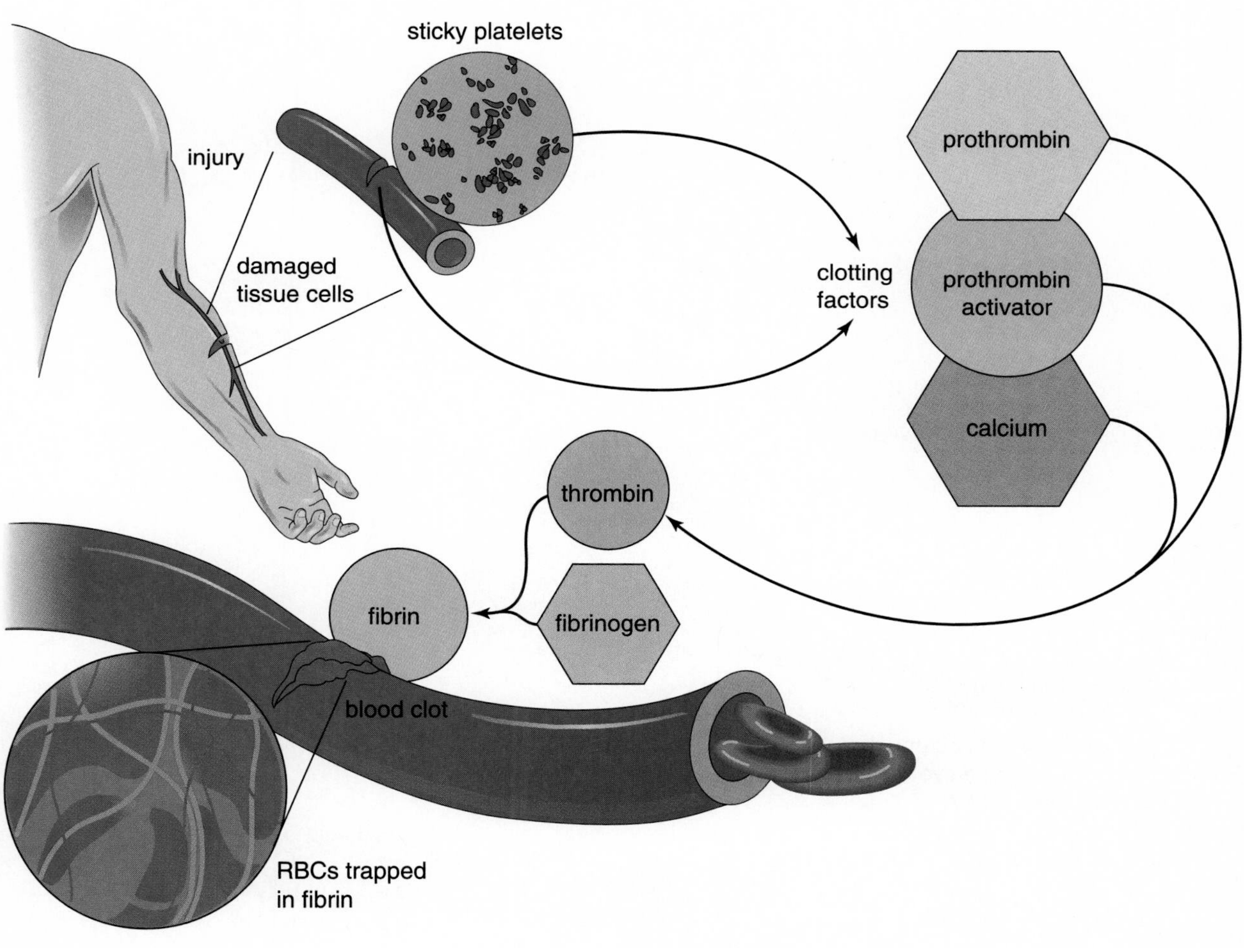

FIGURE 14.4
Blood Clotting Cascade

chemicals in body fluids and tissues). Any abnormality in the clotting cascade can cause problems with clot formation, such as the vaso-occlusive crisis that occurs in sickle-cell anemia (Figure 14.5).

The lymph system works with the blood system to protect the body and remove by-products of cellular processes. Encompassing a network of lymph nodes and vessels plus the spleen, thymus, and tonsils, the lymph system drains fluids from body tissues, particularly waste products, and carries them into the blood.

Cancer is a disease resulting from excessive cell division. Normally, all cells of the body divide and replace themselves in a carefully controlled process. In cancers, the process is disturbed and cell division continues past its normal point. Cancer cells usually do not carry out their intended function. Instead, they eventually invade and overtake normal cells and prevent normal function. There are three main methods for cancer cells to metastasize: (1) by direct extension to surrounding structures; (2) through the lymphatic system; or (3) via the blood system, which is called hematogenous spread.

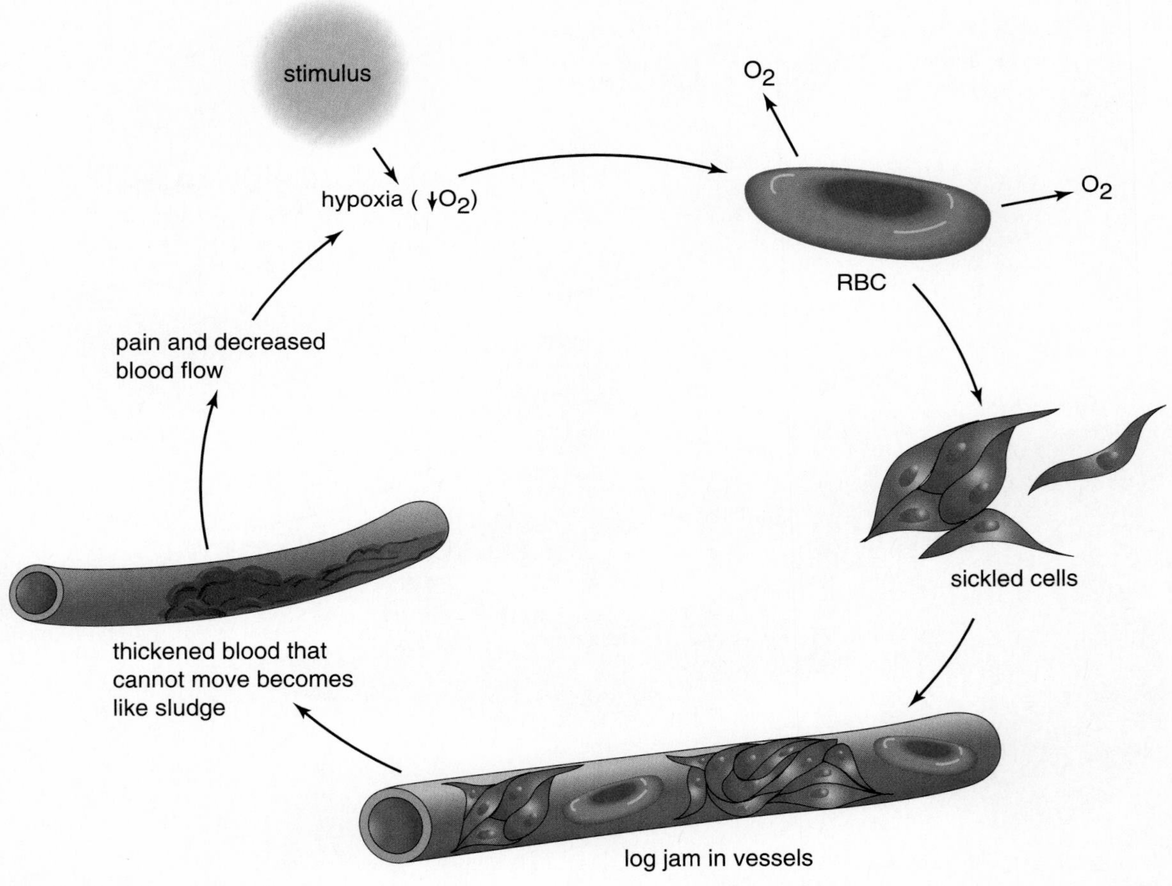

FIGURE 14.5
Vaso-Occlusive Crisis in Sickle Cell Anemia

Physical Assessment

The patient who presents to the hematology-oncology (heme-onc) specialist may be nervous, upset, and often quite ill. The referring physician may have already ordered blood tests that have suggested a blood dyscrasia, hemoglobinopathy, or cancer. Prior x-rays and/or scans may have indicated the possibility of a solid tumor. Sometimes specific symptoms send the person to the hematologist-oncologist. A detailed review of systems and a complete physical examination are essential to planning the patient's care.

Hematologic Diseases and Conditions

Hemophilia is an inherited autosomal disorder that causes bleeding because of the lack of certain clotting factors in the blood.

Sickle cell anemia and thalassemias are inherited hemoglobinopathies that stem from an absence of a globin chain on the red blood cell. Globin chains are named with the letters of the Greek alphabet.

Immune thrombocytopenic purpura (ITP) is characterized by petechiae and ecchymoses as a result of a low platelet count. It is believed that ITP results from a viral organism that has caused the immune system to turn against itself (autoimmune) and coat the platelet cell with an antigen. The body makes antibodies against these antigens, causing the platelets to be destroyed.

Thrombosis is the formation of clots inside the blood vessels rather than in the normal extravascular pathway. Several different kinds of thromboses can occur, including cerebral, coronary, placental, and compression, to name a few. They typically are the result of injury to a vessel wall or reduced blood circulation.

There are several red cell abnormalities that cause hemolysis. These include osmotic fragility, hereditary spherocytosis, and a deficiency of the glucose-6-phosphate dehydrogenase (G6PD) enzyme.

Oncologic Diseases and Conditions

Cancers are classified into two major categories, hematologic tumors and solid tumors. Hematologic tumors involve the blood-forming organs and include lymphomas, leukemias, and multiple myeloma. Solid tumors include sarcomas and carcinomas. Sarcoma describes cancers of the connective tissues, such as muscle, blood vessels, and bone. Carcinomas are subdivided into adenocarcinomas (originating in surface linings of the glands) and squamous cell, or epidermoid, carcinomas (originating in epithelium of a nonglandular nature, such as the surface of the skin or the membranes of the respiratory tract).

Some 90 percent of cancers are solid tumors; 10 percent are hematologic tumors. The leading causes of cancer deaths in adults are lung cancer, colorectal cancer, prostate cancer, and breast cancer. In children, the most prevalent type of cancer is leukemia.

Common Tests, Surgical Procedures, and Treatment Regimens

Methods for treating cancers depend on the specific type of cancer. For solid tumors, the staging or classification is most important for prognosis and treatment. Several classification systems are used, depending on the body area affected. For example, Dukes staging is used for colon cancer, and Jewett staging is used for bladder cancer. The TNM system is the most widely used classification and involves three components and subcategories:

T (T1–T4)	Extent of the primary tumor
N (N0–N3)	Extent of regional lymph node involvement
M (M0–M1)	Presence or absence of distant metastasis

Solid tumors are removed surgically if the tumor is resectable. For hematologic cancers, chemotherapy is usually the first treatment of choice. Another widely used treatment is radiation therapy, which involves directing a radiation beam toward the cancer to rearrange the cellular DNA and kill the cell.

The word *chemotherapy* means chemical therapy and can refer to any pharmacologic agent. However, the term usually refers to the chemical treatment of cancer. Chemotherapeutic agents kill rapidly dividing cells including cancer cells, hair cells, cells of the mucous membranes, and blood cells. The toxicities and side effects associated with chemotherapeutic agents are due to the destruction of the normal cells in these areas. These agents are usually given in combinations and are named with acronyms. The generic name and the brand name may be used to form the acronym. The following list includes some of the most common chemotherapy treatment regimens:

ABV	Adriamycin, bleomycin, vinblastine
CAF	cyclophosphamide, Adriamycin, 5-fluorouracil
CAV	cyclophosphamide, Adriamycin, vincristine
CHOP	cyclophosphamide, hydroxyldaunorubicin, Oncovin, prednisone
COD	cyclophosphamide, Oncovin, DTIC
CytaBOM	cytarabine, bleomycin, Oncovin, methotrexate
DCTER	("doctor") dexamethasone, cytosine arabinoside, thioguanine, etoposide, rubidomycin
DECAL	daunomycin, etoposide, cyclophosphamide, Ara-C, L-asparaginase
FAM	5–fluorouracil, Adriamycin, mitomycin C
HiDAC	("high dak") high dose Ara-C
MACOPB	("May-cop-B") methotrexate, Adriamycin, cyclophosphamide, Oncovin, prednisone, bleomycin
MOPP	mechlorethamine, Oncovin, prednisone, procarbazine
ProMACE	prednisone, methotrexate, Adriamycin, cytarabine, etoposide,
VAD	vincristine, Adriamycin, dexamethasone

Researchers the world over continue to try to find a cure for all cancers. Scientists are experimenting with recombinant DNA technology and biotherapy as well as studying the influence of the mind-body connection, or neuropsychoimmunology. Despite great advances in the treatment of cancer, early detection is still the best weapon against this dreaded disease. Recommended periodic screening methods include breast self-exam (BSE), mammography, prostate exam, and sigmoidoscopy. In addition, certain markers in the blood can predict persons at risk for specific cancers. Those with known genetic risks should be watched closely for the earliest signs of cancer.

Building Language Skills

The following tables list common hematology-oncology terms, drugs, and abbreviations. The list of terms and definitions includes the most difficult words contained in the dictated reports in this chapter. These words are identified in GREEN type. A list of common drugs is found in Appendix D.

Medical Terms and Pharmacologic Agents

additive
(**ad**-i-tiv) (n) a substance which is added in small quantities to improve the qualities of the original

adenopathy
(ad-e-**nop**-a-thee) (n) swelling or enlargement of any gland, especially the lymph nodes

agglutination
(a-gloo-ti-**nay**-shun) (n) the process in which cells group or clump together, especially as a response to a specific antibody; commonly used in blood typing

allogenic
(al-O-**jen**-ik) (adj) describing tissues or cell types that are from different individuals belonging to the same species; describing individuals of the same species

anaphylactic
(**an**-a-fi-**lak**-tik) (adj) describing an allergic hypersensitivity reaction of the body to a substance

apoptosis
(ap-O-**tO**-sis/**ap**-op-**tO**-sis) (n) a cell fragmenting into pieces which are phagocytosed by other cells; programmed cell death

asparaginase
(as-**par**-a-ji-nays) (n) an antineoplastic agent derived from the bacterium *Escherichium coli*

autologous
(aw-**tol**-o-gus) (adj) describing a transplantation where the tissue graft is taken from the same individual receiving it

beta subunit
(**bay**-ta) (n) glycoprotein hormone containing two different polypeptide subunits designated as alpha and beta chains

bilateral
(bI-**lat**-er-al) (adj) affecting or relating to two sides

capillary fragility
(**kap**-i-layr-ee) (n) used in a test to determine the presence of vitamin C deficiency or thrombocytopenia; pressure is applied to the arm, and then the number of petechiae (representing broken capillaries) in a small area are counted

capsular
(**cap**-soo-lar) (adj) pertaining to a sheath of continuous enclosure around an organ or structure

carcinoma
(kar-si-**nO**-ma) (n) a malignant tumor of epithelial cells

cellular
(**sel**-yoo-lar) (adj) composed of or derived from cells

cellular immunity
(n) immunity which is based on the T cells recognizing the antigen itself, rather than the presence of an antibody; cell-mediated immunity

chromic
(**krO**-mik) (adj) relating to or containing chromium, such as chromic acid

coagulation
(kO-ag-yoo-**lay**-shun) (n) process of blood clotting

collagen
(**kol**-le-jen) (n) the gelatin or sticky substance of skin, bone, cartilage, ligaments, and connective tissue

craniotomy
(kray-nee-**ot**-O-mee) (n) surgical incision into the skull, performed to control bleeding, remove tumors, relieve pressure inside the cranium, or insert instruments for diagnosis

dysuria
(dis-**yoo**-ree-a) (n) painful or difficult urination, symptomatic of numerous conditions (e.g., cystitis; urethritis; infection in urinary tract)

ecchymosis
(ek-im-**O**-sis) (n) reddish or purplish flat spot on the skin; a bruise; ecchymoses (pl)

embryo
(**em**-bree-O) (n) in humans, the developing prenatal child from conception to the end of the second month

embryonal
(**em**-bree-O-nal) (adj) relating to an embryo; in an early stage of development

emesis
(**em**-e-sis) (n) vomiting; may be of gastric, systemic, nervous, or reflex origin

eosinophil
(ee-O-**sin**-O-fil) (n) a type of white blood cell readily stained with eosin

erythrocyte
(e-**rith**-rO-sIt) (n) mature red blood cell

erythromycin
(**ee**-rith-rO-**mI**-sin) (n) antibiotic used to treat infections caused by a wide variety of bacteria and other microorganisms

fetoprotein
(fee-tO-**prO**-teen) (n) antigen (substance or organism that produces an antibody) naturally present in the fetus and sometimes present in adults with certain cancers

fibrinogen
(fi-**brin**-O-jen) (n) a substance in the blood plasma that can be converted into fibrin to produce blood clotting

fibrosis
(fI-**brO**-sis) (n) abnormal formation of fibrous tissue

follicle
(**fol**-i-kl) (n) pouch-like cavity, such as a hair follicle in the skin enclosing a hair, or a graafian follicle

follicular
(fo-**lik**-yoo-lar) (adj) pertaining to a follicle or follicles (a small secretory sac or cavity [pouchlike cavity, as that in the skin enclosing a hair])

fundus
(**fun**-dus) (n) the bottom or base of an organ; the part farthest from the opening

gallium
(**gal**-ee-um) (n) a rare metal; a gallium scan after an infusion of gallium provides a better view of lymphatic tissue

granuloma
(gran-yoo-**lO**-ma) (n) a mass of tissue consisting of many newly growing capillaries formed during the healing process; growth may be due to injury, infection, or inflammation

hemangioma
(he-**man**-jee-**O**-ma) (n) a congenital benign tumor consisting of a mass of blood vessels

hemophilia
(hee-mO-**fil**-ee-a) (n) an inherited blood disorder in males characterized by a defect in the clotting process due to a lack of one or more of the clotting factors

hemorrhage
(**hem**-o-rij) (n) loss of a large amount of blood quickly, either externally or internally

hyperdiploid
(**hI**-per-**dip**-loyd) (n) an individual organism or cell that has one or more extra chromosomes; (adj) relating to such an individual or cell

inguinal
(**ing**-gwi-nal) (adj) relating to or located in the groin area (where the abdomen and thighs join)

karyotype
(**kar**-ee-O-tIp) (n) chromosomal makeup of a cell; often displayed as chromosome pairs arranged by size

laparotomy
(lap-a-**rot**-O-mee) (n) a surgical procedure in which an incision is made into the abdominal wall

leukemia
(loo-**kee**-mee-a) (n) production of abnormal white blood cells; a type of cancer of the blood

lumbar
(**lum**-bar) (n) relating to the lower back, between the ribs and pelvis

lymphadenitis
(**lim**-fad-e-**nI**-tis) (n) inflammation of one or more lymph nodes

lymphadenopathy
(lim-fad-e-**nop**-a-thee) (n) any disorder of lymph nodes or of the lymphatic system

lymphatic
(lim-**fat**-ik) (adj) relating to or resembling lymph or lymph nodes

lymphoblastic
(lim-fO-**blas**-tik) (adj) relating to or resembling lymphoblasts, immature white blood cells

lymphocyte
(**lim**-fO-sIt) (n) white blood cell that produces antibodies

mediastinal
(**mee**-dee-as-**tI**-nal) (adj) relating to the space in the chest cavity between the lungs that contains the heart, aorta, esophagus, trachea, and thymus

metastasis
(me-**tas**-ta-sis) (n) spread of a tumor from its site of origin to distant sites

morphology
(mOr-**fol**-O-jee) (n) the shape and structure of an organism or body part

necrosis
(ne-**krO**-sis) (n) death of some or all of the cells in a tissue

neutrophil
(**noo**-trO-fil/**noo**-trO-fIl) (n) the most common type of mature white blood cell; its primary function is phagocytosis; granular leukocyte

orchiectomy
(Or-kee-**ek**-tO-mee) (n) surgical removal of one or both testes

organomegaly
(**Or**-ga-nO-**meg**-a-lee) (n) abnormal enlargement of an organ, particularly an organ of the abdominal cavity, such as the liver or spleen

palliative
(**pal**-ee-a-tiv) (adj) describes a treatment that minimizes symptoms but does not cure the disease

parenchyma
(pa-**reng**-ki-ma) (n) the functional or specific tissue of an organ, not including supporting or connective tissue

pelvis
(**pel**-vis) (n) the bones in the lower portion of the trunk of the body; the bones between the spine and legs

petechial
(pee-**tee**-kee-al/pee-**tek**-ee-al) (adj) relating to or having petechiae, tiny reddish or purplish spots on the skin from broken capillaries

phagocytosis
(**fag**-O-sI-**tO**-sis) (n) the process in which a cell engulfs and destroys bacteria, foreign particles, cellular debris, and other cells

platelet
(**playt**-let) (n) disc-shaped, small cellular element in the blood that is essential for blood clotting

poikilocytosis
(**poy**-ki-lO-sI-**tO**-sis) (n) having poikilocytes (abnormal and irregularly shaped red blood cells) in the blood

porphyrins
(**pOr**-fi-rinz) (n) a group of pigmented compounds essential to life; for example, hemoglobin contains the heme porphyrin

pruritus
(proo-**rI**-tus) (n) itching skin condition

purpura
(**pur**-poo-ra) (n) any of several bleeding disorders in which the escape of blood into tissues below the skin causes reddish or purplish spots

roentgenology
(**rent**-gen-**ol**-o-jee) (n) the study of the use of roentgen rays (x-rays) for diagnosis and therapy

scirrhous
(**skir**-us) (adj) describing or resembling a hard, fibrous, malignant tumor

sclerosis
(skle-**rO**-sis) (n) condition characterized by hardening of a tissue or organ, resulting from inflammation and mineral deposits

scrotal
(**skrO**-tal) (adj) relating to the scrotum

scrotum
(**skrO**-tum) (n) the pouch of skin containing the testes, the male reproductive glands

sequela
(see-**kwel**-a) (n) an abnormal condition resulting from a disease; sequelae (see-**kwel**-ee) (pl)

serous
(**seer**-us) (adj) relating to or having a watery consistency

sessile
(**sess**-il) (adj) attached directly at the base; not on a stalk

sonography
(so-**nog**-ra-fi) (n) ultrasonography; use of high-frequency sound waves to produce an image of an organ or tissue

splenectomy
(sple-**nek**-tO-mee) (n) surgical removal of the spleen

squamous
(**skway**-mus) (adj) scaly; covered with or consisting of scales

staphylococcemia
(**staf**-i-lO-kok-**see**-mee-a) (n) the presence of staphylococci (bacterial microorganisms) in the blood

suppuration
(**sup**-yu-**ray**-shun) (n) the production or discharge of pus

testicular
(tes-**tik**-yoo-lar) (adj) relating to the testes, the male reproductive glands

thrombocytopenia
(**throm**-bO-sI-tO-**pee**-nee-a) (n) an abnormal decrease in platelets in the blood, resulting in bleeding and easy bruising

thrombocytopenic
(**throm**-bO-sI-tO-**pee**-nik) (adj) relating to thrombocytopenia

thrombosis
(throm-**bO**-sis) (n) the formation, development, or existence of a blood clot, or thrombus, within the vascular system

tumor
(**too**-mor) (n) abnormal mass of tissue; neoplasm

tympanic
(tim-**pan**-ik) (adj) pertaining to the middle ear or tympanic cavity

yolk sac
(**yOk** sak) (n) a membranous sac surrounding the food yolk in the embryo

Abbreviations

HEMATOLOGY

AFP	alpha-fetoprotein (tumor marker for liver and germ cells)
AHF	antihemophilic factor VIII
AHG	antihemophilic globulin factor VIII
ANC	absolute neutrophil count
baso	basophil
CA-125	ovarian carcinoma antigen (tumor marker for ovary)
CBC	complete blood count
CEA	carcinoembryonic antigen (tumor marker for colon, lung, breast, others)
diff	differential
eosin/eos	eosinophil
ESR	erythrocyte sedimentation rate
hCG	human chorionic gonadotropin (tumor marker for germ cells)
HCT, Hct	hematocrit
HGB, Hgb	hemoglobin
ITP	idiopathic thrombocytopenic purpura
LDH	lactic dehydrogenase (tumor marker germ cell and lymphoma)
lymphs	lymphocytes
MCH	mean corpuscular hemoglobin
MCHC	mean corpuscular hemoglobin concentration
MCV	mean corpuscular volume
mono	monocyte
plts or PLT	platelets
PMN	polymorphonuclear neutrophil
polys	polymorphonuclear neutrophils
PT	prothrombin time
PTT	partial thromboplastin time
RBC	red blood cell
sed rate	sedimentation rate
segs	segmented neutrophils
WBC	white blood cell

ONCOLOGY

AFP	alpha-fetoprotein
ALL	acute lymphoblastic leukemia
AML	acute myelogenous leukemia
ANLL	acute nonlymphoblastic leukemia
APL, APML	acute promyelocytic leukemia
BCE	basal cell epithelioma
BM	bone marrow (or bowel movement)
BMA	bone marrow aspiration
BMT	bone marrow transplant
BSE	breast self-exam
bx	biopsy
CA	cancer, carcinoma
cGy	centigray
CLL	chronic lymphoblastic leukemia
CML	chronic myelogenous leukemia
DES	diethylstilbestrol
Gy	gray
HD	Hodgkin's disease
PSA	prostate specific antigen (tumor marker for prostate)
RT	radiation therapy
TNM	tumor, nodes, metastasis (refers to tumor staging)

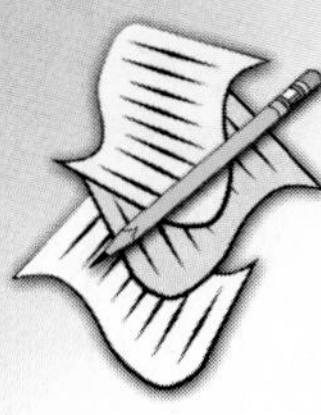

EXERCISE 14.1

Recognizing Look-Alikes and Sound-Alikes

Below is a list of frequently used words that look alike and/or sound alike. Study the meaning and pronunciation of each set of words, then read the following sentences carefully and circle the word in parentheses that correctly completes the meaning.

knot	(n) lump, bump; measurement of nautical speed
naught	(adj) zero
not	(adv) a negative response

acidic	(adj) acid-forming
acetic	(adj) pertaining to acetic acid or vinegar
ascitic	(adj) watery, albumin- and glucose-containing

advice	(n) opinion given
advise	(v) to counsel, to give advice

generic	(adj) nonspecific, nontrademark
genetic	(adj) hereditary

for	(prep) as; to
fore	(adj) front; near
four	(adj) the number "4"

basal	(adj) basic, elemental, forming the base
basil	(n) herb used in cooking

radical	(adj) going to the root of the cause
radicle	(n) small root of a nerve or vessel
free radical	(n) an atom or group of atoms carrying an unpaired electron and no charge

anergy	(n) impaired ability to react to certain antigens
energy	(n) capacity to do work

prostate	(n) male gland
prostrate	(adj) lying face down

presence	(n) attendance
presents	(n) gifts
presents	(v) displays, appears

incidence	occurrence, rate of occurrence
incidents	multiple occurrences
instance	example, sample

1. I (adviced, advised) the patient to return in one week.
2. Medical papers always use the (generic, genetic) name for drugs.
3. The patient (presence, presents) with a two-week history of headaches.
4. I gave the patient (advice, advise) regarding proper diet and exercise.
5. The pathology report states that the lesion is a (basal, basil) cell carcinoma.
6. The patient appears depressed and is complaining of lack of (anergy, energy) and insomnia.
7. The patient had breast cancer, requiring a (radical, radicle) mastectomy.
8. The patient was cautioned regarding greasy, spicy, and (acetic, acidic) foods.
9. The (prostate, prostrate) was smooth and without nodules.
10. When the ambulance arrived, she was found (prostate, prostrate) on her bathroom floor.
11. This is another (incidence, incidents, instance) of a disorder that is increasing in (incidence, incidents, instance).

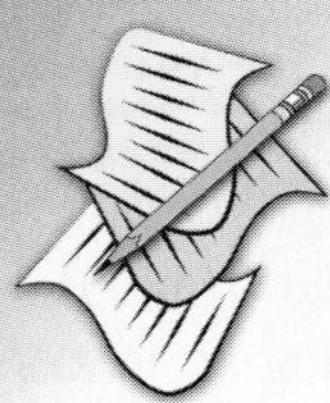

EXERCISE 14.2

Matching Sound and Spelling

The numbered list that follows shows the phonetic spelling of hard-to-spell words. Sound out the word, then write the correct spelling in the blank space provided. Each of the words can be found in the Glossary or in the drug list in Appendix D.

1. ek-i-m-**O**-sis____________________
2. **fag**-O-sI-**tO**-sis ____________________
3. **ses**-il ____________________
4. **pal**-ee-a-tiv____________________
5. lim-**fat**-ik ____________________
6. me-**tas**-ta-sis____________________
7. **rent**-gen-**ol**-o-jee ____________________
8. loo-**kee**-mee-a ____________________
9. a-gloo-ti-**nay**-shun ____________________
10. **skir**-us ____________________
11. **hem**-o-rij ____________________
12. **skway**-mus ____________________
13. **lim**-fO-sIt ____________________
14. **krO**-mik ____________________
15. **staf**-i-lO-kok-**see**-mee-a____________________

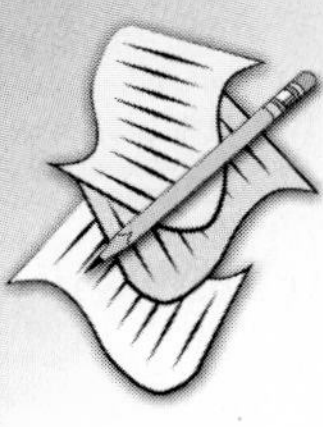

EXERCISE 14.3

Choosing Words from Context

When transcribing dictation, the medical transcriptionist frequently needs to consider the situation when determining the word that correctly completes the sentence. From the list below, select the term that meaningfully completes each of the following statements.

carcinoma	embryo	platelet
lymphadenopathy	pelvis	lumbar
ecchymoses	leukemia	sclerosis
parenchyma	emesis	hemorrhage

1. The most common childhood malignancy is ______________.
2. The patient had a low ______________count, which caused him to bleed profusely after the phlebotomy.
3. Mr. Smith had a hepatic ______________, which required chemotherapy.
4. There was ________________ of the vein after the chemotherapeutic agent infiltrated at the infusion site.
5. After the ________________puncture, Johnny had to lie down for about an hour.
6. Drinking alcohol, using drugs, and smoking during pregnancy are dangerous to the forming ______________.
7. There were __________________all over the child's body, leading to the diagnosis of immune thrombocytopenic purpura (ITP).
8. The __________________ of the left kidney was invaded by the tumor.
9. The physical examination of the child with leukemia revealed cervical ________________.
10. The tumor was invading the ______________, requiring removal of the adjacent hip.
11. Mr. Johnson received medication prior to chemotherapy to prevent________________.
12. If you do not achieve hemostasis during surgery, you can have a serious________________.

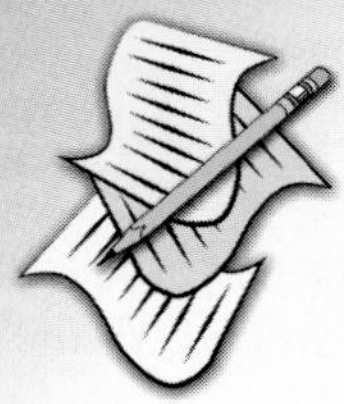

EXERCISE 14.4

Pairing Words and Meanings

From this list, locate the term that best matches each of the following definitions. Write the letter of the term in the space provided by each definition.

A.	ecchymosis	E.	lymphocyte	H.	orchiectomy
B.	gallium	F.	necrosis	I.	phagocytosis
C.	hemophilia	G.	neutrophil	J.	thrombocytopenia
D.	laparotomy				

1. white blood cell __________
2. the process by which certain cells destroy microorganisms __________
3. surgical excision of a testicle __________
4. bruise; purplish spot from accumulation of blood under skin __________
5. a condition with diminished number of platelets, resulting in bleeding and bruising __________
6. a rare metal __________
7. a disorder characterized by excessive bleeding and occurring only in males __________
8. surgical procedure in which an incision is made in abdominal wall __________
9. death of some or all of the cells in a tissue __________
10. leukocytes that increase in the presence of infection __________

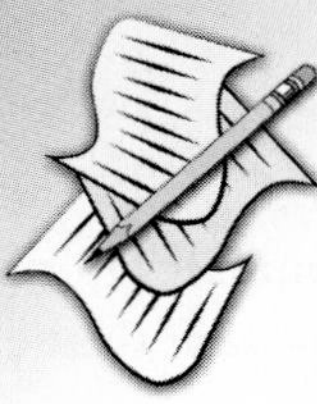

E X E R C I S E 1 4 . 5

Creating Terms from Word Forms

Combine prefixes, root words, and suffixes from this list to create medical words that fit the following definitions. Fill in the blanks with the words you construct.

a-; an-	without, no	basal	base
cyt/o	cell	macro	big
erythr/o	red	micro	small
hem/o; hemat/o	blood	papilla	nipple-like
immun/o	safe, protected against	-logy	study of
leuk/o	white	-oma	tumor
phag/o	eating, swallowing	-osis	increase or condition
plasm/o	formed; plasma	-philia	attraction for
reticul/o	net	-plasia	growth; formation
thromb/o	clot	-poiesis	production

1. no growth ______________________________
2. forms a network of cells, occuring during active blood regeneration______________________________
3. cell clotting ______________________________
4. benign, nipple-like tumor ______________________________
5. blood cell that functions as an anticoagulant ______________________________
6. white blood cell that fights bacteria, stains neutral______________________________
7. study of cells ______________________________
8. ingestion/digestion of cells, bacteria______________________________
9. study of immune system ______________________________
10. abnormally large cells______________________________

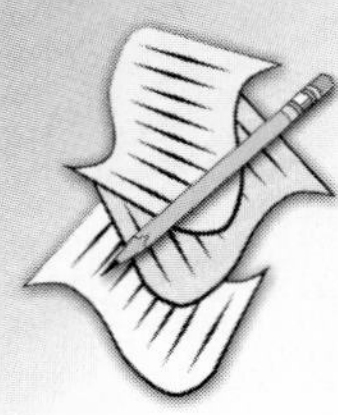

EXERCISE 14.6

Proofreading Review

Read the following partial report and look for errors in form, meaning, capitalization, word choice, punctuation, and spelling. Circle the errors, then key the report with the errors corrected.

Charlotte is a 30 yr old women who first noted a fullness in the right lower anterior cervical region in the late winter. It had gradually groin in size. In early March she was treated with a one week course of erythromycin with out response. the mass 'bothered" her slightly but it was not painful. Their has been no change in her usually good appetite her weight has remained staple.

The outside radiographic studies were reviewed with the radiologist The chest x-ray reveals a relatively small anterior mediastinal mass (approximately 1/4 of the chest diameter). The chest CT scan conforms the presents of the mediastinal mass, without pulmonary parenchymal involvement.

Building Transcription Skills

The Outpatient Visit

The outpatient visit report (Figure 14.6) is a medical document similar in content to a brief history and physical or a chart note.

Required Headings/Content No specific headings are required in the outpatient visit report. The report usually begins with the patient's diagnosis and includes a brief history of the illness, the results of a physical examination, results of laboratory tests, the physician's impression and treatment plan, including lab tests scheduled for subsequent visits, and referrals to other physicians. The format varies considerably from clinic to clinic, since this report is one of the more recent document types in the medical industry.

Turnaround Time The outpatient visit report is generally transcribed within 48 hours after dictation.

Preparing to Transcribe

To prepare for transcribing dictation, review the tables of common hematology-oncology terms, drugs, and abbreviations presented in the Building Language Skills section of this chapter. Then, study the format and organization of the model document shown in Figure 14.6, and key the model document. Proofread the document by comparing it with the printed version. Categorize the types of errors you

1" margins and left justification

PATIENT NAME: Connors, Elizabeth
DATE: (current date)

double-space between all sections

DIAGNOSIS
Immune thrombocytopenic purpura (ITP).

INTERVAL HISTORY
Elizabeth was well until 3 weeks ago when she had a viral URI. She had fevers to 101°. Yesterday, mother noted a "red rash" on her back and legs and many bruises. She was referred by Dr. Sanderson for evaluation.

PHYSICAL EXAMINATION
VITALS: Temperature 98.7°, blood pressure 98/56, weight 22 kg.
GENERAL: The patient appears very well.
SKIN: Petechial rash on arms, back, and thighs. Several large ecchymoses over legs, arms, and abdomen.
HEENT: Within normal limits.
FUNDI: Within normal limits.
NODES: Several small, shotty nodes in submandibular chain.
CHEST: Clear.
HEART: Within normal limits, no murmur.
ABDOMEN: Soft, no palpable masses.
LIVER: Not palpable.
SPLEEN: Not palpable.
GU: Within normal limits.
EXT: Within normal limits.
NEURO: Grossly intact.

LABORATORY DATA
WBC: 6500
HGB/HCT: 12.3/37.1
PLTS: 34,000
SEGS/BANDS: 52/0
EOS/BASOS: 3/2
LYMPHS/ATYP: 43/0
ANC: 3380

(continued)

FIGURE 14.6
Outpatient Visit

OUTPATIENT VISIT
PATIENT NAME: Connors, Elizabeth
DATE: (2 days before transcription date)
Page 2

IMPRESSION
Immune thrombocytopenic purpura.

THERAPY
Will repeat counts tomorrow. If platelets are rising, will continue to watch. If decreasing, will hospitalize for a 3-day course of IVIg.

REFERRALS
None at present.

RETURN TO CLINIC
(1 day after current date).

LAB/PROCEDURES (NEXT VISIT)
Counts.

qs

____
Sandford J. Arnold, MD
ds
SA/XX
ds
C: Lawrence C. Cohen, MD
ds
D: (2 days before transcription date)
T: (current date)

FIGURE 14.6
Outpatient Visit (Continued)

made, and document them on a copy of the Performance Comparison chart provided in Chapter 1. A template of this chart is included on the IRC that accompanies this text.

Patient Studies

Transcribe, edit, and correct each report in the following patient studies. Consult reference books for words or formatting rules that are unfamiliar.

As you work on the transcription assignment for this chapter, fill in the Performance Comparison chart that you started when you keyed the model document. For at least three of the reports, categorize and document the types of errors you made. Answer the document analysis questions on the bottom of the chart. With continuous practice and assessment, the quality of your work will improve.

After you have produced a final version of each transcribed report, complete the Performance Report cover sheet, attach it to the top of the transcripts, and submit them to your instructor for evaluation.

Patient Study 14.A — Elizabeth Connors

Elizabeth Connors is a 5-year-old who was well until three weeks ago when she developed a cold with a fever. She recovered in about a week. Yesterday, her mother noticed that her back and legs were covered with tiny red dots that appeared to be a rash. She also had several large bruises on her body. Her mother took Elizabeth to the pediatrician, who sent her to the Hematology Outpatient Clinic.

REPORT 14.1 Outpatient Visit Report

- IVIg is the acronym for intravenous immunoglobulin.

Patient Study 14.B — Stephanie Aaron

Stephanie Aaron is an 11-year-old who was diagnosed with acute lymphoblastic leukemia (ALL). She completed a 2½-year regimen of chemotherapy and is doing very well off all therapy for 1 year.

REPORT 14.2 Chart Summary

- No special format exists for a chart summary. It is normally a narrative report of one or several paragraphs summarizing the patient's history and treatment. List the patient's name at the top, along with the current date. Key the first paragraph a double-space below the date.
- Listen for these drug terms:
  FAB L1 morphology
  cALLa
  vincristine
  intrathecal
  methotrexate
  PEG-L-asparaginase
  BFM regimen

Patient Study 14.C — Nettie Brandise

Nettie Brandise is a 24-year-old young woman who was diagnosed with leukemia 5 years ago. She was treated with radiation, chemotherapy, and a bone marrow transplant (BMT) and is doing well off all therapy. She is seen at the Brookfield Oncology Group for followup every 3 months.

REPORT 14.3 Outpatient Visit Report

Patient Study 14.D — Linda Eastman

Linda Eastman is a 65-year-old woman who had a right radical mastectomy 3 years ago. She presented to urgent care with fever, chills, abdominal pain, and bloody diarrhea, which had been occurring over the previous 2 days. She was transported by ambulance to the hospital for further evaluation and treatment.

REPORT 14.4 History and Physical

Patient Study 14.E — Charlotte Trent

Charlotte Trent is a 30-year-old woman who noticed that she had a lump on her neck. It caused her no pain so she did not see her physician until it grew bigger. Her internist sent her to the surgeon for a biopsy, which showed Hodgkin disease. She was then referred to the oncologist for further workup and treatment.

REPORT 14.5 Consultation Letter

REPORT 14.6 Pathology Report

- Listen for this cell type name:
  Reed-Sternberg

Patient Study 14.F — Robert Hudson

Robert Hudson is a 35-year-old man with a history of sickle cell anemia. He has been hospitalized several times to receive intravenous fluids, blood transfusions, and pain medications. Recently, he had a flu-like illness and subsequently presented to the ER with severe pain in the lower left leg.

REPORT 14.7 History and Physical

Patient Study 14.G — Belinda Kottke

Belinda Kottke is a 57-year-old woman with colorectal cancer that has metastasized to the liver, lung, and brain. She underwent a craniotomy for resection of a brain lesion that was identified on a CT scan.

REPORT 14.8 Discharge Summary

- Listen for this drug term:
  Pepcid

Using Medical References

Use the appropriate medical reference to locate the correct spelling and additional usage information for the words below. (If the reference is not available, use the Glossary in this text.) Circle the correct spelling; then write a sentence using the word correctly.

1.	reontgenogram	roentgenogram	roentgenagram
2.	hemorrages	hemorhages	hemorrhages
3.	scirrhous	schirrhous	scirhous
4.	adjuviant	adjuvent	adjuvant
5.	metastesis	metastassis	metastasis
6.	leucocytes	leukocytes	luekocytes
7.	karyotype	kariotype	caryotype
8.	poikylocytosis	poiklocytosis	poikilocytosis
9.	paliative	palliative	palleative
10.	mammeogram	mammogram	mammagram

Making Expert Decisions

Circle the correct word from the choices in parentheses.

1. As the patient was 94, the family did not want treatment or invasive procedures done, and the patient was given (adjuvant/palliative) treatment only.
2. DIAGNOSIS: (Basil/Basal) cell carcinoma of the skin of the cheek.
3. This 3-month-old Caucasian male (presents/presence) to the Eagle County Medical Center in the arms of his mother, who rushed the patient here saying the patient is having trouble breathing.
4. Contrast material was injected through the T-tube, and the right hepatic (radical/radicle) was outlined.
5. The patient stated that she could not (breath/breathe) through her nostrils.
6. The mass was (aberrant/apparent) in the left upper outer quadrant of the breast.
7. The patient's symptoms were brought to the (for/fore/four) upon careful questioning during the history and physical.
8. A (cor/core/corps) of bone marrow was obtained on biopsy to rule out aplastic anemia.
9. A tumor was suspected when a mass was felt in the abdomen, but on further testing, this was found to be a (gr3/grade 3) carcinoma.
10. When considering a course of therapy, it is important to use a group of drugs that work together, not as (agonists/antagonists).

Transcribing Professional Documents

Transcribe the document named Chapter 14 Assessment. Before you key, review the appropriate document formatting guidelines. Proofread your transcribed document and revise it until you think it is error-free.

15

Immunology

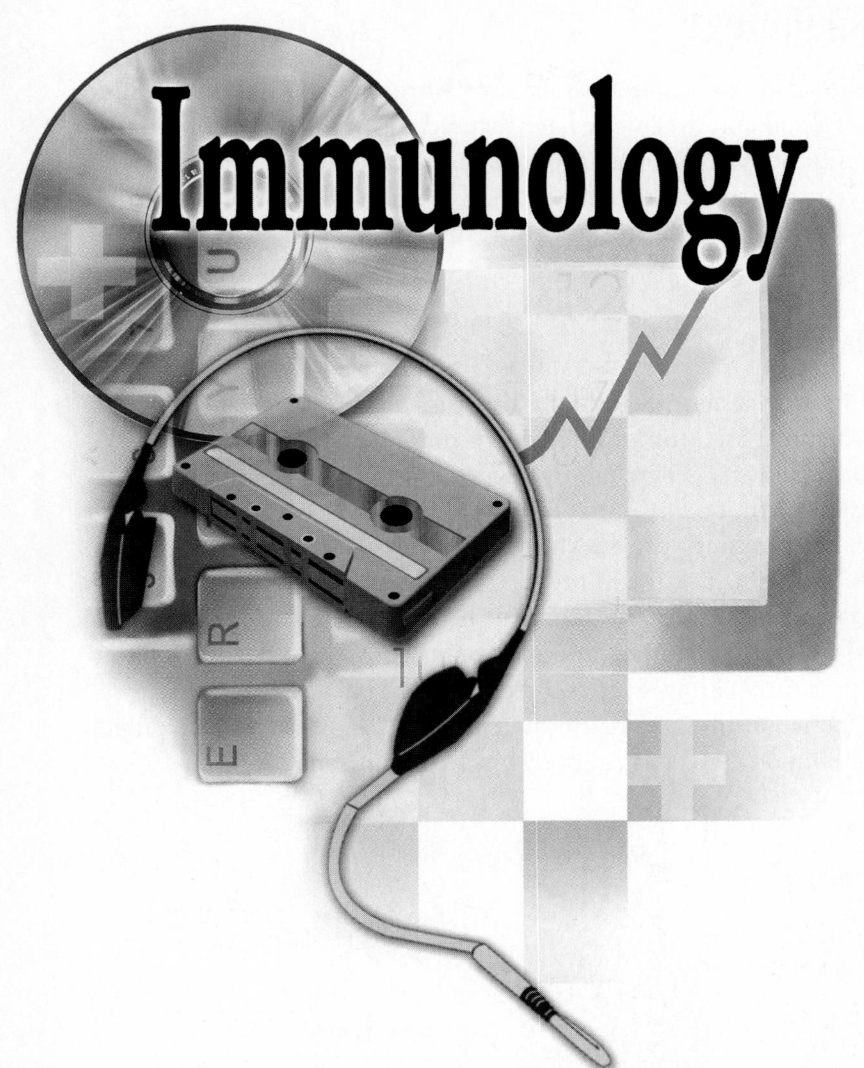

The immune system is a complex system composed of specialized organs, ducts, and cells located throughout the body. It is the body's surveillance system that protects against invading, potentially harmful bacteria, viruses, and parasites, and also threatening cells within the body itself. The area of practice concerned with the functioning of the immune system and the interrelationships between this system and the rest of the body is called immunology. The specialist in the field is called an immunologist. Often the immunologist also specializes in allergy and infectious diseases, as these two specialties relate to the body's immune response to environmental and biological stimuli.

OBJECTIVES

- Use immunology terms correctly according to the context and purpose of the dictation.
- Select and use appropriate general and specialty reference materials.
- Key immunology documents of varying complexity and format.
- Transcribe authentic medical dictation requiring concentration and listening skill.
- Edit medical reports to conform with AAMT style guidelines.
- Proofread and correct transcripts to produce error-free documents.

Exploring Immunology

With the emergence of acquired immunodeficiency syndrome (AIDS) in the 1980s, both the medical profession and the public have focused enormous attention on the functioning of the immune system. Breakthroughs in the treatment of immune system disorders are occurring so quickly that medical support personnel, including medical transcriptionists, must make an extra effort to remain knowledgeable about changes and news in this specialty.

Structure and Function

The organs of the immune system include the thymus, tonsils, lymph nodes, and spleen, as shown in Figure 15.1. Immunity refers to the healthy body's response to foreign substances or organisms. There are two types of immunity: natural immunity, which is present at birth, and acquired immunity, which is specific and develops after birth. Natural immunity provides the body with the ability to recognize "self" from "nonself." The intact skin and mucous membranes are important barriers that are part of natural immunity. The hairs in the nose, the cilia of the respiratory tract, the gastric juices, and other internal mechanisms help to protect the internal body from invading pathogens. Acquired immunity develops as a result of exposure to disease (active immunity) or through immunization (passive acquired immunity). The white blood cells assist in both types of immunity.

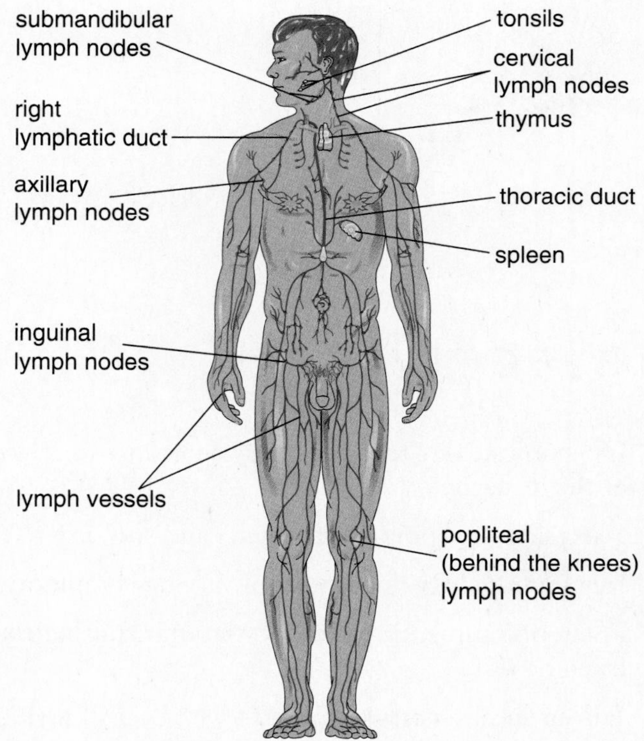

FIGURE 15.1
Components of the Lymphatic System

The immune response begins when the body is invaded by a foreign substance, one the body does not recognize as "self" (Figure 15.2). The first event is phagocytosis of the invading organisms by the granulocytes and macrophages. These white blood cells attack and destroy foreign substances. Next is the humoral or antibody response where B lymphocytes manufacture specific antibodies against the invaders. The third defense mechanism is cellular and involves T lymphocytes, which produce cytotoxic substances to kill the organisms.

The body also produces biologic response modifiers (BRMs), such as interferons, whose complete function is only just being recognized. Cytokines are BRMs that regulate the growth and function of other cells within the immune system. These substances are being investigated for their therapeutic potential as antiviral, anticancer, and acquired immunodeficiency syndrome (AIDS) treatments.

Physical Assessment

The physician assesses the immune system by obtaining a complete history, performing a thorough physical examination, and ordering laboratory tests that include cultures from any secretion that may contain infectious organisms. Frequent illness

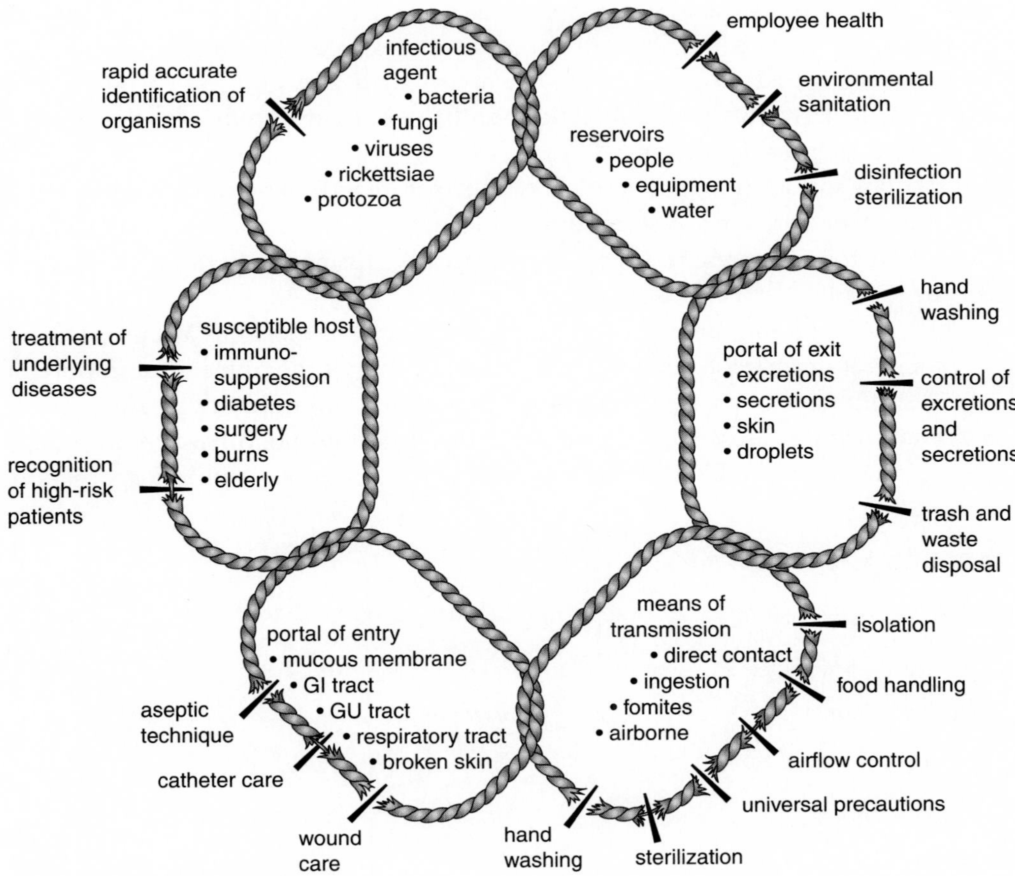

FIGURE 15.2
Interventions That Halt the Transmission of Infections

may suggest that the patient does not have a competent immune system. The very young, the elderly, persons with chronic disease, and persons who are receiving immunosuppressive agents are more susceptible to infection.

The examiner palpates all areas containing superficial lymph nodes. Enlarged lymph nodes, or swollen glands, may indicate an infection. Nodes that have responded to infection or cleared other substances from the body feel spongy, or shotty. Firm, fixed lymph nodes may signal an infection, a serious disorder, or a cancerous node. An enlarged liver or spleen may suggest an abnormality.

Diseases and Conditions

Diseases affecting the immune system can be grouped into five broad categories: infections, allergies, autoimmune disorders, diseases associated with organ transplant, and malignancies.

Infectious disease is any disease that is caused by the growth of a pathogenic organism in the body. There are hundreds of organisms capable of causing disease in humans. Table 15.1 lists a few of the most commonly found pathogens. Note that these scientific names for bacteria include two words. The first is the genus (group) classification, which is always capitalized. The second word is the species within the genus. The species name is never capitalized. When looking up these terms, you may need to first locate the genus name. Species names will be listed beneath as subentries.

Many diseases are contagious, which means they can be passed to other persons. Sexually transmitted diseases (STDs) are a current health problem in the United States, particularly chlamydial infections and the human immunodeficiency virus (HIV), the causative agent for AIDS.

Infections spread through a series of events that include a causative agent, a reservoir, a portal of exit, a mode of transmission, a mode of entry, and a susceptible host. All of these must be present. If any one element is missing, the series is interrupted and the spread of infection is halted.

The most common method of stopping the spread of infectious agents is to stop the mode of transmission (Figure 15.2). Handwashing is the single most important step to stopping the spread of infections. In addition, immunizations are available to prevent certain diseases from spreading. Smallpox and polio have been successfully eliminated in the United States because of a vigorous immunization program.

TABLE 15.1 Common Pathogens

Aspergillus fumigatus	*Klebsiella pneumoniae*
Campylobacter fetus	*Mycobacterium avium*
Candida albicans	*Salmonella choleraesuia*
Diplococcus pneumoniae	*Pneumocystis carinii*
Escherichia coli	*Staphylococcus aureus*
Haemophilus influenzae	*Streptococcus pneumoniae*
Helicobacter pylori	*Staphylococcus viridans*

Allergic reactions result from a hyperactive response to an allergen. Allergens include any substance that produces an allergic response. Examples include inhalants such as dust, perfumes, and pollens; foods such as chocolate, eggs, wheat, and strawberries; drugs such as antibiotics; and contact substances such as wool, chemicals, animals, and plants. In sensitive individuals, the immune system produces antibodies that attack these specialized antigens. Histamine released by the damaged cells will cause symptoms such as runny eyes, sneezing, itching, and a rash. In nonsensitive persons, no significant effects occur.

Autoimmune diseases are disorders resulting from an overactive response to self-antigens, those molecules native to a person's body that the immune system uses to identify "self" components. Examples of autoimmune diseases include rheumatoid arthritis, multiple sclerosis, myasthenia gravis, Graves disease, and systemic lupus erythematosus (SLE).

An excessive reaction to antigens from a different person is the cause of organ transplant disorders, which result in the rejection of grafted tissue. Patients who undergo a kidney, liver, or heart transplant must take antirejection drugs to try to prevent this.

Common Tests and Procedures

Laboratory tests are most important in diagnosing an immune disorder. A common test that is performed includes the measurement of immunoglobulins (Ig), substances necessary for defending the body. Table 15.2 shows the symbol and function of immunoglobulins. The name of each immunoglobulin is pronounced as individual letters and written as follows: IgM, IgG, IgA, IgD, and IgE.

It is also possible to test for immune status through very sophisticated blood tests looking at lymphocyte subsets, particularly helper and suppressor lymphocytes, and natural killer cells. Antibodies from diseases such as polio and CMV can be detected in specific blood tests that measure B-cell function. The presence of HIV is assessed with one of the antibody-detection tests: the enzyme-linked immunosorbent assay (ELISA) or the Western blot.

Allergy testing is a common practice. Scratch tests can determine a person's specific allergies; the radioallergosorbent test (RAST) detects IgE-bound allergens that cause hypersensitivity.

TABLE 15.2 Immunoglobulins and Their Functions

Ig	Function
IgG	crosses the placenta and assists with passive and recall immunity
IgA	protects the gastrointestinal tract and eyes, since secretions may prevent antibody activity
IgM	acts as first line of defense; formed first in response to an antigen
IgD	acts as lymphocyte receptor on activated B cells
IgE	effects the release of agents from cells called mast cells that cause asthma, hay fever, and anaphylaxis

Cultures of urine, blood, sputum, bronchial aspirates, and wounds can help determine the presence of pathogenic organisms. Fecal cultures can reveal the presence of ova and parasites. After a specimen is collected, it is grown on a culture medium and then tested to determine which antibiotics can kill it. This is known as a culture and sensitivity.

Building Language Skills

The following tables list the common immunology terms, drugs, and abbreviations. The list of terms and definitions includes the most difficult words contained in the dictated reports in this chapter. These words are identified in GREEN type. A list of common drugs is found in Appendix D.

Medical Terms and Pharmacologic Agents

aerosolized
(**ayr**-O-sol-Izd) (adj) describing a solution that is dispensed in the form of a mist

allergen
(**al**-er-jen) (n) a substance that produces an allergic reaction

antibody
(**an**-tee-bod-ee) (n) an immunoglobulin produced as an immune response to a specific antigen

antigen
(**an**-ti-jen) (n) a substance that causes the formation of an antibody which will react specifically to the antigen to neutralize, destroy, or weaken it

asthma
(**az**-ma) (n) respiratory disorder with temporary narrowing of the airways, resulting in difficulty in breathing, coughing, gasping, wheezing

atresia
(a-**tree**-zee-a) (n) congenital absence or closure of a normal body opening or tubular structure

autoimmune disease
(aw-tO-i-**myoon**) (n) any disorder in which the body's immune responses produce antibodies that destroy the body's own tissues

B cell
(n) a type of lymphocyte; produces immunoglobulin antibodies in response to antigens

bronchitis
(brong-**kI**-tis) (n) inflammation of the bronchi

choana
(**kO**-an-a) (n) a funnel-shaped opening, especially the posterior opening of the nasal cavity into the nasopharynx

chordae tendineae
(**kOr**-dee ten-**din**-ee-ay) (n) small tendinous cords (strands) that connect the free edges of the atrioventricular valves to the papillary muscles

coagulopathy
(kO-ag-yoo-**lop**-a-thee) (n) defect in the blood clotting mechanisms

communicable
(ko-**myoon**-i-ka-bl) (adj) contagious; capable of being spread with direct or indirect contact

corticomedullary junction
(**kOr**-tee-kO-**med**-yoo-lar-ee **jungk**-shun) (n) coming together (junction) of the cortex and medulla of the kidneys

costal
(**kos**-tal) (adj) relating to or located near a rib; the costal margin is the area at the lower end of the rib cage

costophrenic
(kos-tO-**fren**-ik) (adj) pertaining to the ribs and diaphragm

cytokines
(**sI**-tO-kIns) (n) proteins that are not antibodies but are released on contact with a specific antigen as an immune response

cytomegalovirus
(sI-tO-**meg**-a-lO-**vI**-rus) (n) CMV; one of a group of large-cell, species-specific herpes-type viruses with a wide variety of disease effects

defervescence
(def-er-**ves**-ens) (n) time that marks the decline of fever to normal temperature

diverticula
(dI-ver-**tik**-yoo-la) (n) sacs or pouches in the walls of a canal or organ

duodenum
(doo-O-**dee**-num/doo-**od**-e-num) (n) first part of the small intestine; it receives material from the stomach and passes it to the jejunum, the medial part of the small intestine

ecchymoses
(ek-i-**mO**-sees) (n) small, hemorrhagic, discolored, purplish ("black and blue") spots resulting from an accumulation of blood under the skin's surface

endocardium
(en-dO-**kar**-dee-im) (n) serous lining membrane of inner surface and cavities of the heart

enterovirus
(**en**-ter-O-**vI**-rus) (n) a group of viruses that multiply in the gastrointestinal tract but may cause various diseases, such as polio

epicanthic
(ep-i-**kan**-thik) (adj) pertaining to the vertical fold of skin extending from the root of the nose to the median end of the eyebrow

fibrinopurulent
(**fI**-bri-nO-**pyoo**-roo-lent) (adj) consisting of pus and fibrin

foramen ovale
(fO-**ray**-men O-**val**-ay) (n) hole or opening, especially in a bone or membrane; (particularly the opening between the two atria of the fetal heart that closes after birth)

Graves disease
(n) one type of hyperthyroidism

hematoma
(hee-ma-**tO**-ma/**hem**-a-tO-ma) (n) a swelling or mass of blood confined to an organ, tissue, or space and caused by a break in a blood vessel

hemophagocytosis
(**hee**-mO-**fag**-O-sI-**tO**-sis) (n) ingestion of red blood cells by phagocytes

heparin
(**hep**-a-rin) (n) a naturally occurring anticoagulant (a substance which prevents or slows the clotting of blood)

hepatosplenomegaly
(**hep**-a-tO-splee-nO-**meg**-a-lee) (n) enlargement of the liver and spleen

histiocyte
(**his**-tee-O-sIt) (n) a phagocyte present in connective tissue

hypergammaglobulinemia
(**hI**-per-gam-a-**glob**-yoo-li-**nee**-mee-a) (n) excessive amount of gamma globulins in the blood

immune system
(i-**myoon**) (n) complex interactions that protect the body from pathogenic organisms and other foreign invaders

immunity
(i-**myoo**-ni-tee) (n) one's resistance to disease

immunodeficiency
(**im**-yoo-nO-dee-**fish**-en-see) (n) some part of the body's immune system is inadequate; therefore, the person has decreased resistance to infectious diseases

immunoglobulin
(**im**-yoo-nO-**glob**-yoo-lin) (n) antibody protein

immunology
(im-yoo-**nol**-O-jee) (n) study of the body's response to foreign invasion, such as bacteria or viruses, and allergies

inoculation
(i-nok-yoo-**lay**-shun) (n) the introduction of pathogenic organisms or antigens into the body in order to increase immunity by stimulating the production of antibodies

intercostal
(in-ter-**kos**-tal) (adj) relating to or located between the ribs

in vitro
(in **vee**-trO) (adj, adv) literally, in glass; outside the living organism and in an artificial environment, such as a test tube

in vivo
(in **vee**-vO) (adj, adv) literally, in the living body

isoagglutination
(**I**-sO-a-gloo-ti-**nay**-shun) (n) process in which antibodies (agglutinins) occurring naturally in blood cause clumping of red blood cells of a different group carrying a corresponding antigen (isoagglutinogen)

Kupffer cells
(**koop**-ferz) (n) phagocytes present in the liver

lobule
(**lob**-yool) (n) a small lobe or primary subdivision of a lobe; typical of pancreas and major salivary glands and may be on the surface by bumps and bulges

lymphocyte
(**lim**-fO-sIt) (n) white blood cell that produces antibodies

lymphopenia
(lim-fO-**pee**-nee-a) (n) a decrease in the number of lymphocytes in the blood

macrophage
(**mak**-rO-fayj) (n) any phagocytic cell, such as histiocytes and Kupffer cells

meatus
(**mee**-ay-tus) (n) a passage or opening

mesentery
(**mes**-en-tar-ee) (n) a peritoneal fold encircling the greater part of the small intestines and connecting the intestine to the posterior abdominal wall

neutropenia
(noo-trO-**pee**-nee-a) (n) a decrease in the number of neutrophils in the blood

neutrophil
(**noo**-trO-fil/**noo**-trO-fIl) (n) the most common type of mature white blood cell; its primary function is phagocytosis; granular leukocyte

opportunistic infection
(n) a disease caused by normally harmless microorganisms when the body's resistance to disease is impaired

otitis
(O-**tI**-tis) (n) inflammation of the ear

parenchyma
(pa-**reng**-ki-ma) (n) functional part of an organ, apart from supporting or connective tissue

Parvovirus
(**par**-vO-vI-rus) (n) a genus of viruses; strain B19 can cause anemia in humans

pathogen
(**path**-O-jen) (n) any microorganism or substance that can cause a disease

pericardium
(per-i-**kar**-dee-um) (n) a double-layered sac surrounding the heart and large vessels

petechiae
(pe-**tee**-kee-ee/pe-**tek**-kee-e/pe-**tee**-kee-a) (n) minute red spots appearing on the skin as a result of tiny hemorrhaging

phagocyte
(**fag**-O-sIt/**fAg**O-sIt) (n) a cell able to engulf and destroy bacteria, foreign particles, cellular debris, and other cells

phagocytosis
(**fag**-O-sI-**tO**-sis) (n) the process in which a cell engulfs and destroys bacteria, foreign particles, cellular debris, and other cells

Pneumocystis carinii
(noo-mO-**sis**-tis ka-**rI**-nee-I) (n) a tiny parasite which causes Pneumocystis carinii pneumonia (PCP) in individuals with impaired immune systems

pompholyx
(**pom**-fO-liks) (n) a skin eruption primarily on the hands and feet; may be accompanied by excessive sweating

prophylaxis
(prO-fi-**lak**-sis) (n) prevention of disease or its spread

protease
(**prO**-tee-ays) an enzyme that breaks down proteins

protease inhibitor
(n) an agent that inhibits (prevents or slows down) the release of protease

pyrexia
(pI-**rek**-see-a) (n) fever

retroperitoneal
(**ret**-rO-per-i-tO-**nee**-al) (adj) located behind the peritoneum outside the peritoneal cavity, such as the kidneys

serosanguineous
(**ser**-O-sang-**gwin**-ee-us) (adj) containing or of the nature of serum and blood

sinusitis
(sI-nu-**sI**-tis) (n) inflammation of the nasal sinuses, occurring as a result of an upper respiratory infection, an allergic response, or a defect of the nose

steroid
(**steer**-oyd) (n) any of a large number of similar chemical substances, either natural or synthetic; many are hormones; produced mainly in the adrenal cortex and gonads

substernal
(sub-**ster**-nal) (adj) situated beneath the sternum (breast bone)

systemic lupus erythematosus
(sis-**tem**-ik **loo**-pus er-i-**them**-a-tO-sis/er-i-**thee**-ma-tO-sis) (n) a chronic disease with inflammatory symptoms in various systems of the body; characteristics of the disease and the systems involved may vary widely

T cell
(n) a type of lymphocyte; responsible for cell-mediated immunity

thrombocytopenia
(**throm**-bO-sI-tO-**pen**-ee-a) (n) abnormal decrease in number of the blood platelets

thrush
(n) infection with the fungus Candida, causing white patches in the mouth and throat

titer
(**tI**-ter) (n) strength or concentration of a solution; a unit of measurement usually expressed as a ratio that indicates the minimum concentration of an antibody before losing its power to react to a specific antigen

toxoplasmosis
(**tok**-sO-plaz-**mO**-sis) (n) disease caused by a protozoan parasite

tracheoesophageal
(**trans**-e-sof-a-**gee**-al) (adj) pertaining to the trachea and esophagus

urethral
(yoo-ree-thral) (adj) relating to the urethra, a canal for the discharge of urine from the bladder to the outside of the body

vesicular
(ve-**sik**-yoo-lar) (adj) pertaining to vesicles or small blisters

virus
(**vI**-rus) (n) an organism or the infection caused by the organism; the organism is much smaller than bacteria; it depends completely on the host and is unaffected by common antibiotics

Western blot
(n) a laboratory test to detect the presence of antibodies to specific antigens in the blood

Abbreviations

AFB	acid-fast bacilli	GC	gonorrhea
AIDS	acquired immunodeficiency syndrome; caused by HIV	HIV	human immunodeficiency virus; causes deterioration of the immune system
CMV	cytomegalovirus; one of a group of large species-specific herpes-type viruses with a wide variety of disease effects	PCP	Pneumocystis carinii pneumonia
DPT	diptheria, pertussis, tetanus immunization	PID	pelvic inflammatory disease
EBV	Epstein-Barr virus	SLE	systemic lupus erythematosus
ELISA	enzyme-linked immunosorbent assay (test to determine the amount of a given chemical in a mixture); test for AIDS	STD	sexually transmitted disease
FUO	fever of unknown origin	strep	streptococcus
		TB	tuberculosis
		URI	upper respiratory infection
		VD	venereal disease

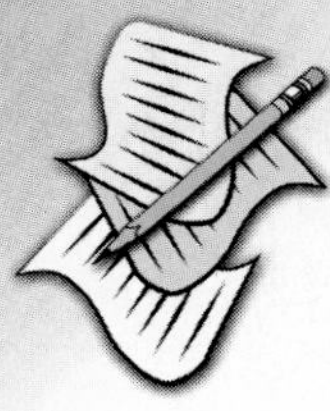

EXERCISE 15.1

Recognizing Look-Alikes and Sound Alikes

Below is a list of frequently used words that look alike and/or sound alike. Study the meaning and pronunciation of each set of words, then read the following sentences carefully and circle the word in parentheses that correctly completes the meaning.

coarse	(adj) composed of large particles; harsh or rough in tone
course	(n) direction, path

except	(v) to eliminate, to exclude
except	(prep) barring, excluding
accept	(v) to receive, to welcome

in vitro	(adj) in a test tube
in vivo	(adj) in the living body

coastal	(adj) relating to area where land and sea meet
costal	(adj) relating to a rib

dose	to give or take a prescribed amount of drug
doze	(v) to nap or to snooze

wait	(v) to remain, to stay
wait	(n) a delay
weight	(n) heaviness, load

allergen	(n) antigen that causes an allergy
antigen	(n) substance causing formation of antibodies

1. After years of infertility, the couple opted for (in vitro, in vivo) fertilization.
2. The patient tolerated every antibiotic in the treatment regimen (accept, except) Ceclor.
3. After taking her sleep medication, she was able to (dose, doze) intermittently.
4. Tests identified the (allergen, antigen) responsible for his itching, watery eyes.
5. She suffered a minor fracture in the (coastal, costal) area of the upper left quadrant.
6. The patient was unable to (accept, except) the limitations imposed by his illness.
7. The hip is a major (wait-, weight-) bearing joint.
8. The treatment (coarse, course) for non-Hodgkin lymphoma is radiation and chemotherapy.
9. After years of careful research, scientists isolated the pathogen in a (coastal, costal) region of the South.
10. All anti-rejection drugs (accept, except) one produced severe reactions in the transplant patient.

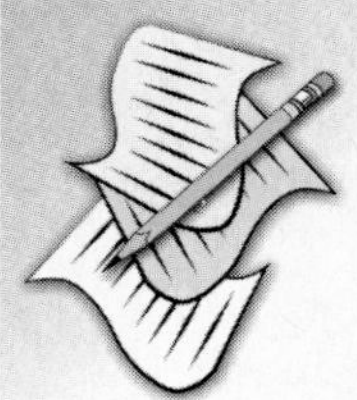

EXERCISE 15.2

Matching Sound and Spelling

The numbered list that follows shows the phonetic spelling of hard-to-spell words. Sound out the word, then write the correct spelling in the blank space provided. Each of the words can be found in the Glossary or in the drug list in Appendix D.

1. **noo**-trO-fil ____________________
2. **path**-O-jen ____________________
3. prO-fi-**lak**-sis ____________________
4. **fag**-O-sIt ____________________
5. pI-**rek**-see-a ____________________
6. ko-**myoon**-i-ka-bl ____________________
7. i-**myoo**-ni-tee ____________________
8. **tI**-ter ____________________
9. lim-fO-**pee**-nee-a ____________________
10. **sef**-a-klor ____________________

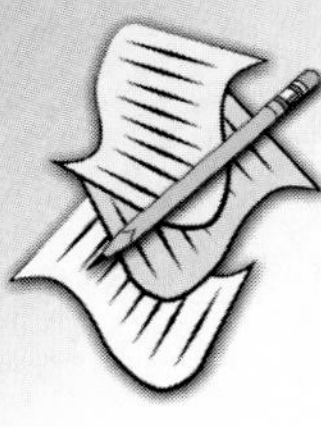

EXERCISE 15.3

Choosing Words from Context

When transcribing dictation, the medical transcriptionist frequently needs to consider the situation when determining the word that correctly completes the sentence. From the list below, select the term that meaningfully completes each of the following statements.

aerosolized	sinusitis	allergens
neutrophil count	immunodeficiency	ecchymoses
antigens	substernal	petechiae
prophylaxis	in vitro	
costal margin	titer	

1. It is necessary for children with sickle cell disease to take penicillin daily as _______________ against life-threatening infection.
2. When examining the abdomen, the physician percusses and palpates around the _______________ for the liver and spleen.
3. New drug therapies are tested ___________________ in the laboratory before being used in vivo.
4. Mr. Rogers had a severe frontal headache. This is often a sign of an infection called ___________________.
5. Joanne caught many colds and viruses; therefore, her doctor was performing laboratory tests to rule out an/a ___________ disorder.
6. When you have a low _______________________, you are susceptible to many bacterial infections.
7. The varicella ___________________was 1:32, indicating a past exposure to chickenpox.
8. If you have allergies, it is often necessary to determine which ________________ cause the allergy.
9. Whenever John took a deep breath, he had ______________ pain.
10. When you have asthma, it is often necessary to have the medications ___________________ through a nebulizer in order for them to reach deep into the lungs.
11. Margaret thought the tiny red dots on her skin were a rash, but Dr. Smith called them ______________.
12. The box banged across John's shins causing several ______________.

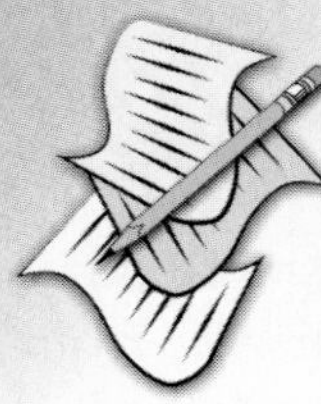

EXERCISE 15.4

Pairing Words and Meanings

From this list, locate the term that best matches each of the following definitions. Write the letter of the term in the space provided by each definition.

A.	bronchitis	E.	immune system	J.	immunology
B.	cytomegalovirus	F.	immunoglobulins	K.	defervesence
C.	enterovirus	G.	neutropenia	L.	in vitro
D.	hypergamma-globulinemia	H.	oral thrush		
		I.	steroid		

1. fungal infection of the mouth ________________
2. antibodies produced in lymph tissues ________________
3. body processes and organs that produce the interactions to protect the body from pathogens and other invaders ________________
4. inflammation of the mucous membranes of the bronchial tubes ________________
5. a virus that multiplies in the intestinal tract ________________
6. abnormally low number of white blood cells in the blood ________________
7. study of the body's response to foreign invasion ________________
8. excessive amount of gamma globulins in the blood ________________
9. a herpes-type virus that produces large cells and causes illness ________________
10. a hormonal substance ________________
11. in glass ________________
12. the time when body temperature returns to normal ________________

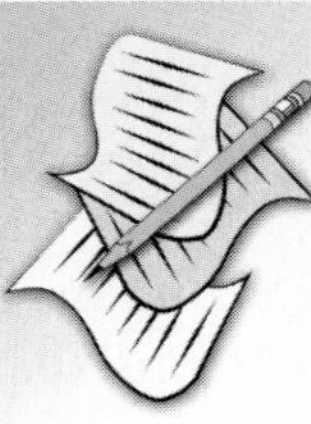

EXERCISE 15.5

Creating Terms from Word Forms

Combine prefixes, root words, and suffixes from this list to create medical words that fit the following definitions. Fill in the blanks with the words you construct.

aden/o	gland	splen/o	spleen
auto-	oneself	globulin	protein
bacteri/o	bacteria	phag/o	eating, swallowing
bronch/o	bronchus	virus	organism
cyt/o	cell	-cyte	cell
enter/o	small intestine	-emia	in the blood
hem/o	blood	-genesis	beginning
immun/o	safe, protected	-itis	inflammation
lymph/o	clear tissue fluid	-megaly	oversized
ot/o	ear	-oma	tumor
ox/o (i)	oxygen	-osis	condition
path/o	disease	-stasis	stop, stand

1. infection of one or more bronchi ______________________
2. protein that protects [the body] ______________________
3. enlarged spleen ______________________
4. imflammation of the lymph nodes ______________________
5. self-protected______________________
6. viral intestinal organism ______________________
7. bacteria in the blood______________________
8. ear infection ______________________
9. oxygen-carrying protein in the erythrocytes ______________________
10. large-cell virus with disease effects______________________
11. the beginning of a disease______________________
12. infected gland______________________

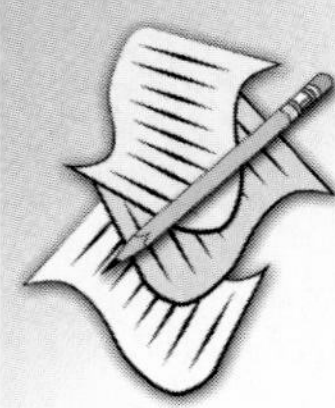

EXERCISE 15.6

Proofreading Review

Read the following partial report and look for errors in form, meaning, capitalization, word choice, punctuation, and spelling. Circle the errors, then key the report with the errors corrected.

This is a nown severe asthmatic patient who has been admitted on numerus occasions. She developed her asthma approximately 2 years ago. She was well up until a weak prior to addmission when she developed a cold which caused her to be a short of breath and conjested. The conjestion continued, and he gave herself some infections of Adrenalin.

Physical examination at the time of admission revealed a lady in moderate distress there were wheezes, rails and ronchi throughout all lung fields. Their were some substernal and intracostal retractions. the throat was somwhat inflammed. The rest of the physical examination at the time of admission was entirely within normal limits.

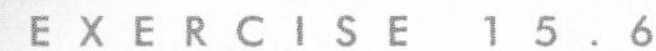

Building Transcription Skills

The Autopsy Report

When a patient dies unexpectedly or if the cause of death is uncertain or needs clarification, the attending physician requests an autopsy. Persons who die at home unexpectedly also will have an autopsy. These specialized pathology reports (Figure 15.4) vary in length and scope. For example, the report may focus on test results for a single organ. Or, if the autopsy concerns a crime victim, the report may detail the results of an extensive examination and studies of all body systems. Often, the autopsy report includes a cover letter that summarizes the results of the postmortem examination.

Required Headings/Content At a minimum, the autopsy report includes these categories:

- Authorization for the procedure
- Date of examination
- Name of the person performing the autopsy
- Names of the managing and consulting physicians
- Summary of the patient's clinical status and any details known to have contributed to the death
- Description of the body and all organs and cavities examined
- Preliminary report based on the gross examination (exam before tissues are removed)

- List of photos and studies completed
- List of microscopic studies
- Diagnosis based on the gross exam and laboratory studies

The report must be signed by the pathologist in compliance with hospital policy and state and federal regulations.

Turnaround Time In a hospital setting, the autopsy report should be completed within 90 days of the patient's death. However, for a criminal investigation, the turnaround time is rapid.

Preparing to Transcribe

To prepare for transcribing dictation, review the tables of common immunology terms, drugs, and abbreviations presented in the Building Language Skills section of this chapter. Then, study the format and organization of the model document shown in Figure 15.4, and key the model document. Proofread the document by comparing it with the printed version. Categorize the types of errors you made, and document them on a copy of the Performance Comparison chart provided in Chapter 1. A template of this chart is included on the IRC that accompanies this text.

Patient Studies

Transcribe, edit, and correct each report in the following patient studies. Consult reference books for words or formatting rules that are unfamiliar.

As you work on the transcription assignment for this chapter, fill in the Performance Comparison chart that you started when you keyed the model document. For at least three of the reports, categorize and document the types of errors you made. Answer the document analysis questions on the bottom of the chart. With continuous practice and assessment, the quality of your work will improve.

After you have produced a final version of each transcribed report, complete the Performance Report cover sheet, attach it to the top of the transcripts, and submit them to your instructor for evaluation.

use letter formatting guidelines

Date

Elgar Lewis, MD
Department of Pediatrics
University Medical School
Fort Worth, TX 78095-1509

Dear Dr. Lewis:

The postmortem examination performed on your patient, Rebecca Arnold, resulted in the following findings:

I. Acute lymphoblastic leukemia, widely disseminated, including bone marrow, spleen, liver, kidneys, lungs, lymph nodes, and other visceral organs.
II. Hemophagocytosis and intravascular coagulopathy within the bone marrow, spleen, liver, and kidneys.
III. Bleeding diathesis (clinical thrombocytopenia)
  A. Massive hemorrhage with hematoma formation in pelvic and lower abdominal retroperitoneal space.
  B. Punctate petechiae within the ascending aorta, heart, and gastrointestinal tract.
  C. Petechiae, with ecchymosis, both extremities.

Based on the above findings, the cause of death is attributed to massive retroperitoneal bleeding with thrombocytopenia (29,000) arising from intravascular coagulopathy and hemophagocytosis-platelet phagocytosis, in a patient with acute lymphoblastic leukemia.

Marvin L. Smith, MD
Pathologist

MS/XX
D: (4 days before today's date)
T: (today's date)

FIGURE 15.4
Autopsy Report (Cover Letter)

1-inch margins
left justification

AUTOPSY #: A-4832
NAME: Arnold, Rebecca
DATE: (4 days before today's date)
MR # 0329415

double-space between sections

This 4-year-old white female was admitted with bruises of a 2-week duration, fever of 1 week, and nose bleeding of 1 day.

On admission hemoglobin was 5.8, platelets 29,000, WBC 30,200 with 85% lymphoblasts. Acute lymphoblastic leukemia with L1 FAB classification was diagnosed after a bone marrow aspiration and biopsy were performed. She received allopurinol for hyperuricemia with a uric acid of 11.9 mg/dL (normal: 2.6-7.0). She was started on vancomycin for fevers. She was transfused single-donor platelets, but experienced a hypersensitivity reaction with chills, intercostal retractions, and nasal flaring with perioral cyanosis. Although the cyanosis improved and the respiratory distress improved, she developed active bleeding from the bone marrow aspiration site.

Shortly thereafter, the patient passed away, 2 days after her admission.

EXTERNAL EXAMINATION: The body is that of a well-developed, moderately nourished, pale female child. The body measures 85 cm from crown to heel, and weighs 15 kg. The facies are normal. The head is covered by a lot of hair. The eyes are of normal size. There are no epicanthic folds. The external ears show normal cartilaginous development; they are in their normal set location. The external auditory canals are patent. The nasal passages are patent. The posterior choanal canal can be probed. The nasal bridge is normal. The tongue is of normal size, and teeth are present. The tongue is free of ulcers and exudate. The palate is normal. There is no peripheral lymphadenopathy. The chest is symmetrical. The abdomen is slightly distended. Muscle development is normal. The genitalia are those of a normal female child. The urethral meatus is patent. The clitoris is not hypertrophied. The anus is patent. The back shows no scoliosis or kyphosis. There are 5 normally formed digits on the hands and feet which are free of edema and cyanosis. The palm lines are examined and are not unusual. The nails are developed. The skin shows pallor, petechiae, and ecchymoses.

(continued)

FIGURE 15.5
Autopsy Report

AUTOPSY #: A-4832
NAME: Arnold, Rebecca
MR #: 0329415
DATE: (4 days before today's date)
Page 2

INTERNAL EXAMINATION: The body is opened through the usual y-shaped incision. Subcutaneous fat is 0.5 cm thick. The umbilicus is removed en bloc with a wide skin margin.

ABDOMINAL CAVITY: The peritoneal cavity contains 50 cc of straw-colored, serosanguinous fluid. The abdominal and pelvic organs are in their normal position. The kidneys are normally located.

THORACIC CAVITY: The great veins are flat. Each pleural space contains 20 ml of clear fluid which is not cultured. No adhesions are found.

PERICARDIAL CAVITY: The pericardium is opened and contains no excess fluid. No adhesions are found. A blood culture is taken.

ORGAN DESCRIPTION
CARDIOVASCULAR SYSTEM **single-space between subsections**
HEART: The apex consists of the right/left ventricle. The aorta and pulmonary artery arise in their normal relation to one another. The pulmonary veins enter the left atrium and no anomalous veins are noted. The heart is opened along the normal blood flow channels. No abnormal valves are noted. The auricular appendage contains no clots or vegetations. The endocardium of the right atrium is of normal thickness. The septum primum covers the foramen ovale adequately and cannot be probed. The tricuspid valve consists of 3 normal, thin leaflets. The right ventricle shows its usual trabecular muscles: the cristae supraventricularis and outflow tract are normal. The pulmonary valve consists of three cusps without thickening. The pulmonary artery cannot be opened into the aorta. The main pulmonary artery measures 4.1 cm in circumference. The right and left pulmonary arteries are identified. The left atrium receives 2 pulmonary veins from each lung. The endocardium of the left atrium is thin. The mitral valve contains 2 normal leaflets, inserted by normal thin chordae tendineae onto the 2 papillary muscles. The mitral valve is continuous with the aortic valve. The outflow tract of the left ventricle is normal: the aortic valve contains 3 normal cusps. The myocardium of the left ventricle is mildly hypertrophied.

(continued)

FIGURE 15.5
Autopsy Report (Continued)

AUTOPSY #: A-4832
NAME: Arnold, Rebecca
MR # 0329415
DATE: (4 days before today's date)
Page 3

The left coronary artery arises from the left coronary cusps, and the right from the right. These pursue their usual course.
MEASUREMENTS

OPEN CIRCUMFERENCE:	Tricuspid 6.2 cm	Mitral 4.8 cm
	Pulmonic 4.1 cm	Aortic 3.5 cm
THICKNESS:	Right Ventricle 0.25 cm	Left Ventricle 1 cm

AORTA AND GREAT VESSELS: The aorta arises from the left ventricle, gives rise to 3 normal branches, and descends along the left side of the vertebral column.
VEINS: The inferior vena cava, superior vena cava, renal veins, and hepatic vein are patent. The splenic vein, inferior mesenteric, superior mesenteric, and portal veins are patent.

RESPIRATORY SYSTEM: The larynx and trachea are free of webs, mucous plugs, foreign bodies, edema, and mucosal ulcerations.
LUNGS: The heart and lungs together weigh 310 g. The pleural surfaces are pale. The bronchial tree is free of mucous plugs and exudate. The pulmonary parenchyma shows consolidation after dissection. The pulmonary arterial tree is free of thromboemboli.

GASTROINTESTINAL SYSTEM: The oral cavity and esophagus are free of fibrinopurulent membranes, vesiculoulcerations, and other lesions. There is no tracheoesophageal fistula, enteric duplication, stenosis, atresia, webs, or diverticula. The stomach is well-rugated and free of ulcers. The mesentery is normally rotated. The small intestine is collapsed. The duodenum, jejunum, ileum, and colon are intact and free of serosal and mucosal lesions. The cecum and appendix are in the right lower quadrant. The colon is normally attached to the posterior abdominal wall. No atresias are noted.
LIVER: The liver weighs 600 g. The capsule is transparent. The liver parenchyma is a normal brown-red and cuts with increased resistance. The lobular pattern is normal.
GALLBLADDER AND BILIARY TREE: The gallbladder contains green bile. Bile stones are absent. The mucosa is green. Bile can be expressed from the gallbladder into the duodenum. The common duct and right and left hepatic ducts are present.

(continued)

FIGURE 15.5
Autopsy Report (Continued)

AUTOPSY #: A-4832
NAME: Arnold, Rebecca
MR #: 0329415
DATE: (4 days before today's date)
Page 4

PANCREAS: The pancreas is cut longitudinally and the pancreatic duct is visualized. The lobular pattern is normal. No necrosis is noted.
GENITOURINARY SYSTEM: The kidneys weigh 150 g together and are left attached to the pelvic organs and aorta. The renal veins are opened and contain no thrombi. The renal arteries are normal. The kidneys show normal lobulations. The capsules strip easily, revealing a smooth surface. On cut surface, the corticomedullary junction is sharp. The parenchyma does not bulge from the cut surface. The pyramids and papillae are normal. Pelves are smooth and ureters arise from these and enter the urinary bladder normally at the trigone. The bladder wall is not hypertrophied. The urethra is opened and no posterior urethral valves are noted. The uterus is normally formed. The ovaries are unremarkable. The fallopian tubes are of average and uniform width.

HEMOLYMPHATIC SYSTEM
SPLEEN: The spleen weighs 145 g. The capsular surface is translucent and contains no wrinkling, exudates, or fibrosis. Cut surface is red and deep purple-brown, and consistency is mushy.
LYMPH NODES: The lymph nodes from the cervical, periaortic, peripancreatic, axillary, and inguinal areas are generally swollen.
THYMUS: The thymus weighs 6 g.
BONE MARROW: The marrow is red, moist, and ample.

ENDOCRINE SYSTEM
THYROID: The red-brown thyroid is normally placed in relation to the larynx. The weight of the bilateral lobes of thyroid is 4 g.
ADRENALS: The adrenals together weigh 6 g; cut surface shows a normal fetal and adult cortex.

MUSCULOSKELETAL SYSTEM
BONE: Two ribs are taken and bisected. The cartilage, epiphysis, and metaphysis are normal.
SKELETAL MUSCLES: Skeletal muscles are grossly normal.
JOINTS: The joints are not remarkable.
CRANIAL CAVITY: The reflected scalp shows no evidence of contusion, hematoma, or other lesion. The calvarium and bones at the base of the skull are not remarkable.

(continued)

FIGURE 15.5
Autopsy Report (Continued)

AUTOPSY #: A-4832
NAME: Arnold, Rebecca
MR #: 0329415
DATE: (4 days before today's date)
Page 5

No fractures or other injuries are present. The dura mater and pia arachnoid and associated spaces are normal in appearance. They are without hemorrhage or evidence of inflammation. The weight of the brain is 1280 g. The cerebral hemispheres are symmetrical and normal in appearance. Cut sections of the brain show symmetry and essentially normal structures throughout. The circle of Willis and other intracranial vessels are normal. The pituitary gland is grossly normal. The pineal gland is present.

SPINAL CORD AND VERTEBRAL COLUMN: Spinal cord and vertebral column are intact.

FINDINGS

I. RESPIRATORY SYSTEM: All lobes of lungs show leukemic cell infiltration around the bronchioles or blood vessels. There is edematous fluid accumulated in air spaces of the left lower lobe.

II. CARDIOVASCULAR SYSTEM: Leukemic cell infiltration with scattered aggregates in subepicardial adipose tissue is seen. Myocardium and endocardium are not remarkable.

III. GASTROINTESTINAL SYSTEM
LIVER: Shows extensive leukemic cell infiltration within all portal areas, but the hepatic architecture is well preserved. No bile stasis is seen. There was a proliferation of histiocytes with ingested platelets. Red blood cells in dilated sinusoids are seen, which is consistent with hemophagocytic syndrome. Atypical leukemic cells are seen infiltrated in the gastrointestinal mucosa and submucosa.

IV. GENITOURINARY SYSTEM
KIDNEYS: Bilateral kidneys show leukemic cell infiltration in the interstitium. Hemophagocytic syndrome is seen with erythrophagocytosis or platelet phagocytosis in the renal tubules.

ADNEXA: Adnexa including uterus, ovaries, and fallopian tubes show leukemic cell infiltration. Retroperitoneum parametrium show hemorrhage admixed with a few atypical cells.

URINARY BLADDER: Shows hematoma formation.

(continued)

FIGURE 15.5
Autopsy Report (Continued)

AUTOPSY #: A-4832
NAME: Arnold, Rebecca
MR#: 0329415
DATE: (4 days before today's date)
Page 6

V. HEMATOLOGICAL SYSTEM
SPLEEN: Shows extensive leukemic cell infiltration with congestion and hemorrhage. Hemophagocytosis is seen, also.

BONE MARROW: Shows leukemic cell infiltration with hemophagocytosis.

VI. LYMPHATIC SYSTEM: All lymph nodes reveal atypical leukemic cell infiltration.

VII. ENDOCRINE SYSTEM: Thymus, adrenal glands, thyroid, and pancreas all show leukemic cell infiltration.

____
Marvin L. Smith, MD

MS/XX
D: (4 days before today's date)
T: (today's date)

FIGURE 15.5
Autopsy Report (Continued)

Patient Study 15.A

June Pringle

June Pringle is a 38-year-old woman who is a severe asthmatic and suffers from chronic sinus problems. She has been to many physicians for treatment of her problems and is on chronic steroid therapy. She is referred to the immunologist for evaluation.

REPORT 15.1 Discharge Summary

- Listen for the following drug terms:
  adrenalin
  Sus-Phrine
  aminophylline (Note that the brand name, Aminophyllin, sounds very similar and is spelled similarly, so you will need to determine if the physician intended to specify the generic or the brand name. In this case, use the generic name.)
  Solu-Cortef
  Slo-Phyllin
  prednisone

REPORT 15.2 Consultation Letter

- Listen for the following drug and laboratory terms:
  Alupent
  immunoglobulins G, A, and M (transcribed as IgG, IgA, and IgM; each is sometimes dictated as the abbreviation)
- Transcribe the blood typing terms (anti-A and anti-B) with a lowercase "a" in "anti" and uppercase letters for the antigens A and B.

Patient Study 15.B **Riza Prince**

Riza Prince is a 15-month-old female who was born to a known HIV-positive mother. She has had several admissions to the hospital since birth and has been referred to the Pediatric AIDS Center in Fort Worth for treatment of AIDS.

REPORT 15.3 Chart Summary

- Listen for the following abbreviations:

FTNSVD	full-term, normal spontaneous vaginal delivery
ANC	absolute neutrophil count
PCP	Pneumocystis carinii
LFTs	liver function tests

- Listen for these drug and disease terms:
  hypergammaglobulinemia
  Bactrim
  pentamidine

REPORT 15.4 Consultation Letter

- Note that data is plural and datum is singular. Today most people use data as a collective term and use the singular verb as in this report.

Patient Study 15.C **Rebecca Arnold**

Rebecca Arnold is a 4-year-old girl who was admitted to the hospital with a fever, nosebleed, and bruises that had been present for 2 weeks. She was diagnosed with acute lymphoblastic leukemia and was treated with allopurinol, vancomycin, and platelet transfusions. Two days after her admission, she died, and an autopsy was performed to confirm the cause of death.

REPORT 15.5 Autopsy Report (Cover Letter)

REPORT 15.6 Autopsy Report

Patient Study 15.D — Courtney Baird

Courtney Baird is a 43-year-old woman with HIV. She reports feeling ill, with a cough and shortness of breath, and presents to her immunologist's office.

REPORT 15.7 History and Physical

Patient Study 15E — Josh Henry

Josh Henry is a 26-year-old man whose 2-year-old daughter was recently diagnosed with chickenpox. Mr. Henry presented to the emergency department with a fever and a vesicular rash covering his body. He was diagnosed with chickenpox, treated with Tylenol and Benadryl, and sent home. However, due to domestic problems, he returned to the hospital and was placed in isolation until the chickenpox lesions crusted.

REPORT 15.8 Discharge Summary

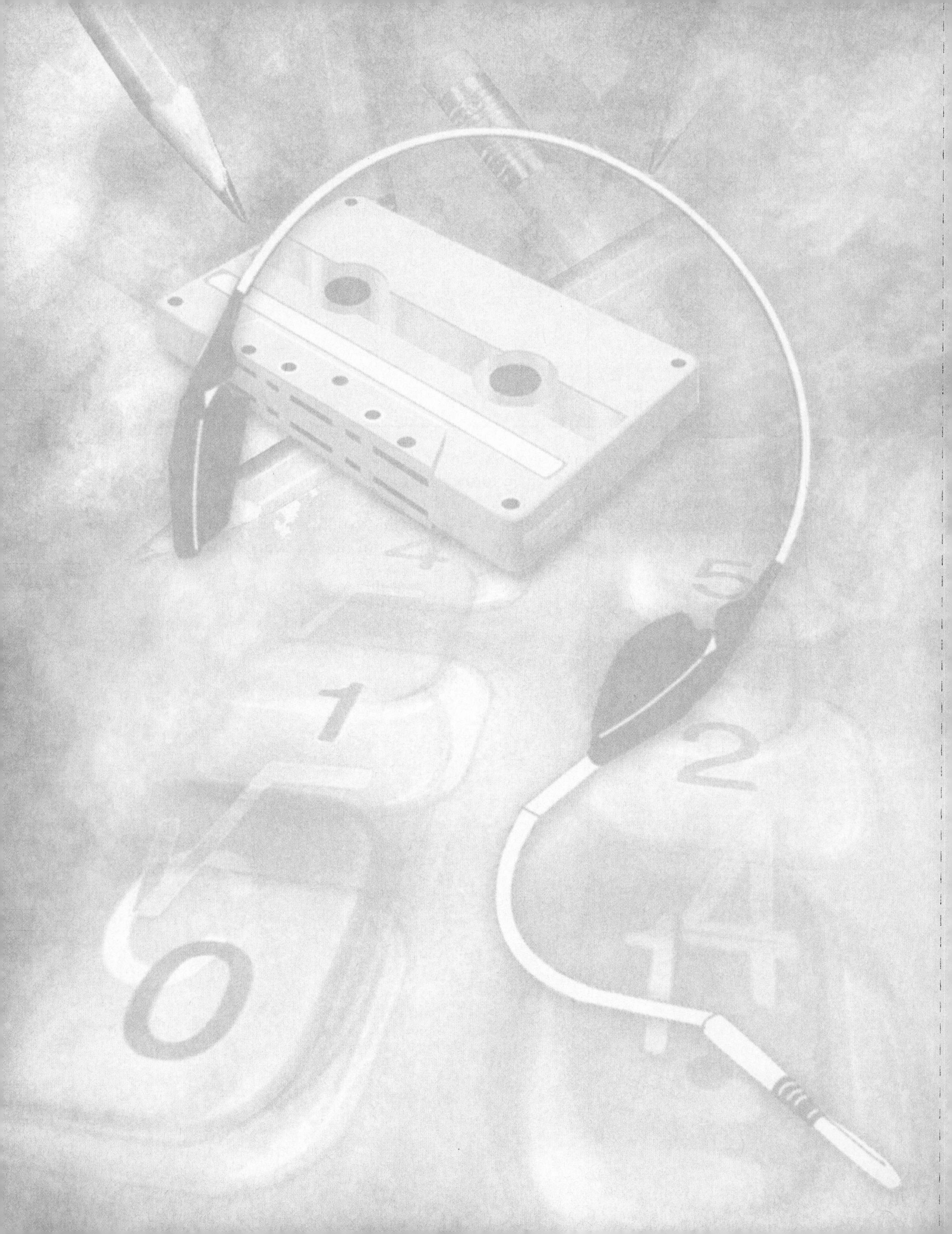

Using Medical References

Use the appropriate medical reference to locate the correct spelling and additional usage information for the words below. (If the reference is not available, use the Glossary in this text.) Circle the correct spelling, then write a sentence using the word correctly.

1.	phagocytosis	phagocytosus	phagoscytosis
2.	azithromycin	azythramiacin	azithrimiacyn
3.	prophylaxcis	prophylaxis	prophalaxis
4.	pyrexia	pryrexia	pyrechsea
5.	isoaglutination	isoagluttination	isoagglutination
6.	nuetropenia	neutrapenia	neutropenia
7.	hyprgammaglobulinemia	hypergamaglobulinemia	hypergammaglobulinemia
8.	streptococcus	streptococus	streptacoccus
9.	immunodeficeincy	imminodeficiency	immunodeficiency
10.	citukynes	cytokines	cytakynnes
11.	asma	aythma	asthma
12.	signusitis	sinusitis	sinisitis

Making Expert Decisions

Circle the correct word from the choices in parentheses.

1. A stool sample was obtained to test for (O&P/ONP).
2. The C3 (complement/compliment) was 33 with a reference range of 80-180.
3. Two units of (packed/pact) red blood cells were given to the patient after surgery.
4. After the exam was over, the patient stated, "Oh, by the way, I've been having rectal bleeding, but (its/it's) nothing really."
5. The CD4 cell count of 250 cells/mm3 (lead/led) to treatment with indinavir plus zidovudine.
6. Obtaining a culture and sensitivity of the urine (preceded/proceeded) the start of antibiotic treatment.
7. The patient had a tendency to (dose/doze) when visiting friends and had a history of sleep apnea, so she was advised to make an appointment with the sleep study clinic.
8. Because of the patient's severely immune-compromised state, a prophylactic (coarse/course) of treatment was recommended to prevent Pneumocystis carinii.
9. The patient was given AZT and would have continued on this course, (accept/except) that he developed severe neutropenia.
10. The patient discussed her fears with her physician, (who's/whose) advice was to contact a support group.

Transcribing Professional Documents

Transcribe the document named Chapter 15 Assessment. Before you key, review the appropriate formatting guidelines. Proofread your transcribed documents and revise it until you think it is error-free.

Appendix A

Endocrinology Job Simulation

Congratulations! Now that you have developed your medical transcription skills to a high level of competency, you are ready to bring your skills to the marketplace.

You have landed a contract to provide transcription services for a professional association of physicians that specializes in disorders of the endocrinology system. You will be expected to be able to recognize the specialized language—the terms, abbreviations, tests, and measurements—used by these professionals.

Medical transcription students generally have developed a professional library by the time they are seeking employment or business. You will need to use your knowledge of medical terminology and combine that with reference materials you own or can access on the Internet.

Your contract starts tomorrow! You have a limited time to research a general knowledge of the specific systems, the most common diseases, and the root words and combining forms that will be most useful to you. As always, you will have access to reference material while you work, but for maximum productivity you should be able to draw upon the resources you carry in your head.

On the first day on the job, you may be given the following tasks:

- A pre-employment spelling test, to be administered by the practice's office manager (your instructor).
- A number of reports to transcribe. The turnaround time will be determined by the office manager.
- Developing 3 lists: a) the 25 terms you would anticipate to occur most frequently (base this list on the endocrine disorders with the highest incidence), b) a list of 25 potentially confusing endocrinology terms, and c) the names and reference values of ten tests of the endocrine system, in table form.

Medical Transcriptionist Job Search

Medical transcriptionists should enjoy excellent job prospects according to the 2000–2001 *Occupational Outlook Handbook.* According to a survey recorded by the director of human resources at one of the top agencies, Headhunter, the market for health services is one of the top ten industries with the fastest wage and salary employment growth.

Overall employment is expected to grow, and the variety of skills that transcriptionists require to be successful enables them to be employed in hospitals, healthcare services, private doctors' offices, clinics, and medical establishments. Individuals can work at home for a medical transcription service, moonlight on the side on short-term projects for extra income, or choose to work part-time. Other options, such as being a supervisor, teaching individuals who want to become medical transcriptionists, or establishing a private business service, are also available to a transcriptionist who has had experience in a medical environment.

If you are interested in finding employment, you must be prepared for the job search. Several of the very basic skills you need are ability to learn, accountability for work performed, adaptability to a diversified work environment, and flexibility. In a medical environment, the transcriptionist must have a knowledge of medical terminology and must be patient, sympathetic, and a good listener when dealing with patients.

Keep in mind that job responsibilities should be compatible with your abilities and that the job should ultimately lead to upward mobility. This section will help you plan your strategies for the job search.

Defining Your Market

How do you get started? Employers generally prefer individuals who have had work experience and job-specific training rather than a novice. As a candidate for a job, you have to prove that you have the skills and qualities required on the job as well as personal attributes and abilities that other persons lack.

There are various steps you should follow. First, you have to decide what you would really like to do and whether or not your skills, knowledge, and other qualifications meet the requirements of the job. Make a list of your major skills.

Decide where you would like to work—hospital, doctor's office, clinic, walk-in health facility center, or organization. Then generate a job prospect list that will include the following traditional ways of finding a job. Develop a network of personal contacts—relatives, friends, church officials, etc.—and ask them to keep you in mind if they are aware of job openings. Join professional organizations, attend meetings, and become friendly with individuals in your profession. Make direct contacts with human resources at hospitals or organizations, read newspaper advertisements and journals, apply to temporary agencies, and use private employment agencies.

Prospective employees are searching for jobs that are posted on the Internet. Statistics show that the usage of the Internet is booming from three million in 1993 to 40 million in 1996, 200 million in 1999, and is expected to be at one billion in 2003. Individuals are going on-line to search for jobs; therefore, the Internet is *the* marketplace.

The Internet is an excellent resource and has several advantages not usually available. (1) You can find the hidden job market, which has unadvertised openings; (2) Major corporations list job openings on the websites because employers can fill jobs faster and less expensively; (3) Resumes can be sent anywhere in short periods of time; (4) Many categories of jobs can be found; and (5) A search can be done at any time, day or evening.

Creating an Effective Resume

A resume is a marketing document by which you hope to make an impression when searching for a job. Two styles of resumes used to get the reader's attention are the traditional, which can be modified to the chronological (Figure B.1a) and the traditional functional (Figure B.1b) formats. Traditional resumes aim to attract the employer by using action verbs, bullets, underlining, and colored paper. The chronological resume lists the dates of employment and educational background in reverse chronological order. This resume focuses on what you have done and have accomplished and what you are now doing. Employers who prefer the chronological resume to the functional resume feel that it clearly depicts the employment history and focuses on increased responsibilities and advancement. The functional format emphasizes skills and accomplishments as they relate to the job the candidate wants. If you lack experience in the job in which you are interested, then you should use the functional resume since the focus is on skills rather than work experience and education. The advantage of using this style of resume is that the applicant can carefully list the core skills and abilities and other areas of expertise that relate to the job. The skills can be stated in categories and supported with facts.

The electronic (online) resume (Figure B.2) must be easily read and understood by the computer. These resumes must be searchable and scannable by the computer. To accomplish this, key words or nouns for database searching must be supplied. Recruiters as well as employers search online for candidates to fill unadvertised job openings. Without knowing if positions are available, you can decide to send a resume to many companies for whom you would like to work. In contrast to traditional style resumes, the online types use plain text style and no italics or underlining. Use capitals, dashes, or asterisks for highlighting.

Interviewing

The interview is the final and most important step in the job-hunting process. Your performance and responses at the interview will be the final opportunity to demonstrate that you are the best candidate for the job. If you made a good impression, you will get the job offer.

Recently, telephone interviews have become the first contact made with an applicant for a job. A human resource person asks the applicant a few questions that pertain to the job. If the applicant makes a good impression, then a face-to-face interview is scheduled.

A computerized interview is also used by many companies. In this situation, the computer asks questions about the background, skills, and previous work experience of the applicant. Good and appropriate responses might lead to a face-to-face interview.

Prepare yourself for the interview by carrying out the following procedures.

- Research the company and gather information about its product, services, growth, culture, and employee/employer relations.
- Consider each interview you had as a learning situation.
- Determine the good points you made at the interview and those that were not so favorable. Study them and prepare yourself for the next interview.
- Make a list of the most frequently asked questions and think about your responses.
- Evaluate yourself, your behavior, your likes and dislikes, previous accomplishments that demonstrate your marketable skills, and your motivation. This will give you the self-confidence you need when responding to questions.
- Be prompt, be cordial, watch your body language, dress conservatively, and keep cell phones closed.

Creating an Application/Cover Letter

The application/cover letter should be included with every resume you send. This letter is actually the first impression you will make. Therefore, it should state the reason you are looking for a new

NAME
Street address
City, State Zip Code
Telephone
E-mail Address

JOB OBJECTIVE Statement of objective in sentence form.

EDUCATION Name of College or University
Street Address
City, State Zip Code
Degree

FIELD OF STUDY - - - - - - - - - - - - - - -

RELATED COURSES____________
____
____
____

SKILLS

WORK EXPERIENCE

Spring, 20XX ____________
College
Duties

Summer, 20XX Institution
Address
City, State Zip Code
Title of Position
Duties

FIGURE B.1a
Model Resumes
(a) The chronological resume would be listed in the following order: job objective, summary of skills, experience (list of names of companies, beginning to final period on staff, duties, education and training (name and major), attendance dates. (b) The functional resume emphasizes skills and accomplishments.

NAME
Street Address
City, State Zip Code
Telephone
E-mail Address

JOB OBJECTIVE Statement of objective in sentence form.

SPECIAL QUALIFICATIONS
- ____________
- ____________

WORK EXPERIENCE

Title____________
Dates ____________

(Use bullets) (Duties)

Title____________
Dates ____________

EDUCATION AND TRAINING

Degree, Major
College
Address

FIGURE B.1b

job, why this job interests you, some aspects of your background, and several important statements that reflect that you are the right person for the position. Indicate where you heard of the opening and how some of your skills and background will show that you are the right person for the job.

In the second paragraph, make a statement focusing on the type of person you are and why you would be an asset to the company. Indicate that the resume outlines your skills, experience, and education, and stress the qualifications that are right for the job. Be sure to make a very positive statement about the company.

In the closing paragraph, indicate your interest in the job and in working for the company. Request an interview and state that you will call on a particular day and at a particular time to set up an appointment. Leave your phone number and/or e-mail address where you can be reached.

Proofread your cover letter carefully. It should reflect you at your best.

NAME
Address
City, State Zip Code
Telephone
E-mail Address

KEYWORDS: medical assistant, pediatric office, transcriptionist, word, excel, telephone, maintains records, reports to work on time

SKILLS

- Operate Word skillfully
- Transcribe recorded dictation
- Computer skills

EMPLOYMENT HISTORY

Supervisor of Training
Inputted correspondence and reports
Transcribe recorded dictation

EDUCATION

A.S. Degree
College
Address
City, State Zip Code

FIGURE B.2
Model Electronic Resumes

Common Laboratory Values

The following list includes the laboratory values that appear most frequently in dictation regarding test results and procedures. These values are provided as a reference only. Each laboratory will have its own normal range.

Abbreviations

dL	deciliter	mcg	microgram	pg	picogram
g	gram	mEq	milliequivalent	mcL	microliter
Hg	mercury	mg	milligram	mcm^3	cubic micron
IU	international unit	m	millimeter		
L	liter	mm^3	cubic millimeter		

Blood Tests	**Normal Range**	
Arterial blood gases		
Partial pressure of oxygen	75–100 mm Hg	
Partial pressure of carbon dioxide	35–45 mm Hg	
pH	7.35–7.42	
Oxygen content	15–23%	
Oxygen saturation	94–100%	
Bicarbonate	22–26 mEq/L	
Blood electrolytes		
Carbon dioxide	22–34 mEq/L	
Calcium	8.9–10.1 mg/dL	
Chloride	100–108 mEq/L	
Magnesium	1.7–2.1 mg/dL	
Phosphates	2.5–4.5 mg/dL	
Potassium	3.5–5.0 mEq/L	
Sodium	135–145 mEq/L	
Blood cell counts		
Erythrocytes		
Men	4.2–5.4 million/mcL	
Women	3.6–5.0 million/mcL	
Children	4.6–4.8 million/mcL	
Erythrocyte sedimentation rate	0–20 mm/hour (increases with age)	
Leukocytes		
Total	4000–10,000 mm^3	
Differential	*Percentage*	*Absolute*
Myelocytes	0	0/mm^3
Band neutrophils	3–5	150–400/mm^3
Segmented neutrophils	54–62	3000–5800/mm^3
Lymphocytes	25–33	1500–3000/mm^3
Monocytes	3–7	300–500/mm^3
Eosinophils	1–3	50–250/mm^3
Basophils	0–0.75	15–50/mm^3

Blood Tests (continued)	**Normal Range**
Mean corpuscular volume (erythro.)	84–99 mcm^3
Mean corpuscular hemoglobin (erythro.)	26–32 pg
Mean corpuscular hemoglobin concentration (erythro.)	30–36%
Hematocrit	
Men	40–54 mL/dL
Women	37–47 mL/dL
Newborns	49–54 mL/dL
Children (varies with age)	35–49 mL/dL
Hemoglobin	
Men	12.4–18 g/dL
Women	11.7–16 g/dL
Newborns	16.5–19.5 g/dL
Children (varies with age)	11.2–16.5 g/dL
Reticulocytes	0.5–2% of total erythrocyte count
Coagulation tests	
Bleeding time (template)	2–8 min
(modified template)	2–10 min
(Ivy method)	1–7 min
(Duke method)	1–3 min
Activated partial thromboplastin time (PTT)	25–36 sec
Prothrombin time (PT)	10–14 sec
Clotting factors II, V, VII, and X	50–150% of normal
Clotting factors VII, IX, XI, and XII	50–150% of normal
Thrombin time	10–15 sec
Fibrin split products (Thrombo-Welco test)	<10 mcg/mL
Fibrinogen (Factor I)	195–365 mg/dL
Platelets	130,000–370,000/mm^3
Blood proteins and pigments	
Haptoglobin	38–270 mg/dL
Phenylalanine, serum	<3 mg/dL
Blood urea nitrogen	8–20 mg/dL
Creatinine	
Men	0.8–1.2 mg/dL
Women	0.6–0.9 mg/dL
Uric acid	
Men	4.3–8.0 mg/dL
Women	2.3–6.0 mg/dL
Bilirubin, serum	
Conjugated	0.1–0.4 mg/dL
Unconjugated	0.2–0.7 mg/dL
Total	0.3–1.1 mg/dL
Coombs' test	
Direct	Negative
Indirect	Negative
Immune system components	
T-cell	68–75% of total white blood cell count
B-cell	10–20% of total white blood cell count
Null cells	5–20% of total white blood cell count

Blood Tests (continued)	**Normal Range**
Immunoglobulins, serum	
IgG	700–1,800 mg/dL
IgA	70–443 mg/dL
IgM	60–290 mg/dL
IgD	0.5–3.0 mg/dL
IgE <500 ng/mL	
Blood enzymes	
Acid phosphatase (thymolphthalein monophosphate substrate), serum	0.5–1.9 IU/L
Alkaline phosphatase	
Men	90–239 IU/L
Women	
(under age 45)	76–196 IU/L
(over age 45)	87–250 IU/L
Blood fats and lipoproteins	
Cholesterol, serum	170–200 mg/dL
HDL	29–77 mg/dL
LDL	62–185 mg/dL
Triglycerides	
Men	40–160 mg/dL
Women	35–135 mg/dL
Plasma and serum values	
Adrenocorticotropin (ACTH), plasma	
6 a.m.	10–80 pg/mL
6 p.m.	<50 pg/mL
Alanine aminotransferase (ALT, SGPT), serum	5–30 U/L
Albumin, serum	3.5–5.5 g/dL
Ammonia nitrogen, plasma	15–49 mcg/dL
Aspartate aminotransferase (AST, SGOT), serum	10–30 U/L
Bile acids, serum	0.3–3.0 mg/dL
Cortisol, plasma	
8 a.m.	6–23 mcg/dL
4 p.m.	3–15 mcg/dL
10 p.m.	<50% of 8 a.m. value
Follicle-stimulating hormone (FSH), plasma	
Men	4–25 mU/mL
Women	4–30 mU/mL
Postmenopausal	40–250 mU/mL
Glucose (fasting), plasma or serum	70–115 mg/dL
Growth hormone (hGH), plasma	0–10 ng/mL
Insulin (fasting), plasma	5–25 mcU/mL
Iron binding capacity, serum	
Total	250–410 mcg/dL
Saturation	20–55%

Blood Tests (continued)	**Normal Range**
Lactate	
Venous blood	4.5–19.8 mg/dL
Arterial blood	4.5–14.4 mg/dL
Lactate dehydrogenase (LD, LDH), serum	100–190 U/L
Lipase, serum	10–140 UL
Luteinizing (LH), serum	
Men	6–18 IU/L
Women	
Premonopausal	5–22 IU/L
Mid-cycle	3 times baseline
Postmenopausal	>30 IU/L
Protein, serum	
Total	6.0–8.0 g/dL
Albumin	3.5–5.5 g/dL
$Alpha_1$ globulin	0.2–0.4 g/dL
$Alpha_2$ globulin	0.5–0.9 g/dL
Beta globulin	0.6–1.1 g/dL
Gamma globulin	0.7–1.7 g/dL
Testosterone, plasma	
Men	275–875 ng/dL
Women	23–75 ng/dL
Pregnant	38–190 ng/dL
Thyroid-stimulating hormone (TSH), serum	0–7 mcU/mL
Thyroxine, free (FT), serum	1.0–2.1 ng/dL
Thyroxine (T_4), serum	4.4–9.9 mcg/dL
Triiodothyronine (T_3), serum	150–250 ng/dL
Triiodothyronine uptake, resin (T_3RU)	25–38% uptake
Urea, serum or plasma	24–49 mg/dL
Viscosity, serum	1.4–1.8 times water
Vitamin A, serum	20–80 mcg/dL
Vitamin B_{12}, serum	180–900 pg/mL

Common Drugs

Capitalized drugs are brand names, and lower-case drugs are generic names.

4-Way Nasal Spray (oxymetazoline hydrochloride)
5-FU (fluorouracil)

A

A-200 (pyrethrins-piperonyl butoxide)
Abelcet (amphotericin B)
Abreva (decosanol)
acarbose (Precose)
Accolate (zafirlukast)
Accupril (quinapril)
acetazolamide (Diamox)
acetohexamide (Dymelor)
acetylcholine chloride (Miochol)
acetylcysteine (Mucomyst)
acetylsalicylic acid (ASA, aspirin)
Achromycin (tetracycline)
Aciphex (rabeprazole)
Actigall (ursodiol)
Actinex (masoprocol)
Activase (alteplase)
activated charcoal
Activella (estradiol-northidrone acetate)
Actonel (risedronate)
Actos (pioglitazone)
Acular (ketorolac)
acyclovir (Zovirax)
Adalat (nifedipine)
adapalene (Differin)
Adderall (amphetamine-dextroamphetamine)
Adrenalin (epinephrine)
Adriamycin (doxorubicin)
Advil (ibuprofen)
AeroBid (flunisolide)
AK-Con (naphazoline)
AK-Dex (dexamethasone)
AK-Spore H.C. (bacitracin-hydrocortisone acetate-neomycin sulfate-polymyxin B)
AK-Sulf (sulfacetamide sodium)
AK-Tracin (bacitracin)
AK-Trol (neomycin-polymyxin B-dexamethasone)
Alamast (pemirolast)
albumin human (Albuminar)
Albuminar (albumin human)
albuterol (Proventil, Proventil HFA, Ventolin, Volmax)
Aldactone (spironolactone)
aldesleukin (Proleukin, Interleukin-2)
alendronate (Fosamax)
alginic acid (Gaviscon)
alitretinoin (Panretin)
Alkeran (melphalan)
allopurinol (Zyloprim)
Alphagan (brimonidine)
alprazolam (Xanax)
alprostadil (Edex, Muse, Caverject)
Alrex (loteprednol)
alteplase (Activase)
altretamine (Hexalen)
aluminum acetate (Burow Solution)
aluminum hydroxide (Amphojel)
aluminum hydroxide-magnesium hydroxide (Maalox, Mylanta)
Alupent (metaproterenol)
amantadine (Symmetrel)
Amaryl (glimepiride)
Ambien (zolpidem)
amcinonide (Cyclocort)
Amen (medroxyprogesterone)
Amicar (aminocaproic acid)
amifostine (Ethyol)
amiloride (Midamor)
aminocaproic acid (Amicar)
aminoglutethimide (Cytadren)
aminolevulinic acid (Levulan)
aminophylline (Truphylline)
amiodarone (Cordarone)
amitriptyline (Elavil)
amoxicillin (Amoxil)
amoxicillin-clavulanic acid (Augmentin)
Amoxil (amoxicillin)
amphetamine-dextroamphetamine (Adderall)
Amphojel (aluminum hydroxide)
amphotericin B (Fungizone, Abelcet)
ampicillin (Omnipen)
Anadrol (oxymetholone)
Ancef (cefazolin)
Androderm (testosterone)
Android (methyltestosterone)
antihemophilic factor, factor VIII (Hemofil)
Antilirium (physostigmine)
antipyrine-benzocaine (Auralgan)
Antivert (meclizine)
Antizol (fomepizole)
Anucort HC (hydrocortisone)
Anusol HC (hydrocortisone)
apomorphine
apraclonidine (Iopidine)
AquaMEPHYTON (vitamin K1)
Aralen phosphate (chloroquine phosphate)
Aricept (donepezil)
Aristocort (triamcinolone)
Armour Thyroid (thyroid)
Artane (trihexyphenidyl)
ASA (acetylsalicylic acid)
Asacol (mesalamine)
asparaginase (Elspar)
aspirin (acetylsalicylic acid)
Atarax (hydroxyzine)
Ativan (lorazepam)
Atropair (atropine)
atropine (Atropair)
Atrovent (ipratropium bromide)
ATS (erythromycin)
attapulgite (Kaopectate)
Augmentin (amoxicillin-clavulanic acid)
Auralgan (antipyrine-benzocaine)
Auro (carbamide peroxide)
Avandia (rosiglitazone)
Aveeno Cleansing Bar (sulphur-salicylic acid)
Aventyl (nortriptyline)
Avonex (interferon beta-1a)
Axid (nizatidine)
azathioprine (Imuran)
azelaic acid (Azelex)
Azelex (azelaic acid)
azithromycin(Zithromax)

Azmacort (triamcinolone)
Azopt (brinzolamide)
Azo-Standard (phenazopyridine)
Azulfidine (sulfasalazine)

B

bacitracin (AK-Tracin)
bacitracin-hydrocortisone acetateneomycin sulfate-polymyxin B (AK-Spore H.C.)
bacitracin-neomycin-polymixin B (Triple Antibiotic)
bacitracin-neomycin-polymyxin B (AK-Spore)
baclofen (Lioresal)
Bactrim (sulfamethoxazole-trimethoprim)
Bactroban (mupirocin)
BAL (dimercaprol)
balsalazide (Colazal)
basiliximab (Simulect)
becalpermin gel (Regranex)
beclomethasone (Beclovent, Vanceril, Vancenase)
Beclovent (beclomethasone)
Bellatal (phenobarbital)
Benadryl (diphenhydramine)
benazepril (Lotensin)
benzalkonium chloride (Zephiran)
benzoyl peroxide
benzthiazide (Hydrex)
benztropine (Cogentin)
beractant (Survanta)
Betadine (providone-iodine)
betamethasone (Diprolene, Diprosone)
Betapace (sotalol)
Betaseron (interferon beta-1b)
betaxolol (Betoptic)
bethanechol (Urecholine)
Betoptic (betaxolol)
Biaxin (clarithromycin)
bicalutamide (Casodex)
Bicillin L-A (penicillin G benzathine)
BiCNU (carmustine)
Biltricide (praziquantel)
bisacodyl (Dulcolax)
bismuth subsalicylate (Pepto-Bismol)
bisoprolol-hydrochlorothiazide (Ziac)
bitolterol (Tornalate)
Blenoxane (bleomycin)
bleomycin (Blenoxane)
Bleph-10 (sulfacetamide sodium)
Blephamide (sulfacetamide-prednisolone)
Bonine (meclizine)
Brethaire (terbutaline)
brimonidine (Alphagan)
brinzolamide (Azopt)
British Anti-Lewisite (dimercaprol)
bromocriptine (Parlodel)
Bronkaid Mist (epinephrine)
Bronkosol (isoetharine)
budesonide (Rhinocort, Pulmicort Turbuhaler, Pulmicort Respules)
bumetanide (Bumex)
Bumex (bumetanide)
bupropion (Zyban)
Burow Solution (aluminum acetate)
BuSpar (buspirone)
buspirone (BuSpar)
busulfan (Myleran)
butenafine (Mentax)

C

Calciferol (ergocalciferol)
calcipotriene (Dovonex)
calcitonin-salmon (Miacalcin)
calcitriol (Rocaltrol)
calcium (Tums, Caltrate, Os-Cal, Titralac, Viactiv)
calcium chloride (CalPlus)
calcium disodium (EDTA)
calfactant (Infasurf)
CalPlus (calcium chloride)
Caltrate (calcium)
camphorated tincture of opium (paregoric)
Camptosar (irinotecan)
Capastat (capreomycin)
capecitabine (Xeloda)
Capoten (captopril)
capreomycin (Capastat)
captopril (Capoten)
Carafate (sucralfate)
carbachol (Isopto)
carbamazepine (Tegretol, Epitol)
carbamide peroxide (Auro, Debrox, Gly-Oxide)
carboplatin (Paraplatin)
Cardizem (diltiazem)
Cardura (doxazosin)
carmustine (BiCNU)
cascara sagrada
Casodex (bicalutamide)
Catapres (clonidine)
Catapres-TTS (clonidine)
Caverject (alprostadil)
CCNU (lomustine, CeeNU)
Ceclor (cefaclor)
CeeNU (lomustine, CCNU)
cefaclor (Ceclor)
cefadroxil (Duricef)
Cefadyl (cephapirin)
cefazolin (Ancef, Kefzol)
cefixime (Suprax)
Cefotan (cefotetan)
cefotaxime (Claforan)
cefotetan (Cefotan)
cefoxitin (Mefoxin)
cefpodoxime (Vantin, Proxetil)
cefprozil (Cefzil)
ceftazidime (Fortaz)
Ceftin (cefuroxime)
ceftriaxone (Rocephin)
cefuroxime (Zinacef, Ceftin)
Cefzil (cefprozil)
CellCept (mycophenolate)
cephalexin (Keflex)
cephalothin (Ceporacin)
cephapirin (Cefadyl)
Cephulac (lactulose)
Ceporacin (cephalothin)
Cerebyx (fosphenytoin)
Cerubidine (daunorubicin)
Cerumenex (triethanolamine polypeptide-oleate condensate)
Chibroxin (norfloxacin)
chlorambucil (Leukeran)
chloramphenicol (Chloromycetin, Chloroptic)
chlorhexidine (Hibiclens)
Chloromycetin (chloramphenicol)
Chloroptic (chloramphenicol)
chloroquine phosphate (Aralen phosphate)
chlorpropamide (Diabinese)
chlorthalidone (Hygroton)
Ciloxan (ciprofloxacin)
cimetidine (Tagamet)
Cipro (ciprofloxacin)
ciprofloxacin (Ciloxan, Cipro)
cisplatin (Platinol)
Citrucel (methylcellulose)
Claforan (cefotaxime)
clarithromycin (Biaxin)
Claritin (ioratadine)
Cleocin T (clindamycin)
Climara (estradiol)

clindamycin (Cleocin T)
clobetasol (Temovate)
clonazepam (Klonopin)
clonidine (Catapres, Catapres-TTS)
Clorox (sodium hypochlorite)
clotrimazole (GyneLotrimin, Lotrimin, FemCare, Mycelex)
clotrimazole-betamethasone (Lotrisone)
clove oil (Eugenol)
coal tar (Tegrin)
cocaine
Cogentin (benztropine)
Cognex (tacrine)
Colace (dioctyl sodium sulfosuccinate)
Colazal (balsalazide)
colfosceril (Exosurf)
Combivent (ipratropium-albuterol)
Compazine (prochlorperazine)
Comtan (entacapone)
conjugated estrogen-medroxyprogesterone (Prempro, Premphase, Premarin)
Copaxone (glatiramer acetate)
Cordarone (amiodarone)
cortisone (Cortone)
Cortisporin (neomycin-polymyxin B-hydrocortisone)
Cortone (cortisone)
Corvert (ibutelide)
Cosmegen (dactinomycin)
Cotazym (pancrelipase)
Coumadin (warfarin)
Creon (pancreatin)
Crolom (cromolyn sodium)
cromolyn sodium (Intal, Nasalcrom, Gastrocrom, Crolom)
Cuprimine (penicillamine)
cyclizine (Marezine)
Cyclocort (amcinonide)
Cyclogyl (cyclopentolate hydrochloride)
Cyclomen (danazol)
cyclopentolate hydrochloride (Cyclogyl)
cyclophosphamide (Cytoxan)
cycloserine (Seromycin)
cyclosporine (Sandimmune)
Cycrin (medroxyprogesterone)
Cylert (pemoline)
Cytadren (aminoglutethimide)
cytarabine (Cytosar-U)
Cytomel (liothyronine)
Cytosar-U (cytarabine)
Cytotec (misoprostol)
Cytoxan (cyclophosphamide)

D

dacarbazine (DTIC-Dome)
daclizumab (Zenapax)
dactinomycin (Cosmegen)
Dalmane (flurazepam)
danazol (Danocrine, Cyclomen)
Danocrine (danazol)
Darvon (propoxyphene)
daunorubicin (Cerubidine)
Daypro (oxaprozin)
DDAVP (desmopressin)
Debrox (carbamide peroxide)
Decadron (dexamethasone)
decosanol (Abreva)
deferoxamine (Desferal)
Deltasone (prednisone)
Demadex (torsemide)
Demulen (ethinyl estradiol-ethynodiol diacetate)
denileukin (Ontak)
Depakene (valproic acid)
Depakote (divalproex)
Depo-Provera (medroxyprogesterone)
Desferal (deferoxamine mesylate)
desipramine (Norpramin)
Desitin (zinc oxide)
desmopressin acetate (DDAVP)
desogestrel-ethinyl estradiol (Ortho-Cept)
desoximetasone (Topicort)
Desoxyn (methamphetamine)
Detrol (tolterodine)
Dexacidin (neomycin-polymyxin B-dexamethasone)
dexamethasone (AK-Dex, Decadron)
Dexedrine (dextroamphetamine)
dexrazoxane (Zinecard)
dextroamphetamine (Dexedrine)
DiaBeta (glyburide)
Diabinese (chlorpropamide)
Dialose (dioctyl potassium sulfosuccinate)
Diamox (acetazolamide)
diazepam (Valium)
diazoxide (Hyperstat)
diclofenac (Voltaren)
Didronel (etidronate)
diethylpropion (Tenuate)
diethylstilbestrol (Stilphostrol)
difenoxin (Motofen)
Differin (adapalene)
diflorasone (Psorcon, Florone)
Diflucan (fluconazole)
digoxin (Lanoxin)
Dilantin (phenytoin)
diltiazem (Cardizem)
dimenhydrinate (Dramamine)
dimercaprol (BAL, British Anti-Lewisite)
dioctyl calcium sulfosuccinate (Surfak)
dioctyl potassium sulfosuccinate (Dialose)
dioctyl sodium sulfosuccinate (Colace)
Dipentum (olsalazine)
diphenhydramine (Benadryl)
diphenoxylate-atropine (Lomotil)
dipivefrin (Propine)
Diprolene (betamethasone)
Diprosone (betamethasone)
dipyridamole (Persantine)
Ditropan (oxybutynin)
divalproex (Depakote)
Dizymes (pancreatin)
dobutamine hydrochloride
docusate-casanthranol (PeriColace)
donepezil (Aricept)
Donnatal (hyoscyamine-atropine-scopolamine-phenobarbital)
dopamine (Intropin)
Dopar (levodopa)
dornase alfa (Pulmozyme)
Doryx (doxycycline)
dorzolamide (Trusopt)
Dovonex (calcipotriene)
doxazosin (Cardura)
doxepin (Zonalon)
doxorubicin (Adriamycin)
doxycycline (Doryx)
Dramamine (dimenhydrinate)
DTIC-Dome (dacarbazine)
Dulcolax (bisacodyl)
Duphalac (lactulose)
Duratest (testosterone)
Duricef (cefadroxil)
Dyazide (triamterene-hydrochlorothiazide)
Dyclone (dyclonine)
dyclonine (Dyclone)
Dymelor (acetohexamide)
Dyrenium (triamterene)

E

echothiophate iodide (Phospholine Iodide)
econazole (Spectazole)
Edecrin (ethacrynic acid)
Edex (alprostadil)
edrophonium (Tensilon)
EDTA (calcium disodium)
Efudex (fluorouracil)
Elavil (amitriptyline)
Eldepryl (selegiline)
Elimite (permethrin)
Ellence (epirubicin)
Elmiron (pentosan polysulfate sodium)
Elocon (mometasone)
Elspar (asparaginase)
Emcyt (estramustine)
enalapril (Vasotec)
Enduron (methyclothiazide)
entacapone (Comtan)
epinephrine (Adrenalin, Primatene Mist, Bronkaid Mist, EpiPen)
EpiPen (epinephrine)
epirubicin (Ellence)
Epitol (carbamazepine)
epoetin alfa (Epogen, Procrit, erythropoietin)
Epogen (epoetin alpha)
Epsom salts (magnesium sulfate)
Ergamisol (levamisole)
ergocalciferol (vitamin D, Calciferol)
EryDerm (erythromycin)
erythromycin (T-Stat, ATS, EryDerm)
erythropoietin (epoetin alfa, Epogen, Procrit)
erythropoietin beta (Marogen)
esomeprazole (Nexium)
Estinyl (ethinyl estradiol)
Estrace (estradiol)
Estraderm (estradiol)
estradiol (Estrace, Estraderm, Vivelle, Climara)
estradiol-norgestimate (Ortho-Prefest)
estradiol-northidrone acetate (Activella)
estramustine (Emcyt)
estropipate (Ogen)
ethacrynic acid (Edecrin)
ethambutol (Myambutol)
Ethamolin (ethanolamine)
ethanolamine (Ethamolin)
ethinyl estradiol (Estinyl)
ethinyl estradiol-ethynodiol diacetate (Demulen)
ethinyl estradiol-norethindrone acetate (Femhrt)
ethionamide (Trecator-SC)
ethosuximide (Zarontin)
Ethyol (amifostine)
etidronate (Didronel)
etodolac (Lodine)
etoposide (VePesid)
Eugenol (clove oil)
Eulexin (flutamide)
Evista (raloxifene)
Exelderm (sulconazole)
Exosurf (colfosceril)

F

factor IX complex human (Koyne, Profilnine, Proplex)
famotidine (Pepcid)
Fastin (phentermine)
FemCare (clotrimazole)
Femhrt (ethinyl estradiol-norethindrone acetate)
FiberTrim (methylcellulose)
filgrastim (Neupogen)
finasteride (Proscar)
Flagyl (metronidazole)
flavoxate (Urispas)
Fleet (glycerin)
Fleet Phospho-Soda (sodium phosphate)
Flomax (tamsulosin)
Flonase (fluticasone)
Florone (diflorasone)
Flovent (fluticasone)
Floxin (ofloxacin)
floxuridine (FUDR)
fluconazole (Diflucan)
Fludara (fludarabine)
fludarabine (Fludara)
flumazenil (Romazicon)
flunisolide (AeroBid)
fluocinonide (Lidex)
fluoride
fluorometholone (FML Forte)
fluorouracil (5-FU, Efudex)
fluoxetine (Prozac, Sarafem)
flurazepam (Dalmane)
flurbiprofen (Ocufen)
flutamide (Eulexin)
fluticasone (Flovent, Flonase)
FML Forte (fluorometholone)
Folex (methotrexate)
folic acid (vitamin B9, Folvite)
folinic acid (leucovorin, Wellcovorin)
Folvite (folic acid)
fomepizole (Antizol)
fomivirsen sodium (Vitravene)
Fortaz (ceftazidime)
Fosamax (alendronate)
fosphenytoin (Cerebyx)
FUDR (floxuridine)
Fulvicin (griseofulvin)
Fungizone (amphotericin B)
furfuryladenine (Kinerase)
furosemide (Lasix)

G

gabapentin (Neurontin)
Gammagard (immune globulin)
Gastrocrom (cromolyn sodium)
Gas-X (simethicone)
Gaviscon (alginic acid)
Gelusil (magnesium trisilicate)
Gentak (gentamicin)
gentamicin (Gentak)
Gesterol (hydroxyprogesterone)
gingko
glatiramer acetate (Copaxone)
glimepiride (Amaryl)
glipizide (Glucotrol, Glucotrol XL)
Glucophage (metformin)
Glucotrol (glipizide)
Glucotrol XL (glipizide)
glyburide (DiaBeta, Glynase, Micronase)
glycerin (Fleet)
Glynase (glyburide)
Gly-Oxide (carbamide peroxide)
Glyset (miglitol)
GoLYTELY (polyethylene glycol-electrolyte solution)
goserelin (Zoladex)
goserelin acetate implant (Zoladex)
granisetron (Kytril)
griseofulvin (Fulvicin)
guaifenesin-dextromethorphan (Robitussin, Humibid)
GyneLotrimin (clotrimazole)

H

Habitrol (nicotine)
halcinonide (Halog)
halobetasol (Ultravate)

Halog (halcinonide)
HCTZ (hydrochlorothiazide)
Head and Shoulders (pyrithione zinc)
Helidac (tetracycline-metronidazole-bismuth)
Hemofil (antihemophilic factor, factor VIII)
heparin
Herplex (idoxuridine)
hexachlorophene (pHisoHex)
Hexalen (altretamine)
HFA (albuterol)
Hibiclens (chlorhexidine)
Hiprex (methenamine)
Humalog (lispro)
Humatrope (somatropin)
Humibid (guaifenesin-dextromethorphan)
Humulin (insulin)
Hycamtin (topotecan)
Hydrea (hydroxyurea)
Hydrex (benzthiazide)
hydrochlorothiazide (HCTZ, Esidrix, HydroDIURIL)
hydrocodone-acetaminophen (Lortab)
hydrocortisone (Anusol HC, Anucort HC, Solu-Cortef)
HydroDIURIL (hydrochlorothiazide)
hydrogen peroxide (Peridex, Peroxyl)
hydroxyprogesterone (Hylutin, Gesterol)
hydroxyurea (Hydrea)
hydroxyzine (Atarax, Vistaril)
Hygroton (chlorthalidone)
Hylutin (hydroxyprogesterone)
hyoscyamine-atropine-scopolamine-phenobarbital (Donnatal)
Hyperstat (diazoxide)
Hytrin (terazosin)

I

ibuprofen (Advil, Motrin)
ibutelide (Corvert)
Idamycin (idarubicin)
idarubicin (Idamycin)
idoxuridine (Herplex)
Ifex (ifosfamide)
ifosfamide (Ifex)
imipenem-cilastatin (Primaxin)
imipramine (Tofranil)
immune globulin (Gammagard)
Immunex (thiotepa)
Imodium (loperamide)
Imuran (azathioprine)
indapamide (Lozol)
Indocin (indomethacin)
indomethacin (Indocin)
Infasurf (calfactant)
INFeD (iron dextran injection)
infliximab (Remicade)
INH (isoniazid)
insulin aspart (Norvolog)
insulin glargine (Lantus)
Intal (cromolyn sodium)
interferon alfa-2a (Roferon)
interferon alfa-2b (Intron)
interferon alfa-n1 (Wellferon)
interferon beta-1a (Avonex)
interferon beta-1b (Betaseron)
Interleukin-2 (aldesleukin)
Intron (interferon alfa-2b)
Intropin (dopamine)
Iopidine (apraclonidine)
ioratadine (Claritin)
ipecac syrup
ipratropium bromide (Atrovent)
ipratropium-albuterol (Combivent)
irinotecan (Camptosar)
iron dextran injection (INFeD)
isoetharine (Bronkosol)
isoniazid (INH, Laniazid, Nydrazid, Rifamate, Rifater)
isopropyl (alcohol)
isoproterenol (Isuprel)
Isoptin (verapamil)
Isopto (carbachol)
Isopto Carpine (pilocarpine)
Isuprel (isoproterenol)

K

K Dur (potassium chloride)
Kaopectate (attapulgite)
Keflex (cephalexin)
Kefzol (cefazolin)
Keppra (levetiracetam)
ketoconazole (Nizoral)
ketorolac (Acular)
ketotifen (Zaditor)
Kinerase (furfuryladenine)
Klonopin (clonazepam)
Koyne (factor IX complex human)
Kwell (lindane)
Kytril (granisetron)

L

lactulose (Duphalac, Cephulac)
Lamictal (lamotrigine)
Lamisil (terbinafine)
lamotrigine (Lamictal)
Laniazid (isoniazid)
Lanoxin (digoxin)
lansoprazole (Prevacid)
Lantus (insulin glargine)
Larodopa (levodopa)
Lasix (furosemide)
latanoprost (Xalatan)
leucovorin (folinic acid, Wellcovorin)
Leukeran (chlorambucil)
Leukine (sargramostim)
leuprolide (Lupron Depot)
levalbuterol (Xopenex)
levamisole (Ergamisol)
levetiracetam (Keppra)
levodopa (Dopar, Larodopa)
levodopa-carbidopa (Sinemet)
levonorgestrel (Norplant)
levonorgestrel-ethinly estradiol (Triphasil 21)
Levothroid (levothyroxine, T_4)
levothyroxine (T_4, Synthroid, Levothroid, Lovoxyl)
Levulan (aminolevulinic acid)
Lidex (fluocinonide)
lidocaine-diphenhydramine-Maalox (Magic Swizzle)
lindane (Kwell)
Lioresal (baclofen)
liothyronine (Cytomel)
liotrix (Thyrolar)
lispro (Humalog)
Lodine (etodolac)
Lomotil (diphenoxylate-atropine)
lomustine (CCNU, CeeNU)
loperamide (Imodium)
lorazepam (Ativan)
Lortab (hydrocodone-acetaminophen)
Lotemax (loteprednol)
Lotensin (benazepril)
loteprednol (Alrex, Lotemax)
Lotrimin (clotrimazole)
Lotrisone (clotrimazole-betamethasone)
lovastatin (Mevacor)
Lovoxyl (levothyroxine, T_4)
Lozol (indapamide)
Luminal (phenobarbital)

Lupron Depot (leuprolide)
Lysodren (mitotane)

M

Maalox (aluminum hydroxide-magnesium hydroxide
Macrodantin (nitrofurantoin)
mafenide acetate (Sulfamylon)
Magic Swizzle (lidocaine-diphenhydramine-Maalox)
magnesium hydroxide (Milk of Magnesia)
magnesium sulfate (Epsom salts)
magnesium trisilicate (Gelusil)
mannitol (Osmitrol, Resectisol)
Marezine (cyclizine)
Marogen (erythropoietin beta)
masoprocol (Actinex)
Matulane (procarbazine)
Maxair (pirbuterol)
Maxitrol (neomycin-polymyxin B-dexamethasone)
Maxzide (triamterene-hydrochlorothiazide)
Mazanor (mazindol)
mazindol (Mazanor)
mebendazole (Vermox)
mechlorethamine (Mustargen)
meclizine (Antivert, Bonine)
Medrol (methylprednisolone)
medroxyprogesterone (Amen, Depo-Provera)
Mefoxin (cefoxitin)
Megace (megestrol)
megestrol (Megace)
melphalan (Alkeran)
Mentax (butenafine)
mequinol-tretinoin (Solage)
mercaptopurine (Purinethol)
Meridia (sibutramine)
mesalamine (Rowasa, Asacol, Pentasa)
Mestinon (pyridostigmine)
Metamucil (psyllium hydrophilic mucolloid)
metaproterenol (Alupent)
metformin (Glucophage)
methamphetamine (Desoxyn)
methazolamide (Neptazane)
methenamine (Urex, Hiprex)
methimazole (Tapazole)
methotrexate (Rheumatrex, Folex)
methyclothiazide (Enduron)
methylcellulose (FiberTrim, Citrucel)
methylene blue (Urolene Blue, Trac 2-X)
methylphenidate (Ritalin)
methylprednisolone (Medrol, Solu-Medrol)
methyltestosterone (Android, Testred)
metoclopramide (Reglan)
metolazone (Zaroxolyn)
Metro-Gel (metronidazole)
metronidazole (Metro-Gel, Flagyl)
Mevacor (lovastatin)
Miacalcin (calcitonin-salmon)
miconazole (Monistat)
Micronase (glyburide)
Midamor (amiloride)
miglitol (Glyset)
Milk of Magnesia (magnesium hydroxide)
Minipress (prazosin)
Mintezol (thiabendazole)
Miochol (acetylcholine chloride)
Mirapex (pramipexole)
misoprostol (Cytotec)
Mithracin (plicamycin)
mitomycin C (Mutamycin)
mitotane (Lysodren)
mitoxantrone (Novantrone)
Mitrolan (polycarbophil)
mometasone (Elocon)
Monistat (miconazole)
montelukast (Singulair)
Motofen (difenoxin)
Motrin (ibuprofen)
Mucomyst (acetylcysteine, N-Acetyl-L-Cysteine)
multiple vitamins (MVI)
mupirocin (Bactroban)
muromonab-CD3 (Orthoclone OKT3)
Muse (alprostadil)
Mustargen (mechlorethamine)
Mutamycin (mitomycin C)
MVI (multiple vitamins)
Myambutol (ethambutol)
Mycelex (clotrimazole)
Mycolog II (nystatin)
mycophenolate (CellCept)
Mycostatin (nystatin)
Mylanta (aluminum hydroxide-magnesium
Mylanta (simethicone)
Myleran (busulfan)
Mylicon (simethicone)
Mysoline (primidone)

N

nabumetone (Relafen)
N-Acetyl-L-Cysteine (Mucomyst)
naloxone (Narcan)
naphazoline (AK Con, Naphcon, Vasocon A)
Naphcon (naphazoline)
Naqua (trichlormethiazide)
Narcan (naloxone)
Nasalcrom (cromolyn sodium)
Natacyn (natamycin)
natamycin (Natacyn)
nedocromil (Tilade)
neomycin-polymyxin B (Neosporin)
neomycin-polymyxin B-dexamethasone (AK-Trol, Dexacidin, Maxitrol)
neomycin-polymyxin B-hydrocortisone (Cortisporin)
Neosporin (neomycin-polymyxin B)
neostigmine (Prostigmin)
Neptazane (methazolamide)
Nestrex (pyridoxine)
Neupogen (filgrastim)
Neurontin (gabapentin)
Nexium (esomeprazole)
Niclocide (niclosamide)
niclosamide (Niclocide)
Nicoderm (nicotine)
Nicorette (nicotine)
nicotine (Habitrol, Nicoderm, Nicorette, Nicotrol, Nicotrol NS, ProStep)
Nicotrol (nicotine)
Nicotrol NS (nicotine)
nifedipine (Adalat, Procardia)
Nilandron (nilutamide)
Nilstat (nystatin)
nilutamide (Nilandron)
nimodipine (Nimotop)
Nimotop (nimodipine)
Nitro-Bid (nitroglycerin)
nitrofurantoin (Macrodantin)
nitroglycerin (Nitrostat, Nitro-Bid)
Nitrostat (nitroglycerin)
Nix (permethrin)
nizatidine (Axid)
Nizoral (ketoconazole)
Nolvadex (tamoxifen)

norethindrone-mestranol (OrthoNovum)
norfloxacin (Chibroxin)
Norplant (levonorgestrel)
Norpramin (desipramine)
nortriptyline (Aventyl, Pamelor)
Norvolog (insulin aspart)
Novantrone (mitoxantrone)
Novolin (insulin)
Nutropin (somatropin)
Nydrazid (isoniazid)
nystatin (Mycolog II, Mycostatin, Nilstat)

O

Ocufen (flurbiprofen)
Ocuflox (ofloxacin)
Ocuserts (pilocarpine)
ofloxacin (Floxin, Ocuflox)
Ogen (estropipate)
olsalazine (Dipentum)
omeprazole (Prilosec)
Omnipen (ampicillin)
Oncovin (vincristine)
ondansetron (Zofran)
Ontak (denileukin)
Orinase (tolbutamide)
orlistat (Xenical)
Orthoclone OKT3 (muromonab-CD3)
OrthoNovum (norethindrone-mestranol)
Ortho-Prefest (estradiol-norgestimate)
Ortho-Cept (desogestrel-ethinyl estradiol)
Os-Cal (calcium)
Osmitrol (mannitol)
oxaprozin (Daypro)
oxcarbazepine (Trileptal)
oxiconazole (Oxistat)
Oxistat (oxiconazole)
oxybutynin (Ditropan)
oxycodone-acetaminophen (Percocet, Tylox)
oxymetazoline hydrochloride (4-Way Nasal Spray)
oxymetholone (Anadrol)

P

paclitaxel (Taxol)
Pamelor (nortriptyline)
Pancrease (pancrelipase)
pancreatin (Creon, Dizymes)
pancrelipase (Cotazym, Pancrease, Zymase)
Panretin (alitretinoin)
pantoprazole (Protonix)
papaverine (Pavabid)
Paraplatin (carboplatin)
paregoric (camphorated tincture of opium)
Parlodel (bromocriptine)
paroxetine (Paxil)
Pavabid (papaverine)
Paxil (paroxetine)
Pediapred (prednisolone)
pemirolast (Alamast)
pemoline (Cylert)
penicillamine (Cuprimine)
penicillin G benzathine (Bicillin L-A)
penicillin V (Veetids)
Pentasa (mesalamine)
pentosan polysulfate sodium (Elmiron)
Pepcid (famotidine)
Pepto-Bismol (bismuth subsalicylate)
Percocet (oxycodone-acetaminophen)
pergolide (Permax)
PeriColace (docusate-casanthranol)
Peridex (hydrogen peroxide)
Permax (pergolide)
permethrin (Nix, Elimite)
Peroxyl (hydrogen peroxide)
Persantine (dipyridamole)
Phazyme (simethicone)
phenazopyridine (Pyridium, Azo-Standard, Urogesic)
Phenergan (promethazine)
phenobarbital (Solfoton, Bellatal, Luminal)
phenol sodium borate-sodium bicarbonate-glycerin (Ulcer Ease)
phentermine (Fastin)
phentolamine (Regitine)
phenytoin (Dilantin)
pHisoHex (hexachlorophene)
Phospholine Iodide (echothiophate iodide)
physostigmine (Antilirium)
pilocarpine (Isopto Carpine, Ocuserts, Salagen)
pioglitazone (Actos)
pirbuterol (Maxair)
Pitressin (vasopressin)
Platinol (cisplatin)
plicamycin (Mithracin)
polycarbophil (Mitrolan)
polyethylene glycol-electrolyte solution (GoLYTELY)
potassium chloride (K Dur)
pralidoxime (Protopam)
pramipexole (Mirapex)
Pravachol (pravastatin)
pravastatin (Pravachol)
praziquantel (Biltricide)
prazosin (Minipress)
Precose (acarbose)
prednisolone (Pediapred)
prednisone (Deltasone)
Premarin (conjugated estrogen-medroxyprogesterone)
Premphase (conjugated estrogen-medroxyprogesterone)
Prempro (conjugated estrogen-medroxyprogesterone)
Prevacid (lansoprazole)
Priftin (rifapentine)
Prilosec (omeprazole)
Primatene Mist (epinephrine)
Primaxin (imipenem-cilastatin)
primidone (Mysoline)
Pro-Banthine (propantheline)
procainamide (Procan, Pronestyl)
Procan (procainamide)
procarbazine (Matulane)
Procardia (nifedipine)
prochlorperazine (Compazine)
Procrit (erythropoietin, epoetin alpha)
Profenal (suprofen)
Profilnine (factor IX complex human)
Prograf (tacrolimus)
Prokine (sargramostim)
Proleukin (aldesleukin)
promethazine (Phenergan)
Pronestyl (procainamide)
propantheline (Pro-Banthine)
Propine (dipivefrin)
Proplex (factor IX complex human)
propoxyphene (Darvon)
propylthiouracil (PTU)
Proscar (finasteride)
ProStep (nicotine)
Prostigmin (neostigmine)
Protonix (pantoprazole)
Protopam (pralidoxime)
Protropin (somatrem)

Proventil (albuterol)
Provera (medroxyprogesterone)
providone-iodine (Betadine)
Proxetil (cefpodoxime)
Prozac (fluoxetine)
pseudoephedrine sulphate (Sudafed)
Psorcon (diflorasone)
psyllium hydrophilic mucolloid (Metamucil)
PTU (propylthiouracil)
Pulmicort (budesonide)
Pulmicort Respules (budesonide)
Pulmozyme (dornase alfa)
Purinethol (mercaptopurine)
pyrazinamide (Tebrazid)
pyrethrins-piperonyl butoxide (Rid, A-200)
Pyridium (phenazopyridine)
pyridostigmine (Mestinon)
pyridoxine (vitamin B6, Nestrex)
pyrithione zinc (Head and Shoulders)

Q

quinapril (Accupril)

R

rabeprazole (Aciphex)
radioactive iodine (^{131}I)
raloxifene (Evista)
ranitidine (Zantac)
ranitidine-bismuth-citrate (Tritec)
Rapamune (sirolimus)
Regitine (phentolamine)
Reglan (metoclopramide)
Regranex (becalpermin gel)
Relafen (nabumetone)
Remicade (infliximab)
Renagel (sevelamer)
Renova (tretinoin)
Requip (ropinirole)
Resectisol (mannitol)
Retin-A (tretinoin)
Rheumatrex (methotrexate)
Rhinocort (budesonide)
Rid (pyrethrins-piperonyl butoxide)
Rifadin (rifampin)
Rifamate (isoniazid)
rifampin (Rifadin, Rimactane)
rifapentine (Priftin)
Rifater (isoniazid)
Rilutek (riluzole)
riluzole (Rilutek)
Rimactane (rifampin)
risedronate (Actonel)
Ritalin (methylphenidate)
Robitussin (guaifenesin-dextromethorphan)
Rocaltrol (calcitriol)
Rocephin (ceftriaxone)
Roferon (interferon alfa-2a)
Romazicon (flumazenil)
ropinirole (Requip)
rosiglitazone (Avandia)
Rowasa (mesalamine)

S

Salagen (pilocarpine)
salmeterol (Serevent)
Sandimmune (cyclosporine)
Sarafem (fluoxetine)
sargramostim (Prokine, Leukine)
selegiline (Eldepryl)
selenium sulfide (Selsun Blue)
Selsun Blue (selenium sulfide)
senna (Senokot)
Senokot (senna)
Septra (sulfamethoxazole-trimethoprim)
Serevent (salmeterol)
Seromycin (cycloserine)
sertraline (Zoloft)
sevelamer (Renagel)
sibutramine (Meridia)
sildenafil (Viagra)
Silvadene (silver sulfadiazine)
silver nitrate
silver sulfadiazine (Silvadene)
simethicone (Phazyme, Gas-X, Mylicon, Mylanta)
Simulect (basiliximab)
simvastatin (Zocor)
Sinemet (levodopa-carbidopa)
Singulair (montelukast)
sirolimus (Rapamune)
Slo-Phyllin (theophylline)
sodium hypochlorite (Clorox)
sodium phosphate (Fleet Phospho-Soda)
Solage (mequinol-tretinoin)
Solfoton (phenobarbital)
Solu-Cortef (hydrocortisone)
Solu-Medrol (methylprednisolone)
somatrem (Protropin)
somatropin (Humatrope, Nutropin)
sotalol (Betapace)
Spectazole (econazole)
spironolactone (Aldactone)
Stilphostrol (diethylstilbestrol)
streptomycin
streptozocin (Zanosar)
sucralfate (Carafate)
Sudafed (pseudoephedrine sulphate)
sulconazole (Exelderm)
sulfacetamide sodium (AK-Sulf, Bleph-10)
sulfacetamide-prednisolone (Blephamide)
sulfamethoxazole-trimethoprim (Bactrim, Septra)
Sulfamylon (mafenide acetate)
sulfasalazine (Azulfidine)
sulfate-polymyxin B (AK-Spore H.C.)
sulphur-salicylic acid (Aveeno Cleansing Bar)
Sultrin (triple sulfa)
Suprax (cefixime)
suprofen (Profenal)
Surfak (dioctyl calcium sulfosuccinate)
Survanta (beractant)
Symmetrel (amantadine)
Synthroid (levothyroxine, T_4)
syrup of ipecac

T

Tabloid (thioguanine)
tacrine (Cognex)
tacrolimus (Prograf)
Tagamet (cimetidine)
tamoxifen (Nolvadex)
tamsulosin (Flomax)
Tapazole (methimazole)
Tasmar (tolcapone)
Taxol (paclitaxel)
Tebrazid (pyrazinamide)
Tegretol (carbamazepine)
Tegrin (coal tar)
Temodar (temozolamide)
Temovate (clobetasol)
temozolamide (Temodar)
Tensilon (edrophonium)
Tenuate (diethylpropion)
terazosin (Hytrin)
terbinafine (Lamisil)
terbutaline (Brethaire)
testosterone (Androderm, Duratest)
Testred (methyltestosterone)
tetracycline (Achromycin,

Topicycline)
tetracycline-metronidazole-bismuth (Helidac)
Theo-dur (theophylline)
theophylline (Theo-dur, Slo-Phyllin)
thiabendazole (Mintezol)
thiethylperazine (Torecan)
thioguanine (Tabloid)
thiotepa (Immunex)
thyroid (Armour Thyroid)
Thyrolar (liotrix)
Tigan (trimethobenzamide)
Tilade (nedocromil)
timolol (Timoptic)
Timoptic (timolol)
Tinactin (tolnaftate)
tioconazole (Vagistat)
Titralac (calcium)
tizanidine (Zanaflex)
TobraDex (tobramycin-dexamethasone)
tobramycin-dexamethasone (TobraDex)
Tofranil (imipramine)
tolazamide (Tolinase)
tolbutamide (Orinase)
tolcapone (Tasmar)
Tolinase (tolazamide)
tolnaftate (Tinactin)
tolterodine (Detrol)
Topamax (topiramate)
Topicort (desoximetasone)
Topicycline (tetracycline)
topiramate (Topamax)
topotecan (Hycamtin)
Torecan (thiethylperazine)
Tornalate (bitolterol)
torsemide (Demadex)
Trac 2-X (methylene blue)
Trecator-SC (ethionamide)
tretinoin (Retin-A, Renova)
triamcinolone (Aristocort, Azmacort)
triamterene (Dyrenium)
triamterene-hydrochlorothiazide (Dyazide, Maxzide)
trichlormethiazide (Naqua)
triethanolamine polypeptide-oleate condensate (Cerumenex)
triflupromazine (Vesprin)
trifluridine (Viroptic)
trihexyphenidyl (Artane)
Trileptal (oxcarbazepine)
trimethobenzamide (Tigan)
Triphasil 21 (levonorgestrel-ethinly estradiol)
Triple Antibiotic (bacitracin-neomycin-polymixin B)
triple sulfa (Sultrin, Trysul)
Tritec (ranitidine-bismuth-citrate)
Truphylline (aminophylline)
Trusopt (dorzolamide)
Trysul (triple sulfa)
T-Stat (erythromycin)
Tums (calcium)
Turbuhaler (budesonide)
Tylox (oxycodone-acetaminophen)

U

Ulcer Ease (phenol sodium borate-sodium bicarbonate-glycerin)
Ultravate (halobetasol)
Urecholine (bethanechol)
Urex (methenamine)
Urispas (flavoxate)
Urogesic (phenazopyridine)
Urolene Blue (methylene blue)
ursodiol (Actigall)

V

Vagistat (tioconazole)
valacyclovir (Valtrex)
Valium (diazepam)
valproic acid (Depakene)
valrubicin (Valstar)
Valstar (valrubicin)
Valtrex (valacyclovir)
Vancenase (beclomethasone)
Vanceril (beclomethasone)
Vantin (cefpodoxime)
Vasocon A (naphazoline)
vasopressin (Pitressin)
Vasotec (enalapril)
Veetids (penicillin V)
Velban (vinblastine)
Ventolin (albuterol)
VePesid (etoposide)
verapamil (Isoptin)
Vermox (mebendazole)
Vesprin (triflupromazine)
Viactiv (calcium)
Viagra (sildenafil)
vidarabine (Vira-A)
vinblastine (Velban)
vincristine (Oncovin)
Vira-A (vidarabine)
Viroptic (trifluridine)
Vistaril (hydroxyzine)
vitamin B6 (pyridoxine)
vitamin B9 (folic acid)
vitamin D (ergocalciferol)
vitamin K1 (AquaMEPHYTON)
Vitravene (fomivirsen sodium)
Vivelle (estradiol)
Volmax (albuterol)
Voltaren (diclofenac)

W

warfarin (Coumadin)
Wellcovorin (leucovorin)
Wellferon (interferon alfa-n1)

X

Xalatan (latanoprost)
Xanax (alprazolam)
Xeloda (capecitabine)
Xenical (orlistat)
Xopenex (levalbuterol)

Z

Zaditor (ketotifen)
zafirlukast (Accolate)
Zanaflex (tizanidine)
Zanosar (streptozocin)
Zantac (ranitidine)
Zarontin (ethosuximide)
Zaroxolyn (metolazone)
Zenapax (daclizumab)
Zephiran (benzalkonium chloride)
Ziac (bisoprolol-hydrochlorothiazide)
zileuton (Zyflo)
Zinacef (cefuroxime)
zinc oxide (Desitin)
Zinecard (dexrazoxane)
Zithromax (azithromycin)
Zocor (simvastatin)
Zofran (ondansetron)
Zoladex (goserelin acetate implant)
Zoladex (goserelin)
Zoloft (sertraline)
zolpidem (Ambien)
Zonalon (doxepin)
Zonegran (zonisamide)
zonisamide (Zonegran)
Zovirax (acyclovir)
Z-Pak (azithromycin)
Zyban (bupropion)
Zyflo (zileuton)
Zyloprim (allopurinol)
Zymase (pancrelipase)

Abbreviations and Symbols

Medical Abbreviations

A

AB or Ab	abortion
ABG	arterial blood gas
a.c.	before meals
AC	air conduction
ACC	accommodation
ACG	angiocardiography
ACS	American Cancer Society
ACTH	adrenocorticotropic hormone
AD	right ear (auris dextra)
ADH	antidiuretic hormone
ad lib	as desired
AE	above the elbow (amputation)
AFB	acid-fast bacillus (organism that causes tuberculosis)
AFP	alpha-fetoprotein (tumor marker for liver and germ cells)
A/G	albumin/globulin ratio
AGN	acute glomerulonephritis
AHF	antihemophilic factor VIII
AHG	antihemophilic globulin factor VIII
AICA	anterior inferior communicating artery
AIDS	acquired immuno deficiency syndrome; caused by HIV
AK	above the knee (amputation)
ALL	acute lymphoblastic leukemia
ALS	amyotrophic lateral sclerosis
a.m.	morning
AMA	American Medical Association
AML	acute myelogenous leukemia
ANC	absolute neutrophil count; antigen neutralizing capacity
ANLL	acute nonlymphoblastic leukemia
ANS	autonomic nervous system
AOM	acute otitis media
A&P	auscultation and percussion
AP	anterior posterior (used in radiology)
APL or APML	acute promyelocytic leukemia
ARDS	acute respiratory distress syndrome
AROM	active range of motion
AS	aortic stenosis; left ear (auris sinistra)
ASD	atrial septal defect
ASHD	arteriosclerotic heart disease
ATN	acute tubular necrosis
AV	atrioventricular; arteriovenous

B

BaE or BE	barium enema
baso	basophil
BBB	bundle-branch block
BBT	basal body temperature (temperature in the morning before doing anything muscular)
BCE	basal cell epithelioma
BCM	below costal margin
BE	barium enema (also BaE); below the elbow (amputation)
BFM	Berlin-Frankfurt-Munster (chemotherapy); biceps femoral muscle
BID or b.i.d.	twice a day
BiPAP	bilevel positive airway pressure
BK	below the knee (amputation)
BM	bowel movement; bone marrow (in oncology)
BMA	bone marrow aspiration
BMR	basal metabolic rate
BMT	bone marrow transplant
BOOP	bronchiolitis obliterans–organizing pneumonia
BP	blood pressure
BPH	benign prostatic hypertrophy
BSE	breast self-exam
BSO	bilateral salpingo-oophorectomy (removal of both ovaries and fallopian tubes)
BTL	bilateral tubal ligation (sterilization by cutting or cauterizing the fallopian tubes)
BUN	blood urea nitrogen (blood test)
BX or bx	biopsy

C

C	Celsius or centigrade
C1, C2, etc.	cervical vertebra (number)
CA	cancer or carcinoma
CA-125	ovarian carcinoma antigen (tumor marker for ovary)
CAD	coronary artery disease
CALLA or cALLa	common acute lymphocytic leukemia antigen
CAT scan	computerized axial tomography scan
CBC	complete blood count
CC	chief complaint; cardiac catheterization
cc	cubic centimeter
CCU	coronary care unit
CDC	Centers for Disease Control
CDH	congenital dislocation of the hip
CEA	carcinoembryonic antigen (tumor marker for colon, lung, breast, others)
CF	circumflex (artery)
cGy	centigray
CHF	congestive heart failure
CLL	chronic lymphoblastic leukemia
cm	centimeter
CML	chronic myelogenous leukemia
CMV	cytomegalovirus; one of a group of large species-specific herpes-type viruses with a wide variety of disease effects
CNS	central nervous system
C/O or c/o	complained of
CO2	carbon dioxide
COLD	chronic obstructive lung disease
contra	against
COPD	chronic obstructive pulmonary disease
CP	cerebral palsy
CPAP	continuous positive air pressure
CPD	cephalopelvic disproportion
CPR	cardiopulmonary resuscitation
C&S	culture and sensitivity
CS or C section	cesarean section
CSF	cerebrospinal fluid
CT scan	computerized tomography scan
CV	cardiovascular
CVA	cerebrovascular accident (stroke); costovertebral angle
CXR	chest radiograph; chest x-ray
cysto	cystoscopy; cystoscopic examination

D

D	diopter (strength of lens in eyeglass prescription)
d	day
db	decibel
D&C	dilatation (or dilation) and curettage (instrumental expansion of the cervix and scraping of the uterine cavity)
DC	discharge
DDS	Doctor of Dental Surgery
D&E	dilation and evacuation
derm	dermatology
DES	diethylstilbestrol
DI	diabetes insipidus
diff	differential (describes cells in the white blood count)
DIP	desquamative intersitial pneumonia
DIP joint	distal interphalangeal joint
DJD	degenerative joint disease
DM	diabetes mellitus
DNA	deoxyribonucleic acid
DNR	do not resuscitate
DO	Doctor of Osteopathy
DOA	date of admission; dead on arrival
DOB	date of birth
DOS	date of service
DPT	diphtheria-pertussis-tetanus (immunization)
DTR	deep tendon reflexes
DUB	dysfunctional uterine bleeding
DVM	Doctor of Veternary Medicine
DVT	deep vein thrombosis
DX or Dx	diagnosis

E

EAC	external ear canal
EBV	Epstein-Barr virus
ECG or EKG	electrocardiogram
EDC	estimated or expected date of confinement
EEG	electroencelphalogram or electroencephalography
EENT	eye, ear, nose, throat
EGD	esophagogastroduodenoscopy
ELISA	enzyme-linked immunoabsorbent assay (test to determine the amount of a given chemical in a mixture)
Em	emmetropia
EMG	electromyogram or electromyography

ENT	ear, nose, throat
EOM	extraocular movement
EOMI	extraocular muscle intact
eos or eosin	eosinophil (type of white blood cell)
ER	emergency room
ESR	erythrocyte sedimentation rate (blood test)
EST	electric shock therapy
ESWL	extracorporeal shock-wave lithotripsy
et al.	and others
EXT or ext	extremities

F

F	Fahrenheit
FAAP	Fellow of the Academy of Pediatrics
FAB L1	French-American-British Level 1
FACP	Fellow of the American College of Physicians
FACS	Fellow of the American College of Surgeons
FBS	fasting blood sugar
FDA	Food and Drug Administration
FEF	forced expiratory flow
FEF25-75%	forced midexpiratory flow
FEKG	fetal electrocardiogram
FEV	forced expiratory volume
FEV1	forced expiratory volume in one second
FEV3	forced expiratory volume in three seconds
FH	family history
FHR	fetal heart rate
FHT	fetal heart tone
FS	frozen section (pathology)
FSH	follicle stimulating hormone
FTI	free thyroxine index
FTND	full term normal delivery
FTNSVD	full term normal spontaneous delivery
FUO	fever of unknown origin
FVC	forced vital capacity
FVL	flow volume loop
FX or Fx	fracture

G

GB	gallbladder
GC	gonorrhea (gynococcal)
GERD	gastroesophageal reflux disease
GFR	glomerular filtration rate
GH	growth hormone
GI	gastrointestinal
g	gram (measurement)
gr	grain (measurement)
GTT	glucose tolerance test
gtt or gtts	drop or drops (measurement)
GU	genitourinary
Gy	gray
GYN or Gyn	gynecology

H

h	hour
HAL	hyperalimentation
HCG or hCG	human chorionic gonadotropin (a hormone; tumor marker for germ cells)
HCl	hydrochloric acid
HCT or Hct or hct	hematocrit
HD	hip disarticulation; Hodgkin disease
HDL	high-density lipoprotein (a type of cholesterol)
HEENT	head, eyes, ears, nose, throat
Hg	mercury
HGB or hgb or hb	hemoglobin
HIV	human immunodeficiency virus; causes deterioration of the immune system
HNP	herniated nucleus pulposus (disc); hemagglutinin neuroaminidase protein
HP	hemipelvectomy
HPI	history of present illness
HRT	hormone replacement therapy
h.s.	hour of sleep (at bedtime)
HSG	hysterosalpingography
HSV-1	herpes simplex virus Type 1
HSV-2	herpes simplex virus Type 2

I

ICA	internal carotid artery
ICP	intracranial pressure
ICU	intensive care unit
I&D	incision and drainage
ID	intradermal; infectious disease; internal development (ortho)
Ig	immunoglobulin
IICP	increased intracranial pressure
IM	intramuscular
IMA	internal mammary artery

I&O	intake and output
IOL	intraocular lens
IOP	intraocular pressure
IPPB	intermittent positive-pressure breathing
IQ or I.Q.	intelligence quotient
IS	intracostal space; incentive spirometry
ITP	immune thrombocytopenic purpura
IU	international unit
IUD	intrauterine device
IV or I.V.	intravenous (intravenously)
IVC	intravenous cholangiography
IVDA	intravenous drug abuser
IVIG	intravenous immunoglobulin
IVP	intravenous pyelogram

K

KD	knee disarticulation
kg	kilogram
KOH	potassium hydroxide
KUB	kidney, ureter, bladder (x-ray examination)

L

L or l	liter
L1, etc.	first lumbar vertebra, etc.
L&A	light and accommodation
LAD	left anterior descending coronary artery
LAT or lat	lateral
lb	pound
LCA	left coronary artery
LCF	left circumflex
LDH	lactic dehydrogenase (tumor marker germ cell and lymphoma)
LDL	low-density lipoprotein (a type of cholesterol)
LE	left eye
leuk	leukocytes (white blood cells)
LH	luteinizing hormone
LIMA	left internal mammary artery
LLQ	left lower quadrant
LMCA	left main coronary artery
LMP	last menstrual period
LOC	loss of consciousness; level of consciousness
LP	lumbar puncture (spinal tap)
LPA	left pulmonary artery
LPN	Licensed Practical Nurse
LRQ	lower right quadrant
LUQ	left upper quadrant
lymphs	lymphocytes (a type of white blood cell)

M

m	meter
mcg	microgram
MCH	mean corpuscular hemoglobin
MCHC	mean corpuscular hemoglobin concentration
MCP joint	metacarpophalangeal joint
MCV	mean corpuscular volume
MCL	midclavicular line
MD or M.D.	Medical Doctor or Doctor of Medicine
MDI	metered dose inhaler
mEq	milliequivalents
mets	metastases
mg	milligram
MI	myocardial infarction
ml or mL	milliliter
mm	millimeter
mn or m	minum
mono	monocyte (a type of white blood cell)
MPA	main pulmonary artery
MRI	magnetic resonance imaging
MS	mitral (valve) stenosis; multiple sclerosis; musculoskeletal
MVP	mitral valve prolapse
MYOP or myop	myopia

N

NAD	no acute distress; no appreciable disease
NB	newborn
NB or N.B.	note well or notice (nota bene)
neuts	neutrophils (a type of white blood cell)
NKDA	no known drug allergy
NL or N.L.	normal limits
NPH	neutral protamine Hegedron (a type of insulin)
NPO or n.p.o.	nothing by mouth
NSAID	nonsteroidal anti-inflammatory drug

O

O2	oxygen
OA	osteoarthritis
OB	obstetrics

OD	right eye (oculus dexter); doctor of optometry; overdose (drug)
od	once a day
OM	obtuse marginal coronary artery
OR	operating room
ortho	orthopedics
os	mouth
OS	left eye (oculus sinister)
Oto	otology
OU or ou	both eyes (oculi unitas)
oz	ounce

P

P	pulse
PA	physician's assistant; posterior anterior view in an x-ray; pulmonary artery
P&A	percussion and auscultation
PAM	potential acuity meter
PAN	periodic alternating nystagmus; periarteritis nodosa
Pap	Papanicolaou smear
PAP	positive airway pressure
PAT	paroxysmal atrial tachycardia
Path	pathology
PBI	proteinbound iodine
PC or pc or P.C. or p.c.	after meals
PCP	Pneumocystis carinii pneumonia
PCV	packed cell volume
PD	patent ductus; peritoneal dialysis; postprandial (after meals)
PDA	posterior descending artery; patent ductus arteriosis
PE	physical examination
PE tubes	pressure-equalizing tubes
PEEP	positive end expiratory pressure
PEF	peak expiratory flow
per	through or by
PERRLA	pupils equal, round, and reactive to light and accommodation
pH	hydrogen ion concentration
PICA	posterior inferior communicating artery
PID	pelvic inflammatory disease
PIP joint	proximal interphalangeal joint
PKU	phenylketonuria (an amino acid)
plts or PLT	platelets
p.m.	afternoon or evening
PMD	primary medical doctor
PMH	past medical history
PMI	point of maximal impulse
PMN	polymorphonuclear neutrophil
PMP	previous menstrual period
PND	paroxysmal nocturnal dyspnea
PNH	paroxysmal nocturnal hematuria
PNS	peripheral nervous system
PO or po or P.O or p.o.	by mouth (per os)
poly	polymorphonuclear neutrophil
PP or pp	postprandial (after meals)
PROM	passive range of motion
prn or p.r.n.	as needed
PSA	prostate specific antigen (tumor marker for prostate)
PT	prothrombin time
PT or P/T	physical therapy
PTA	prior to admission
PTH	parathyroid hormone
PTT	partial thromboplastin time
PVC	premature ventricular contraction

Q

q	every
qd or q.d.	every day
qh or q.h.	every hour
q. 2 h or q 2h	every 2 hours
QID or Q.I.D. or q.i.d.	four times a day
qns or q.n.s.	quantity not sufficient
q.o.d.	every other day

R

R	respiration
rad	radiation dose
RAI	radioactive iodine
RBC	red blood cell
RCA	right coronary artery
RDS	respiratory distress syndrome
RE	right eye
REM	rapid eye movement
Rh	rhesus blood factor (a factor within the blood)
RLQ	right lower quadrant
RN or R.N.	Registered Nurse
RNA	ribonucleic acid
ROJM	range of joint movement
ROM	range of motion
RP	retrograde pyelogram (a kidney test)
RPA	right pulmonary artery

RRR	regular rate and rhythm
RT or R/T	radiation therapy
RUQ	right upper quadrant
Rx or RX	prescription

S

S1, etc.	first sacral vertebra, etc.
S-A	sinoatrial node
SAR	seasonal allergic rhinitis
SC or SQ or Subcu	subcutaneous
SD	shoulder disarticulation
sed rate	sedimentation rate
seg	segmented neutrophil
SFA	superficial femoral artery
SIDS	sudden infant death syndrome
SLE	systemic lupus erythematosus
SMR	submucosal resection
SNS	somatic nervous system
SOB	shortness of breath
sp. gr.	specific gravity
SQ or SC or Subcu	subcutaneous
ST	esotropia
staph	staphylococcus
Stat	immediately
STD	sexually transmitted disease
strep	streptococcus
Subcu or SC or SQ	subcutaneous

T

T	temperature
T1, etc.	first thoracic vertebra, etc.
T3	triiodothyronine
T4	thyroxine
T&A	tonsillectomy and adenoidectomy
tab	tablet
TAH	total abdominal hysterectomy
TAH/BSO	total abdominal hysterectomy with bilateral salpingo-oophorectomy
TB	tuberculosis
tbs or tblsp	tablespoonful
TENS	transcutaneous electric nerve stimulation
THA	total hip arthroplasty
TIA	transient ischemic attack
T.I.D. or tid or t.i.d.	three times a day
TM	tympanic membrane
TMJ	temporomandibular joint
TNM	tumor, nodes, metastasis (refers to tumor staging)
TPN	total parenteral nutrition
TPR	temperature, pulse, respiration
TSH	thyroid stimulating hormone
tsp	teaspoonful
TTH	thyrotrophic hormone
TUR; TURP	transurethral resection (prostatectomy)
Tx	treatment

U

UA or U/A	urinalysis
UC	uterine contractions
UGI	upper gastrointestinal
ULQ	upper left quadrant
ung	ointment
UPPP	uvulopalatophryngoplasty
URI	upper respiratory infection
URQ	upper right quadrant
USP	United States Pharmacopeia
UTI	urinary tract infection
UV	ultraviolet

V

VA	visual acuity
VAH	vaginal hysterectomy
VBAC	vaginal birth after cesarean section
VC	vital capacity
VD	venereal disease
VDRL	Venereal Disease Research Laboratory (test for syphilis)
VF	visual field
VH	vaginal hysterectomy
VHD	ventricular heart disese
VLDL	very lowdensity lipoprotein
VSD	ventricular septal defect

W

WBC	white blood cell
WDWN	well-developed, well-nourished
Wgt or wt	weight
WNL or W.N.L.	within normal limits

X

x	by (size as in 5 x 5 inches)
XRT	x-ray therapy or radiation therapy
XT	exotropia
XX	female sex chromosomes
XY	male sex chromosomes

Medical Symbols

p̄	after
α	alpha, is proportional to, particle
≈	approximately equal to
@	at
↑↑	Babinski sign, extensor response (neurologic examination)
↓↓	Babinski sign, plantar response (neurologic examination)
ā	before
β	beta
Δ	change, prism diopter
✔c̄	check with
©	copyright
↓ or ↘	decrease, below, falling
°	degree
°C	degrees Centigrade
°F	degrees Fahrenheit
Λ	diastolic blood pressure
→ or ←	direction of reaction
⊗	end of anesthesia (used in anesthesia records)
⊗	end of operation
=	equals
♀	female
fʒ	fluid ounce
'	foot, minute, primary accent, univalent
γ	gamma
>	greater than; from which is derived
≥	greater than or equal to
"	inch, second, secondary accent, bivalent
↑ or ↗	increase, elevated, rising
(–)	insignificant
++++ or 4+	large amount or pronounced reaction
Ⓛ	left
<	less than; derived from
≤	less than or equal to
♂	male
μ	micron
–	minus, negative, alkaline reaction; deficiency
+++ or 3+	moderate amount of reaction
Ⓜ	murmur
-	negative
≠	not equal to
≯	not greater than
≮	not less than
#	number, pound(s), gauge, weight, fracture
/	of, per
1×	once
ī	one
ʒ	ounce
¶	paragraph
%	per cent
π	pi
+	plus, positive, acid reaction, excess
±	plus or minus
(±)	possibly significant
℞	prescription
1°	primary, first degree
●	pulse rate (used in anesthesia records)
?	questionable, possible
:	ratio, is to
○	respirations (used in anesthesia records)
®	right, registered trademark
2d	second
2ndry	secondary
2°	secondary, second degree
(+)	significant
≃	similar
+ or 1+	slight trace or reaction
X	start of anesthesia (used in anesthesia records)
⊙	start of operation
S	suction (used in anesthesia records)
V	systolic blood pressure
Δ	temperature (used in anesthesia records)
↓↓	testes descended
↑↑	testes undescended
∴	therefore
3°	third degree
īīī	three
++ or 2+	trace or noticeable reaction
24°	24 hours
2× or ×2	twice
īī	two
™	trademark
↑	up
±	very slight trace or reaction
c̄	with
s̄	without

Postal Abbreviations

TWO-LETTER ABBREVIATIONS FOR U.S. STATES AND DEPENDENCIES

State	Abbr.	State	Abbr.	State	Abbr.	State	Abbr.
Alabama	AL	Idaho	ID	Montana	MT	Rhode Island	RI
Alaska	AK	Illinois	IL	Nebraska	NE	South Carolina	SC
Arizona	AZ	Indiana	IN	Nevada	NV	South Dakota	SD
Arkansas	AR	Iowa	IA	New Hampshire	NH	Tennessee	TN
California	CA	Kansas	KS	New Jersey	NJ	Texas	TX
Canal Zone	CZ	Kentucky	KY	New Mexico	NM	Utah	UT
Colorado	CO	Louisiana	LA	New York	NY	Vermont	VT
Connecticut	CT	Maine	ME	North Carolina	NC	Virginia	VA
Delaware	DE	Maryland	MD	North Dakota	ND	Virgin Islands	VI
District of Columbia	DC	Massachusetts	MA	Ohio	OH	Washington	WA
Florida	FL	Michigan	MI	Oklahoma	OK	West Virginia	WV
Georgia	GA	Minnesota	MN	Oregon	OR	Wisconsin	WI
Guam	GU	Mississippi	MS	Pennsylvania	PA	Wyoming	WY
Hawaii	HI	Missouri	MO	Puerto Rico	PR		

ABBREVIATIONS FOR CANADIAN PROVINCES AND TERRITORIES

Province/Territory	Abbr.	Province/Territory	Abbr.
Alberta	AB	Nova Scotia	NS
British Columbia	BC	Ontario	ON
Labrador	LB	Prince Edward Island	PE
Manitoba	MB	Quebec	PQ
New Brunswick	NB	Saskatchewan	SK
Newfoundland	NF	Yukon Territory	Y
Northwest Territories	NT		

Glossary

A

abdomen (ab-**dO**-men/**ab**-dO-men) (n) that part of the body between the chest and the pelvis (the lower part of the trunk of the body)

abduction (ab-**duk**-shun) (n) the lateral movement of a limb away from the median plane of the body

abrasion (a-**bray**-zhun) (n) scraping away of skin or mucous membrane by friction

abscess (**ab**-ses) (n) a pus-filled cavity, usually because of a localized infection

accommodation (ah-kom-o-**day**-shun) (n) the eye's ability to focus or see

acne (**ak**-nee) (n) an eruption of papules or pustules on the skin, involving the oil glands

acyanotic (ay-sI-a-**not**-ik) (adj) pertaining to the absence of cyanosis (slightly bluish, grayish, slatelike, or dark purple discoloration of the skin due to a reduction of oxygenated blood

additive (**ad**-i-tiv) (n) a substance which is added in small quantities to improve the qualities of the original

adduction (ad-**duk**-shun) (n) movement of a leg or arm toward the middle of the body

adenitis (ad-e-nI-tis) (n) inflammation of a lymph node or gland

adenocarcinoma (ad-en-O-**kar**-si-**nO**-ma) (n) malignant tumor of epithelial cells arising from the glandular structures which are a part of most organs of the body

adenoidectomy (**ad**-e-noy-**dek**-tO-mee) (n) surgical removal of the adenoids from the nasopharynx

adenopathy (ad-e-**nop**-a-thee) (n) swelling or enlargement of any gland, especially the lymph nodes

adenosis (ad-e-**nO**-sis) (n) any disease of a gland, especially of a lymphatic gland

adipose (**ad**-i-pOz) (adj) containing fat

adnexal (ad-**nek**-sal) (adj) relating to appendages or accessory parts of an organ

adrenarche (**ad**-ren-ar-kee) (n) the beginning of hormonal activity that leads up to puberty and the associated sexual development

aerosol (**ayr**-O-sol) (n) a liquid or solution dispensed as a fine mist or a product dispensed from a pressurized container as a fine mist

aerosolized (**ayr**-O-sol-Izd) (adj) describing a solution that is dispensed in the form of a mist

afebrile (ay-**feb**-ril) (adj) without fever

afferent (**af**-er-ent) (adj) inward or toward a center, as a nerve; carrying a sensory impulse

agglutination (a-gloo-ti-**nay**-shun) (n) the process in which cells group or clump together, especially as a response to a specific antibody; commonly used in blood typing

agnosia (ag-**nO**-see-a) (n) unable to perceive or recognize sensory stimuli

agraphia (a-**graf**-ee-a) (n) impairment of the ability to write

akinesis (ay-ki-**nee**-sis/ay-kI-**nee**-sis) (n) absence or loss of the power of voluntary motion; partial or incomplete paralysis

ala nasi (**a**-la **nay**-sI) (adj) the outer flare of each nostril; alae nasi (**a**-lee) (pl)

albinism (**al**-bi-nizm/al-**bin**-izm) (n) a congenital lack of melanin in the skin, hair, and eyes

albumin (al-**byoo**-min) (n) a type of simple protein, varieties of which are widely distributed throughout the tissues and fluids

albuterol (al-**byoo**-ter-ol) (n) bronchodilator available in oral and inhalent forms to be used in asthma, emphysema, and other lung conditions

alimentary canal (al-i-**men**-ter-ee ka-**nal**) (n) gastrointestinal tract; tube-like structure through which food passes and is digested and absorbed

allergen (**al**-er-jen) (n) a substance that produces an allergic reaction

allogenic (al-O-**jen**-ik) (adj) describing tissues or cell types that are from different individuals belonging to the same species; describing individuals of the same species

alopecia (al-O-**pee**-shee-a) (n) partial or total loss of hair

alopecic (al-O-**pee**-sik) (adj) relating to alopecia

alveolus (al-**vee**-O-lus) (n) tiny chambers of the lungs where the exchange of oxygen and carbon dioxide takes place; alveoli (al-**vee**-O-lI) (pl)

amblyopia (am-blee-**O**-pee-a) (n) decreased vision in one or both eyes; not correctable

ambulation (am-byoo-**lay**-shun) (n) walking or moving about

amenorrhea (a-men-O-**ree**-a) (n) stoppage or absence of menses

amnesia (am-**nee**-zee-a) (n) a disturbance of long-term memory; total or partial inability to recall past experiences

amniocentesis (**am**-nee-O-sen-**tee**-sis) (n) taking a sample of amniotic fluid

amnion (**am**-nee-on) (n) the inner of the fetal membranes; a thin transparent sac that holds the fetus

amphotericin (**am**-fO-tear-a-sin) (n) a toxic antibiotic reserved for use in serious, potentially fatal infections of fungi and protozoa; amphotericin B

amplitude (**am**-pli-tood) (n) the extent of a vibrating or alternating movement or wave from the average to the extreme; a louder sound has a greater amplitude

anagen (**an**-a-jen) (n) the actively growing phase of the hair growth cycle

anaphylactic (**an**-a-fi-**lak**-tik) (adj) describing an allergic hypersensitivity reaction of the body to a substance

anastomosis (a-**nas**-tO-mO-sis) (n) a natural or surgical connection between two blood vessels, spaces, or organs

anesthesia (**an**-es-**thee**-zee-a) (n) absence of sensation, especially pain; usually applied to the medical technique of reducing or eliminating a person's sensation of pain to enable surgery to be performed

anesthetic (**an**-es-**thet**-ik) (n) the medications used to produce anesthesia

aneurysm (**an**-yoo-rizm) (n) bulging out of an arterial wall due to a weakness in the wall

angina pectoris (**an**-ji-na/an-**jI**-na **pek**-tO-ris) (n) an attack of intense chest pain; also known as stenocardia

angiodysplasia (**an**-jee-O-dis-**play**-zee-a) (n) degenerative stretching or enlarging of the blood vessels in an organ

angioedema (an-jee-O-e-**dee**-ma) (n) periodically recurring episodes of noninflammatory swelling

angiography (an-jee-**og**-ra-fee) (n) an x-ray taken after a radiopaque dye is given to visualize the vessels

angioma (an-jee-**O**-ma) (n) a swelling or tumor composed primarily of blood vessels; spider, strawberry, cherry angiomas

anhidrosis (an-hI-**drO**-sis) (n) the suppression or absence of perspiration

anicteric (an-ik-**ter**-ik) (adj) without jaundice or icterus (a yellowing of the skin and whites of the eyes)

ankylosis (**ang**-ki-**lO**-sis) (n) stiffening or rigidity of a joint either as a result of a disease process or from surgery

ankylotic (ang-ki-**lot**-ik) (adj) relating to or having ankylosis

annulus (**an**-yoo-lus) (n) a circular structure or opening

anorexia (an-O-**rek**-see-a) (n) diminished appetite; aversion to food

anovulation (an-ov-yoo-**lay**-shun) (n) absence of egg production or release from the ovary

anovulatory (an-**ov**-yoo-la-tOr-ee) (adj) not accompanied by production of or discharge of an ovum (egg) or suppressing ovulation

antecubital (an-te-**kyoo**-bi-tal) (adj) front of the elbow; often the site for drawing blood

anteflexion (an-te-**flek**-shun) (n) the abnormal position of an organ that is bent forward over itself

anterior (an-**teer**-ee-or) (adj) front of a part, organ, or structure

antibody (**an**-tee-bod-ee) (n) an immunoglobulin produced as an immune response to a specific antigen

antiemetic (**an**-ti-ee-**met**-ik) (n) pharmacologic agent used to decrease nausea and/or vomiting

antigen (**an**-ti-jen) (n) a substance that causes the formation of an antibody which will react specifically to the antigen to neutralize, destroy, or weaken it

aorta (ay-**Or**-ta) (n) the main artery leaving the heart

aortic root (ay-**Or**-tik) (n) the opening of the aorta in the left ventricle of the heart

aortogram (ay-**Or**-tO-gram) (n) x-ray of the aorta after injection of a radiopaque substance

Apgar score (n) scoring system to assess newborn's physical condition

aphagia (a-**fay**-jee-a) (n) inability to swallow

aphasia (a-**fay**-zee-a) (n) difficulty with using and understanding words

aphonia (a-**fO**-nee-a) (n) loss of the voice as a result of disease or injury

aphthous stomatitis (**af**-thus stO-ma-**tI**-tis) (n) small ulcers of the mucous membrane of the mouth

apocrine (**ap**-O-krin) (adj) relating to sweat glands

apophyseal (a-pO-**fiz**-ee-al) (adj) relating to or having an apophysis

apophysis (a-**pof**-i-sis) (n) a projection or outgrowth of a bone

apoptosis (ap-O-**tO**-sis/**ap**-op-**tO**-sis) (n) a cell fragmenting into pieces which are phagocytosed by other cells; programmed cell death

arachnoid (a-**rak**-noyd) (n) the middle of the three membranes covering the brain; it is a delicate fibrous membrane, resembling a cobweb

arrhythmia (a-**rith**-mee-a) (n) disturbance of normal rhythm; irregular heartbeat

arteriosclerosis (ar-**teer**-ee-O-skler-**O**-sis) (n) hardening of the arteries

arteritis (**ar**-tur-**I**-tis) (n) inflammation of one or more arteries

artery (**ar**-ter-ee) (n) a vessel that carries blood away from the heart to other tissues throughout the body

arthralgia (ar-**thral**-jee-a) (n) joint pain

arthritis (ar-**thrI**-tis) (n) inflammation of one or more joints

arthroplasty (**ar**-thrO-plas-tee) (n) surgical repair of a joint; creation of a new joint

articulation (ar-tik-yoo-**lay**-shun) (n) the connecting of bones as a joint

arytenoid (ar-i-**tee**-noyd) (n) cartilage and muscles of the larynx; (adj) resembling a ladle or pitcher mouth

ascending aorta (n) the beginning section of the aorta, rising from the left ventricle of the heart to the arch

asepsis (a-**sep**-sis) (n) lack of germs; a state of sterility; methods used to create or maintain a sterile environment

aseptic (a-**sep**-tik/ay-**sep**-tik) (adj) sterile; being without infection or contamination

asparaginase (as-**par**-a-ji-nays) (n) an antineoplastic agent derived from the bacterium *Escherichium coli*

assessment (as-**ses**-ment) (n) a complete evaluation of the patient; diagnosis

astereognosis (a-**steer**-ee-og-**nO**-sis) (n) loss of the ability to judge the form of an object by touch

asthma (**az**-ma) (n) respiratory disorder with temporary narrowing of the airways, resulting in difficulty in breathing, coughing, gasping, wheezing

astigmatism (a-**stig**-ma-tizm) (n) visual condition in which light rays entering the eye are bent unequally, preventing a sharp focus point on the retina

asymmetry (ay-**sim**-e-tree) (n) lack of symmetry of parts or organs on opposite sides of body

asymptomatic (ay-simp-tO-**mat**-ik) (adj) without symptoms

ataxia (a-**tak**-see-a) (n) muscular incoordination

atelectasis (at-e-**lek**-ta-sis) (n) incomplete expansion of the lungs at birth or collapse of the adult lung

atherosclerosis (**ath**-er-O-skler-**O**-sis) (n) buildup of fatty plaques inside arteries; a type of arteriosclerosis

atraumatic (ay-traw-**mat**-ik) (adj) without injury or trauma

atresia (a-**tree**-zee-a) (n) congenital absence or closure of a normal body opening or tubular structure

atrial (**ay**-tree-al) (adj) relating to the atrium

atrioventricular (**ay**-tree-O-ven-**trik**-yoo-lar) (adj) relating to both the atria (upper chambers) and the ventricles (lower chambers) in the heart, or blood flow between them

atrioventricular groove (n) a groove visible on the outside of the heart between the atria and the ventricles

atrium (**ay**-tree-um) (n) one of the two upper chambers of the heart

atrophy (**at**-rO-fee) (n) a decrease in size of a part or organ; a wasting away of tissue as a result of disuse, radiation therapy, surgery, disease

attenuation (a-ten-yoo-**ay**-shun) (n) process of weakening, such as the potency of a drug or the virulence of a disease-causing germ

audiologic (aw-dee-O-**loj**-ik) (adj) pertaining to hearing disorders or loss

audiometry (aw-dee-**om**-e-tree) (n) test used to measure hearing (using an audiometer)

aura (**aw**-ra) (n) a sensation, as of light or warmth, that may precede an attack of migraine or a seizure

aural (**aw**-ral) (adj) relating to the ear

auricle (**aw**-ri-kl) (n) external ear; pinna

auscultation (aws-kul-**tay**-shun) (n) process of listening for sounds produced in some of the body cavities, especially chest and abdomen, in order to detect abnormal conditions

autoimmune disease (aw-tO-i-**myoon**) (n) any disorder in which the body's immune responses produce antibodies that destroy the body's own tissues

autologous (aw-**tol**-O-gus) (adj) something that has its origin within an individual, especially a factor present in tissues or fluids; a transplantation where the tissue graft is taken from the same individual receiving it

axial (**ak**-see-al) (adj) situated in or relating to an axis

axilla (**ak**-sil-a) (n) the armpit

axillary node (**ak**-sil-ayr-ee nOd) (n) any of the lymph glands of the armpit that help to fight infection in the neck, chest, and arm area

B

B cell (n) a type of lymphocyte; produces immunoglobulin antibodies in response to antigens

Babinski reflex (bab-**in**-skeez **ree**-fleks) (n) an extension or moving of the big toe upward or toward the head, with the other toes fanned out and extended when the sole of the foot is stimulated

bacteremia (bak-te-**ree**-mee-a) (n) the presence of bacteria in the blood

bedsore (**bed**-sor) (n) an infected wound on the skin that occurs at pressure points in patients confined to bed

benign (bee-**nIn**) (adj) describing a mild illness or a nonmalignant tumor

beta subunit (**bay**-ta) (n) glycoprotein hormone containing two different polypeptide subunits designated as alpha and beta chains

bibasilar (bI-**bays**-i-lar) (adj) occurring in both bases

bifurcation (bI-fer-**kay**-shun) (n) forking into two branches

bilateral (bI-**lat**-er-al) (adj) affecting or relating to two sides

bile (bIl) (n) a thick, yellow-green-brown fluid secreted by the liver

biliary (**bil**-ee-ayr-ee) (adj) relating to bile or the gallbladder and its ducts

bilirubin (bil-i-**roo**-bin) (n) a red bile pigment, formed from hemoglobin during normal and abnormal destruction of erythrocytes

biopsy (**bI**-op-see) (n) the removal of tissue and/or fluid from the body for microscopic examination; the specimen obtained

bleomycin (blee-O-**mI**-sin) (n) antitumor agents

blepharectomy (blef-ar-**ek**-tO-mee) (n) excision of a lesion of the eyelid

blepharitis (blef-a-**rI**-tis) (n) inflammation of the eyelid

bolus (**bO**-lus) (n) a mass of something such as masticated (chewed) food or substance that is ready to be swallowed; an amount of medication

brachial (**bray**-kee-al) (adj) pertaining to the arm

Braxton Hicks sign (n) irregular contractions of the uterus after the first trimester of pregnancy

breech presentation (n) fetal position in which the feet or buttocks appear first in the birth canal

bronchial (**brong**-kee-al) (adj) relating to the bronchi

bronchiectasis (brong-kee-**ek**-ta-sis) (n) persistent, abnormal widening of the bronchi, with an associated cough and spitting up of mucus

bronchiole (**brong**-kee-Ol) (n) one of the smaller subdivisions of the bronchi

bronchitis (brong-**kI**-tis) (n) inflammation of the bronchi

bronchovesicular (**brong**-kO-ve-**sik**-yoo-lar) (adj) relating to the bronchioles and alveoli in the lungs

bronchus (**brong**-kus) (n) the divisions of the trachea leading to the lungs; bronchi (**brong**-kI) (pl)

Brudzinski sign (n) in meningitis, if a leg is passively flexed, a similar movement occurs in the other leg; if the neck is passively flexed, the legs also flex

bruit (**broo**-ee/broot) (n) an adventitious sound of venous or arterial origin heard on auscultation

buccal (**buk**-al) (adj) relating to the area inside the cheek

bulbar (**bul**-bar) (adj) bulb-shaped or relating to the medulla oblongata in the brain

bulimia (boo-**lim**-ee-a) (n) a chronic disorder involving repeated and secretive bouts of binge eating followed by self-induced vomiting, use of laxatives, or vigorous exercise in order to prevent weight gain

bulla (**bul**-a) (n) large bleb in the skin that contains fluid; bullae (pl)

bullae (**bul**-ee) (n, pl) blisters of the skin containing clear fluid

C

cachexia (ka-**kek**-see-a) (n) a general weight loss and wasting occurring in the course of a chronic disease or emotional disturbance

café-au-lait spots (kaf-ay-O-**lay** spots) (n) light brown spots of patchy pigmentation of the skin

calcaneus (kal-**kay**-nee-us) (n) heel bone; calcanei (kal-**kay**-nee-I) (pl)

calcification (**kal**-si-fi-**kay**-shun) (n) a hardening of tissue resulting from the formation of calcium salts within it

calculus (**kal**-kyoo-lus) (n) stone; a hard stone-like mass formed in the body; calculi (pl)

caliber (**kal**-i-ber) (n) diameter of a tube or vessel, such as a blood vessel

callous (**kal**-us) (adj) being hardened and thickened, having calluses; also feeling no emotion or sympathy.

callus (**kal**-us) (n) thickened skin which develops at points of pressure or friction; the bony substance which develops around the broken ends of bone during healing

candidal rash (**kan**-di-dal rash) (n) a rash which usually includes itching, a white discharge, peeling, and easy bleeding; caused by the yeastlike fungus *Candida;* common examples are diaper rash, thrush, and vaginitis

cannula (**kan**-yoo-la) (n) a tube for insertion into a duct or cavity to allow the escape of fluid

cannulate (**kan**-yoo-layt) (v) to introduce a cannula through a passageway

capillary (kap-i-**layr**-ee) (n) tiny blood vessel connecting arterioles and venules

capillary fragility (**kap**-i-layr-ee) (n) used in a test to determine the presence of vitamin C deficiency or thrombocytopenia; pressure is applied to the arm, and then the number of petechiae (representing broken capillaries) in a small area are counted

capsular (**cap**-soo-lar) (adj) pertaining to a sheath of continuous enclosure around an organ or structure

carbuncle (**kar**-bung-kl) (n) subcutaneous, pus-filled interconnecting pockets, caused by staphylococcal infection; eventually discharges through an opening in the skin

carcinoma (kar-si-**nO**-ma) (n) malignant growth of epithelial cells that occurs in the linings of the body parts and in glands

cardiac tamponade (**kar**-dee-ak tam-po-**nayd**) (n) compression of the venous return to the heart by fluid or blood in the pericardium

cardiomyopathy (**kar**-dee-O-mI-**op**-a-thee) (n) disease of the heart muscle

carotid (ka-**rot**-id) (n) paired arteries (right and left) that arise from the aorta and provide the principal blood supply to the head and neck

carpal tunnel (**kar**-pul **tun**-nul) (n) where the median nerve and flexor tendons pass through the wrist

caruncle (**kar**-ung-kl) (n) small, fleshy outgrowth

cataract (**kat**-a-rakt) (n) clouding of the lens of the eye, resulting in loss of transparency

catheter (**kath**-e-ter) (n) a tube inserted into the body for removing or instilling fluids for diagnostic or therapeutic purposes

catheterization (**kath**-e-ter-I-**zay**-shun) (n) the insertion of a catheter

causalgia (kaw-**zal**-jee-a) (n) persistent severe burning sensation of the skin, usually following injury of a sensory nerve

cauterization (kaw-ter-i-**zay**-shun) (n) destroying tissue by burning for medical reasons

cautery (**kaw**-ter-ee) (n) a means of destroying tissue by electricity, freezing, heat, or corrosive chemicals

cavernous sinus thrombosis (**kav**-er-nus **sI**-nus throm-**bO**-sis) (n) a group of symptoms caused by an obstruction in the cavernous intracranial sinus

cecum (**see**-kum) (n) any part ending in a cul-de-sac; specifically the closed, pocket-like beginning of the large intestine in the lower right part of the abdomen

ceftazidime (sef-**taz**-i-deem) (n) antibiotic used in the treatment of moderate to severe infections

cellular (**sel**-yoo-lar) (adj) composed of or derived from cells

cellular immunity (n) immunity which is based on the T cells recognizing the antigen itself, rather than the presence of an antibody; cell-mediated immunity

cellulitis (sel-yoo-**lI**-tis) (n) inflammation of the connective tissue caused by infection

centimeter (**sen**-ti-mee-ter) (n) unit of measurement; one hundredth of a meter; approximately 0.4 inches

central nervous system (CNS) (n) portion of the nervous system consisting of the brain and spinal cord

cephalad (**sef**-a-lad) (adv) toward the head

cephalalgia (**sef**-al-**al**-jee-a) (n) headache

cephalocaudal (**sef**-a-lO-**caw**-dal) (adj) relating to the axis of the body from the head to the base of the spine

cerclage (sair-**klazh**) (n) procedure to encircle tissues with a ligature, wire, or loop

cerebellar (ser-e-**bel**-ar) (adj) relating to the cerebellum, the part of the brain concerned with the coordination and control of voluntary muscular activity

cerebrospinal (**ser**-e-brO-spI-nal/se-**ree**-brO-spI-nal) (adj) relating to the brain and spinal cord

cerebrovascular (**ser**-e-brO-**vas**-kyoo-lar) (adj) relating to the blood vessels of the brain, especially to pathological changes

cerumen (se-**roo**-men) (n) earwax

cervical (**ser**-vi-kal) (adj) relating to a neck or cervix

cervical (**ser**-vi-kal) (adj) relating to a neck, or cervix, especially the neck (cervix) of the uterus

cervix (ser-viks) (n) the neck or part of an organ resembling a neck, such as the cervix of the uterus

chancre (**shang**-ker) (n) hard sore; the sore that develops at the site of entry of a pathogen

chemosis (kee-**mO**-sis) (n) an accumulation of fluid in the eye, causing swelling around the cornea

chemotherapy (kem-O-**thayr**-a-pee/**keem**-O-thayr-a-pee) (n) treatment of disease with drugs

chloasma (klO-**as**-ma) (n) light brown patches on the face and elsewhere; commonly associated with pregnancy

choana (**kO**-an-a) (n) a funnel-shaped opening, especially the posterior opening of the nasal cavity into the nasopharynx

cholangiography (kO-lan-jee-**og**-ra-fee) (n) x-ray examination of the bile ducts

cholecystectomy (**kO**-lee-sis-**tek**-tO-mee) (n) excision of the gallbladder

cholecystitis (**kO**-lee-sis-tI-tis) (n) inflammation or irritation of gallbladder, usually caused by the presence of gallstones

choledocholithiasis (kO-**led**-O-kO-lith-**I**-a-sis) (n) presence of calculi (stones) in the common bile duct

cholelithiasis (**kO**-lee-lith-**I**-a-sis) (n) formation or presence of gallstones in the gallbladder which may not cause any symptoms or perhaps only vague abdominal discomfort and intolerance to certain foods

cholesteatoma (kO-les-tee-a-**tO**-ma) (n) a tumor-like mass of scaly epithelium and cholesterol in the middle ear

chondral (**kon**-drul) (adj) relating to cartilage

chondritis (kon-**drI**-tis) (n) inflammation of cartilage

chondromalacia (**kon**-drO-ma-**lay**-shee-a) (n) softening of cartilage

chordae tendineae (**kOr**-dee ten-**din**-ee-ay) (n) small tendinous cords (strands) that connect the free edges of the atrioventricular valves to the papillary muscles

choroid (**kO**-royd) (n) a vascular membrane surrounding the eyeball, between the retina and sclera

chromic (**krO**-mik) (adj) relating to or containing chromium, such as chromic acid

chromosome (**krO**-mO-sOm) (n) the structure in the cell nucleus that transmits genetic information; consists of a double strand of DNA in the form of a helix; there are normally 46 in humans

Chvostek sign (**khvosh**-teks) (n) an abnormal spasm of facial muscles when the facial nerve is tapped lightly

cicatrix (**sik**-a-triks) (n) scar

ciliary action (sil-ee-ar-ee) (n) the lashing movement of a group of cilia, which can produce a current of movement in a fluid

cilium (**sil**-ee-um) (n) a short hair-like extension of a cell surface, capable of lashlike movement, which aids in the movement of unicellular organisms and in the movement of fluids in higher organisms; eyelash; cilia (pl)

circumflex (**ser**-kum-fleks) (adj) bending around; describes anatomical structures that are shaped like an arc of a circle

circumscribed (**ser**-kum-skrIbd) (adj) having a boundary; confined

cirrhosis (sir-**rO**-sis) (n) a chronic degenerative liver disease characterized by damaged cell function and impaired blood flow

cirrhotic (sir-**rot**-ik) (adj) affected with cirrhosis

claudication (klaw-di-**ka**-shun) (n) limping; painful cramps in calf of leg due to poor blood circulation

clavicle (**klav**-i-kl) (n) clavicula; collar bone

clavicula (kla-**vik**-yoo-la) (n) clavicle; collar bone

clavicular (kla-**vik**-yoo-lar) (adj) pertains to the clavicle, or collarbone

clonus (**klO**-nus) (n) abnormal condition in which a skeletal muscle alternately contracts and relaxes

clubbing (**klub**-ing) (n) condition of the fingers and toes in which their ends become wide and thickened; often a sign of disease, especially heart or lung disease

coagulation (kO-ag-yoo-**lay**-shun) (n) process of blood clotting

coagulopathy (kO-ag-yoo-**lop**-a-thee) (n) defect in the blood clotting mechanisms

cochlea (**kok**-lee-a) (n) a spiral-shaped cavity in the internal ear

collagen (**kol**-a-jen) (n) the protein which forms the tough white fibers of connective tissue, cartilage, and bone

collaterals (ko-**lat**-er-als) (n) accompanying, as side by side; blood vessels that branch from larger vessels

colonic (ko-**lon**-ic) (adj) pertaining to the colon

colostomy (kO-**los**-to-mee) (n) surgical creation of an opening in the abdominal wall to allow material to pass from the bowel through that opening rather than through the anus

colostrum (kO-**los**-trum) (n) the first milk secreted after childbirth

colposcopy (kol-**pos**-ko-pee) (n) examination of the tissues of the vagina and cervix with a lighted instrument that magnifies the cells

comedo (**kom**-i-dO) (n) in a hair follicle or oil gland, a plug of dead cells and oily secretions; blackhead; comedones (com-i-**dO**-neez) (pl)

communicable (ko-**myoon**-i-ka-bl) (adj) contagious; capable of being spread with direct or indirect contact

compressible (kom-**pres**-i-bl) (adj) pressed together; made more compact by or as by pressure

concha (**kon**-ka) (n) a shell-shaped anatomical structure, such as the auricle of the ear; conchae (pl)

concussion (kon-**kush**-un) (n) an injury of a soft structure resulting from violent striking or shaking, especially an injury to the brain

conductive deafness (n) hearing impairment due to obstruction of sound waves; the sound waves are not passed on to the inner ear

condyle (**kon**-dil) (n) the rounded projecting end of a bone where ligaments are attached

condyloma (kon-di-**lO**-ma) (n) warty growth in the genital area

confluent (**kon**-floo-ent) (adj) merging together; connecting

congenital (kon-**jen**-I-tal) (adj) present at birth

congestive heart failure (CHF) (kon-**jes**-tiv) (n) condition in which the heart is unable to pump adequate blood to the tissues and organs, often due to myocardial infarction

conjunctiva (kon-junk-**ti**-va) (n) the mucous membrane covering the front of the eyeball and inside the eyelids; conjunctivae (pl)

conjunctival (kon-**junk**-ti-val (adj) pertaining to the conjunctiva

conjunctivitis (kon-junk-ti-**vI**-tis) (n) inflammation of the conjunctiva

consolidation (kon-sol-i-**day**-shun (n) solidification into a firm, dense mass

contusion (kon-**too**-zhun) (n) a bruise

cornea (**kor**-nee-a) (n) the outer, transparent portion of the eye through which light passes to the retina

corneal (**kor**-nee-al) (adj) the clear, transparent, anterior portion of the fibrous coat of the eye composing about one-sixth of its surface

coronal (ka-**rO**-nal) (adj) pertaining to a corona, a structure resembling a crown

coronary bypass surgery (**kOr**-o-nayr-ee) (n) vein grafts or other surgical methods are used to carry blood from the aorta to branches of the coronary arteries in order to increase the flow beyond a local obstruction

coronary cusp (n) one of the triangular parts of a heart valve

cortex (**kOr**-teks) (n) the outer part of an organ, such as the brain or kidney, as distinguished from the inner portion, or medulla

cortical (**kOr**-ti-kal) (adj) relating to a cortex

corticomedullary junction (**kOr**-tee-kO-**med**-yoo-lar-ee **jungk**-shun) (n) coming together (junction) of the cortex and medulla of the kidneys

coryza (ko-**rI**-za) (n) acute rhinitis; acute head cold; inflammation of the mucous membrane of the nose with sneezing, tearing, and watery nasal discharge

costal (**kos**-tal) (adj) relating to or located near a rib; the costal margin is the area at the lower end of the rib cage

costophrenic (kos-tO-**fren**-ik) (adj) pertaining to the ribs and diaphragm

Coumadin (**coo**-mah-din) (n) Brand name for warfarin, an agent to prevent blood clots

craniotomy (kray-nee-**ot**-O-mee) (n) surgical incision into the skull, performed to control bleeding, remove tumors, relieve pressure inside the cranium, or insert instruments for diagnosis

cranium (**kray**-nee-um) (n) the bony skull that holds the brain

crepitus (**krep**-i-tus) (n) grating sound or vibration made by movement of fractured bones (bone fragments); crepitation

cribriform (**krib**-ri-fOrm) (adj) perforated with small holes of uniform size; (n) a polyporous structure

cricoid cartilage (**krI**-koyd) (n) a ring-shaped cartilage in the lower part of the larynx

Crohn disease (krOn) (n) chronic inflammatory condition affecting the colon and/or terminal part of the small intestine and producing frequent episodes of diarrhea, abdominal pain, nausea, fever, weakness, and weight loss

cryosurgery (**krI**-O-ser-jer-ee) (n) the use of extreme cold to destroy tissue

cryptitis (crip-**tI**-tis) (n) inflammation of a crypt or follicle

culture (**kul**-chur) (n) propagation of microorganisms in a solid or liquid medium

curettage (**kyoo**-re-tahzh) (n) surgical scraping or cleaning, usually of the interior of a cavity or tract, for removal or sampling of tissue

cutaneous (koo-**tay**-nee-us) (adj) pertaining to the skin

cuticle (**kyoo**-ti-kl) (n) the edge of thickened skin around the bed of a nail; the sheath surrounding the base of a hair follicle

cyanosis (cI-a-**nO**-sis) (n) bluish discoloration of the skin and/or mucous membranes due to decreased amount of oxygen in the blood cells

cyanotic (sI-a-**not**-ik) (adj) pertaining to cyanosis

cyst (sist) (n) a bladder or an abnormal sac containing gas, fluid, or a semisolid material

cystic (**sis**-tik) (adj) relating to a cyst

cystic duct (n) the duct of the gallbladder which unites with the hepatic duct from the liver to form the common bile duct

cystic fibrosis (**sis**-tik fI-**brO**-sis) (n) an inherited disease, in which the mucus- producing glands become clogged with thick mucus; digestion zand respiration are affected

cystitis (sis-**tI**-tis) (n) inflammation of the urinary bladder

cystoscopy (sis-**tos**-ko-pee) (n) examination of the inside of the urinary bladder with a lighted instrument inserted through the urethra

cystostomy (sis-**tos**-tO-mee) (n) surgical creation of an opening in the bladder

cytokines (**sI**-tO-kIns) (n) proteins that are not antibodies but are released on contact with a specific antigen as an immune response

cytomegalovirus (sI-tO-**meg**-a-lO-**vI**-rus) (n) CMV; one of a group of large-cell, species-specific herpes-type viruses with a wide variety of disease effects

D

dacryocystorhinostomy (**dak**-ree-O-**sis**-tO-rI-**nos**-tO-mee) (n) a surgical opening to provide drainage between the tear duct and the nasal mucosa

dactylomegaly (dak-til-O-**meg**-a-lee) (n) abnormal enlargement of one or more fingers or toes

debride (da-**breed**/dee-**brId**) (v) to remove unhealthy tissue and foreign material to prevent infection and permit healing

decelerations (dee-cel-er-**ay**-shunz) (n) decreases in speed or rate (of contractions)

decompression (**dee**-kom-presh-un) (n) removal of bone to relieve pressure

deep vein (or venous) thrombosis (deep vayn throm-**bO**-sis) (n) a clump of various blood components in a blood vessel, forming an obstruction

defervescence (def-er-**ves**-ens) (n) time that marks the decline of fever to normal temperature

defibrillator (dee-**fib**-ri-lay-ter) (n) an agent, measure, or machine, e.g., an electric shock, that stops fibrillation of the ventricular muscle and restores the normal beat

degenerative (di-**jen**-er-a-tiv) (adj) relating to or causing deterioration or worsening of a condition

dehydration (dee-hI-**dray**-shun) (n) extreme loss of water from the body tissues

dementia (dee-**men**-shee-a) (n) a general mental deterioration due to organic or psychological factors

Demerol (**dem**-err-all) (n) Brand name for meperidine, a narcotic analgesic

dermabrasion (**der**-ma-bray-zhun) (n) peeling of skin done by a mechanical device with sandpaper or wire brushes

dermatitis (der-ma-**tI**-tis) (n) inflammation of skin often evidenced by itching, redness, and lesions

dermatology (der-ma-**tol**-o-jee) (n) the study of the skin, hair, and nails

dermatophyte (**der**-ma-tO-fIt) (n) a parasitic fungus that causes skin disease

desiccate (**des**-i-kayt) (v) to dry out

Dexedrine (**dex**-a-dreen) brand name for dextroamphetamine, a CNS stimulant

diabetes insipidus (dI-a-**bee**-tez in-**sip**-i-doos) (n and adj) disease caused by insufficient secretion of antidiuretic hormone (AHD) from the posterior pituitary gland

diagnosis (dI-ag-**nO**-sis) (n) deciding the nature of a medical condition by examination of the symptoms; diagnoses (pl)

diaphoresis (**dI**-a-fO-ree-sis) (n) profuse perspiration or sweating

diaphragm (**dI**-a-fram) (n) the muscle that separates the thoracic (chest) and abdominal cavities

diaphysis (dI-**af**-i-sis) (n) shaft of a long bone

diathesis (dI-a-**thee**-sis) (n) unusual predisposition to certain disease conditions

diffuse (di-**fyoos**) (adj) spreading, scattered

digital (**dij**-i-tal) (adj) relating to or resembling a finger or toe

digoxin (di-**jok**-sin) (n) a heart stimulant

Dilantin (dill-**ann**-tin) brand name for phenytoin, used for the prevention and management of seizures

dilatation (dil-a-**tay**-shun) (n) stretching or enlarging; dilation

dilation (dI-**lay**-shun) (n) expansion of an organ or vessel

diltiazem (dil-**tie**-a-zem) (n) a generic calcium channel blocker, used for hypertension

diplopia (di-**plO**-pee-a) (n) double vision; may be monocular

discrete (dis-**kreet**) (adj) separate; distinct

distal (**dis**-tal) (adj) away from the center, toward the far end of something

distally (**dis**-ta-lee) (adv) occurring farthest from the center, from a medial line, or from the trunk

distention (dis-**ten**-shun) (n) the state of being stretched out or inflated

distress (n) trouble; mental or physical suffering

diverticula (dI-ver-**tik**-yoo-la) (n) sacs or pouches in the walls of a canal or organ

diverticulosis (**dI**-ver-tik-yoo-**lO**-sis) (n) presence of diverticula (pouches) in the intestinal tract

Doppler (**dop**-ler) (n) a diagnostic instrument that emits an ultrasonic beam into the body

dorsal (**dOr**-sal) (adj) relating to the back; posterior

dorsum (**dOr**-sum) (n) the back or posterior surface of a part

ductus arteriosus (**duk**-tus ar-ter-ee-**O**-sus) (n) blood vessel in the fetus connecting the pulmonary artery directly to the ascending aorta, thus bypassing the pulmonary circulation

duodenum (doo-O-**dee**-num/doo-**od**-e-num) (n) first part of the small intestine; it receives material from the stomach and passes it to the jejunum, the medial part of the small intestine

dura mater (**doo**-ra **may**-ter/**mah**-ter) (n) the outermost of the three membranes surrounding the brain and spinal cord; it is tough and fibrous

dural (**doo**-ral) (adj) pertaining to the dura mater, the outer membrane covering the spinal cord and brain

dysfunction (dis-**funk**-shun) (n) abnormal or impaired function

dysgerminoma (dis-jer-mi-**nO**-ma) (n) a rare cancerous ovarian tumor

dyslexia (dys-**lek**-see-a) (n) impairment of ability to read in which letters and words are reversed

dysmenorrhea (dis-men-Or-**ee**-a) (n) painful menstruation

dyspareunia (dis-pa-**roo**-nee-a) (n) painful sexual intercourse

dyspepsia (dis-**pep**-see-a) (n) imperfect digestion; epigastric discomfort

dysphagia (dis-**fay**-jee-a) (n) difficulty swallowing

dyspnea (disp-**nee**-a) (n) shortness of breath; difficulty in breathing

dysuria (dis-**yoo**-ree-a) (n) difficult or painful urination

E

ecchymoses (ek-i-**mO**-sees) (n) small, hemorrhagic, discolored, purplish ("black and blue") spots resulting from an accumulation of blood under the skin's surface

eccrine (**ek**-rin) (adj) relating to sweat glands

echocardiogram (ek-O-**kar**-dee-O-gram) (n) a sound-wave image of the heart's size, position, and motion

echolalia (ek-O-**lay**-lee-a) (n) involuntary repetition of a word or sentence just spoken by another person

ectopic pregnancy (ek-**top**-ik) (n) pregnancy in which a fertilized ovum is implanted outside the uterus, often in a fallopian tube

eczema (**ek**-si-ma/**eg**-ze-ma) (n) inflammatory condition of the skin characterized by blisters, redness, and itching

edema (e-**dee**-ma) (n) excessive accumulation of fluid in tissues, especially just under the skin or in a given cavity

edematous (e-**dem**-a-tus) (adj) having edema

effusion (e-**fyoo**-zhun) (n) escape of fluid into a cavity or tissues; the fluid itself

egophony (ee-**gof**-O-nee) (n) an abnormal voice sound, like the bleating of a goat

electrocardiogram (ee-**lek**-trO-**kar**-dee-**O**-gram) (n) a graphic record of electrical waves within the heart

electrocautery (ee-**lek**-trO-**caw**-ter-ee) (n) application of a needle or snare heated by an electric current to destroy tissue

electrodesiccation (el-ek-trO-de-si-**kay**-shun) (n) destruction of tissue by the use of electrical current; fulguration

electrolysis (el-ek-**trol**-i-sis) (n) destruction of a hair follicle by passing an electrical current through it

electrolyte (ee-**lek**-trO-lIt) (n) an ionized chemical capable of conducting an electric current; the body contains many different electrolytes in specific amounts to keep it functioning properly

electron (ee-**lek**-tron) (n) a subatomic particle with a negative charge

electrophoresis (ee-lek-trO-fO-**ree**-sis) (n) the movement of charged suspended particles through a liquid medium in response to changes in an electric field; for example, a hemoglobin electrophoresis measures the types of hemoglobin in the blood

ellipse (el-**lipz**) (n) a conic section taken either parallel to an element or parallel to the axis of the intersected cone; an oval

embolism (**em**-bO-lizm) (n) blockage of a blood vessel by an abnormal object, such as a clot

embryo (**em**-bree-O) (n) in humans, the developing prenatal child from conception to the end of the second month

embryonal (**em**-bree-O-nal) (adj) relating to an embryo; in an early stage of development

emesis (**em**-e-sis) (n) vomiting; may be of gastric, systemic, nervous, or reflex origin

emetic (e-**met**-ik) (n) pharmacologic agent used to induce vomiting and eliminate toxic substances

en bloc (ahn blok) (adj) as a whole, in one piecez

encephalopathy (en-**sef**-a-**lop**-a-thee) (n) disease or dysfunction of the brain

encopresis (en-cO-**pree**-sis) (n) inability to control bowel movements, fecal incontinence

endocapillary (**en**-dO-**cap**-layr-ee (n) within one of the tiny blood vessels

endocarditis (**en**-dO-kar-**dI**-tis) (n) inflammation of the endocardium and/or the heart valves

endocardium (en-dO-**kar**-dee-im) (n) serous lining membrane of inner surface and cavities of the heart

endocervical (en-dO-**ser**-va-cal) (adj) pertaining to the lining of the canal of the cervix uteri

endometrial (en-do-**mee**-tree-al) (adj) pertaining to the mucous membrane lining of the uterus

endometrium (**en**-dO-**mee**-tree-um) (n) lining of the womb, composed of three layers and shed during menstruation

endoscope (**en**-dO-skOp) (n) a lighted instrument for examining the inside of a body cavity or organ

endotracheal tube (**en**-dO-**tray**-kee-al toob) (n) a catheter inserted through the mouth or nose into the trachea to maintain an open airway to deliver oxygen to permit suctioning of mucus or to prevent aspiration of foreign materials

engorged (en-**gOrjd**) (adj) filled to the limit of expansion

enterovirus (**en**-ter-O-**vI**-rus) (n) a group of viruses that multiply in the gastrointestinal tract but may cause various diseases, such as polio

enucleation (ee-noo-klee-**ay**-shun) (n) removal of a tumor or structure as a whole, as in removal of the eyeball

enuresis (en-yoo-**ree**-sis) (n) bed-wetting; involuntary urination, especially at night in bed

eosinophil (ee-O-**sin**-O-fil) (n) a type of white blood cell readily stained with eosin

ephelides (ef-**ee**-lI-deez) (n, pl) freckles

epicanthic (ep-i-**kan**-thik) (adj) pertaining to the vertical fold of skin extending from the root of the nose to the median end of the eyebrow

epidermis (ep-i-**der**-mis) (n) the top or outer layer of the skin

epididymis (ep-i-**did**-i-mis) (n) one of a pair of long, coiled ducts in the scrotum; they carry and store spermatozoa between the testes and ductus deferens

epidural (ep-i-**doo**-ral) (adj) located over or under the dura

epiglottis (**ep**-i-**glot**-is) (n) flap of elastic cartilage at the back of the mouth that covers the opening to the windpipe during swallowing, thereby preventing choking.

epiglottitis (ep-i-glot-**tI**-tis) (n) inflammation of the epiglottis, causing potentially fatal airway obstruction, especially in small children

epilepsy (**ep**-i-**lep**-see) (n) convulsive disorder

epileptiform (ep-i-**lep**-ti-fOrm) (adj) having the form of epilepsy

epinephrine (ep-I-**nef**-rin) (n) a hormone of the adrenal medulla that acts as a strong stimulant and blood vessel constrictor

epiphora (ee-**pif**-O-ra) (n) overflow of tears

epiphyseal (ep-i-**fiz**-ee-al) (adj) relating to an epiphysis

epiphysis (e-**pif**-i-sis) (n) end of a long bone, separated by cartilage from the shaft until the bone stops growing when the shaft and end are joined

epiploic (**ep**-i-**plO**-ik) (adj) relating to the omentum, a fold of peritoneum attached to the stomach and connecting it with the adjacent organs

episiotomy (e-peez-ee-**ot**-O-mee) (n) incision of perineum to facilitate delivery and prevent laceration (jagged tear)

epistaxis (**ep**-i-**stak**-sis) (n) nosebleed

epithelial (ep-i-**thee**-lee-al) (adj) relating to or consisting of epithelium

epithelium (ep-i-**thee**-lee-um) (n) cell layers covering the outside body surfaces as well as forming the lining of hollow organs (e.g., the bladder) and the passages of the respiratory, digestive, and urinary tracts

eructation (ee-ruk-**tay**-shun) (n) belching

erythema (er-i-**thee**-ma) (n) redness of the skin; inflammation

erythema infectiosum (er-i-**thee**-ma in-fek-shee-**O**-sum) (n) a mild, infectious disease characterized by an erythematous rash; also called fifth disease

erythematous (er-i-**them**-a-tus/er-i-**thee**-ma-tus) (adj) relating to or having erythema; reddened; inflamed

erythrocyte (e-**rith**-rO-sIt) (n) mature red blood cell

erythroderma (e-rith-rO-**der**-ma) (n) any skin condition associated with unusual redness of the skin

erythromycin (**ee**-rith-rO-**mI**-sin) (n) antibiotic used to treat infections caused by a wide variety of bacteria and other microorganisms

esophagus (ee-**sof**-a-gus) (n) the muscular canal that connects the pharynx and stomach

esotropia (es-O-**trO**-pee-a) (n) a condition in which one or both eyes appear to turn inward; cross eye(s)

estradiol (es-tra-**dI**-ol) (n) a hormone produced by the ovary; often used to treat menopausal symptoms

ethmoidal (eth-**moy**-dal) (adj) relating to the ethmoid bone or ethmoid sinus

eustachian tube (yoo-**stay**-shun/yoo-**stay**-kee-an) (n) a tube leading from the middle ear to the nasopharynx; thus air pressure is equalized on both sides of the tympanic membrane

eversion (ee-**vur**-zhun) (n) turning out or inside out

exacerbation (eg-zas-er-**bay**-shun) (n) aggravation of symptoms or increase in the severity of a disease

exanthema (eg-zan-**thee**-ma) (n) a disease, such as measles or chickenpox, accompanied by a general rash on the skin, which may have particular characteristics specific to the disease

excision (ek-**si**-zhun) (n) cutting out; surgical removal of all or part of a lesion, structure, or organ

excisional biopsy (ek-**sizh**-un-al **bI**-op-see) (n) surgical removal of a tissue for microscopic examination

excoriation (eks-kO-ree-**ay**-shun) (n) a scratching or scraping injury to the skin

excrescence (eks-**kres**-ens) (n) abnormal projection or outgrowth; such as a wart

exophthalmos (ek-sof-**thal**-mos) (n) protrusion of the eyeball(s)

exotropia (ek-sO-**trO**-pee-a) (n) outward turning of one eye relative to the other

expectoration (ek-spek-tO-**ray**-shun) (n) expelling by mouth; spitting

expiratory (ek-**spI**-ra-**tO**-ree) (adj) relating to expiration, or breathing out air from the lungs

extensor (eks-**ten**-ser, eks-**ten**-sOr) (n) muscle that, when flexed, causes extension of a joint or straightening of an arm or leg

extrahepatic (eks-tra-he-**pat**-ik) (adj) unrelated to or located outside the liver

extraocular (eks-tra-**ok**-yoo-lar) (adj) outside the eye

extravasation (eks-**trav**-a-**say**-shun) (n) a leakage of fluid (e.g., blood) to the tissues outside the vessel normally containing it, which may occur in injuries, burns, and allergic reactions

exudate (**eks**-oo-dayt) (n) any fluid that has oozed out of a tissue, usually due to inflammation or injury

exudated (eks-yoo-**day**-ted) (adj) pertaining to any fluid that has exuded out of a tissue or its capillaries

exudates (**eks**-oo-daytz) (n) accumulations of fluid in a cavity; matter that penetrates through vessel walls into adjoining tissues

exudative (**eks**-oo-dayt-iv) (adj) relating to exudate

F

facial (**fay**-shul) (adj) relating to the face

fallopian tubes (fa-**lO**-pee-an) (n) passageways from ovaries to uterus

familial (fa-**mi**-lee-al) (adj) pertaining to a disease or characteristic that is present in some families

fascia (**fash**-ee-a) (n) a thin layer of fibrous connective tissue that supports soft organs and covers structures such as muscles; fasciae (pl)

fascial (**fash**-ee-al) (adj) relating to fascia

femoral (**fem**-o-ral) (adj) relating to the thigh bone or femur

femoralis (fem-or-**awl**-is) (adj) pertaining to the femur, the longest and strongest bone in body, going from hip to knee

fenestra ovalis (fe-**nes**-tra O-**val**-is) (n) an oval opening between the middle ear and the vestibule; closed by the base of the stapes

fetal distress (**fee**-tal) (n) life-threatening condition affecting the fetus

fetoprotein (fee-tO-**prO**-teen) (n) antigen (substance or organism that produces an antibody) naturally present in the fetus and sometimes present in adults with certain cancers

fibrinogen (fi-**brin**-O-jen) (n) a substance in the blood plasma that can be converted into fibrin to produce blood clotting

fibrinopurulent (**fI**-bri-nO-**pyoo**-roo-lent) (adj) consisting of pus and fibrin

fibrinous (**fI**-brin-us) (adj) pertaining to, of the nature of, or containing fibrin (a whitish filamentous protein)

fibrosis (fI-**brO**-sis) (n) a condition marked by thickening and scarring of connective tissue

fifth disease (n) erythema infectiosum; a mild, infectious disease characterized by an erythematous rash

fissure (**fish**-ur) (n) a deep furrow, cleft, or slit; e.g., in the liver, lungs, ligaments, brain, or teeth

fistula (**fis**-tyoo-la) (n) abnormal opening or channel connecting hollow organs or leading from an internal organ to the outside or a cavity; such as a urinary fistula

fixation (fik-**say**-shun) (n) process of securing a part, as by suturing

flaring (**flayr**-ing) (adj) widening of an area, as the nostrils; a spreading area of redness around a lesion

flatulence (**flat**-yoo-lens) (n) presence of an excessive amount of gas in the stomach and intestines

flexion (**flek**-shun) (n) the act of bending or the condition of being bent, in contrast to extending

flexor (**flek**-ser, **flek**-sOr) (n) muscle that bends a joint

flexure (**flek**-sher) (n) a bend, as in an organ or structure

floater (**flO**-ter) (n) spot in the visual screen when one stares at a blank wall; caused by bits of protein and other debris moving in front of the retina

fluorescein (**floor**-ess-scene) (n) a yellow dye which glows in visible light

follicle (**fol**-i-kl) (n) pouch-like cavity, such as a hair follicle in the skin enclosing a hair

follicular (fo-**lik**-yoo-lar) (adj) pertaining to a follicle or follicles (a small secretory sac or cavity [pouchlike cavity, as that in the skin enclosing a hair])

folliculitis (fol-i-kyoo-**lI**-tis) (n) inflammation of the hair follicles

foramen (fO-**ray**-men) (n) hole or opening, especially in a bone or membrane

foramen ovale (fO-**ray**-men O-**val**-ay) (n) hole or opening, especially in a bone or membrane; (particularly the opening between the two atria of the fetal heart that closes after birth)

foramina (for-**ray**-mi-na) (n) apertures or perforations through a bone or a membrane structure; plural of foramen

fossa (**fos**-a) (n) channel or shallow depression; fossae (pl)

fracture (**frak**-chur) (v) to break; (n) a broken bone

fremitus (**frem**-i-tus) (n) a vibration that can be felt by the hand on the chest

fulguration (ful-gyoo-**ra**-shun) (n) destruction of tissue by the use of electrical current; electrodessication

fundus (**fun**-dus) (n) the bottom or base of an organ; the part farthest from the opening; that part of the interior of the eyeball exposed to view through the ophthalmoscope; fundi (pl)

funduscopic (fun-dus-**skop**-ik) (adj) relating to funduscopy

funduscopy (fun-dus-**kop**-ee) (n) examination of the fundus of the eye using a funduscope; ophthalmoscopy

fungal (**fung**-gal) (adj) caused by fungus or pertaining to fungus

fungating (**fung**-gayt-ing) (adj) growing rapidly like a fungus, applied to certain tumors

furuncle (**fyoo**-rung-kl) (n) a localized, pus-forming infection in a hair follicle or gland

G

gadolinium (gad-O-**lin**-ee-um) (n) a rare earth metallic element

gallbladder (**gawl-blad**-er) (n) pear-shaped organ that is located on the lower surface of the liver and is a reservoir for bile until discharged through the cystic duct

gallium (**gal**-ee-um) (n) a rare metal; a gallium scan after an infusion of gallium provides a better view of lymphatic tissue

ganglion (**gang**-glee-on) (n) a group of nerve cell bodies located in the peripheral nervous system

gangrene (**gang**-green) (n) death of cells or tissue due to obstruction of blood supply

gastritis (gas-**trI**-tis) (n) inflammation of the gastric (stomach) mucosa

gastroenteritis (**gas**-trO-en-ter-**I**-tis) (n) inflammation of the gastric mucosa and intestine

gastroesophageal (**gas**-trO-ee-soph-a-**jee**-al) (adj) related to both stomach and esophagus

Gastrografin (Gas-tro-**graf**-in) (n) brand name for an oral contrast medium used for radiographic examination of the alimentary tract

genital (**jen**-i-tal) (adj) relating to reproduction or the organs of reproduction

genitalia (jen-i-**tay**-lee-a) (n) the genitals; male or female reproductive organs, especially the external ones

gestation (jes-**tay**-shun) (n) the intrauterine development of an infant; pregnancy

gestational age (ges-**tay**-shun-al aj) (n) age of a fetus or newborn, usually expressed in weeks since the onset of the mother's last menstrual period

gingiva (**jin**-ji-va) (n) the gum; the tissue that attaches the teeth to the jaws

gingival (**jin**-ji-val) (adj) relating to the gums

girdle (**ger**-dl) (n) a zone or belt

gland (n) organ that secretes one or more substances not needed by the organ itself

glans (n) the head of the penis; "glans penis"

Glasgow coma scale (**glas**-gO/**glaz**-gO) (n) a clinical scale to assess impaired consciousness; assessment includes motor responsiveness, verbal performance, and eye opening

glaucoma (glaw-**kO**-ma) (n) disease of the eye in which intraocular pressure increases, damaging the optic nerve; can lead to blindness

glomerulus (glO-**mayr**-yoo-lus) (n) a cluster of capillaries at the beginning of each nephron (the functional unit of the kidney); glomeruli (pl)

glossopharyngeal neuralgia (**glos**-O-fa-**rin**-jee-al noo-**ral**-jee-a) (n) a condition of sharp spasmic pain in the throat or palate

glove-stocking anesthesia (**an**-es-**thee**-see-a) (n) glove or gauntlet anesthesia is loss of sensation in the hand; stocking anesthesia is loss of sensation in the area covered by a stocking

Goldmann perimeter screen test (n) assesses patient response when a light comes into view

gonioplasty (gO-ni-O-**plas**-tee) (n) procedure that contracts the peripheral iris to eliminate contact with the trabecular meshwork

gonioscopy (gO-ni-**O**-skOp-ee) (n) procedure that allows viewing of the anterior chamber angle using a slit lamp and a goniolens, a special mirror contact lens

gonorrhea (gon-O-**ree**-a) a contagious disease usually affecting the genitourinary tract; transmitted chiefly by sexual intercourse

graafian follicle (**graf**-ee-an) (n) a mature follicle on the ovary in which an oocyte matures and is released at ovulation

granuloma (gran-yoo-**lO**-ma) (n) a granular tumor or growth, usually of lymphoid and epitheloid cells

Graves disease (n) one type of hyperthyroidism

gravida (**grav**-i-da) (n) a pregnant woman; may be used in combination with a number or prefix to indicate the number of pregnancies and their outcome

gross (grOs) (adj) visible to the naked eye

guttural (**gut**-er-al) (adj) relating to the throat, or guttur

H

helix (**hee**-liks) (n) the folded edge of the external ear

hemangioma (he-man-jee-**O**-ma) (n) a congenital benign tumor consisting of a mass of blood vessels

hemarthrosis (**hee**-mar-**thrO**-sis/**hem**-ar-**thrO**-sis) (n) accumulation of blood in a joint

hematemesis (hee-ma-**tem**-e-sis) (n) vomiting of blood

hematochezia (**hee**-ma-tO-**kee**-zee-a) (n) passage of bloody stools

hematocrit (**hee**-ma-tO-krit/**hem**-a-tO-krit) (n) centrifuge for separating solids from plasma in the blood; measure of the volume of red blood cells as a percentage of the total blood volume

hematology (hee-ma-**tol**-o-jee) (n) the study of blood

hematoma (hee-ma-**tO**-ma/**hem**-a-tO-ma) (n) a swelling or mass of blood confined to an organ, tissue, or space and caused by a break in a blood vessel

hematuria (hee-ma-**too**-ree-a) (n) presence of blood in the urine

hemifocal (hem-i-**fO**-kal) (adj) refers to half of the body; usually a type of seizure

hemiparesis (hem-ee-pa-**ree**-sis, hem-ee-**par**-e-sis) (n) muscular weakness of one half of the body

hemodynamic (**hee**-mO-dI-**nam**-ik) (adj) relating to the mechanics of blood circulation

hemoglobin (hee-mO-**glO**-bin) (n) the iron-containing pigment of the red blood cells

hemophagocytosis (**hee**-mO-**fag**-O-sI-**tO**-sis) (n) ingestion of red blood cells by phagocytes

hemophilia (hee-mO-**fil**-ee-a) (n) an inherited blood disorder in males characterized by a defect in the clotting process due to a lack of one or more of the clotting factors

hemoptysis (hee-**mop**-ti-sis) (n) expectoration of blood; spitting or coughing up blood

hemorrhage (**hem**-o-rij) (n) loss of a large amount of blood quickly, either externally or internally

hemorrhagic (hem-O-**raj**-ik) (adj) relating to or experiencing a hemorrhage

hemorrhoid (**hem**-a-royd) (n) varicose vein of anal opening

hemosiderin (hee-mO-**sid**-er-in) (n) an iron-containing pigment derived from hemoglobin when red blood cells disintegrate

hemostasis (**hee**-mO-stay-sis/hee-**mos**-ta-sis) (n) cessation of bleeding either naturally through the blood coagulation process, mechanically (with surgical clamps), or chemically (with drugs)

hemostatic (**hee**-mO-**stat**-ik) (adj) relating to procedure, device, or substance that stops flow of blood

hemothorax (hee-mO-**thOr**-aks) (n) blood in the chest cavity

heparin (**hep**-a-rin) (n) a naturally occurring anticoagulant (a substance which prevents or slows the clotting of blood)

hepatic (he-**pat**-ik) (adj) pertaining to the liver

hepatitis (hep-a-**tI**-tis) (n) acute or chronic inflammation of the liver

hepatoduodenal (**hep**-at-O-doo-O-**dee**-nal) (adj) referring to the portion of the lesser omentum (fold of peritoneal tissue attaching and supporting the stomach and adjacent organs) between the liver and the duodenum

hepatosplenomegaly (**hep**-a-tO-**meg**-a-lee, hee-**pat**-O-**meg**-a-lee) (n) enlargement of both liver and spleen

hernia (**her**-nee-a) (n) protrusion of an organ or part of an organ or other structure through the muscle wall of the cavity that normally contains it

herpes zoster (**her**-peez **zos**-ter) (n) a viral infection causing inflammation along the path of nerve with associated painful vesicles (blisters) on the skin above; shingles

hiatal (hI-**ay**-tal) (adj) pertaining to a hernia of part of the stomach into the opening in the diaphragm, through which the esophagus passes

hilar (**hI**-lar) (adj) pertaining to a hilum, the part of an organ where the nerves and vessels enter and leave

hippocampus (hip-O-**kam**-pus) (n) structure within the brain

hirsutism (**hur**-soot-izm) (n) excessive body hair

histiocyte (**hiss**-tee-O-cyte) (n) a cell that participates in the body's reaction to infection or injury; found in connective tissue

histology (his-**tol**-O-jee) (n) a science of tissues, including their cellular composition and organization

HMS drops (ach-**em**-ess) (n) a brand name of eye drops containing Medrysone, a corticosteroid

homeostasis (**hO**-mee-O-**stay**-sis/**hO**-mee-**os**-ta-sis) (n) equilibrium in the internal environment of the body, such as temperature and electrolyte balance

humeral (hyoo-mer-al) (adj) pertaining to the humerus, the upper bone of arm extending from the elbow to the shoulder joint where it articulates with the scapula

humerus (**hyoo**-mer-us) (n) the long bone of the upper arm

hydrocephalic (hI-drO-se-**fal**-ik) (adj) relating to or having hydrocephalus

hydrocephalus (hI-drO-**sef**-a-lus) (n) increased accumulation of cerebrospinal fluid within the ventricles of the brain

hydrocephaly (hI-drO-**sef**-a-lee) (n) the condition of having hydrocephalus

hyperdiploid (**hI**-per-**dip**-loyd) (n) an individual organism or cell that has one or more extra chromosomes; (adj) relating to such an individual or cell

hyperemesis (hI-per-**em**-e-sis) (n) excessive vomiting

hyperemia (hI-per-**ee**-mee-a) (n) increased blood in part of the body, caused by inflammatory response or blockage of blood outflow

hyperemic (hI-per-**ee**-mik) (adj) showing hyperemia

hypergammaglobulinemia (**hI**-per-gam-a-**glob**-yoo-li-**nee**- mee-a) (n) excessive amount of gamma globulins in the blood

hyperglycemic (**hI**-per-glI-**see**-mic) (adj) pertaining to or characterized by hyperglycemia, an abnormally large concentration of glucose in the circulating blood

hypermenorrhea (**hI**-per-men-O-ree-a) (n) lengthy or heavy menses; menorrhagia

hyperopia (hI-per-**O**-pee-a) (n) farsightedness

hyperpigmentation (hI-per-pig-men-**tay**-shun) (n) darkening of the skin due to excessive pigment in the skin

hyperplasia (hI-per-**play**-see-a) (n) increase in size of a tissue or organ due to an increase in the number of cells (not including tumor formation)

hyperplastic (hI-per-**plas**-tik) (adj) relating to hyperplasia

hyperreflexia (**hI**-pur-re-**flek**-see-a) (n) condition in which deep tendon reflexes are abnormally strong

hypertrophy (hI-**per**-trO-fee) (n) increase in size

hypertropia (hI-per-**trO**-pee-a) (n) a type of squint in which the eye looks upward

hyphae (**hI**-fay) (n) cells forming the filaments of mold

hypokinesis (**hI**-pO-ki-**nee**-sis) (n) decreased or slow motor reaction to stimulus

hypomenorrhea (**hI**-pO-men-O-**ree**-a) (n) decreased menses

hypometabolism (**hI**-pO-me-**tab**-O-lizm) (n) lowered metabolism

hypoperfusion (**hI**-pO-per-**fyoo**-zhun) (n) lower-than-normal passage of a liquid through an organ or body part

hypotropia (hI-pO-**trO**-pee-a) (n) a type of squint in which the eye looks downward

hysterectomy (his-ter-**ek**-tO-mee) (n) surgical removal of the uterus

I

ichthyosis (ik-thee-**O**-sis) (n) condition in which the skin is dry and scaly, resembling fish skin

ictal (**ik**-tal) (adj) referring to the onset of a seizure

icteric (ik-**ter**-ik) pertaining to jaundice

idiopathic (**id**-ee-O-**path**-ik) (adj) of unknown cause; describes a disease for which no identifiable cause can be determined

idiopathy (id-ee-**op**-a-thee) (n) any disease of unknown cause

ileitis (il-ee-**I**-tis) (n) inflammation of the ileum (lower-three-fifths of the small intestines)

ileostomy (**il**-ee-**os**-tO-mee) (n) surgical formation of an opening of the ileum (distal portion of the small intestine) onto the abdominal wall through which feces pass

ileum (**il**-ee-um) (n) the third portion of the small intestine, about 12 feet in length, extending from the junction with the jejunum to the ileocecal opening

ileus (**il**-ee-us) (n) obstruction of the intestines

ilium (**il**-ee-um) (n) the broad, flaring portion of the hip bone

immune system (i-**myoon**) (n) complex interactions that protect the body from pathogenic organisms and other foreign invaders

immunity (i-**myoo**-ni-tee) (n) one's resistance to disease

immunodeficiency (**im**-yoo-nO-dee-**fish**-en-see) (n) some part of the body's immune system is inadequate; therefore, the person has decreased resistance to infectious diseases

immunoglobulin (**im**-yoo-nO-**glob**-yoo-lin) (n) antibody protein

immunohistochemistry (**im**-yoo-nO-**his**-tO-**kem**-is-tree) (n) special techniques used on cells to identify certain characteristics, especially the presence of specific antigens

immunology (im-yoo-**nol**-O-jee) (n) study of the body's response to foreign invasion, such as bacteria or viruses, and allergies

impetigo (im-pe-**tI**-gO) (n) a streptococcal or staphylococcal infection of the skin characterized by lesions, usually on the face, which rupture and become covered with a thick yellow crust; highly contagious

in situ (in **sI**-too) (adj, adv) in position; at the original location, or site

in vitro (in **vee**-trO) (adj, adv) literally, in glass; outside the living organism and in an artificial environment, such as a test tube

in vivo (in **vee**-vO) (adj, adv) literally, in the living body

incise (in-**sIzd**) (v) to cut with a knife

incised (in-**sIzd**) (adj) cut with a knife

incision and drainage (n) commonly dictated "I and D"; procedure of cutting through an infected lesion and allowing it to drain

incisional biopsy (in-**si**-zhun-al **bI**-op-see) (n) removal of part of a lesion for microscopic examination

incus (**ing**-kus) (n) the anvil-shaped bone in the middle ear

Indocin (in-doe-sin) (n) Brand name for indomethacin, an analgesic nonsteroidal anti-inflammatory drug

infarction (in-**fark**-shun) (n) formation of dead tissue as a result of diminished or stopped blood flow to the tissue area

inferior (in-**fee**-ree-Or) (adj) lower; below; of lesser value

infiltrate (in-**fil**-trayt) (v) to pass into or through a substance or a space

infraumbilical (**in**-fra-um-**bil**-i-kal) (adj) below the umbilicus (navel)

infundibulopelvic (in-fun-**dib**-yoo-lO-**pel**-vik) (adj) relating to or located in the infundibulum (the end of the fallopian tube farthest from the uterus) and the pelvis

infundibulum (in-fun-**dib**-yoo-lum) (n) a funnel-shaped opening

inguinal (**ing**-gwi-nal) (adj) relating to or located in the groin area (where the abdomen and thighs join)

inoculation (i-nok-yoo-**lay**-shun) (n) the introduction of pathogenic organisms or antigens into the body in order to increase immunity by stimulating the production of antibodies

inspiratory (in-**spI**-ra-tO-ree) (adj) relating to inhalation, drawing air into the lungs

integumentary (in-teg-yoo-**men**-ta-ree) (adj) relating to the skin

intercostal (in-ter-**kos**-tal) (adj) relating to or located between the ribs

interictal (in-ter-**ik**-tal) (adj) between seizures

interstitial (in-ter-**stish**-al) (adj) relating to or located in the space between tissues, such as interstitial fluid

intestine (in-**tes**-tin) (n) the portion of the alimentary canal extending from the pyloric opening of the stomach to the anus (opening of the rectum)

intimal (**in**-ti-mal) (adj) relating to the innermost lining of a part, especially of a blood vessel; (n) intima

intraductal (adj) inside a duct

intrahepatic (**in**-tra-he-**pat**-ik) (adj) within the liver

intraocular pressure (in-tra-**ok**-yoo-lar **presh**-er) (n) the pressure of the fluid within the eye

intrauterine (in-tra-**yoo**-ter-in) (adj) within the uterus

intravenous (IV) (**in**-tra-**vee**-nus) (adj) within or by way of a vein

introitus (in-**trO**-i-tus) (n) an opening or entrance into a canal or cavity, such as the vagina

intussusception (**in**-tus-su-**sep**-shun) (n) taking up or receiving one part within another, especially the infolding of one segment of the intestine within another

inversion (in-**vur**-shun) (n) reversal of position, as upside down or inside out

iris (**I**-ris) (n) colored portion of the eye that regulates the amount of light entering through the pupil; irides (**ir**-i-deez) (pl)

ischemia (is-**kee**-mee-a) (n) decreased blood supply due to obstruction, such as narrowing of the blood vessels

ischium (**is**-kee-um/**ish**-ee-um) (n) bone upon which body rests when sitting; fuses with the ilium and pubis to form the pelvis; ischia (**is**-kee-a) (pl)

isoagglutination (**I**-sO-a-gloo-ti-**nay**-shun) (n) process in which antibodies (agglutinins) occurring naturally in blood cause clumping of red blood cells of a different group carrying a corresponding antigen (isoagglutinogen)

J

jaundice (**jawn**-dis) (n) yellowish skin and whites of the eyes

jugular (**jug**-yoo-lar) (adj) relating to the throat or neck

K

karyotype (**kar**-ee-O-tIp) (n) chromosomal makeup of a cell; often displayed as chromosome pairs arranged by size

keloid (**kee**-loyd) (n) a mass of scar tissue

keratin (**ker**-a-tin) (n) a tough, fibrous protein in skin, hair, and nails

keratoplasty (**ker**-a-tO-**plas**-tee) (n) surgery on the cornea, especially transplant of a cornea

keratosis (ker-a-**tO**-sis) (n) a condition in which the skin thickens and builds up with excessive keratin

keratotic (ker-a-**tot**-ik) (adj) relating to keratosis

kidneys (**kid**-neez) (n) a pair of bean-shaped organs near the spinal column that filter blood and produce urine

knuckle (**nuk**-l) (n) a finger joint; an abnormal kink or loop

Kupffer cells (**koop**-ferz) (n) phagocytes present in the liver

kyphosis (kI-**fO**-sis) (n) abnormal curving of the spine causing a hunchback

L

labial (**lay**-bee-al) (adj) relating to the lips

labyrinth (**lab**-i-rinth) (n) an anatomical structure made up of a complex of cavities, such as the inner ear

labyrinthitis (**lab**-i-rin-**thI**-tis) (n) inflammation of the inner ear (labyrinth) or ethmoidal labyrinth (nose)

lacrimation (**lak**-ri-**may**-shun) (n) secretion of tears

lamina (**lam**-i-na) (n) thin membrane or plate-like structure, such as the two parts of a vertebra that join to hold the spinous process of the vertebra over the spinal cord (pl laminae)

laminar (**lam**-i-nar) (adj) relating to lamina

laparoscope (**lap**-a-rO-skOp) (n) a device for observing the inside of an organ or cavity

laparotomy (lap-a-**rot**-O-mee) (n) a surgical procedure in which an incision is made into the abdominal wall

laryngectomy (**lar**-in-**jek**-tO-mee) (n) surgical removal of the larynx

laryngostomy (**lar**-ing-**gos**-tO-mee) (n) surgically creating an opening into the larynx

larynx (**lar**-ingks) (n) the voice box, located between the pharynx and the trachea

laser iridotomy (ir-i-**dot**-O-mee) (n) cutting some of the fibers of the iris with a laser

lateral (**lat**-er-al) (adj) relating to a side, away from the center plane; e.g., cheeks are lateral to the nose

latissimus (la-**tis**-i-mus) (n) denoting a broad anatomical structure, such as a muscle

leiomyoma (lI-O-mI-**O**-ma) (n) tumor in smooth muscle tissue

lesion (**lee**-zhun) (n) general term for any visible, circumscribed injury to the skin; such as, a wound, sore, rash, or mass

lethargy (**leth**-ar-jee) (n) state of sluggishness, stupor, unresponsiveness

leukemia (loo-**kee**-mee-a) (n) production of abnormal white blood cells; a type of cancer of the blood

leukocyte (**loo**-kO-sIt) (n) white blood cell

leukoplakia (loo-kO-**play**-kee-a) (n) a precancerous change in a mucous membrane, such as the mouth or tongue

levator (le-**vay**-ter/le-**vay**-tOr) (n) muscle that lifts or raises the body part to which it is attached

ligament (**lig**-a-ment) (n) band of fibrous connective tissue that binds joints together and connects bones and cartilage

linear (**lin**-ee-ar) (adj) pertaining to or resembling a line

lipping (**lip**-ing) (n) excessive growth in a liplike shape at the edge of a bone

lithotomy (li-**thot**-O-mee) (n) surgical removal of a stone, especially from the urinary tract

lithotripsy (**lith**-O-trip-see) (n) procedure using a laser to break apart stones (calculi)

lobe (lOb) (n) rounded part of an organ, separated from other parts of the organ by connective tissue or fissures

lobectomy (lOb-**ek**-tO-mee) (n) the removal of a lobe from an organ or gland

lobule (**lob**-yool) (n) a small lobe or primary subdivision of a lobe; typical of pancreas and major salivary glands and may be on the surface by bumps and bulges

lochia (**lO**-kee-a) (n) vaginal discharge occurring after childbirth

loop (n) a curve or bend forming a complete or almost complete oval or circle

lordosis (lOr-**dO**-sis) (n) abnormal curving of the spine causing a swayback

loupe (loop) (n) a magnifying lens

lucency (**loo**-sen-see) (n) giving off light; being luminous or translucent

lumbar (**lum**-bar) (adj) relating to the lower back, between the ribs and pelvis

lumen (**loo**-men) (n) cavity, canal, or channel within an organ or tube; the space inside a structure; lumina or lumens (pl)

luminal (**loo**-min-al) (adj) related to the lumen of a tubular structure, such as a blood vessel

lymph (limf) (n) a thin fluid that bathes the tissues of the body, circulates through lymph vessels, is filtered in lymph nodes, and enters the blood stream through the thoracic duct

lymphadenitis (lim-**fad**-e-**nI**-tis) (n) inflammation of one or more lymph nodes

lymphadenopathy (lim-fad-e-**nop**-a-thee) (n) any disorder of lymph nodes or of the lymphatic system

lymphatic (lim-**fat**-ik) (adj) relating to or resembling lymph or lymph nodes

lymphoblastic (lim-fO-**blas**-tik) (adj) relating to or resembling lymphoblasts, immature white blood cells

lymphocyte (**lim**-fO-sIt) (n) white blood cell that produces antibodies

lymphocytic (lim-fO-**sit**-ik) (adj) relating to or characteristic of lymphocytes

lymphoid (**lim**-foyd) (adj) resembling lymph or relating to the lymphatic system

lymphoma (lim-**fO**-ma) (n) a general term for various types of tumors of the lymphatic system

lymphopenia (lim-fO-**pee**-nee-a) (n) a decrease in the number of lymphocytes in the blood

lytic (**lit**-ik) (adj) pertaining to lysis, a gradual subsidence of the symptoms of an acute disease

M

macrophage (**mak**-ro-fayj) (n) a large scavenger cell (phagocyte) that digests microorganisms and cell debris

macula (**mak**-yoo-la) (n) small discolored spot on the retina

macule (**mak**-yool) (n) a small discolored spot on the skin

maculopapular (mak-yoo-lO-**pap**-yoo-lar) (adj) describing skin lesions that are raised in the center

malaise (ma-**layz**) (n) a feeling of general discomfort or uneasiness, often the first indication of an infection or other disease

malformation (mal-for-**may**-shun) (n) abnormal development or structure of the body or a part

malignancy (ma-**lig**-nan-see) (n) a cancer that is invasive and spreading

malleolus (ma-**lee**-O-lus) (n) either of the two bumplike projections on each side of the ankle; malleoli (pl)

malleus (**mal**-ee-us) (n) the largest of the three inner ear bones; club-shaped; attached to the tympanic membrane

mammary (**mam**-a-ree) (adj) relating to the breast

mammogram (**mam**-O-gram) (n) x-ray of the breast

mandibular (man-**dib**-yoo-lar) (adj) relating to the lower jaw

mastication (mas-ti-**kay**-shun) (n) process of chewing food

mastoiditis (mas-toy-**dI**-tis) (n) inflammation of the mastoid process (part of the temporal bone behind the ear)

maxilla (mak-**sil**-a) (n) the upper jaw

maxillary sinus (**mak**-si-layr-ee **sI**-nus) (n) an air cavity in the body of the upper jaw bone; connects with the middle passage (meatus) of the nose

meatus (mee-**ay**-tus) (n) a passage or channel, especially with an external opening

meconium (mee-**kO**-nee-um) (n) first bowel movement of a newborn, which are thick, sticky, greenish to black and composed of bile pigments and gland secretions

mediastinum (**mee**-dee-as-**tI**-nal) (n) relating to the space in the chest cavity between the lungs that contains the heart, aorta, esophagus, trachea, and thymus

mediastinal (mee-dee-as-**tI**-nal (adj) related to the mediastinum, a septum or cavity between two principal portions of an organ

mediolateral (**mee**-dee-O-**lat**-er-al) (adj) relating to the middle and side of a structure

medulla oblongata (me-**dool**-a ob-long-**gah**-ta) (n) the lowest part of the brain, connecting to the spinal cord; contains the cardiac, vasomotor, and respiratory centers of the brain

melanin (**mel**-a-nin) (n) naturally-occurring dark brown or black pigment found in the hair, skin, and eyes

melanocyte (**mel**-an-O-sIt) (n) a cell that produces melanin

melanocytic (mel-a-nO-**sit**-ik) (adj) pertaining to or composed of melanocytes

melena (me-**lee**-na) (n) passage of dark, tarry stool

melitis (mee-**lI**-tis) (n) inflammation of the cheek

menarche (me-**nar**-kee) (n) the initial menstrual period

Meniere disease (mayn-**yairz**) (n) a disease of the inner ear with attacks of dizziness, nausea, ringing in the ear, and increasing deafness

meninges (me-**nin**-jeez) (n) membranes covering the brain and spinal cord

meningitis (men-in-**jI**-tis) (n) inflammation of the meninges

meningocele (me-**ning**-gO-seel) (n) protrusion of the brain or spinal cord through a defect in the skull or spinal column

menometrorrhagia (**men**-O-mee-trO-**rah**-jee-a) (n) excessive menstrual bleeding or bleeding between menstrual periods

menopause (**men**-O-pawz) (n) the end of a woman's reproductive period of life and cessation of menses

menorrhagia (men-O-**ray**-jee-a) (n) prolonged or heavy menses; hypermenorrhea

menorrhalgia (men-O-**ral**-jee-a) (n) painful menstruation or pelvic pain accompanying menstruation

menses (**men**-seez) (n) monthly flow of bloody fluid from the uterus

menstruation (men-stroo-**ay**-shun) (n) the discharge of a bloody fluid from the uterus at regular intervals during the life of a woman from puberty to menopause

mesentery (**mes**-en-tar-ee) (n) a peritoneal fold encircling the greater part of the small intestines and connecting the intestine to the posterior abdominal wall

mesial (**mee**-zee-al; **mes**-ee-al) (adj) situated toward the midline of the body or the central part of an organ or tissue (also called medial)

mesosalpinx (**mez**-O-**sal**-pinks) (n) free end of the broad ligament which supports the fallopian tubes

metaphyseal (met-a-**fiz**-ee-al) (adj) relating to a metaphysis

metaphysis (me-**taf**-i-sis) (n) a conical section of bone between the epiphysis and diaphysis of long bones

metaplasia (me-ta-**play**-zee-a) (n) conversion of a tissue into a form that is not normal for that tissue

metastasis (me-**tas**-ta-sis) (n) the shifting of a disease from one part of the body to another, especially in cancer; metastases (pl)

metastatic (met-a-**stat**-ic) (n) pertaining to metastasis (movement of cells, especially cancer cells, from one part of the body to another

metatarsal (**met**-a-**tar**-sal) (adj) relating to a metatarsus; (n) a metatarsal bone

metatarsus (**met**-a-**tar**-sus) (n) any of the five long bones of the foot between the ankle and the toes

metrorrhagia (mee-trO-**rah**-jee-a) (n) bleeding from the uterus between menstrual periods

microscopy (mI-**kros**-kO-pee) (n) use of a microscope to magnify and examine objects

milia (**mil**-ee-a) (n, pl) whiteheads, due to obstruction of the outlet of hair follicles or sweat glands

miliaria (mil-ee-**ay**-ree-a) (n) a skin eruption of small vesicles and papules; heat rash

millicuries (**mil**-i-**kyoo**-rees) (n) a unit of radioactivity, abbreviated mc

mitotic (mI-**tot**-ik) (adj) pertaining to mitosis, a type of cell division in which a cell divides into two genetically identical daughter cells

mitral (**mI**-tral) (adj) relating to the bicuspid or mitral valve of the heart, between the atrium and the ventricle on the left side of the heart

morphology (mOr-**fol**-O-jee) (n) the shape and structure of an organism or body part

motility (mO-**til**-i-tee) (n) ability to move spontaneously

mucoperiosteum (**myoo**-kO-per-ee-**os**-tee-um) (n) the mucous membrane covering the hard palate at the front of the roof of the mouth

mucosa (myoo-**kO**-sa) (n) mucous membrane

mucosal (myoo-**kO**-sal) (adj) concerning any mucous membrane

mucous (**myoo**-kus) (adj) having the nature of or resembling mucus

mucus (**myoo**-kus) (n) viscous (sticky, gummy) secretions of mucous membranes and glands

multinucleated (mul-ti-**noo**-klee-ay-ted) (adj) possessing several nuclei

multipara (mul-**tip**-a-ra) (n) a woman who has given birth to two or more children

murmur (**mer**-mer) (n) abnormal heart sound

myasthenia gravis (mI-as-**thee**-nee-a **grav**-is) (n) a chronic progressive muscular weakness, beginning usually in the face and throat, due to a defect in the conduction of nerve impulses

mycosis (mI-**kO**-sis) (n) disease caused by a fungus

myelocyte (**my**-e-lo-cyte) (n) immature granulocytic leukocyte normally found in bone marrow and present in the circulatory blood in certain diseases, e.g., myelocytic anemia

myocardial (mI-O-**kar**-dee-al) (adj) relating to the myocardium, the heart muscle

myopia (mI-**O**-pee-a) (n) nearsightedness; visual defect in which parallel rays come to a focus

myringitis (mir-in-**jI**-tis) (n) inflammation of the tympanic membrane; tympanitis

myringoplasty (mi-**ring**-gO-**plas**-tee) (n) surgical repair of the eardrum

myringotomy (mir-ing-**got**-o-mee) (n) surgical incision into the tympanic membrane

N

nafcillin (naf-**sill**-in) (n) an antibiotic; one of the varieties of penicillin

naris (**nay**-ris) (n) nostril; nares (**nay**-rees) (pl)

nasopharynx (**nay**-zO-**far**-ingks) (n) open chamber behind the nose and above the palate

nausea (**naw**-zee-a, **naw**-zha) (n) an inclination to vomit

nauseous (**naw**-zee-us; **naw**-shus) (adj) causing nausea or feeling nausea

nebulization (**neb**-yoo-li-**zay**-shun) (n) production of fine particles, such as a spray or mist, from liquid

necrosis (ne-**krO**-sis) (n) death of some or all of the cells in a tissue

necrotic (ne-**krot**-ik) (adj) relating to or undergoing necrosis

neoadjuvant (nee-O-**ad**-joo-vant) (adj) used in conjunction with other types of therapy

neoplasm (**nee**-O-plazm) (n) any abnormal growth of tissue, usually malignant; tumor

neoplastic (nee-O-**plas**-tik) (adj) pertaining to the nature of new, abnormal tissue formation; usually refers to cancer

nephrectomy (ne-**frek**-tO-mee) (n) surgical removal of a kidney

nephrolithiasis (**nef**-rO-li-**thI**-a-sis) (n) presence of stones (calculi) in the kidney(s)

nephrolithotomy (**nef**-rO-li-**thot**-O-mee) (n) surgical incision into a kidney to remove stones (calculi)

nephron (**nef**-ron) (n) the functional unit of the kidney that filters the blood

nephrostomy (ne-**fros**-tO-mee) (n) surgical creation of an opening in the kidney for drainage

neural (**noo**-ral) (adj) relating to nerves or the nervous system

neuralgia (noo-**ral**-jee-a) (n) pain of a severe, throbbing, or stabbing character along the course of a nerve

neurapraxia (noor-a-**prak**-see-a) (n) loss of conduction in a nerve without structural degeneration

neurasthenia (noor-as-**thee**-nee-a) (n) a condition, commonly accompanying or following depression, characterized by fatigue believed to be brought on by psychological factors

neurilemma (noor-i-**lem**-a) (n) a cell that enfolds one or more axons of the peripheral nervous system

neuroblastoma (**noor**-O-blas-**tO**-ma) (n) malignant (cancerous) tumor containing embryonic nerve cells

neuroectodermal (**noo**-rO-ek-tO-**der**-mal) (adj) embryonic tissue that gives rise to nerve tissue

neuromuscular (noor-O-**mus**-kyoo-lar) (adj) pertains to the muscles and nerves

neuron (**noor**-on) (n) nerve cell; the morphological and functional unit of the nervous system, consisting of the nerve cell body, the dendrites, and the axon

neuropathy (noo-**rop**-a-thee) (n) disorder affecting the cranial or spinal nerves

neutropenia (noo-trO-**pee**-nee-a) (n) a decrease in the number of neutrophils in the blood

neutrophil (**noo**-trO-fil/**noo**-trO-fIl) (n) the most common type of mature white blood cell; its primary function is phagocytosis; granular leukocyte

nevus (**nee**-vus) (n) congenital discoloration of the skin; birthmark or mole; nevi (pl)

nocturia (nok-**too**-ree-a) (n) frequent urination during the night

node (nOd) (n) a small knot of tissue, distinct from surrounding tissue; a lymph node

nodular (**nod**-yoo-lar) (adj) containing or resembling nodules; having small, firm, knotty masses

nodule (**nod**-yool) (n) a small mass, distinct from surrounding tissue

nuchal (**noo**-kal) (adj) pertaining to the neck, or nucha (nape of neck)

nulligravida (nul-i-**grav**-i-da) (n) a woman who has never been pregnant

nystagmus (nis-**tag**-mus) (n) involuntary, rhythmic oscillation of the eyeballs

O

obese (o-**bees**) (adj) very fat

oblique (ob-**leek**) (adj) slanting

obstipation (ob-sti-**pay**-shun) (n) severe constipation

obturator (**ob**-too-ray-tor) (n) device or body structure that closes up or covers an opening

obtuse (ob-**toos**) (adj) dull or blunt; not pointed or acute

occiput (**ok**-si-put) (n) the back part of the skull

occlusion (o-**kloo**-zhun) (n) blockage, such as coronary occlusion

ocular (**ok**-yoo-lar) (adj) concerning the eye or vision

odontoid process (O-**don**-toyd **pros**-es) (n) the toothlike projection from the upper surface of the second cervical vertebra on which the head rotates

oligohydramnios (**ol**-i-gO-hI-**dram**-nee-os) (n) abnormally small amount of amniotic fluid

oligomenorrhea (**ol**-i-gO-men-O-**ree**-a) (n) infrequent or very light menstrual bleeding

omental (O-**men**-tal) (adj) relating to the omentum

omentum (O-**men**-tum) (n) fold of peritoneal tissue attaching to and supporting the stomach and intestines

onycholysis (on-ee-**kol**-i-sis) (n) loosening of the nails from their beds

oophorectomy (O-of-Or-**ek**-tO-mee) (n) surgical removal of one or both ovaries

opacification (O-**pas**-i-fi-kay-shun) (n) clouding or loss of transparency, especially of the cornea or lens of the eye

opacity (O-**pas**-i-tee) (n) state of being opaque, impenetrable by visible light rays or by forms of radiant energy, such as x-rays

ophthalmologist (of-thal-**mol**-o-jist) (n) a physician specializing in diseases of the eye

ophthalmoscopy (of-thal-**mos**-ko-pee) (n) procedure used to examine the optic nerve head for color, shape, and vascularization

ophthalmus (of-**thal**-mus) (n) the eye

opportunistic infection (n) a disease caused by normally harmless microorganisms when the body's resistance to disease is impaired

optic (**op**-tik) (adj) pertaining to the eye or sight

optic chiasm (**op**-tik **kI**-azm) (n) the point of crossing of the optic nerves

optometrist (op-**tom**-e-trist) (n) a professional who tests visual acuity and prescribes corrective lenses

orbital cellulitis (**or**-bit-al sel-yoo-**lI**-tis) (n) inflammation of tissue around or behind the eye

orchidopexy (Or-ki-**dop**-eks-ee) (n) surgical procedure in which an undescended testicle is sutured into place; also orchiopexy

orchiectomy (Or-kee-**ek**-tO-mee) (n) surgical removal of one or both testes

orchiocele (**Or**-kee-O-seel) (n) scrotal hernia; tumor of a testis

organism (**or**-ga-nizm) (n) a living plant, animal, or microorganism

organomegaly (**Or**-ga-nO-**meg**-a-lee) (n) abnormal enlargement of an organ, particularly an organ of the abdominal cavity, such as the liver or spleen

orifice (**or**-i-fis) (n) an opening; the mouth, entrance, or outlet of any aperture

orthopnea (Or-thop-**nee**-a) (n) difficulty in breathing when lying down

oscilloscope (o-**sil**-O-scOp) (n) an instrument which displays electrical oscillations (waves) on a screen

osseous (**os**-ee-us) (adj) bony; resembling bone; osteal

ossicles (os-i-kls) (n) small bones, such as the auditory ossicles (the three bones of the inner ear)

osteal (**os**-tee-ul) (adj) bony; resembling bone; osseous

ostealgia (os-tee-**al**-jee-a) (n) pain in a bone

ostectomy (os-**tek**-tO-mee) (n) surgical removal of all or part of a bone

osteophyte (**os**-tee-O-fIt) (n) a bony outgrowth; projection or bone spur

osteoporosis (os-tee-O-pO-**rO**-sis) (n) abnormal loss of bone tissue, causing fragile bones that fracture easily

osteosarcoma (os-tee-O-sar-**ko**-ma) (n) a tumor of the bone, usually highly malignant

ostial (**os**-tee-ul) (adj) relating to any opening (ostium)

otalgia (**Otal**-jeea) (n) earache

otitis (O-**tI**-tis) (n) inflammation of the ear

otitis externa (O-**tI**-tis eks-**ter**-na) (n) inflammation of the external ear

otitis media (O-**tI**-tis **mee**-dee-a) (n) inflammation of the middle ear

otorhinolaryngology (**O**-tO-**rI**-nO-lar-in-**gol**-o-jee) (n) study of the ears, nose, and throat

otosclerosis (**O**-tO-sklee-**rO**-sis) (n) a growth of sponge-like bone in the inner ear, eventually leading to deafness

otoscope (**O**-tO-skOp) (n) an instrument for examining the eardrum

otoscopy (O-**tos**-kO-pee) (n) visual examination of the ear with an otoscope

ototoxic (O-to-**tok**-sic) (adj) harmful to the organs of hearing or auditory nerve

oximetry (ok-**sim**-e-tree) (n) measuring the amount of oxygen combined with the hemoglobin in a blood sample

P

palate (**pal**-at) (n) the roof of one's mouth, composed of the hard palate (front) and the soft palate (back)

palliative (**pal**-ee-a-tiv) (adj) describes a treatment that minimizes symptoms but does not cure the disease

pallor (**pal**-or) (n) abnormal paleness of the skin; deficiency of color

palpable (**pal**-pa-bl) (adj) perceivable by touch

palpate (**pal**-payt) (v) to examine by touch; to feel

palpation (pal-**pay**-shun) (n) technique of examination in which the examiner feels the firmness, texture, size, shape, or location of body parts

palpitations (pal-pi-**tay**-shuns) (n) stronger and more rapid heartbeats as felt by the patient; pounding or throbbing of the heart

palsy (**pawl**-zee) (n) an abnormal condition characterized by partial paralysis

pancreas (**pan**-kree-as) (n) gland lying behind the stomach that produces and secretes insulin, glucagon, and digestive enzymes

pancrelipase (pan-kree-**lip**-ase) (n) standardized preparation of enzymes with amylase and protease, obtained from the pancreas of hogs

papilledema (pa-pill-e-**dee**-ma) (n) edema and inflammation of the optic nerve at its point of entrance into the eyeball

papillopathy (pap-i-**lop**-a-thee) (n) the blood supply to the optic disk and retina is obstructed; often producing low-tension glaucoma

papule (**pap**-yool) (n) a small, solid, raised skin lesion, as in chickenpox

para (**par**-a) (n) a woman who has given birth to one or more children; the term may be used in combination with a number or prefix to indicate how many times a woman has given birth

paraplegia (par-a-**plee**-jee-a) (n) paralysis of the lower portion of the body and of both legs

parasite (**par**-a-sIt) (n) an organism that lives on or in another and draws its nourishment therefrom

parenchyma (pa-**reng**-ki-ma) (n) functional part of an organ, apart from supporting or connective tissue

parenchymal (pa-**reng**-ki-mal) (adj) pertaining to the distinguishing or specific cells of a gland or organ contained in and supported by the connective tissue framework

parenteral (pa-**ren**-ter-al) (adj) not through the digestive system, such as introduction of nutrients into the veins or under the skin

parietal (pa-**rI**-e-tal) (adj) relating to the inner walls of a body cavity; a section (lobe) of the brain

paronychia (par-O-**nik**-ee-a) (n) infected skin around the nail

paroxysmal (par-ok-**siz**-mal) (adj) relating to or recurring in paroxysms (sudden, severe attacks of symptoms or convulsions)

Parvovirus (**par**-vO-vI-rus) (n) a genus of viruses; strain B19 can cause anemia in humans

patent (**pa**-tent) (adj) open; unblocked

pathogen (**path**-O-jen) (n) any microorganism or substance that can cause a disease

pathologic (path-O-**loj**-ik) (adj) pertaining to pathology, the medical science concerned with all aspects of disease, especially with the structural and functional changes caused by disease

pectoriloquy (pek-tO-**ril**-O-kwee) (n) voice sounds transmitted through the pulmonary structures, clearly audible on auscultation

pectus carinatum (**pek**-tus kar-i-**nay**-tum) (n) forward protusion of the sternum; pigeon breast

pectus excavatum (**pek**-tus eks-ka-**vay**-tum) (n) markedly sunken sternum; funnel breast

pedal (**ped**-al or **pE**dal) (adj) relating to the foot

pedicle (**ped**-i-kl) (n) the stem that attaches a new growth

pedunculated (pee-**dung**-Q-late-ed) (adj) possessing a stalk

pelvic (**pel**-vik) (adj) relating to or located near the pelvis

pelvis (**pel**-vis) (n) the bones in the lower portion of the trunk of the body; the bones between the spine and legs

pemphigus (**pem**-fi-gus) (n) a distinctive group of diseases marked by successive crops of bullae

pendulous (**pen**-ju-lus) (adj) loosely hanging

percussion (per-**kush**-un) (n) a technique of physical examination in which the sound of fingers or a small tool tapping parts of the body is used to determine position and size of internal organs and to detect the presence of fluid

percutaneous (per-kyoo-**tay**-nee-us) (adj) through the skin

perforation (per-fO-**ray**-shun) (n) abnormal opening or hole in a hollow organ

perfusion (per-**fyoo**-zhun) (n) passing of a fluid through spaces

periauricular (**per**-ee-aw-**rik**-yoo-lar) (adj) around the ear

pericardial (per-i-**kar**-dee-al) (adj) surrounding the heart; relating to the pericardium

pericarditis (per-i-kar-**dI**-tis) (n) an inflammatory disease of the pericardium (tough outer layer of the heart wall and lining of the pericardial sac that surrounds the heart)

pericardium (per-i-**kar**-dee-um) (n) a double-layered sac surrounding the heart and large vessels

pericolonic (per-ee-ko-**lon**-ik) (adj) pertaining to the region around the colon

perihilar (per-i-**hI**-lar) (adj) occurring near the hilum, the part of an organ where the nerves and vessels enter and leave

perineum (**per**-i-**nee**-um) (n) the external region between the vulva and the anus in women and between the scrotum and the anus in men

peripheral iridectomy (per-**if**-er-al ir-i-**dek**-tO-mee) (n) procedure that creates a hole in the iris; used to relieve high intraocular pressure

peripheral nervous system (per-**if**-er-al) (n) portion of nervous system that connects the CNS to other body parts

peripheral vascular disease (pe-**rif**-e-ral **vas**-kyoo-lar)(n) any disorder affecting the blood circulatory system, except the heart

peristalsis (per-i-**stal**-sis) (n) the movement of the intestine or other tubular structure, characterized by waves of alternate circular contraction and relaxation of the tube by which the contents are propelled onward

peritoneal (**per**-i-tO-**nee**-al) (adj) relating to the peritoneum

peritoneum (per-i-tO-**nee**-um) (n) lining of the abdominal cavity

petechia (pe-**tee**-kee-a/pee-**tek**-ee-a) (n, sing.) tiny reddish or purplish flat spot on the skin as a result of a tiny hemorrhage within the skin (usually used in the plural form, petechiae)

petechiae (pe-**tee**-kee-ee/pe-**tek**-kee-e/pe-**tee**-kee-a) (n) minute red spots appearing on the skin as a result of tiny hemorrhaging

petechial (pee-**tee**-kee-al/pee-**tek**-ee-al) (adj) relating to or having petechiae, tiny reddish or purplish spots on the skin from broken capillaries

petit mal (pe-**tee** mahl) (n) a type of seizure characerized by a brief blackout of consciousness with minor rhythmic movements, seen especially in children

phacoemulsification (fak-O-ee-mul-si-fi-**kay**-shun) (n) process that disintegrates a cataract using ultrasonic waves

phagocyte (**fag**-O-sIt/**fAg**O-sIt) (n) a cell able to engulf and destroy bacteria, foreign particles, cellular debris, and other cells

phagocytosis (**fag**-O-sI-**tO**-sis) (n) the process in which a cell engulfs and destroys bacteria, foreign particles, cellular debris, and other cells

pharyngitis (far-in-jI-tis) (n) inflammation of the pharynx

pharynx (**far**-ingks) (n) throat; passageway for air from nasal cavity to larynx, and food from mouth to esophagus

phasic (**fay**-sic) (adj) pertaining to a phase, a stage of development

phlebitis (fle-**bI**-tis) (n) inflammation of a vein

phlebotomy (fle-**bot**-O-mee) (n) incision into a vein for drawing blood

phonation (fO-**nay**-shun) (n) process of uttering vocal sounds

photon (**fO**-ton) (n) a unit of radiant energy or light intensity

photophobia (fO-tO-**fO**-bee-a) (n) marked intolerance to light

pia mater (**pI**-a **may**-ter/**pee**-a **mah**-ter) (n) the innermost of the three membranes surrounding the brain and spinal cord; it carries a rich supply of blood vessels

pigment (**pig**-ment) (n) any organic coloring substance in the body

pigmented (**pig**-men-ted) (v) colored by a pigment

pineal gland (**pin**-ee-al) (n) small, cone-shaped gland in the brain thought to secrete melatonin

pinna (**pin**-a) (n) the external ear; auricle; pinnae (**pin**-ee) (pl)

Pitocin (pit-toe-sin) (n) Brand name for oxytocin, a synthetically produced, naturally-occurring hormone

pituitary gland (pi-**too**-i-tayr-ee) (n) gland suspended from the base of the hypothalamus

plantar (**plan**-tar) (adj) relating to the undersurface (sole) of the foot

platelet (**playt**-let) (n) disc-shaped, small cellular element in the blood that is essential for blood clotting

pleura (**ploor**-a) (n) membrane lining the chest cavity and covering the lungs

pleural (**ploor**-al) (adj) relating to the pleura

pleurisy (**ploor**-I-see) (n) inflammation of the pleura; pleuritis

plexus (**plek**-sus) (n) a network of intersecting nerves and blood vessels or of lymphatic vessels

Pneumocystis carinii (noo-mO-**sis**-tis ka-**rI**-nee-I) (n) a tiny parasite which causes Pneumocystis carinii pneumonia (PCP) in individuals with impaired immune systems

pneumonia (noo-**mO**-nee-a) (n) inflammation and congestion of the lung, usually due to infection by bacteria or viruses

pneumonitis (noo-mO-**nI**-tis) (n) inflammation of the lungs

pneumoperitoneum (**noo**-mO-per-i-ton-**ee**-um) (n) condition in which air or gas is collected in the peritoneal cavity

pneumothorax (noo-mO-**thor**-aks) (n) abnormal presence of air or gas in the chest cavity

poikilocytosis (**poy**-ki-lO-sI-**tO**-sis) (n) having poikilocytes (abnormal and irregularly shaped red blood cells) in the blood

polycystic (pol-ee-**sis**-tik) (adj) having or consisting of many cysts

polydipsia (pol-ee-dip-**see**-a) (n) excessive thirst

polyp (**pol**-ip) (n) a general descriptive term used with reference to any mass of tissue that bulges or projects outward or upward from the normal surface level

polyphagia (pol-ee-**fay**-jee-a) (n) eating abnormally large amounts of food at a meal

polyuria (pol-ee-**yoo**-ree-a) (n) excessive urinary output

pompholyx (**pom**-fO-liks) (n) a skin eruption primarily on the hands and feet; may be accompanied by excessive sweating

popliteal (pop-**lit**-ee-al) (adj) concerning the posterior surface of the knee

porphyrins (**pOr**-fi-rinz) (n) a group of pigmented compounds essential to life; for example, hemoglobin contains the heme porphyrin

postictal (pOst-**ik**-tal) (adj) relating to the period following a seizure

precordial (pree-**kor**-dee-al) (adj) pertaining to the precordium (region of the chest over the heart)

presbycusis (**prez**-bee-**koo**-sis) (n) the loss of hearing acuity due to aging

presbyopia (prez-bee-**O**-pee-a) (n) farsightedness associated with aging

presents (pre-**sents**) (v) appears; shows; displays; the symptoms displayed are the presenting symptoms

Prilosec (**pry**-low-sec) (n) Brand name for omeprazole, a gastric acid secretion inhibitor

primipara (prE-**mip**-ah-ra) (n) a woman who has had one pregnancy that produced a living infant

prognosis (prog-**nO**-sis) (n) the expected outcome of a disease

prolapse (prO-**laps**) (n) dropping of an organ from its normal position, a sinking down

pronator (**prO**-nay-ter, **prO**-nay-tOr) (n) muscle that moves a part into the prone position

prophylaxis (prO-fi-**lak**-sis) (n) prevention of disease or its spread

proprioception (**prO**-pree-O-**sep**-shun) (n) sensation due to receiving stimuli from muscles, tendons, or other internal tissues which provides a sense of movement and position of the body

prostate gland (**pros**-tayt) (n) a gland located at the base of the bladder and surrounding the beginning of the urethra in the male

prostatic (pros-**tat**-ik) (adj) relating to the prostate gland

prosthesis (pros-**thee**-sis) (n) artificial replacement for a diseased or missing part of the body, such as artificial limbs; prostheses (pl)

protease (**prO**-tee-ays) an enzyme that breaks down proteins

protease inhibitor (n) an agent that inhibits (prevents or slows down) the release of protease

proteinaceous (**prO**-tee-**nay**-shus/**prO**-tee-i-**nay**-shus) (adj) relating to or resembling proteins

proteinuria (prO-tee-**noo**-ree-a) (n) presence of abnormally large amounts of protein in the urine

proton (**prO**-ton) (n) a positively charged particle that is a fundamental component of the nucleus of all atoms; used in radiotherapy

protuberant (prO-**too**-ber-ant) (adj) pertaining to a part that is prominent beyond a surface, like a knob

proximal (**prok**-si-mal) (adj) nearest the point of attachment, center of the body, or point of reference

proximally (**prok**-si-mal-lee) (adv) occurring nearest to the point of attachment, center of the body, or point of reference

pruritic (pru-**ri**-tic) (adj) itching

pruritus (proo-**rI**-tus) (n) itching skin condition

Pseudomonas (soo-dO-**mO**-nas) (n) a genus of bacteria commonly found in soil and water and which may cause infection

psoriasis (sO-**rI**-a-sis) (n) chronic skin disease in which reddish scaly patches develop

psychosomatic (**sI**-kO-sO-mat-ik) (adj) relating to the influence of the mind upon the functions of the body

pterygium (ter-**ij**-ee-um) (n) web eye; an outward growth of tissue of the eye

pterygoid plate (**ter**-i-goyd) (n) wing-shaped bones at the back of the nasal cavity

ptosis (**tO**-sis) (n) sagging of the upper eyelid

punch biopsy (punch **bI**-op-see) (n) a special instrument is used to take a small cylindrical piece of tissue for microscopic examination

pupil (**pyoo**-pil) (n) the round opening in the center of the iris which opens or closes to adjust to light

pupillary (**pyoo**-pi-layr-ee) (adj) relating to the pupil of the eye

purpura (**pur**-poo-ra) (n) any of several bleeding disorders in which the escape of blood into tissues below the skin causes reddish or purplish spots

purulent (**pyoor**-u-lent) (adj) relating to, containing, or forming pus

pustular (**pus**-choo-lar) (adj) relating to or having pustules

pustule (**pus**-chool) (n) small pus-containing elevation on the skin

pyelogram (**pI**-el-O-gram) (n) x-ray of the kidney and ureters; usually a radiopaque dye is injected into the patient to show the outline of the kidney and associated structures

pyrexia (pI-**rek**-see-a) (n) fever

pyrosis (pI-**rO**-sis) (n) heartburn

Q

quadriceps (**kwah**-dri-seps) (adj) four-headed, as a quadriceps muscle; one of the extensor muscles of the legs

quadriparesis (kwod-ri-pa-**ree**-sis) (n) paralysis of both arms and both legs

R

radial keratotomy (**ray**-dee-al ker-ah-**tot**-O-mee) (n) incision(s) in the cornea radiating out from the center

radiculopathy (ra-**dik**-yoo-**lop**-a-thee) (n) disease of the spinal nerve roots

radiograph (**ray**-dee-O-graf) (n) an image produced through exposure to x-rays

radiopaque (ray-dee-O-**payk**) (adj) opaque to x-rays or other radiation; an injection of a radiopaque dye or substance may be used to visualize areas of the body by x-ray

radiotherapy (ray-dee-O-**thayr**-a-pee) (n) the treatment of disease by application of radium, ultraviolet, and other types of radiation

rales (rahls) (n) abnormal sounds, such as rattling or bubbling, heard on auscultation of the lungs

ramus (**ray**-mus) (n) branch, especially of a nerve or blood vessel

recession (ree-**sesh**-un) (n) the withdrawal of a part from its normal position

rectal (**rek**-tal) (adj) relating to the rectum, the lower part of the large intestine

rectovaginal (**rek**-tO-**vaj**-i-nal) (adj) relating or located near the rectum and vagina

rectus (**rec**-tus) (adj) relating to the rectus muscle of the eye

referral (ree-**fer**-al) (n) a physician's sending of a patient to another physician

reflex (**ree**-fleks) (n) an involuntary response to a stimulus

reflux (**ree**-fluks) (n) a return or backward flow

refractory (ree-frak-tO-ree) (adj) obstinate, stubborn; resistant to ordinary treatment

regimen (**rej**-i-men) (n) plan of therapy, including drugs

regression (ree-**gresh**-un) (n) returning to an earlier condition

regurgitation (ree-**ger**-ji-**tay**-shun) (n) a backward flowing, as a backflow of blood through a defective heart valve or the bringing up of gas or undigested food from the stomach

regurgitation (ree-gur-ji-**tay**-shun) (n) the return of gas or small amounts of food from the stomach

renal (**ree**-nal) (adj) related to the kidney

renal failure (**ree**-nal) (n) inability of the kidneys to function

resection (ree-**sek**-shun) (n) surgical removal of a portion of a structure or organ

residual (re-**zid**-yoo-al) (adj) related to a residue which is left behind

respiration (res-pi-**ray**-shun) (n) inhalation and exhalation; the exchange of gases—oxygen and carbon dioxide—between an organism and the environment

respiratory (**res**-per-a-tOr-ee) (adj) relating to respiration

respiratory distress syndrome (**res**-pi-ra-tOr-ee dis-**tres sin**-drOm) (n) acute lung disease, especially in premature newborn babies, caused by a lack of surfactant in the lung tissue

reticulocyte (re-**tik**-yoo-lO-sIt) (n) a red blood cell containing a network of granules representing an immature stage in development

retina (**ret**-i-na) (n) innermost layer of the eyeball that receives images formed by the lens and transmits visual impulses through the optic nerve to the brain; composed of three types of nerves

retinal hemorrhage (**ret**-i-nal **hem**-or-age) hemorrhage of the retina

retinitis pigmentosa (ret-in-**I**-tis pig men **toe** saw) (n) a inflammation of the retina with pigment changes, eventually leading to blindness

retinoblastoma (**ret**-i-nO-blas-**tO**-ma) (n) malignant sarcoma or neoplasm of the retina; hereditary and generally occurring in young children

retinopathy (re-ti-**nop**-a-thee) (n) one of many disorders of the retina

retinoscopy (ret-i-**nos**-ko-pee) (n) light beam test used to detect refractive errors

retraction (ree-**trak**-shun) (n) the act of pulling back

retrograde (**ret**-rO-grayd) (adj) moving or going backward

retroperitoneal (**ret**-rO-per-i-tO-**nee**-al) (adj) located behind the peritoneum outside the peritoneal cavity, such as the kidneys

rhabdomyosarcoma (**rab**-dO-**mI**-O-sar-**kO**-ma) (n) highly malignant tumor developing from striated muscle cells

rheumatic fever (roo-**mat**-ik **fee**-ver) (n) fever following infection with *Streptococcus* bacteria; may affect the joints, skin, and heart

rheumatoid (**roo**-ma-toyd) (adj) resembling rheumatism, with pain, inflammation, and deformity of the joints

rhinitis (rI-**nI**-tis) (n) inflammation of the mucous membrane of the nose

rhinophyma (rI-nO-**fI**-ma) (n) enlargement of the nose from severe rosacea

rhinoplasty (**rI**-nO-plas-tee) (n) surgery to correct a defect in the nose or to change its shape

rhinorrhea (rI-nO-**ree**-a) (n) a watery discharge from the nose

rhonchus (**rong**-kus) (n) abnormal sound heard on auscultation of the chest, usually during expiration; rhonchi (pl)

rigidity (ri-**jid**-i-tee) (n) stiffness; inflexibility

Rinne test (**rin**-ne) (n) also Rinne's (**rin**-ez); a hearing test comparing perception of air and bone conduction in one ear with a tuning fork; normally air conduction is more acute

roentgenology (**rent**-gen-**ol**-o-jee) (n) the study of the use of roentgen rays (x-rays) for diagnosis and therapy

rubella (roo-**bel**-a) (n) a contagious viral disease with fever and a red rash; German measles

S

sac (sak) (n) pouch

sagittal (**saj**-i-tal) (adj) relating to a line from front to back in the middle of an organ or the body

salivary gland (**sal**-i-vayr-ee) (n) a gland that secretes saliva into the mouth

saphenous vein (sa-**fee**-nus vayn) (n) either of two main veins in the leg that drain blood from the foot

scabies (**skay**-beez) (n) contagious rash with intense itching; caused by mites

scan (n) scanning a tissue, organ, or system using a special apparatus that displays and records its image, such as computer tomography (CAT scan); the image so obtained

scapula (**skap**-yoo-la) (n) a large, triangular, flattened bone lying over the ribs

sciatica (sI-**at**-i-ka) (n) pain in the lower back and hip radiating down the back of the thigh into the leg, usually due to herniated lumbar disk

scirrhous (**skir**-us) (adj) describing or resembling a hard, fibrous, malignant tumor

sclera (**skleer**-a) (n) a fibrous coat that covers approximately five-sixths of the outer tunic of the eye; sclerae (pl)

sclerosis (sklee-**rO**-sis) (n) hardening or induration of an organ or tissue, especially that due to excessive growth of fibrous tissue

sclerostomy (skle-**ros**-tO-mee) (n) surgical formation of an opening in the sclera

sclerotic (sklee-**rot**-ic) (adj) pertaining to or affected with sclerosis, a condition that shows hardness of tissue resulting from inflammation, mineral deposits, or other causes; in neuropathy, induration of nervous and other structures by a hyperplasia of the interstitial fibrous atructures

scoliosis (skO-lee-**O**-sis) (n) abnormal curvature of the spine to one side

scotoma (skO-**tO**-ma) (n) a blind spot; a small area of defective vision

scrotal (**skrO**-tal) (adj) relating to the scrotum

scrotum (**skrO**-tum) (n) the pouch of skin containing the testes, the male reproductive glands

sebaceous (see-**bay**-shus) (adj) relating to sebum

seborrhea (seb-O-**ree**-a) (n) overactivity of the oil glands of the skin

sebum (**see**-bum) (n) an oily secretion of the oil glands of the skin

seed (n) as related to oncology, it is the beginning of a tumor

seeding (n) the local spreading of immature tumor cells

semicircular canals (**sem**-ee-**sir**-kyoo-lar ka-**nals**) (n) three fluid-filled loops in the labyrinth of the inner ear, associated with the body's sense of balance

sensorineural deafness (**sen**-sOr-i-**noor**-al) (n) hearing impairment due to nerve disturbance

sentinel node (**sen**-ti-nal nOd) (n) an enlarged, supraclavicular lymph node infiltrated with cancer cells that have metastasized from an obscurely located primary cancer

septal (**sep**-tal) (adj) pertaining to a dividing partition

septum (**sep**-tum) (n) division between two cavities or two masses of tissue, such as the nasal septum; septa (pl)

sequela (see-**kwel**-a) (n) a condition following and resulting from a disease; sequelae (see-kwel-ee) (pl)

serosanguineous (**see** row sang win ess) (adj) characterized by blood and serum

serous (**seer**-us) (adj) relating to or having a watery consistency

serous otitis media (**seer**-us O-**tI**-tis **mee**-dee-a) (n) inflammation of the middle ear accompanied by production of a watery fluid (serum)

sessile (**sess**-il) (adj) attached directly at the base; not on a stalk

Seton procedure (n) placing of a tube in the anterior chamber to drain fluid and decrease the intraocular pressure

sheath (n) structure surrounding an organ, body part, or object

shotty (**shot**-ee) (adj) resembling shot (hard pellets) to the touch; as shotty nodes

shunt (shunt) (v) to turn away from; to divert

sickle cell anemia (**sik**-l sel a-**nee**-mee-a) (n) hereditary blood disease in which abnormal hemoglobin causes red blood cells to become sickle-shaped, fragile and nonfunctional, leading to many acute and chronic complications

sigmoid colon (**sig**-moyd **kO**-lon) (n) that part of the colon extending from the end of the descending colon to the rectum

sigmoidoscopy (**sig**-moy-**dos**-ko-pee) (n) the inspection of the rectum and colon via endoscope

sinus (**sI**-nus) (n) a passageway or hollow in a bone or other tissue

sinus rhythm (**si**-nus **rith**-um) (n) normal cardiac rhythm

sinusitis (sI-nu-**sI**-tis) (n) inflammation of the nasal sinuses, occurring as a result of an upper respiratory infection, an allergic response, or a defect of the nose

situs (**sI**-tus) (n) a position

sleep apnea syndrome (**ap**-nee-a) (n) breathing stops, briefly and periodically, due to partial upper airway obstruction during sleep

slit-lamp (n) instrument consisting of a microscope and a thin, bright beam of light; used to examine the eye

sonography (so-**nog**-ra-fi) (n) ultrasonography; use of high-frequency sound waves to produce an image of an organ or tissue

sonometer (**son**-O-mee-ter) (n) a bell-shaped instrument used to measure hearing

speculum (**spek**-yoo-lum) (n) an instrument used for examining canals or the interior of a cavity

sphenoidal (sfee-**noy**-dal) (adj) concerning the sphenoid bone

sphenoidal sinus (sfee-**noy**-dal) (n) one of two sinuses in the sphenoid bone opening to the nasal cavity

sphincter (**sfingk**-ter) (n) a muscle that encircles a duct, tube, or opening in such a way that its contraction constricts the opening

sphincterotomy (sfink-tur-**ot**-O-mee) (n) procedure that produces cuts in the iris sphincter muscle to allow pupillary enlargement

spinous (**spI**-nus) (adj) pertaining to or resembling a spine, a short, sharp process of bone

splenectomy (sple-**nek**-tO-mee) (n) surgical removal of the spleen

splenic (**splen**-ik) (adj) referring to the spleen

spondylitis (spon-di-**lI**-tis) (n) inflammation of one or more vertebrae

sporadic (spO-**rad**-ik) (adj) occurring occasionally or in isolated situations

sprain (n) injury to a joint by overstretching the ligaments; (v) to injure a joint and sometimes the nearby ligaments or tendons

sputum (**spyoo**-tum) (n) spit; expectorated material

squamous (**skway**-mus) (adj) scaly; covered with or consisting of scales

stapes (**stay**-peez) (n) the smallest and innermost of the three auditory bones in the inner ear; stirrup

staphylococcemia (**staf**-i-lO-kok-**see**-mee-a) (n) the presence of staphylococci (bacterial microorganisms) in the blood

Staphylococcus aureus (staf-il-O-**kok**-us **awr**-ee-us) (n) a common species of Staphylococcus (a bacteria), present on nasal mucous membranes and skin that causes pus-producing infections

stenocardia (sten-O-**kar**-dee-a) (n) an attack of intense chest pain; also called angina pectoris

stenosis (ste-**nO**-sis) (n) narrowing or constriction of a passageway or opening, such as a blood vessel

sterile (**ster**-il) (adj) free from living microorganisms

sternocleidomastoid (**ster**-nO-**klI**-dO-**mas**-toyd) (n) one of two muscles arising from the sternum and the inner part of the clavicle

sternum (**ster**-num) (n) the breast bone

steroid (**steer**-oyd) (n) any of a large number of similar chemical substances, either natural or synthetic; many are hormones; produced mainly in the adrenal cortex and gonads

strabismus (stra-**biz**-mus) (n) improper alignment of eyes; crossed eye(s)

strain (n) injury, usually to muscle, caused by overstretching or overuse; (v) to injure muscles by overstretching or overuse

strep (n) short form of Streptococcus, a genus of bacteria; many species cause disease in humans

Streptococcus (strep-tO-**kok**-us) (n) a genus of bacteria; many species cause disease in humans

stress incontinence (stres in-**kon**-ti-nens) (n) inability to retain urine under tension, such as sneezing or coughing

sty (stI) (n) an infection of a marginal gland of the eyelid; stye

subcutaneous (sub-kyoo-**tay**-nee-us) (adj) under the skin

subcuticular (sub-kyoo-**tik**-yoo-lar) (adj) beneath the cuticle of epidermis

subdural hematoma (sub-**doo**-ral hee-ma-**tO**-ma/hem-a-**tO**-ma) (n) an accumulation of blood under the dura mater surrounding the brain

subjective data (sub-**jek**-tiv **day**-tah) (n) information revealed by the patient to the health care provider

sublingual (sub-**ling**-gwahl) (adj) beneath the tongue

submandibular (sub-man-**dib**-yoo-lar) (adj) under the lower jaw

substernal (sub-**ster**-nal) (adj) situated beneath the sternum (breast bone)

subxiphoid (sub-**zif**-oyd) (adj) below a sword-shaped structure, as the xiphoid process, a structure beneath the lowest portion of the sternum

supine (soo-**pIn**) (adj) lying on the back

suppuration (**sup**-yu-**ray**-shun) (n) the production or discharge of pus

supraglottic (soo-pra-**glot**-ik) (adj) located above the glottis, the sound-producing apparatus of the larynx

suprapubic (soo-pra-**pyoo**-bik) (adj) above the pubic bones

suprapubic (soo-pra-**pyoo**-bik) (adj) above the pubic arch

supratentorial (**soo**-pra-ten-**tO**-ree-al) (adj) located above the tentorium, a tentlike structure

suture (**soo**-chur) (n and v) natural seam, border in the skull formed by the close joining of bony surfaces; closing a wound with a sterile needle and thread

symphysis (**sim**-fi-sis) (n) joint in which fibrocartilage firmly unites the bones

syncopal (**sin**-kO-pal) (adj) relating to fainting

syncope (**sin**-ko-pee) (n) fainting

syndrome (**sin**-drOm) (n) the signs and symptoms that constitute a specific disease

synovial fluid (si-**nO**-vee-al **floo**-id) (n) protective lubricating fluid around joints

systemic lupus erythematosus (sis-**tem**-ik **loo**-pus er-i-**them**-a-tO-sis/er-i-**thee**-ma-tO-sis) (n) a chronic disease with inflammatory symptoms in various systems of the body; characteristics of the disease and the systems involved may vary widely

systolic (sis-**tol**-ik) (adj) pertaining to systole, the part of the heart cycle in which the heart is in contraction

T

T cell (n) a type of lymphocyte; responsible for cell-mediated immunity

tachycardia (**tak**-e-**kar**-dee-a) (n) an abnormally rapid heart rate

tachycardic (**tak**-e-**kar**-dik) (adj) relating to or suffering from an abnormally rapid heart rate

tachypnea (tak-ip-**nee**-a) (n) rapid rate of breathing

tangent screen test (n) maps the field of vision using a marker

Tanner staging (n) method of indicating the sexual development of a child or adolescent

telogen (**tel**-O-jen) (n) the resting phase of the hair growth cycle

temporal (**tem**-po-ral) (adj) pertaining to the temple of the head or the corresponding lobe of the brain

testicular (tes-**tik**-yoo-lar) (adj) relating to the testes, the male reproductive glands

texture (**teks**-chur) (n) character, structure, and feel of parts of the body

thecal (**thee**-kal) (adj) referring to a covering or enclosure

thelarche (thee-**lar**-kee) (n) the beginning of breast development in girls

theophylline (thee-**of**-i-lin) (n) a drug used in chronic obstructive lung disease

thermodilution (**ther**-mO-di-**loo**-shun) (n) method of determining cardiac output; involves injecting a cold liquid into the bloodstream and measuring the temperature change downstream

thoracoscopy (thOr-a-**kos**-kO-pee) (n) diagnostic examination of the pleural cavity with an endoscope

thoracotomy (thOr-a-**kot**-O-mee) (n) surgical incision of the chest wall

thorax (**thor**-aks) (n) the chest

thrombocytopenia (**throm**-bO-cy-to-**pee**-nee-a) (n) abnormal decrease in the number of blood platelets

thrombocytopenic (**throm**-bO-sI-tO-**pee**-nik) (adj) relating to thrombocytopenia

thrombophlebitis (**throm**-bO-fle-**bI**-tis) (n) inflammation of a vein with clot formation (thrombus)

thrombosis (throm-**bO**-sis) (n) the formation, development, or existence of a blood clot, or thrombus, within the vascular system

thrombus (**throm**-bus) (n) blood clot attached to the interior wall of a vein or artery

thrush (n) infection with the fungus Candida, causing white patches in the mouth and throat

thyroid (**thI**-royd) (n) a gland in the neck that secretes thyroid hormone

thyromegaly (thI-rO-**meg**-a-lee) (n) enlargement of the thyroid gland

tibia (tib-ee-a) (n) inner and thicker of the two bones of the human leg between the knee and the ankle

tibial (**tib**-ee-al) (adj) relating to the tibia

tinea (**tin**-ee-a) (n) fungal infection; such as tinea pedis or athlete's foot

tinnitus (ti-**nI**-tus) (n) noise, such as ringing, in the ears

titer (**tI**-ter) (n) strength or concentration of a solution; a unit of measurement usually expressed as a ratio that indicates the minimum concentration of an antibody before losing its power to react to a specific antigen

tobramycin (tO-bra-**mI**-sin) (n) an antibiotic drug

tomographic (tO-**mog**-ra-feek) (adj) referring to an x-ray technique which displays an organ or tissue at a particular depth

tonometry (tO-**nom**-et-ree) (n) a test that measures intraocular pressure

tonsils (**ton**-silz) (n) lymphoid tissue structures in the oropharynx

torso (**tor**-sO) (n) trunk of the body

toxoplasmosis (**tok**-sO-plaz-**mO**-sis) (n) disease caused by a protozoan parasite

trabeculectomy (tra-bek-yoo-**lek**-tO-mee) (n) surgical removal of a section of the cornea to decrease intraocular pressure in patients with severe glaucoma

trabeculoplasty (tra-**bek**-yoo-lO-**plas**-tee) (n) surgical procedure that decreases intraocular pressure in open-angle glaucoma

trachea (**tray**-kee-a) (n) the windpipe

tracheoesophageal (**trans**-e-sof-a-**gee**-al) (adj) pertaining to the trachea and esophagus

tracheostomy (tray-kee-**os**-tO-mee) (n) a surgically created opening into the trachea (windpipe)

tracheotomy (**tray**-kee-**ot**-O-mee) (n) the surgical procedure in which a tracheostomy is created

tragus (**tray**-gus) (n) the small projection of cartilage in front of the external opening to the ear canal

transaminase (trans-**am**-i-nays) (n) an enzyme that catalyzes transamination, the transfer of an animo group from one compound to another or the transposition of an animo group within a single compound

transesophageal (tranz-ee-sof-a-**jee**-al) (adj) pertaining to an abnormal opening between the trachea and esophagus

transmural (trans-**myoo**-ral) (adj) relating to the entire thickness of the wall of an organ

transperineal (trans-per-i-**nee**-al) (adj) across or through the perineal region between the urethral opening and the anus, including the skin and underlying tissues

transurethral (trans-yoo-**ree**-thral) (adj) through the urethra, such as a surgical procedure

transverse (trans-**vers**) (adj) at right angles to the long axis of the body or an organ; crosswise; side to side

trocar (**trO**-kar) (n) sharply pointed surgical instrument used for aspiration or removal of fluids from cavities

trochanter (trO-**kan**-ter) (n) one of the projections at the upper end of the femur (thigh bone)

trochanteric (trO-kan-**ter**-ik) related to a trochanter, either of the two bony processes below the neck of the femur)

tumor (**too**-mor) (n) abnormal mass of tissue; neoplasm

turbinate (**ter**-bi-nayt) (n) one of several thin, spongy, bony plates within the walls of the nasal cavity

turbinates (**ter**-bi-naytz) (n) three scroll-shaped bones that form the sidewall of the nasal cavity

turgor (**ter**-gOr) (n) fullness; the normal resiliency of the skin; normal tension in a cell; swelling

tympanic (tim-**pan**-ik) (adj) pertaining to the middle ear or tympanic cavity

tympanic membrane (tim-**pan**-ik) (n) eardrum

tympanometric (**tim**-pa-nO-**met**-rik) (adj) pertaining to tympanometry, a procedure for evaluation of motility of eardrum and middle ear disorders

tympanoplasty (**tim**-pa-nO-plas-tee) (n) surgical repair of the middle ear

Tzanck's smear (tsangks smeer) (n) a method to help diagnose skin lesions by the miscroscopic examination of material from them

U

ulcerative colitis (**ul**-ser-a-tiv kO-**lI**-tis) (n) a chronic disease characterized by ulcers in the colon and rectum

ultrasound (**ul**-tra-sownd) (n) sound waves at very high frequencies used in the technique of obtaining images for diagnostic purposes

umbo (**um**-bO) (n) the inner surface of the tympanic membrane where it connects with the malleus in the middle ear

unilateral (yoo-ni-**lat**-e-ral) (adj) affecting or occurring on only one side

unremarkable (adj) nothing unusual is noted

upper respiratory infection (URI) (n) an infection of the upper respiratory tract such as the common cold, laryngitis, sinusitis, and tonsillitis

ureter (yoo-**ree**-ter/**yoo**-ree-ter) (n) either of a pair of tubes that carry urine from the kidney to the urinary bladder

ureteral (yoo-**ree**-te-ral) (adj) relating to the ureters

urethra (yoo-**ree**-thra) (n) a tube that drains urine from the bladder to the outside

urethral (yoo-ree-thral) (adj) relating to the urethra, a canal for the discharge of urine from the bladder to the outside of the body

urethroscopy (yoo-ree-**thros**-ko-pee) (n) an examination of the inside of the urethra with a urethroscope, a lighted instrument

urticaria (er-ti-**kar**-ee-a) (n) hives; an eruption of itching red, raised lesions

urticarial (er-ti-**kar**-ee-al) (adj) relating to or having urticaria

uterine (**yoo**-ter-in/**yoo**-ter-In) (adj) relating to the uterus (the female reproductive organ where the fertilized egg develops before birth; the womb)

uveitis (yoo-vee-**I**-tis) (n) inflammation of the uvea, including the choroid and the iris

uvula (**yoo**-vyoo-la) (n) small, fleshy mass hanging from the soft palate in the mouth

uvulitis (yoo-vyoo-**lI**-tis) (n) inflammation of the uvula

uvulopalatopharyngoplasty (**yoo**-vyoo-lO-**pal**-a-tO-fa-**rin**-gO-plas-tee) (n) UPPP for short; a surgical treatment for sleep apnea for patients who cannot tolerate or respond to medical therapies

V

varicella (var-i-**sel**-a) (n) chickenpox; a highly contagious viral disease

varicose veins (var-I-kOs vaynz) (n) veins that become distended, swollen, knotted, tortuous, and painful because of poor valvular function

vascular (**vas**-kyoo-lar) (adj) relating to the blood vessels

vascularity (vas-kyoo-**lar**-i-tee) (n) the blood vessels in a part of the body

vasectomy (va-**sek**-tO-mee) (n) excision of a portion of the vas deferens, in association with prostatectomy or to produce sterility

vena cava (**vee**-na **kav**-a) (n) one of the largest veins of the body; venae cavae (pl)

veno-occlusive (**vee**-nO O-**kloo**-siv) (adj) concerning obstruction of veins

venous (**vee**-nus) (adj) relating to a vein or veins

ventricle (**ven**-tri-kl) (n) either of the two lower chambers of the heart; areas of the brain that produce and drain cerebrospinal fluid (CSF)

ventriculogram (ven-**trik**-yoo-lO-gram) (n) an x-ray of the ventricles

ventriculography (ven-trik-yoo-**log**-ra-fee) (n) x-ray visualization of heart ventricles after injection of a radiopaque substance

vertebral (ver-**tee**-bral) (adj) relating to a vertebra or the vertebrae

vertex (**ver**-teks) (n) the crown or top of the head

vertigo (**ver**-tigO) (n) dizziness

vesical (**ves**-i-kul) (adj) referring to the bladder or gallbladder

vesicle (**ves**-i-kl) (n) blister; small, raised skin lesion containing clear fluid

vesicouterine (**ves**-i-kO-**yoo**-ter-in) (adj) pertaining to the urinary bladder and uterus

vesicular (ve-**sik**-yoo-lar) (adj) pertaining to vesicles or small blisters

vesiculopustular (ves **ick** you low **pus** to ler) (adj) characterized by vesicles and pustules

vestibulum (ves-**tib**-yoo-lum) (n) the central cavity of the labyrinth in the inner ear, between the cochlea and the semicircular canals

viable (**vI**-a-bl) (adj) capable of surviving; living

vibrissae (vI-**bris**-a) (n) nose hairs

villi (**vil**-I) (n) many tiny projections, occurring over the mucous membrane of the small intestine that accomplish the absorption of nutrients and fluids; villus (sing)

villous (**vil**-us) (adj) relating to villi

vincristine (vin-**kris**-teen) (n) an antineoplastic drug that disrupts cell division and is used to treat many cancers, especially those of the lymphatic system.

virus (**vI**-rus) (n) an organism or the infection caused by the organism; the organism is much smaller than bacteria; it depends completely on the host and is unaffected by common antibiotics

viscera (**vis**-er-a) (n) main internal organs within the trunk of the body, especially those in the abdominal cavity

visceral (**vis**-er-al) (adj) relating to or located near the viscera

visceromegaly (**vis**-er-O-**meg**-a-lee) (n) generalized enlargement of the abdominal organs

Vistaril (viss-ta-rill) (n) Brand name for hydroxyzine, used for the treatment of anxiety and nausea

visual acuity (**vizh**-yoo-al a-**kyoo**-i-tee) (n) clearness of vision, e.g., 20/20 visual acuity

visualization (**vich**-oo-al-I-**zay**-shun) (n) the act of viewing an object, especially the picture of a body structure as obtained by x-ray study

vitiligo (vi-ti-**lee**-gO) (n) white patches, due to loss of pigment, appearing on the skin

vitreous humor (**vit**-ree-us **hyoo**-mer) (adj) glassy; gelatin-like substance within the eyeball

vortex (**vOr**-teks) (n) whirlpool; resembling a whirlpool

vulva (**vul**-va) (n) external female genital organs; vulvae (pl)

vulvar (**vul**-var) (adj) relating to the vulva

W

Weber test (**web**-er) (n) a hearing test performed with a tuning fork placed at points in the middle of the skull to determine where the vibration is heard (not where it is felt)

Western blot (n) a laboratory test to detect the presence of antibodies to specific antigens in the blood

wheal (hweel) (n) a raised, red circumscribed lesion usually due to an allergic reaction; usually accompanied by intense itching; welt

wheezing (**hweez**-ing) (n) breathing with difficulty and with a whistling sound; can be heard aloud and/or on auscultation

Wright peak flow (n) maximum flow of expired air as measured by the Wright flowmeter

X

xanthoma (zan-**thO**-mah) (n) yellowish nodules in or under the skin, especially in the eyelids

xanthopsia (zan-**thop**-see-a) (n) yellow vision; a condition in which everything seen appears yellowish

xeromammogram (**zeer**-O-**mam**-o-gram) (n) type of x-ray of the breast

xerostomia (zeer-O-**stO**-mee-a) (n) dryness of the mouth

xiphoid (**zif**-oyd) (adj) referring to the xiphoid process, the cartilage at the lower end of the sternum (breast bone); also spelled xyphoid

Xylocaine (**zI**-lO-kayn) (n) trade name for lidocaine hydroxhloride

Y

yolk sac (**yOk** sak) (n) a membranous sac surrounding the food yolk in the embryo

Index

E

F

G

P

Q

R